The Desktop Guide to

INCLUDES CD-ROM.   and

icine

For Elsevier:
Commissioning Editor: Karen Morley
Development Editor: Louise Allsop
Project Manager: Caroline Horton
Design Direction: Jayne Jones

The Desktop Guide to Complementary and Alternative Medicine

An evidence-based approach

Second edition

Editors

Edzard Ernst MD PhD FRCP FRCPEd
Professor of Complementary Medicine, Peninsula Medical School, Universities of Exeter and Plymouth, Exeter, UK

Max H Pittler MD PhD
Senior Research Fellow in Complementary Medicine, Peninsula Medical School, Universities of Exeter and Plymouth, Exeter, UK

Barbara Wider MA
Research Fellow in Complementary Medicine, Peninsula Medical School, Universities of Exeter and Plymouth, Exeter, UK

Assistant Editor

Kate Boddy MA
Academic Assistant in Complementary Medicine, Peninsula Medical School, Universities of Exeter and Plymouth, Exeter, UK

Forewords by

David Eisenberg MD
Director of the Osher Institute, Division for Research and Education in Complementary and Integrative Medical Therapies, Harvard Medical School, Boston, Massachusetts, USA

Brian M Berman MD
Professor of Family Medicine, University of Maryland Center for Integrative Medicine, Baltimore, Maryland, USA

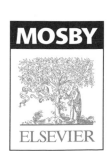

MOSBY
ELSEVIER

An imprint of Elsevier Limited

First published 2006

ISBN 0-723-43383-6
1   British Library Cataloguing in Publication Data
A catalogue record for this book is available from the British Library

2   Library of Congress Cataloging in Publication Data
A catalog record for this book is available from the Library of Congress

The
Publisher's
policy is to use
**paper manufactured
from sustainable forests**

Printed in China

Contents

Foreword to the first edition

It is a rare physician these days who has not had a patient ask about an unconventional treatment for their medical condition. In fact, many physicians are themselves wondering if there might be some value to an alternative treatment, particularly when grappling with treating a chronically ill patient who is not responding well to conventional care. The surge of interest in complementary and alternative medicine is well documented in many Western countries but, despite the fact that many of these therapies have been around for hundreds if not thousands of years and are the primary source of health care for over 70% of the world's population, we have had very little access to good information about whether they work or are safe. Physician and consumer are caught in the same bind. With an abundance of claims being made about the curative powers of any number of complementary therapies and a similar number of disclaimers being made about 'quackery', how is either to know where the truth lies?

The authors of this book have been a formidable force in turning these tables and bringing the light of scientific understanding to complementary medicine. Since taking on the first chair position to be created in complementary medicine, Professor Edzard Ernst, more than any other single person, has tackled the impressive task of systematically reviewing the world's research literature on complementary medicine. Dr David Eisenberg, with the publication of his surveys on complementary medicine use in the USA, has helped to identify what therapies people are using and for what problems.

In this book they draw together this information to give us an understanding of the main complementary therapies – their origins, underlying concepts, scientific rationale and method of clinical practice – as well as looking at the main conditions for which the therapies are used. Most important of all, they give us access to the most up-to-date, evidence-based information on safety and effectiveness.

Throughout health care there has been an increasing emphasis on the practice of evidence-based medicine. The premise of the movement is that clinical practice should integrate the expertise of the practitioner with the wishes of the patient and the best available evidence. The evidence-based movement saw a similar growth to that of complementary medicine over the last couple of decades of the old millennium. However, a common criticism of complementary medicine is that it cannot be part of evidence-based medicine because little or no research exists in the field. I would dispute this as an outright claim and am indebted to the authors of this book for their exhaustive work in bringing together and evaluating the evidence that does exist. Although sparse in many areas and often of poor quality, a body of scientific research does exist in complementary medicine that merits examination. As responsible and, above all, caring practitioners, it behoves us to familiarise ourselves with this information so we better comprehend the potential role complementary therapies may play in helping our patients to heal and to maintain health. Complementary medicine is a strong consumer-driven movement. Patients are telling us that this is something that they want. Armed with an understanding of what the therapies are, how they are practiced, and the current best evidence, patients can better define their own wishes and practitioners can better use their own expertise, allowing both to work together and make informed clinical decisions.

Brian M Berman,
Baltimore, 2001

Foreword to the second edition

One generation ago (think of the 1970s), a compendium of scientific research involving therapies such as acupuncture, herbal medicines, chiropractic, massage, meditation, etc, was unimaginable. A decade ago (think mid-1990s) the phrase 'evidence-based approach to complementary and alternative medicine' was a bit of an oxymoron. The perception on the part of the medical and scientific elite was that 'these approaches do not work therefore they cannot work'. Over several years, this reflexive dismissiveness softened somewhat and evolved into the notion that 'these approaches are all placebo'. That position shifted to 'they are not all placebo, but some are dangerous'. As well-designed clinical trials were published, the perception shifted yet again to 'they are not all placebo and they are not all dangerous but they don't lend themselves to rigorous scientific assessment of efficacy or safety'. *The Desktop Guide to Complementary and Alternative Medicine, an Evidenced-Based Approach*, unequivocally demonstrates that these therapeutic approaches can and must be rigorously and systematically evaluated. This second edition also demonstrates the extraordinary pace with which the international scientific community has been engaged in this important line of inquiry.

Thanks to Edzard Ernst, Max Pittler, Barbara Wider, Kate Boddy and their colleagues, this reference thoughtfully and systematically summarises the evidence to date regarding the clinical efficacy, safety or lack thereof regarding the most commonly used complementary and alternative medical therapies. To their credit, the authors have developed procedures which allow for the systematic location, selection, appraisal and synthesis of information which is currently available. Importantly, they have distilled and presented an enormous spectrum of clinically relevant information in a highly user-friendly and accessible fashion. Evidence for a given therapy or condition is summarised in a transparent and reproducible fashion; the reader is provided with 'Overall Recommendations', 'a Risk–Benefit Assessment' and an easily readable 'Summary of Evidence'. Importantly, and wisely, the authors have emphasised that 'the absence of evidence of effectiveness does not imply absence of effectiveness'. They have also, wherever possible, accepted the truism that 'safety trumps efficacy'. Whenever information regarding risks and benefits is presented, the authors have deliberately 'erred on the side of safety'. Special attention to interactions involving herbs and herb–drug combinations are also conveniently highlighted.

In many ways, this Desktop Guide helps address a fundamental premise shared by the co-authors of the recently published Institute of Medicine (IOM) report on Complementary and Alternative Medicine (CAM) in the United States,[1] namely that 'patients, health professionals and public officials need evidence of effectiveness, safety, and costs to make sound decisions about the use or avoidance of all health care interventions, including CAM'.[2] That report recommends that 'the same principles and standards of evidence of treatment effectiveness apply to all treatments, whether currently labeled as conventional medicine or CAM'.[3] Moreover, a goal shared by this book's authors and the authors of the Institute of Medicine report is to create a health care delivery system that is comprehensive, patient-centered, and evidence-based.

Clearly, the 'evidence-base' has mushroomed since the publication of the first Desktop Guide five years ago. It is apt to rapidly expand in quantity and improve in quality over the next five years. This is, in part, due to the fact that the US National Institutes of Health currently spends in excess of $300 million per year[4] in support of scientific research involving complementary and alternative medical therapies; and, that other governments worldwide are also beginning to invest in this line of sponsored research investigation.

In addition to complimenting Ernst and colleagues for compiling this remarkable update on the weight of evidence regarding efficacy and safety of complementary and alternative medical therapies, allow me to make some predictions as to how the 'evidence' in this field is likely to evolve between now and the publication of what I hope will be a 'Third Edition' of this resource five or more years hence. My first prediction is that over the next five years more and more research in this area will be aimed at mechanism and not simply at efficacy or safety. It is understandable that over the past decade the research community has invested its resources in the design and implementation of clinical trials to address the question, 'Does this (CAM) therapy work relative to no therapy or a credible sham therapy or compared to 'conventional' therapy?' Those of us professionally involved in this research recognise that, to a certain extent, 'mechanism is king' and that evidence of efficacy in the absence of a plausible explanatory scientific model will be insufficient to change behaviour or satisfactorily change the opinions of the skeptical elite. As such, those therapies identified as clinically effective are most apt to be studied mechanistically. Examples include mechanisms whereby acupuncture induces changes in pain perception in the brain and peripheral nervous system; mechanisms whereby hypnosis, meditation, guided-imagery and other mind-body techniques alter brain function, immune function, etc, and explorations of genetic predisposition to individual CAM therapies paralleling research aimed at identifying genetic predispositions to responsiveness to individual drugs. As the mechanism of action of individual complementary and alternative medical therapies are uncovered, scientific discoveries will follow and these, in turn, will increase the momentum in support of further clinical research. If we think the pace of research in this area is fast currently, just wait until the basic scientists add their collective weight to this process.

Second, I share with Ernst and colleagues the view that cost-effectiveness research in this area remains in its infancy. The fundamental question as to whether access to complementary and alternative medical therapies increases costs, decreases costs, or is cost neutral is critically important for policy makers, employers, and health care providers intent on advising their patients appropriately. It is my prediction, shared by many others, that future clinical trials can and must incorporate an assessment of costs and that between now and the publication of the next edition of this book, such data will help guide us in our collective clinical and policy recommendations.

Finally, and importantly, as mentioned in the recent Institute of Medicine report, studies currently show that patients frequently use more than one therapeutic modality to treat their principal symptom or medical condition and this behaviour has implications for future research design. 'Therefore, it is important to understand how CAM and conventional medical treatments (and providers) interact with each other and to study models of how CAM and conventional treatments can be provided in integrated and coordinated ways'.[5] These findings have implications for the design of future clinical trials to assess the safety, efficacy and cost-effectiveness of CAM therapies used by adults. Specifically, the Institute of Medicine report argues that, 'Although it is still important to evaluate individual therapies for individual conditions, a research portfolio that is limited to this approach may not adequately simulate CAM therapy use by the adult population. It may therefore be important methodologically to design some studies that offer patients access to multiple CAM therapies across multiple CAM professional groups, as this would be closer to real life experience'.[6] As such, we can predict that the next edition of this Desktop Guide will likely require another section summarising research which evaluates combinations of therapeutic modalities (i.e. 'integrative models of care') and which goes beyond the assessment of individual therapeutic options.

There is a proverb in Chinese which says 'Real gold is not afraid of the heat of the hottest fire'. Ernst and colleagues have deftly applied modern scientific rules of evidence to help distinguish useful from useless and safe from unsafe. They have, through their systematic approach, constructed a unique crucible into which the existing evidence base of complementary and alternative medicine has been plunged, heated and brought to a slow boil. Thankfully, Ernst and colleagues have searched for and strained out much of the 'gold'. They have also identified the 'silver' and the 'bronze' from this cauldron of information. They have placed these valuable findings against a black velvet backdrop for all to see. The transparency, clarity and breadth of their 'presentation' are what distinguish this compendium of evidence from its many rivals. On behalf of clinicians, researchers and consumers of complementary and alternative medicine, I offer them my thanks for this extraordinary contribution.

David Eisenberg,
Boston, 2005

REFERENCES

1 Committee on the Use of Complementary and Alternative Medicine by the American Public, Board on Health Promotion and Disease Prevention, Institute of Medicine of the National Academies. Complementary and Alternative Medicine in the United States. Washington DC: The National Academies Press; 2005.

2 Eisenberg DM. The Institute of Medicine report on CAM in the US. Altern Ther Health Med 2005;11:10-15

3 IOM report, p 125

4 IOM report, p 27

5 IOM report, p 221

6 IOM report, p 62

Preface to the first edition

An epitaph to opinion-based medicine

Complementary and alternative medicine (CAM) is becoming more relevant to mainstream healthcare professionals so the option of CAM will increasingly need to be considered when making clinical decisions. Although much advice on CAM has in the past been based on opinion, both patients and their advisers recognise the need for information based on evidence.

The whole thrust of this book is to help establish an evidence base for CAM. Evidence for the most important parts of our book means data from controlled (preferably randomised) clinical trials or preferably systematic reviews of such studies. But what about expert opinion? Surely years of experience reflected in such opinions must be of considerable value? In a way, this statement amounts to a testable hypothesis – so we decided to test it.

We selected seven recent, general CAM books from our shelves[1-7] which contained chapters devoted to specific medical conditions. From these books, we extracted the CAM treatments which were recommended for specific medical conditions. For the purpose of this exercise a 'recommendation' was defined as a mention in a positive context. CAM treatments were recommended for about 300 different conditions. Thus we derived lists of 'opinion-based' recommendations for CAM treatments according to each condition. Where possible, we then compared this collective opinion with the evidence from our systematic reviews as summarised in the condition chapters of this book.

The results are both fascinating and disappointing; most of all, they are somewhat worrying. The first striking finding was that an extremely broad range of CAM treatments was recommended for many conditions (Table 1). The second, perhaps more surprising result was the lack of agreement between the authors of the seven books. Most treatments were recommended for a given condition only by one or two, rarely by more than four and never by all authors.

Obviously opinion and evidence can differ without either being wrong. One therapy could, for instance, be recommended without the back-up of trial evidence simply because trials are not yet available. However, we found several instances where a

Table I **Some conditions for which numerous (> 50) CAM treatments were recommended**

Condition	Number of treatments recommended
Acne	61
Addictions	120
AIDS/HIV	69
Allergies	57
Anxiety	54
Arthritis	131
Asthma	119
Back pain	65
Cancer	133
Coronary heart disease	71
Chronic fatigue syndrome	64
Common cold	96
Cystitis	57
Depression	87
Dermatitis	57
Diabetes mellitus	89
Eczema	55
Emphysema	54
Fungal infection	75
Hay fever	65
Headache	78
Haemorrhoids	54
Herpes	69
Hypertension	95
Infections	55
Insomnia	74
Irritable bowel syndrome	69
Menopausal problems	68
Pneumonia: bacterial, mycoplasmal and viral	52
Premenstrual syndrome	59
Prostate disorders	63
Psoriasis	57
Sciatica	55
Sinusitis	64
Varicose veins	56

given therapy was being recommended while conclusive trial evidence (i.e. more than one reliable RCT or a systematic review of RCTs) showed that it was not effective for that particular condition. Examples are:

- chelation therapy for cardiovascular disease
- chiropractic for asthma
- guar gum for body weight reduction.

And there were other most remarkable differences between opinion and evidence. For instance, treatments which were supported by compelling evidence from metaanalyses and systematic reviews were not consistently included by all the authors in their recommendation. Examples are:

- acupuncture for nausea
- biofeedback for constipation
- relaxation for anxiety
- saw palmetto for benign prostatic hyperplasia.

One could argue that the books were written before this evidence became available. We checked this notion and found that it did not apply in the above instances.

Truly worrying discrepancies were noted in relation to recommendations for treating a certain condition with a given therapy where the evidence suggests that this therapy should be contraindicated in this particular situation. Examples are:

- chiropractic for osteoporosis
- ginger for morning sickness.

We find such contradictions deeply disturbing. They may exist in other areas of medicine as well but certainly not in such abundance as found here. We believe that they are a reflection of the relative youth of CAM research and of the fact that an evidence-based approach is still a novel concept in CAM. The discrepancies, inconsistencies and contradictions certainly show that opinions, even when originating from CAM 'experts', are not reliable or valid.

We feel that this point is of considerable importance as it touches the core concept of this book. Opinions in various guises seem to dominate CAM. Because they are unreliable, they also have the potential of misleading healthcare professionals and (more importantly) harming patients. The issue here is not to point an accusing finger at any one book or any one author (in fact, not all the examples used above apply to all the books cited). The issue is rather that CAM (and its literature) is presently far from being evidence-based and ought to become evidence-based sooner rather than later. The best way forward, as far as we can see, lies in objectively and reproducibly establishing and updating the evidence – and this is precisely what our book aims to achieve.

Our main aim was to provide state-of-the-art information and evidence on CAM as a practical reference resource, in a way that is accessible to busy physicians and other healthcare professionals. Despite persistent suggestions that the RCT is not an appropriate or feasible method for testing CAM, we have found large numbers of RCTs that cover almost every form of therapy, demonstrating that CAM can be tested in a rigorous manner. As in all branches of medicine, inevitably some evidence is negative. But the overriding conclusions are that some forms of CAM are frequently supported by evidence and therefore do have a role in modern health care.

Edzard Ernst, Max H Pittler,
Clare Stevinson and Adrian White
Exeter, 2001

REFERENCES

1 Pelletier K R. The best alternative medicine. New York: Simon Schuster, 2000

2 Spencer J W, Jacobs J J. (eds) Complementary/alternative medicine. An evidence-based approach. St Louis: Mosby; 1999

3 Springhouse. Nurse's handbook of alternative and complementary medicine. Springhouse, PA: Springhouse; 1998

4 The Burton Goldberg Group. Alternative medicine: the definitive guide. Payallup, WA: Future Medicine; 1994

5 Jamil T. Complementary medicine: a practical guide. Oxford: Butterworth Heinemann; 1997

6 Time-Life. The medical advisor. Alexandria, VA: Time-Life Books; 1997

7 Pizzorno J E, Murray M T (eds). Textbook of natural medicine. Edinburgh: Churchill Livingstone; 1999

Contributors

Michael H Cohen JD MBA
Assistant Clinical Professor of Medicine at Harvard Medical School Osher Institute, Boston, Massachusetts, Senior Lecturer at the College of the Bahamas, Nassau, Bahamas, and Principal in the Law Offices of Michael H. Cohen, Cambridge, Massachusetts, USA. (Chapter Legal and ethical issues regarding evidence-based complementary, alternative, and integrative medical therapies)

Peter Canter BSc PhD
Research Fellow, Complementary Medicine, Peninsula Medical School, Universities of Exeter and Plymouth, UK. (Chapters Meditation and Bilberry)

Clare Stevinson DSc MSc PhD
Research Fellow, Behavioural Medicine, University of Alberta, Edmonton, Canada. (Chapter Why patients use complementary and alternative medicine)

Acknowledgements

The following organisations were invited to comment on the 1st edition of this book. We would like to thank the organisations marked with an asterisk for responding. Inclusion in this list does not imply approval of the text by the individual or the organisation or that all their comments were included in the update.

Acupuncture Association of Chartered Physiotherapists
American Academy of Medical Acupuncture
American Association of Oriental Medicine
British Acupuncture Association & Register
*Mike Cummings, British Medical Acupuncture Society
*Nicky Robinson, The British Acupuncture Council
*Daniel Maxwell, The British Acupuncture Council
Society for Acupuncture Research
Society of Auricular Acupuncturists
The College of Traditional Acupuncture
Society of Teachers of the Alexander Technique
Aromatherapy and Allied Practitioners' Association
*Carole Preen, Aromatherapy Consortium
Association of Medical Aromatherapists
Institute of Classical Aromatherapy
International Society of Professional Aromatherapists
International Federation of Aromatherapists
The Aromatherapists' Society
*Jane Bird, The British Autogenic Society
*Judy Ramsell Howard, Dr Edward Bach Centre
*Stefan Ball, The Edward Bach Foundation
*Donald Moss, Mark Schwartz, Association for Applied Psychophysiology and Biofeedback
Biofeedback Foundation of Europe
*The Lord Colwyn, Arterial Health Foundation
American Chiropractic Association
*Sue Wakefield, British Chiropractic Association
*Grayden Bridge, Canadian Chiropractic Association
European Chiropractors' Union
*Phillippa Barton-Hanson, General Chiropractic Council
McTimoney Chiropractic College
*George Haig, Scottish Chiropractic Association
International Cranial Association
*Michael Kern, CranioSacral Therapy Association UK
British Alliance of Healing Associations

British Association of Therapeutic Touch
National Federation of Spiritual Healers
*Kevin Taylor, World Federation of Healing
General Osteopathic Council
American Herbal Products Association
European Herbal Practitioners Association
International Herb Association
National Institute of Medical Herbalists
Österreichische Gesellschaft für Phytotherapie
*Tony Booker, Register of Chinese Herbal Medicine
The American Herbalists Guild
The Institute of Traditional Herbal Medicine and Aromatherapy
Homoeopathic Medical Research Council
Faculty of Homeopathy and British Homeopathic Association
*Melanie Oxley, Society of Homoeopaths
*UK Homoeopathic Medical Association
American Society for Clinical Hypnosis
Association of Qualified Curative Hypnotists
*Keith Jones, British Association of Therapeutical Hypnotists
British Society of Clinical Hypnosis
*Geoff Callow, British Society of Experimental and Clinical
Hypnosis
*Mike Heap, British Society of Experimental and Clinical Hypnosis
British Society of Hypnotherapists
*Fiona Biddle, National Council for Hypnotherapy
*Shaun Brookhouse, National Council for Hypnotherapy
UK Confederation of Hypnotherapy Organisations
American Massage Therapy Association
Association of Massage Therapists
*Greg Morling, Australian Association of Massage Therapists
British Association of Massage Therapy
General Council for Massage Therapists
*Ian Macwhinnie, Shiatsu Society
American Association of Naturopathic Physicians
General Council and Register of Naturopaths
Incorporated Society of Registered Naturopaths
*Sarah Eldred, General Osteopathic Council
*Karl-Ludwig Resch, Saxon Balneology and Spa Medicine
Research Institute, Germany
Association of Reflexologists
*Nicola Hall, The British Reflexology Association
*Renée Tanner, International Federation of Reflexologists
The Reflexologists' Society
*Patricia Rockwood, American Yoga Association
British Wheel of Yoga
T'ai Chi Union
UK T'ai Chi Association

We wish to thank the following individuals for revising parts of the 1st edition of this book:
H Boon (Toronto, Canada)
D Eisenberg (Boston, USA)
A Huntley (Exeter, UK)
L Long (Exeter, UK)
R März (Neumarkt, Germany)
V Schulz (Berlin, Germany)
W Weiger (Boston, USA).

We are also indebted to R Clark, J Morgan and N Watson for secretarial work on both editions.

All unauthored chapters of the first edition were jointly written by E Ernst, M H Pittler, C Stevinson and A R White, all from the Department of Complementary Medicine, School of Postgraduate Medicine and Health Sciences, University of Exeter, UK.

The second edition was jointly revised, updated and expanded by E Ernst, M H Pittler and B Wider, all from Complementary Medicine, Peninsula Medical School, Universities of Exeter and Plymouth, UK. K Boddy performed the literature searches.

Glossary and abbreviations

Glossary

Cochrane Review

Cochrane Reviews are systematic summaries of evidence of the effects of healthcare interventions prepared and maintained by the Cochrane Collaboration. The reviews employ specific methods, are prepared using Review Manager (RevMan) software, adhere to a structured format and are regularly updated (*http://www.cochrane.org*)

Confidence interval (CI)

Quantifies the uncertainty in measurement. Usually reported as 95% CI, which is the range of values within which one can expect to find the true value in 95% of cases.

Controlled clinical trial (CCT)

Control is a standard against which experimental observations may be evaluated. In clinical trials, one group of participants is given an experimental intervention, while another group (i.e. the control group) is given either a standard treatment for the disease, a placebo or no treatment at all.

Crossover

Participants in the intervention group receive the control treatment upon completion of the treatment cycle. Similarly those in the control group 'crossover' and receive the experimental intervention.

Double-blind trial

A clinical trial design in which neither the participating individuals nor the study staff knows which participants are receiving the experimental treatment and which are receiving the control treatment or placebo. Double-blind trials are thought to produce objective results, since the expectations of the participant and study staff about the experimental drug do not affect the outcome.

Meta-analysis

A quantitative statistical method to pool trial data in a single estimate. Can be part of a systematic review.

P-value

Probability that an observed difference between groups occurred by chance alone. A result is conventionally regarded as 'statistically significant' if the likelihood that it is due to chance alone is less than five times out of 100 (p < 0.05).

Randomisation

The process by which patients in a clinical trial are randomly assigned to experimental intervention or control treatment. Randomisation minimises the differences among groups by equally distributing participants with particular characteristics (known or unknown) amongst all the trial arms.

Randomised clinical trial (RCT)

Study where participants are randomly allocated to receive experimental or control treatment.

Systematic review

Review in which literature from multiple sources is systematically searched for, assessed and evaluated to answer clearly formulated questions.

Abbreviations of frequently used terms

The following abbreviations are used throughout this book:

CAM complementary and alternative medicine
RCT randomised clinical trial
CCT controlled clinical trial
CI confidence intervals (95% unless otherwise stated).

The following abbreviations are used in the boxes and tables in Section 2 only:

min	minute(s)	mo	month(s)
h	hour(s)	y	year(s)
d	day(s)	m	metre(s)
w	week(s)	g	gram(s)
wkly	weekly	mg	milligram(s).

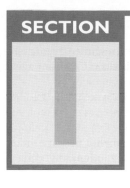

SECTION

1

Using the book

THE BOOK AT A GLANCE

- The purpose of the Desktop Guide is to present relevant, reliable, thorough and up-to-date information on CAM in a clear concise format with a focus on clinical evidence.
- The clinical evidence is retrieved through systematic searches in six general and specialist literature databases carried out up to May 2005 (see *Methods* p 4).
- Studies are selected according to the following priority order: systematic reviews and meta-analyses, randomised clinical trials, controlled clinical trials, uncontrolled trials (see *Methods* p 4).
- Assessment of trials is a combination of the methodological quality of the body of evidence, the level of evidence and the volume of evidence resulting in an indication of the weight of the evidence (low O – high OOO) and the direction of the evidence (clearly positive ⇧ to clearly negative ⇩) (see *How to use this book* p 8).
- Key information and an application of judgement are presented in the 'Summary of clinical evidence tables' and 'Overall recommendation' (Section 2), and the 'Risk–benefit assessments' (Sections 3 and 4) (see *Methods* p 5).
- Absence of evidence of effectiveness does not imply absence of effectiveness.
- Safety issues: the precautionary principle has been applied, so a treatment is not considered risk-free unless evidence suggests otherwise: a simple Yes/No descriptor alerts the reader in a general way to the existence (however rare) of potentially serious safety concerns (see *Methods* p 5).
- Pregnancy and lactation are cited as contraindications for all medicines included in this book unless there is positive evidence of safety in these situations (see *Methods* p 5).

METHODS

The intention of this book is to provide relevant, reliable, thorough and up-to-date information in a clear, concise format. In order to achieve this, a systematic approach was used to locate, select, appraise and present information. This chapter describes the procedures followed.

Definition of complementary and alternative medicine

For the purposes of this book complementary and alternative medicine (CAM) was defined as 'diagnosis, treatment and/or prevention which complements mainstream medicine by contributing to a common whole, satisfying a demand not met by orthodoxy, or diversifying the conceptual framework of medicine'.[1] What constitutes CAM may vary according to national differences and individual viewpoints. The list below indicates many of the treatments that we considered mainstream rather than CAM and were therefore not generally covered in this book. However, some of these treatments are mentioned in Section 2 (Conditions) for particular non-mainstream indications.

- Behavioural therapy
- Cognitive therapy
- Counselling
- Diets and nutritional advice
- Electromagnetic therapy
- Electrotherapy
- Exercise
- Hydrotherapy
- Lifestyle approaches
- Low-dose laser therapy
- Spa therapy
- Specific herbs, e.g. senna (*Cassia* spp), castor oil (*Ricinus communis*), Cayenne pepper (*Capsicum frutescens*)
- Transcranial magnetic stimulation
- Transcutaneous electrical nerve stimulation (TENS)
- Ultrasound
- Vitamins and minerals

Selection of topics

The conditions covered by Section 2 are those which are commonly seen in primary care, frequently treated with CAM and for which the most evidence relating to effectiveness is available.

Sections 3 and 4 cover CAM treatments (therapies and medicines) that are popular with patients. Treatments for which evidence relating to effectiveness is available are the subject of individual chapters. Other treatments where there is only some evidence of effectiveness are covered in tables.

Provisional lists of potential topics for chapters and tables were produced during discussion and amended after inspecting the results of literature searches (see *Literature searches* below) and internal review (see *Review process* below). Thirteen additional chapters have been included in this 2nd edition of the Desktop Guide.

Sources and referencing

A number of sources were used to compile information for this book. These included reference books, our own files, contact with other experts, a survey of CAM organisations (see *Survey* below) and systematic literature searches (see *Literature searches* below). Since a considerable amount of information is compressed into each chapter it was decided to keep referencing to a minimum. Comprehensive referencing would involve lengthy and repetitive reference lists distracting the reader from quick access to clear information. For example, information on risks presented in Sections 3 and 4 is largely based on a vast number of case reports and individual referencing would have been more of a hindrance than a help to the reader. Therefore a bibliography of the main reference sources for the book is provided at the end of this section, which indicates the principal sources of the information. The exception to this is information relating to *Clinical evidence* which provides the major focus of this book. In Sections 2, 3, and 4 key references are provided for the evidence cited at the end of each chapter to allow the interested reader to trace the source.

Survey of CAM professional bodies

In order to obtain information about the forms of CAM covered in this book, a survey of professional bodies of CAM was conducted.[2] A list of addresses of 526 CAM organisations was compiled, comprising all 364 addresses of UK CAM organisations (generated by a systematic survey sponsored by the UK Department of Health[3]) and an additional 162 addresses of organisations outside the UK, which have had previous direct contact with our department. Those professional bodies that were dedicated to individual forms of CAM (223 in total) were sent questionnaires asking about indications and contraindications of therapies and training requirements of practitioners. Although the response rate was low (36%), the information obtained was used to supplement material from other sources.

Literature searches for clinical evidence

Systematic searches were carried out in the databases Medline, Embase, Amed, the Cochrane Database of Systematic Reviews, Natural Standard, and the Natural Medicines Comprehensive Database. Each database was searched from its respective inception until March 2000 for the 1st edition and update searches were run until May 2005. The search strategy used to locate relevant literature was developed and refined. In addition, our own files, the bibliographies of relevant papers and the contents pages of all issues of the review journal FACT (Focus on Alternative and Complementary Therapies; London: Pharmaceutical Press, *www.pharmpress.com/fact*) were searched for further studies. No language restrictions were imposed. Studies in languages other than English were translated in-house.

Selection of clinical evidence

Each author selected relevant studies on a particular topic by scrutinising the abstracts. Systematic reviews and meta-analyses of clinical trials were given priority and copies of originals obtained. Where systematic reviews or meta-analyses were not located, the evidence from RCTs and CCTs was considered next. In their absence uncontrolled studies were considered. In most cases, original reports were obtained.

Appraisal of clinical evidence

All authors were familiar with the process of systematic reviews and consistently evaluated the methodological quality of the studies by assessing important criteria such as randomisation, blinding, and description of withdrawals and dropouts in an informal review process. For systematic reviews and meta-analyses, the assessment of the methodological quality of included trials by the original authors was accepted. The quality of the review itself was assessed informally. In the *Summary of clinical evidence* tables (Section 2), the methodological quality of the body of evidence of a particular treatment for a particular condition was combined with the level of the evidence and the volume of the evidence to produce a measure of 'weight'. This is intended to indicate the degree of confidence that can be placed on the evidence. Details are given in *How to use this book* (see p 8).

Application of judgement

Clinical judgement was used by the authors in two specific areas: the *Overall recommendation* (Section 2) and the *Risk–benefit assessment* of each treatment (Sections 3 and 4). These judgements are based on experience and current medical practice as well as the evidence. In an attempt to minimise bias and achieve standardisation, the process was subjected to internal and external review (see *Review process* below). It should be noted that stating that there is a lack of compelling evidence for a treatment does not imply that the treatment is ineffective.

Presentation of information

In most parts of each chapter, the information is presented in a concise narrative form in a predefined format (see *How to use this book*, p 7). However, for *Clinical evidence* in Section 2 key information is displayed in the *Summary of evidence* tables. Additionally, the most authoritative systematic review or meta-analysis on a subject has been abstracted into a box. Selected clinical trials are sometimes presented in standardised tables; usually these are the most scientifically rigorous or clinically relevant. Data have been extracted according to predefined criteria into tables which also provide additional information or a critical comment. At the end of Sections 3 and 4, tables are presented containing brief information on other treatments that were not included as full chapters.

Information on safety

Information on safety is central to the assessment of a treatment's value. Hence this material is an important component of the book. Unfortunately, there is often only fragmentary knowledge on safety in CAM. The treatment chapters (Sections 3 and 4) address risks as fully as is possible from available data. In general, the precautionary principle has been applied, so a treatment is not considered risk-free unless evidence suggests otherwise. In our view, this is prudent and follows the most important axiom of medicine: *primum nihil nocere* – first do no harm. Unless there is positive evidence for safety pregnancy and lactation are cited as contraindications for all medicines included in this book. Allergic reactions have been mentioned where they have been reported but should be assumed possible for all herbs and many supplements, with the potential to be serious.

For the *Summary of clinical evidence* tables in Section 2, many different ways of summarising safety data were considered, but it proved impossible to provide sufficient useful detail. It was therefore decided to use a simple Yes/No descriptor to alert the reader in a general way to the existence (however rare) of potentially serious safety concerns, cross-referencing to the sections providing specific details (see *How to use this book*, p 9). Even when a treatment is apparently innocuous, the table entry is 'Yes' if there is insufficient information available to establish safety and serious risks are considered possible. This applies to all herbs and some supplements. Other supplements are marked 'Yes' because overdose is associated with serious consequences. Most products derived from natural sources carry the risk of allergic reactions (see above). In the case of homeopathic remedies, this is unlikely at non-material dilutions, hence homeopathy is marked 'No'. Aromatherapy, on the other hand, is marked 'Yes', due to the allergic reactions possible with essential oils. Therapies marked 'Yes' that cannot be cross-referenced to a specific chapter or table are hydrotherapy (for which cardio-respiratory decompensation and bacterial infections have been reported), exercise (where sudden death has been recorded), electrotherapy (for which psychological disturbance and local injury from electrodes are possible) and fasting and particular diets (where malnutrition can occur). Our intention is not to be alarmist, but clearly the priority must be to minimise all possible risks for the patient.

Review process

All information presented in this book was subjected to an internal review by all three authors. Chapters were revised accordingly and additional information was incorporated. Regular consensus conferences were held to ensure a standardised approach. This was performed particularly with a view to minimising bias in areas where a degree of personal judgement was introduced (see *Application of judgement* above). Any disputes that appeared during the consensus conferences were resolved through discussion.

For the 1st edition international experts on CAM were involved in an external review process, in particular the US editor. Information on herbs has been reviewed by three independent experts from Germany and Canada. Specific chapters were reviewed by individuals with relevant expertise (see *Acknowledgements*, p xix). The second edition was thoroughly revised, updated throughout and expanded. Criticism and praise from book reviews and any other feedback received on the first edition were systematically collated, internally discussed and each point addressed in the second edition. Also, the chapters of Section 3 were sent to 79 professional organisations of the respective therapies and comments invited (see *Acknowledgements*, p xix). Their replies were reviewed and discussed internally and, where appropriate, incorporated.

The ultimate review, however, remains with you, the reader. We welcome constructive criticism on all aspects of this publication and invite readers to contact us via the publisher.

REFERENCES

1 Ernst E, Resch K L, Mills S *et al.* Complementary medicine – a definition. Br J Gen Pract 1995;309: 107–111

2 Long L, Huntley A, Ernst E. Which complementary and alternative therapies benefit which condition? A survey of 223 professional organisations. Complement Ther Med 2001;9:178–185

3 Mills S, Peacock W. Professional organisations of complementary and alternative medicine in the United Kingdom 1997: a report to the Department of Health. Centre for Complementary Health Studies, University of Exeter

HOW TO USE THIS BOOK

This book is divided into four main sections:

- Conditions
- Therapies
- Herbal and non-herbal medicines
- General topics.

Standardised structures have been adopted for the chapters within the first three sections. To help the reader understand and make the best use of the information in the individual chapters, there are brief explanations of the material provided under each subheading, with the help of examples taken from the book.

For further details on the methods employed for writing these sections, see p 2.

**Section 2
Conditions**

This section includes chapters on conditions commonly seen in primary care for which CAM is popular. Chapters are presented in alphabetical order and are subdivided according to the subheadings shown in the example below (hay fever).

USING THE BOOK

Quoted from BMJ Clinical Evidence (see p 16) where available

Information on the use of CAM by patients with the condition

An evidence-based summary of the data relating to the effectiveness of different forms of CAM for the condition. Priority is given to systematic reviews/meta-analyses and RCTs. Treatments are listed in alphabetical order (except Other therapies; see below)

Optional standardised tables of RCTs. **NB:** When several exist, only a few examples appear in the table, selected for their rigour or clinical relevance

Brief overview of the evidence relating to a treatment for the condition

140 CONDITIONS

HAY FEVER

Synonyms/ subcategories

Seasonal allergic rhinitis, pollenosis.

Definition

Type I immediate hypersensitivity reaction mediated by specific IgE antibody to a seasonal allergen, leading to mucosal inflammation characterised by sneezing, itching, rhinorrhoea, nasal blockage and conjunctivitis.

CAM usage

The best treatment for allergic rhinitis is, of course, to avoid allergens but this is not usually practical. Allergies are one of the main reasons for using complementary therapies, according to a US survey,[1] almost half of patients with allergies try a natural product with herbal medicine and relaxation used the most. A German survey found that hay fever was the allergy most commonly treated with CAM (62%) and that only four treatment modalities accounted for almost the entire usage: homeopathy, autologous blood injection, acupuncture and bioresonance.[2]

Clinical evidence

Acupuncture

Uncontrolled studies have previously suggested that acupuncture has value in the management of hay fever, but the evidence from RCTs (Table 2.38) is mixed and suggests that effects may be attributable to non-specific factors. Three RCTs found acupuncture to be superior in preventing[3] or treating[4,5] hay fever symptoms yet three found no difference between acupuncture and sham groups for either prevention[6] or treatment.[7,8]

Table 2.38 **RCTs of acupuncture for hay fever**

Reference	Sample size	Interventions [regimen]	Result	Comment
Williamson[3]	30	A) Acupuncture [1 session/w for 3 w] B) Conventional medication	A superior to B for prevention	Conclusion unclear statistics uncertain
Xue[4]	26	A) Acupuncture [three sessions/w for 4 w] B) Sham acupuncture	A superior to B for treatment	Superior for subjective symptoms but not for relief medication scores

Diet

One RCT assessed the effects of an antigen avoidance diet during infancy on later development of atopy.[9] Common allergens such as cow's milk, egg and peanuts were avoided during gestation and first 3 years of life (n = 165). Prevalence of hay fever or other allergies was no different from the control group at age 7 years.

Herbal medicine

Four out of five RCTs of **butterbur** (*Petasites hybridus*) (Table 2.39) report positive findings. Two found it to be more effective than placebo,[10,11] one superior to placebo and equally effective as fexofenadine,[12] and one equally effective as cetirizine.[13] One small RCT found it not to be clinically effective.[14]

Homeopathy

Seven placebo-controlled RCTs of *Galphimia glauca* from one research group were subjected to meta-analysis by the same researchers (Box 2.47).[21] Collectively the results suggested that the remedy is effective for both ocular and nasal symptoms. The success rate of 79% is comparable to conventional treatments, with minimal adverse events reported. Encouraging results were reported from a small pilot RCT (n = 36) of homeo-

CONDITIONS 141

pathic grass pollens versus placebo.[22] The same research team conducted a larger (n = 144) double-blind placebo-controlled RCT testing homeopathic dilutions of specific antigens identified for each hay fever patient by skin tests.[23] Symptom scores and use of antihistamines were reduced more in the homeopathic group. A double-blind RCT compared a homeopathic nasal spray with a conventional one (cromolyn sodium) over 42 days in 146 hay fever sufferers.[24]

Box 2.47
Meta-analysis
Homeopathic
Galphimia glauca
for hay fever
Lüdtke[21]

- Seven randomised double-blind placebo-controlled trials and four not placebo-controlled trials involving 1038 patients (752 in placebo-controlled trials)

- Overall rate of improved eye-symptoms is about 1.25 (CI 1.09 to 1.43) times higher in the verum than in the placebo group

- Verum success rate is estimated by 79.3% (CI 74.1% to 85.0%) comparable with those of conventional antihistaminics

- No side effects occurred

- Conclusion: a significant superiority of *Galphimia glauca* over placebo is demonstrated. However, as not all of the single studies were analysed by intention to treat analysis the results may be biased

Summary details of any authoritative systematic review/meta-analysis on a subject

Hypnotherapy
An RCT (n = 47) tested the effects of hypnotic suggestion on skin reactions to allergen prick tests in individuals with hay fever and asthma.[26] Hypnosis was associated with smaller weals, but specific suggestions had no influence. An RCT (n = 79) reported improvements of symptoms with self-hypnosis in patients with moderate to severe allergic rhinitis to grass or birch pollen.[27]

Supplements
Fish oil supplementation was investigated in a double-blind placebo-controlled RCT (n = 37) involving pollen-sensitive individuals with hay fever and asthma.[28] Various outcomes measured over a pollen season revealed no differences between the fish oil and pulsatic groups.

Treatments for which there is only minimal evidence. **NB:** Other therapies do not appear in *Summary of clinical evidence* table

Other therapies
Encouraging results have been reported in CCTs of imagery,[29,30] and pulsatic electromagnetic therapy.[31]

**Overall
recommendation**

Encouraging evidence exists for a homeopathic preparation of *Galphimia glauca*. Whether it is as effective as conventional medication still needs to be directly investigated. Adverse events are rare with homeopathic remedies, so it might be an option for patients dissatisfied with their orthodox medication. The results for butterbur are also encouraging and it seems to be associated with fewer adverse events than conventional medication. There is not convincing evidence from clinical trials for the effectiveness of any other complementary therapy in the prevention or treatment of hay fever.

An evidence-based judgement evaluating the benefits and risks of CAM for the condition in relation to conventional treatments. **NB:** A lack of compelling evidence is not the same as ineffectiveness

USING THE BOOK

143 CONDITIONS

For each treatment, the totality of available evidence is assessed and presented according to three criteria: 1) weight of evidence; 2) direction of evidence; 3) serious safety concerns (see p 5 for explanations)

Table 2.40
Summary of clinical evidence for hay fever

Treatment	Weight of evidence	Direction of evidence	Serious safety concerns
Acupuncture			
(prevention)	O	⇨	Yes (see p 294)
(treatment)	OOO	⇨	Yes (see p 294)
Diet (prevention)	O	⇩	No (see p 5)
Herbal medicine			
Butterbur	OO	⬈	Yes (see p 477)
Chinese herbal formula	OO	⬈	Yes (see p 5)
Grapeseed	O	⇩	Yes (see p 414)
Nettle	O	⬈	Yes (see p 443)
Tinaspora cordifolia	O	⇧	Yes (see p 5)
Homeopathy	OO	⇧	No (see p 327)
Hypnosis	OO	⬈	Yes (see p 331)
Supplements			
Fish oil	O	⇩	Yes (see p 483)
Vitamin E	O	⬈	Yes (see p 5)

REFERENCES

1 Zuckerman G B, Bielory L. Complementary and alternative medicine herbal therapies for atopic disorders. Am J Med 2002;113 suppl:47S–51S
2 Schafer T, Riehle A, Wichmann H E, Ring J. Alternative medicine in allergies – prevalence, patterns of use, and costs. Allergy 2002;57:694–700
3 Williamson L. Hay fever prophylaxis using single point acupuncture: a pilot study. Acup Med 1994;12:84–87
4 Xue C C, English R, Zhang J J, Da Costa C, Li C G. Effect of acupuncture in the treatment of seasonal allergic rhinitis: a randomized controlled clinical trial. Am J Chin Med 2002;30:1–11

**Section 3
Therapies**

This section includes chapters on forms of CAM that are identified as therapeutic modalities and excludes medicines such as herbs or food supplements. Chapters are presented in alphabetical order and are subdivided according to the headings shown in the example below (aromatherapy).

Other therapies with some evidence of effectiveness are presented in a table at the end of this section. Brief information is provided for each one, including a description, its main uses and any concerns about its safety.

THERAPIES **300**

AROMATHERAPY

Definition	The controlled use of plant essences for therapeutic purposes.
Related techniques	Massage.
Background	The medicinal use of plant oils has a long history in ancient Egypt, China and India. The development of modern aromatherapy is attributed to French chemist René Gattefosse, who burned his hand while working in a perfume laboratory and immediately doused it in some nearby lavender oil. The burn healed quickly without scarring, leading him to study the potential curative powers of plant oils. He coined the term aromatherapy in 1937.
Traditional concepts	Essential oils can be applied directly to the skin through massage or a compress, added to baths, inhaled with steaming water or spread throughout a room with a diffuser. The oils have effects at the psychological, physiological and cellular levels. These effects can be relaxing or stimulating depending on the chemistry of the oil and also the previous associations of the individual with a particular scent.
Scientific rationale	The scent from the oil activates the olfactory sense. This triggers the limbic system, which governs emotional responses and is involved with the formation and retrieval of learned memories. Essential oils are also absorbed through the skin via the dermis and layer of subcutaneous fat to the bloodstream. Laboratory studies suggest that molecules of the oil can affect organ function, although the clinical relevance of these findings is not clear.
Practitioners	In most countries aromatherapy is largely unregulated. In the UK it is in the process of being regulated. Various aromatherapy associations offer courses with the number of hours of training required ranging from 180 to 500. Many nurses and other healthcare professionals routinely seek aromatherapy qualifications.
Conditions frequently treated	Anxiety, headaches, insomnia, musculoskeletal pain, and other stress related conditions. Some therapists recommend regular aromatherapy as a means of maintaining general health and well-being. A US survey suggests that stress, musculoskeletal problems and pain are the most common conditions treated by aromatherapists.[1]
Typical session	During an initial session the aromatherapist will ask about a client's medical history, health and lifestyle and which aromas are liked or disliked. The therapist will then select essential oils deemed appropriate for the client according to this information. Treatment would usually consist of an aromatherapy massage and advice may be given about home treatments involving the use of oils in baths or a diffuser. The initial session may last up to 2 hours. Subsequent sessions would typically last 1 hour.
Course of treatment	For chronic conditions, one weekly session would be recommended for several weeks, with fortnightly or monthly follow-ups.
Clinical evidence	A systematic review of all RCTs of aromatherapy was conducted.[2] Based on six trials with hospitalised patients, it was concluded that aromatherapy massage has mild, transient anxiolytic effects. Due to lack of independent replication, the results of six other trials were not considered conclusive. These included positive findings for the treatment of alopecia areata[3] and prevention of bronchitis[4] and negative results for postnatal perineal discomfort.[5] Another systematic review included four RCTs of topical applications of tea tree oil.[6]

SECTION THREE

Other forms of treatment that share important features with the therapy

Brief introduction to the origins of the therapy, its cultural context and historical development

Summary of the underlying principles of the therapy.
NB: Not all practitioners use the traditional concepts

Evaluation of the principles of the therapy and mechanism of action from a scientific perspective

Persons employing the therapy. Patients should ensure that any therapist used is a member of a recognised body or association, holds professional liability insurance cover and that the recognised body has a code of ethics and conduct and a complaints and disciplinary procedure.
NB: Many therapies are practised by more than one professional group

In alphabetical order

Evidence-based summary of the data relating to the effectiveness of the therapy. In cases where a considerable amount of evidence exists, only the most important is presented. Priority is given to systematic reviews/meta-analyses and RCTs

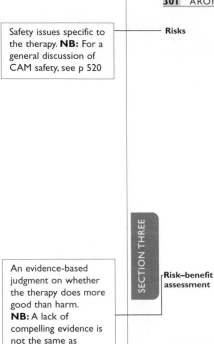

301 AROMATHERAPY

Risks

Safety issues specific to the therapy. **NB:** For a general discussion of CAM safety, see p 520

Contraindications
Pregnancy, contagious diseases, epilepsy, local venous thrombosis, varicose veins, broken skin, recent surgery, circulatory disorders.

Precautions/warnings
Essential oils should not be taken orally or used undiluted on the skin. Some oils cause photosensitive reactions and some have carcinogenic potential. Allergic reactions are possible with all oils. Aromatherapy should generally be considered an adjunctive treatment, not an alternative to conventional care.

Adverse effects
Allergic reactions, phototoxic reactions, nausea, headache.

Interactions
Many essential oils are believed to have the potential to either enhance or reduce the effects of prescribed medications including antibiotics, tranquillisers, antihistamines, anticonvulsants, barbiturates, morphine, quinidine.

Quality issues
Products marketed as 'aromatherapy oils' may be synthetic or adulterated rather than the pure essential oil.

Risk–benefit assessment

An evidence-based judgment on whether the therapy does more good than harm. **NB:** A lack of compelling evidence is not the same as ineffectiveness

The trial evidence on aromatherapy is confusingly contradictory. Aromatherapy appears to have some benefits as a palliative or supportive treatment, particularly in reducing anxiety. In the hands of a responsible therapist there seem to be few risks. Aromatherapy may thus be worth considering as an adjunctive treatment for chronically ill patients or individuals with psychosomatic illness.

SECTION THREE

REFERENCES
1 Osborn C E, Barlas P, Baxter G D, Barlow J H. Aromatherapy: a survey of current practice in the management of rheumatic disease symptoms. Complement Ther Med 2001;9:62–67
2 Cooke B, Ernst E. Aromatherapy: a systematic review. Br J Gen Pract 2000;50:493–496
3 Hay I C, Jamieson M, Ormerod A D. Randomised trial of aromatherapy. Successful treatment for alopecia areata. Arch Dermatol 1998;134:1349–1352
4 Ferley J P, Poutignat N, Zmirou D et al. Prophylactic aromatherapy for supervening infections in patients with chronic bronchitis. Statistical evaluation conducted in clinics against a placebo. Phytother Res1989;3:97–100
5 Dale A, Cornwell S. The role of lavender oil in relieving perineal discomfort following childbirth: a blind randomised clinical trial. J Adv Nurs 1994;19:89–96

Section 4 Herbal and non-herbal medicines

This section includes chapters on forms of CAM that are considered medications such as herbal and non-herbal supplements. Vitamins and minerals are not included (see p 2). Chapters are presented in alphabetical order of the common name and are subdivided according to the headings in the example below (valerian). It was decided to use the common name of herbs due to the frequent uncertainties of terminology in the original articles. Exact taxonomic names is an area which requires attention in future studies.

Other herbs and non-herbal supplements with some evidence of effectiveness are presented in tables at the end of this section. Brief information is provided, including a description, main uses and safety concerns. There are also tables relating to the safety of herbs.

HERBAL AND NON-HERBAL MEDICINE   **468**

VALERIAN
(*Valeriana officinalis, Valeriana edulis*)

Plant taxonomy
according to GRIN
(see p 17)

Source	Rhizome.

Main constituents	Alkaloids, amino acids (gamma-aminobutyric acid), iridoids/valepotriates, phenylpropanoids, sesquiterpenoids volatile oils.

In alphabetical order

Background	*Valeriana officinalis* is one of over 200 members of the *Valerianaceae* family. A herbaceous perennial, it is native to most of Europe and Asia and grows in damp swampy areas. The name *Valeriana* derives from the Latin word *valere* meaning well-being. Its use as a medicinal herb dates back to Hippocrates' time. *Valeriana edulis* is widely used in South America for insomnia and anxiety.

For herb: brief
description of
historical background,
etymology and botany.
For supplement:
rationale for its use

Examples of traditional uses	Digestive problems, flatulence, urinary tract disorders.

Pharmacologic action	Sedative, anxiolytic. Mechanisms are unclear, but gamma-aminobutyric acid receptors may be involved.

Conditions frequently treated	Anxiety, insomnia.

Conditions and
purposes for which the
medicine was
traditionally used; in
alphabetical order.
NB: May be
unsupported or even
contraindicated by
current evidence

Clinical evidence	The hypnotic effects of valerian have been investigated in several double-blind placebo-controlled RCTs. Improvements following single doses have been reported (e.g.[1]) as well as with repeated administration (e.g.[2]). A systematic review of the subject concluded that the evidence was promising but not conclusive, due to inconsistent results and methodological limitations.[3] RCTs published subsequently found valerian to be effective as oxazepam in enhancing the sleep quality of insomniacs after 4 weeks.[4] A sizeable (n = 202) RCT with patients suffering from insomnia confirmed that valerian extract (600 mg/day) is at least as effective as oxazepam (10 mg/day) in increasing sleep quality when taken for 6 weeks.[5]

Pharmacologic effects
demonstrated.
NB: Mention is made
of mechanisms only if
considered relevant

In alphabetical order

Dosage	400–900 mg of extract 30–60 minutes before bedtime.

Evidence-based
summary of the data
relating to the
effectiveness of the
medicine. In cases where
a considerable amount
of evidence exists, only
the most important is
presented. Priority is
given to systematic
reviews/meta-analyses
and RCTs

Risks	**Contraindications** Pregnancy and lactation (see p 5), known allergy, hepatic impairment. **Precautions/warnings** Care should be taken if driving or operating machinery when taking valerian. Long-term risks are under-researched. **Adverse effects** Headache and gastrointestinal symptoms are occasionally reported. Morning hangover reported occasionally although RCTs investigating safety factors have found no impairment of reaction time or alertness the morning after intake. Hepatotoxicity has been reported from herbal preparations in which valerian was combined with other herbs, including skullcap. The trial data suggest that adverse effects of valerian are less frequent than those of benzodiazepines.[4,5] **Overdose** Symptoms of tachycardia, nausea, vomiting, dilated pupils, drowsiness, confusion, visual hallucinations, blurred vision, cardiac disturbance, excitability, headache, hypersensitivity reactions and insomnia have been reported following acute overdoses, with full recoveries made in all cases. **Interactions** Potentiation of the effects of sedatives, hypnotics or other central nervous system depressants is possible at high doses.[18] RCTs have shown no potentiation of alcohol.

Usual therapeutic dose,
where possible based
on clinical trial data.
NB: Due to scarce
data, no attempt is
made to suggest
optimum duration of
treatment. The effects
of some herbs may
take several weeks to
appear. There is
generally a lack of
adequate data regarding
long-term use

USING THE BOOK

Saftey issues specific to the medicine. **NB:** For a general discussion of CAM saftey, see p 520

An evidence-based judgement on whether the medicine does more good than harm. **NB:** A lack of compelling evidence is not the same as ineffectiveness

SECTION FOUR

470 VALERIAN

Quality issues
Composition and purity of extracts vary greatly. Standardised extracts often use valepotriates as the marker substance although valerenic acid is considered more reliable due to its stability. Aqueous extracts are devoid of valepotriates.

Risk–benefit assessment
Even though the evidence is not entirely uniform, the majority of the sound clinical trials suggest efficacy for insomnia. For that indication, valerian may offer advantages over benzodiazepines. It is unclear whether herbal combinations have advantages over single valerian extracts. Indications other than insomnia require further study. The risks of short-term valerian monotherapy seem to be acceptable. Therefore valerian can be recommended as a short-term solution to insomnia.

REFERENCES
1 Leathwood P D, Chauffard F, Heck E, Munoz-Box R. Aqueous extract of valerian root (Valeriana officinalis L) improves sleep quality in man. Pharmacol Biochem Behav 1982;17:65–71
2 Vorbach E U, Gortelmeyer R, Bruning J. Therapie von Insomnien: Wirksamkeit und Verträglichkeit eines Baldrianpräparats. Psychopharmakotherapie 1996;3:109–115

3 Stevinson C, Ernst E. Valerian for insomnia: systematic review of randomized placebo-controlled trials. Sleep Med 2000;1:91–99
4 Dorn M. Baldrian versus oxazepam: efficacy and tolerability in non-organic and non-psychiatric insomniacs: a randomized, double-blind, clinical comparative study. Forsch Komplementärmed Klass Naturheilkd 2000;7:79–84

Significance levels

When reporting research results, only differences that are statistically significant ($p < 0.05$) are mentioned; p values and the term 'significant' are omitted for conciseness.

Weight of evidence

The weight of the evidence refers to the level of confidence (see pp 4–5) that can be placed on it. There are three discrete categories of weight:

Low	0
Moderate	00
High	000

The judgement of weight is based on a combination of three largely independent factors:

- the level of evidence (the highest level being systematic review/meta-analysis, followed by RCT, CCT and uncontrolled study)
- the methodological quality of the investigations (the validity and reliability of the studies)
- the volume of information (the number of studies and their sample sizes).

Judgements take into account all three of these dimensions of weight. Therefore a treatment where volume and level are high (e.g. meta-analysis of 50 studies) will not necessarily receive a high weight if the quality is low (e.g. methodologically flawed studies). Similarly, even if quality and level are high (e.g. a rigorous RCT), weight can only be considered low if there is a low volume of evidence (only a single trial).

Direction of evidence

The direction of the evidence refers to the collective positive or negative outcome of the studies for that treatment. Direction can be reported in one of five ways:

> Clearly positive ⇧
> Tentatively positive ⬈
> Uncertain ⇨
> Tentatively negative ⬊
> Clearly negative ⇩

Direction is largely judged independently of weight of evidence. The reader must interpret the direction of the evidence in the light of its weight. For example, a clearly positive result based on evidence with low weight (e.g. a single, small, non-randomised trial) may not be as informative as a tentatively positive finding backed by a body of evidence with high weight (e.g. a systematic review of RCTs).

Serious safety concerns

Cases where a treatment has been, or may potentially be, associated with life-threatening consequences, hospitalisation or sustained harm, even if rare.

No = reports of serious events were not located and are considered unlikely

Yes = serious events have been reported or are considered possible

Whenever possible, page references are provided for the treatment's own chapter or relevant table. In some cases, information is not available about safety. The general principle is to err on the side of caution; so when in doubt, a treatment is marked Yes. This applies to all herbs and some supplements (see *Methods*, p 5).

NB

- It is imperative that the reader refers to the treatment chapter or table. Even where a treatment is marked No, there may be contraindications and precautions which, if ignored, could have potentially serious consequences.
- Even where a therapy is not associated with serious complications, indirect risks may exist and could have serious consequences. CAM practitioners may not be medically qualified and should not therefore be expected to have competence in orthodox medical management.
- Many of the reported serious adverse events are avoidable by good clinical practice.

For a general discussion of CAM safety, see p 520.

BIBLIOGRAPHY OF MAIN REFERENCE SOURCES

SECTION 2 CONDITIONS

British Medical Journal. Clinical evidence. British Medical Journal Publishing Group; 2005. Online. Available: http://www.clinicalevidence.com

Stedman T. Stedman's medical dictionary. 27th edn. Baltimore: Williams and Wilkins; 2003

SECTION 3: THERAPIES

Barnett H. The Which? guide to complementary therapies. London: Which?; 2002

Callahan D. (ed). The role of complementary and alternative medicine. Washington: Georgetown University Press; 2002

Freeman, L. Mosby's complementary and alternative medicine evidence-based approach. St Louis: Mosby; 2001

Fugh-Berman A. Alternative medicine: what works. Tucson: Odonian; 1996

Jonas W B, Levin J S (eds). Essentials of complementary and alternative medicine. Baltimore: Lippincott Williams and Wilkins; 1999

Kelner M J, Wellman B, Saks M (eds). Complementary and alternative medicine: challenge and change. Reading: Harwood Academic Publishers; 2000

Lewith G, Jonas WB, Walach H. Clinical research in complementary therapies. Edinburgh: Churchill Livingstone; 2001

Mac Beckner W, Berman B M. Complementary therapies on the internet. St Louis: Churchill Livingstone, USA; 2003

Micozzi, M S. Fundamentals of complementary and alternative medicine. Edinburgh: Churchill Livingstone; 2000

Novey DW (ed). Clinician's complete reference to complementary and alternative medicine. St. Louis: Mosby; 2000

Peters D, Woodham A. The complete guide to integrated medicine. London: Dorling Kindersley; 2000

Peters D, Woodham A. The complete guide to integrated medicine. the best of complementary and conventional care. London: Dorling Kindersley; 2000

Schimmel K C (ed). Lehrbuch der Naturheilverfahren. Stuttgart: Hippokrates; 1990

Spencer J W, Jacobs J. Complementary and alternative medicine: an evidence-based approach. 2nd edn. St. Louis: Mosby; 2003

Stone J. An ethical framework for complementary and alternative therapies. London: Routledge; 2002

Yuan C S, Bieber E J. Textbook of complementary and alternative medicine. New York: Parthenon; 2003

Zollman C, Vickers A. ABC of complementary medicine. London: BMJ Books; 2000

SECTION 4 HERBAL AND NON-HERBAL MEDICINES

Barnes J, Anderson L A, Phillipson J D. Herbal medicines. 2nd edn. London: Pharmaceutical Press; 2002

Basch E, Ulbricht C E (eds). Natural standard herb and supplement handbook: the clinical bottom line. St Louis, MO: Elsevier Mosby; 2005

Blumenthal M (ed). The ABC clinical guide to herbs. Austin: American Botanical Council; 2003

Blumenthal M, Goldberg A, Brinckmann J (eds). Herbal medicine. expanded commission E monographs. Austin: American Botanical Council; 2000

Boon H, Smith M. The botanical pharmacy. Kingston: Quarry Press; 1999

Boon H, Smith M. The complete natural medicine guide to the 50 most common medicinal herbs. Toronto: Robert Rose; 2004

Bratman S, Gitman A M. Mosby's handbook of herbs and supplements and their therapeutic uses. St Louis: Mosby; 2003

Braun L, Cohen M. Herbs and natural supplements. An evidence-based guide. Sydney: Elsevier; 2005

Brinker F. Herb contraindications and drug interactions. Sandy: Eclectic Medical Publications; 1998

Capasso F, Gaginella T S, Grandolini G, Izzo A A. Phytotherapy: a quick reference to herbal medicine. Berlin: Springer-Verlag; 2003

Cupp M J. Toxicology and clinical pharmacology of herbal products. Totowa: Humana Press; 2000

Dukes M N G, Aronson J K (eds). Meyler's side effects of drugs. 14th edn. Amsterdam: Elsevier; 2000

Ernst E. Herb–drug interactions – an update. Perfusion 2003;16:175–194

Fetrow C, Avila J. The complete guide to herbal medicines. Springhouse: Springhouse Corporation; 2000

Fetrow C W, Avila J R. Professional's handbook of complementary and alternative medicines. Springhouse, PA: Springhouse; 1999

Fugh-Berman A. Herb–drug interactions. Lancet 2000;355:134–138

Fugh-Berman A. The 5-minute herb and dietary supplement consult. Philadelphia: Lippincott Williams & Wilkins; 2003

Hänsel R, Keller K, Rimpler H, Schneider G. Hagers Handbuch der pharmazeutischen Praxis. Berlin: Springer; 1994

Harkness R, Bratman S. Mosby's handbook of drug–herb and drug–supplement interactions. St Louis: Mosby; 2003

Hildebrandt H (ed). Psychrembel Wörterbuch Naturheilkunde und alternative Heilverfahren. Berlin: deGruyter; 1996

Lininger S W (ed). A–Z guide to drug-herb-vitamin interactions. Rocklin; CA: Prima; 1999

Mahady G B, Fong H H S, Farnsworth N R. Botanical, dietary supplements: quality, safety and efficacy. Rotterdam: AA Balkema Publishers; 2001

Mason P. Dietary supplements. 2nd edn. London: Pharmaceutical Press; 2001. Online. Available: *http://www.medicinescomplete.com/mc/*

Meletis C D, Jacobs T. Interactions between drugs and natural medicines. Sandy: Eclectic Medical Publications; 1999

Murray M T. Encyclopedia of nutritional supplements. Rocklin: Prima; 1996

Jellin J M (ed). Natural Medicines Comprehensive Database, Online. Available: *www.naturaldatabase.com*

Natural Standard Database, Online. Available: *www.naturalstandard.com*

Rapport L, Lockwood B. Nutraceuticals. London: Pharmaceutical Press; 2002

Ross I A. Medicinal plants of the world, Vol. 2. Totowa: Humana Press; 2001

Rotblatt M, Ziment I. Evidence-based herbal medicine. Philadelphia: Hanley & Belfus; 2002.

Royal Pharmaceutical Society of Great Britain (ed). British national formulary. London: Pharmaceutical Press; 2005. Online. Available: *http://www. medicinescomplete.com/mc/*

Schulz V, Hänsel R, Blumenthal M, Tyler V E. Rational phytotherapy: a reference guide for physicians and pharmacists. 5th edn. Berlin: Springer Verlag; 2004

Skidmore-Roth L. Mosby's handbook of herbs & natural supplements. St. Louis: Mosby; 2001.

Stockley I H (ed). Stockley's interaction alert. London: Pharmaceutical Press; 2005. Online. Available: *http://www.medicinescomplete.com/mc/*

Reynolds Sweetman S J E F (ed). Martindale: the complete drug reference. Martindale: the extra pharmacopoeia. London: Pharmaceutical Press; 2005. Online. Available: *http://www.medicinescomplete.com/mc/*

Ulbricht C E, Basch E (eds). Natural Standard herb and supplement reference: evidence-based clinical reviews. St Louis, MO: Elsevier Mosby; 2005

USDA, ARS, National Genetic Resources Program. Germplasm Resources Information Network (GRIN) Online Database. National Germplasm Resources Laboratory, Beltsville, Maryland. Available: *http://www.ars-grin.gov2/cgi-bin/npgs/html/index.pl*

Wichtl M (ed). Herbal drugs and phytopharmaceuticals. 3rd edn. Stuttgart: Medpharm Scientific Publishers; 2004

World Health Organisation. Monographs on selected medicinal plants. Geneva: WHO; 1999

Conditions

ACNE

Synonyms/ subcategories	Acne vulgaris, cystic acne, pimples, comedones.
Definition	Acne is a skin disorder of the sebaceous follicles that presents as lesions which are either inflamed (i.e. papules, pustules and nodules) or non-inflamed (i.e. open or closed comedones, papules, pustules and nodules). It is one of the most common skin conditions requiring medical treatment, yet its pathophysiology is poorly understood. The characteristic localisation of acne to the face and upper trunk is a result of the distribution of oil-secreting structures known as sebaceous glands within the hair follicles. Most common type is acne vulgaris, but approximately 20 subtypes are recognised.
CAM usage	Herbal medicines are most commonly used to control infection, stop itching and improve symptoms.
Clinical evidence	*Herbal medicine* Oral and topical application of **Ayurvedic herbal** preparations containing *Aloe barbadensis*, *Azardirachta indica*, *Curcuma longa*, *Hemidesmus indicus*, *Terminalia chebula*, *Terminalia arjuna* and *Withania somnifera*, and *Piper longum* was tested in a double-blind RCT (n = 53).[1] The combined use of internal and external preparation was more effective in treating acne than the oral formulation alone. Sunder Vati was reported to be more effective in reducing the lesion count compared with three other Ayurvedic formulations and placebo in a double-blind RCT (n = 82).[2] Three RCTs found encouraging results for various **Chinese herbal mixtures** in the treatment of acne vulgaris. Fu Fang She She Cao He Ji (Compound Oldenlandis Mixture) was found to be more effective than Dang Gui Ku Shen Wan,[3] Quingre Cuochuang tablets were as effective as standard medication antisterone, tetracycline and metronidazole[4] and Xiao Cuo Fang combined with adapalene gel was more effective in reducing skin injury and had fewer adverse events than retinoic acid cream.[5] In all three trials the patient groups receiving the Chinese herbal medicines were almost twice as large as the control groups which might have confounded the results. In an RCT (n = 20) oral **gugulipid** (*Commiphora mukkul*) was comparable to oral tetracycline in the treatment of nodulocystic acne in decreasing inflammation and the number of relapses.[6] An individualised dose of juice from *Ocimum basilicum* was tested against standard treatment with oral tetracycline and topical sulfur lotion in a single-blind controlled trial (n = 51).[7] Improvement was similar in both groups.

A range of concentrations of *Ocimum gratissimum* oil was compared with 10% benzoyl peroxide and placebo in an RCT (n = 126) with 16 parallel groups. The 2% and 5% *O. gratissimum* oil in alcohol and 5% oil in cetamocrogol base were more effective than benzoyl peroxide while 2% oil in cetamocrogol had similar effects to the reference product. Sample sizes of the individual groups were however too small to make any firm conclusions.[8]

In an investigator-blind RCT including 124 patients with mild to moderate acne **tea tree** (*Melaleuca alternifolia*) oil was compared with benzoyl peroxide.[9] Both treatments showed an improvement from baseline in treating lesions but the lack of placebo or power calculation limits the conclusions.

The combination of **Toto** (including *Elaeis guineesis* and *Butyrospermum paradoxum*) ointment and soap was reported to be more effective than either of them alone or sulfur ointment.[10] The fact that 30 out of the 36 acne patients received the combined treatment, however, limits the findings.

Supplements

In a double-blind RCT of 139 patients, the **yeast** preparation *Saccharomyces cerevisiae* Hansen CBS 5926 (Perenterol) was found to be more effective than placebo in the treatment of various forms of acne.[11]

Several small placebo-controlled trials suggested that **zinc** (Table 2.1) can improve acne[12-16] yet two found no beneficial effects.[17,18] Comparative trials with tetracycline have yielded conflicting results.[19,20] These findings are confirmed by an unsystematic review.[21] Topically, in combination with erythromycin, zinc also seems to be beneficial.[22-24]

Other therapies

A small RCT (n = 30) of a combination of **biofeedback-assisted relaxation** and cognitive imagery reported a reduction in acne severity when compared with attention-comparison and medical control groups.[25]

Overall recommendation Since there is no cure for acne, treatment or prevention modalities that are not associated with the adverse effects of some conventional acne treatments are desirable. Zinc seems an option particularly when tetracyclines are contraindicated; its effectiveness compared with standard treatment is however unclear. Some other herbals or supplements such as yeast, have yielded encouraging results but the evidence is not strong enough to make any recommendations.

CONDITIONS

Table 2.1 **Controlled clinical trials of zinc for acne**

Reference	Sample size	Interventions [regimen]	Result	Comment
Goransson[12]	54	A) Oral zinc sulfate [0.6 g daily for 6 w] B) Placebo	A superior to B in reducing number of lesions	Photographic assessment of acne vulgaris showed no improvement but acne load did
Hillstrom[13]	91	A) Oral zinc sulfate [0.4 g daily for 12 w] B) Placebo	A superior to B	Acne vulgaris; subjective parameters measured only
Michaelsson[14]	64	A) Oral zinc sulfate [corresponding to 135 mg zinc daily for 3 mo] B) As A plus Vitamin A [300 000 IU] C) Vitamin A D) Placebo	A better than D, no additional benefits with B or C	Mixed types of acne included
Verma[15]	56	A) Zinc sulfate [600 mg daily for 3 mo] B) Placebo	A superior to B	Isolated inflammatory acne only, no response at all in placebo group
Dreno[16]	66	A) Zinc gluconate [200 mg daily corresponding to 30 mg zinc metal] B) Placebo	A superior to B in inflammatory score	Inflammatory acne, low doses used
Orris[17]	22	A) Zinc sulfate monohydrate [411 mg/daily for 8 w] B) Placebo	No differences in lesion counts between A and B	Male patients with moderate mixed acne, more comedones than inflammatory elements
Weismann[18]	39	A) Oral zinc sulphate [60 mg daily for 4, 8 or 12 w] B) Placebo	No differences between A and B	No effect on larger infiltrates, treatment times differed between patients
Cunliffe[19]	48	A) Oral zinc sulphate/ citrate complex [dose not stated, for 3 mo] B) Tetracycline hydrochloride [500 mg daily for 3 mo]	B superior to A in reducing grade and number of non-inflamed lesions, pupules and pustules	Moderately severe acne
Michaelsson[20]	37	A) Oral zinc B) Tetracyclines	A equally effective as B on acne scores	Moderate and severe acne

Reference	Sample size	Interventions [regimen]	Result	Comment
Feucht[22]	141	A) 4% erythromycin liquid plus 1.2% zinc acetate [2 × day for 10 w] B) Oral tetracycline [250 mg] C) Placebo	A equally effective as B and superior to C	
Schachner[23]	73	A) 4% erythromycin liquid plus 1.2% zinc acetate [for 12 w] B) Placebo	A superior to B in acne severity grade and number	Placebo group patients received verum after 12 weeks for 1 year and duplicated improvement reported in group A
Habbema[24]	122	A) 4% erythromycin lotion plus zinc [for 12 w] B) 2% erythromycin lotion	A superior to B in reducing number of acne lesions and severity grade	

Table 2.2
Summary of clinical evidence for acne

Treatment	Weight of evidence	Direction of evidence	Serious safety concerns
Herbal medicine			
Ayurvedic herbal medicine	OO	⬀	Yes (see p 5)
Chinese herbal medicine	OO	⬀	Yes (see p 5)
Gugulipid	O	⬀	Yes (see p 5)
Ocimum basilicum	O	⬀	Yes (see p 5)
Ocimum gratissimum	O	⬀	Yes (see p 5)
Tea tree	O	⬀	Yes (see p 466)
Toto	O	⇨	Yes (see p 5)
Supplements			
Yeast	O	⬆	Yes (see p 5)
Zinc	OOO	⬀	Yes (see p 5)

REFERENCES

1 Lalla J K, Nandedkar S Y, Paranjape M H, Talreja N B. Clinical trials of ayurvedic formulations in the treatment of acne vulgaris. J Ethnopharmacol 2001;78:99–102
2 Paranjpe P, Kulkarni P H. Comparative efficacy of four Ayurvedic formulations in the treatment of acne vulgaris: a double-blind randomised placebo-controlled clinical evaluation. J Ethnopharmacol 1995;49:127–132
3 Liu W, Shen D, Song P, Xu X. Clinical observation in 86 cases of acne vulgaris treated with Compound Oldenlandis Mixture. J Tradit Chin Med 2003;23:255–256
4 Ma X H, Zhu S L, Zhou G M. [Clinical observation on treatment of female delayed acne vulgaris with qingre cuochuang tablet]. Zhongguo Zhong Xi Yi Jie He Za Zhi 2004;24:115–117 Chinese

CONDITIONS

5   Biyun C. [The clinical observation of treating acne vulgaris with 'xiao cuo fang'] Zhong Yao Cai 2004;27:308–310 Chinese

6   Thappa D M, Dogra J. Nodulocystic acne: oral gugulipid versus tetracycline. J Dermatol 1994;21:729–731

7   Balambal R, Thiruvengadam K V, Kameswarant L, Janaki V R, Thambiah A S. *Ocimum basilicum* in acne vulgaris – a controlled comparison with a standard regime. J Assoc Physicians India 1985;33:507–508

8   Orafidiya L O, Agbani E O, Oyedele A O, Babalola O O, Onayemi O. Preliminary clinical tests on topical preparations of *Ocimum gratissimum* Linn leaf essential oil for the treatment of acne vulgaris. Clin Drug Investig 2002;22:313–319

9   Bassett I B, Pannowitz D L, Barnetson RS. A comparative study of tea-tree oil versus benzoylperoxide in the treatment of acne. Med J Aust 1990;153:455–458

10 Alebiosu C O, Ogunledun A, Ogunleye D S. A report of clinical trial conducted on Toto ointment and soap products. J Natl Med Assoc 2003;95:95–105

11 Weber G, Adamczyk A, Freytag S. [Treatment of acne with a yeast preparation] Fortschr Med 1989;107:563–566

12 Goransson K, Liden S, Odsell L. Oral zinc in acne vulgaris: a clinical and methodological study. Acta Derm Venereol 1978;58: 443–448.

13 Hillstrom L, Pettersson L, Hellbe L, Kjellin A, Leczinsky C G, Nordwall C. Comparison of oral treatment with zinc sulphate and placebo in acne vulgaris. Br J Dermatol 1977;97:681–684.

14 Michaelsson G, Juhlin L, Vahlquist A. Effects of oral zinc and vitamin A in acne. Arch Dermatol 1977;113:31–36

15 Verma K C, Saini A S, Dhamija S K. Oral zinc sulphate therapy in acne vulgaris: a double-blind trial. Acta Derm Venereol 1900;60:337–340

16 Dreno B, Amblard P, Agache P, Sirot S, Litoux P. Low doses of zinc gluconate for inflammatory acne. Acta Derm Venereol 1989;69:541–543

17 Orris L, Shalita A R, Sibulkin D, London S J, Gans E H. Oral zinc therapy of acne. Absorption and clinical effect. Arch Dermatol 1978; 114:1018–1020

18 Weismann K, Wadskov S, Sondergaard J. Oral zinc sulphate therapy for acne vulgaris. Acta Derm Venereol 1977;57:357–360

19 Cunliffe W J, Burke B, Dodman B, Gould D J. A double-blind trial of a zinc sulphate/citrate complex and tetracycline in the treatment of acne vulgaris. Br J Dermatol 1979;101:321–325

20 Michaelsson G, Juhlin L, Ljunghall K. A double-blind study of the effect of zinc and oxytetracycline in acne vulgaris. Br J Dermatol 1977;97:561–566

21 Stephan F, Revuz J. [Zinc salts in dermatology] Ann Dermatol Venereol 2004;131:455–460

22 Feucht C L, Allen B S, Chalker D K, Smith J G Jr. Topical erythromycin with zinc in acne. A double-blind controlled study. J Am Acad Dermatol 1980;3:483–491

23 Schachner L, Eaglstein W, Kittles C, Mertz P. Topical erythromycin and zinc therapy for acne. J Am Acad Dermatol 1990;22:253–260

24 Habbema L, Koopmans B, Menke H E, Doornweerd S, De Boulle K. A 4% erythromycin and zinc combination (Zineryt) versus 2% erythromycin (Eryderm) in acne vulgaris: a randomized, double-blind comparative study. Br J Dermatol 1989;121:497–502

25 Hughes H, Brown B W, Lawlis G F, Fulton J E Jr. Treatment of acne vulgaris by biofeedback relaxation and cognitive imagery. J Psychosom Res 1983;27:185–191

AIDS/HIV INFECTION

Definition   Infection with human immunodeficiency virus (HIV) type 1 or type 2. Clinically characterised by 8–10 years of asymptomatic infection followed by episodes of varying type and severity of illness.

CAM usage   The prevalence of CAM use in AIDS patients and HIV-positive individuals is high.[1] There is no uniformity as to which treatments are used most. National differences exist and 'flavour of the month' treatments abound. One study examining the prevalence of CAM use in an ethnically diverse, gender-balanced sample of persons living with HIV/AIDS reported that more than two thirds (67%) of the participants who were taking HIV-related medications were also taking CAM supplement. Multivitamins, mineral supplements, Chinese herbs and other medicinal herbs, acupuncture, massage, and meditation were most commonly used to specifically treat HIV-related symptoms.[2] A large number of complementary therapies are relevant in relation to the treatment or palliative/supportive care of AIDS patients.

Clinical evidence

It is helpful to differentiate between alleged CAM 'AIDS cures' (including treatments which are claimed to delay the clinical course of the disease or decrease viral load) and CAM therapies used in palliative or supportive care.

Acupuncture

RCTs tested the effectiveness of acupuncture to treat HIV-related peripheral neuropathic pain.[3,4] No evidence for effectiveness was found.

Exercise

A systematic review of ten RCTs of regular aerobic exercise found that this approach is effective in decreasing depressive symptoms in HIV positive individuals.[5]

Guided imagery

An RCT tested guided imagery or progressive muscle relaxation versus no intervention in 69 HIV-positive individuals.[6] There were no beneficial effects in terms of quality of life but perceived health status was best in the group treated with guided imagery.

Herbal medicine

An RCT tested two different doses of boxwood (*Buxus sempervirens*) against placebo in HIV-infected, asymptomatic patients.[7] Results were encouraging but not compelling: 'CD4 counts fell in the low dose group but not in the high-dose group'.

A placebo-controlled, double-blind RCT of a complex **Chinese herbal mixture** of eight different herbs yielded encouraging results:[8] 'life satisfaction' improved in the experimental group but CD4 counts did not. A follow-up study attempted to overcome these problems; 68 HIV-infected adults were randomised to receive either placebo or standardised preparation of 38 Chinese herbs for 6 months.[9] No differences in terms of viral load, CD4 cell count, symptoms or psychometric parameters emerged.

St John's wort (*Hypericum perforatum*) has antiretroviral activity in vitro. When 30 HIV-infected individuals were given high-dose intravenous hypericin, no positive effects were seen on virologic markers or CD4 counts.[10] However, a significant degree of phototoxicity was noted.

An RCT of **tea tree oil** *(Melaleuca alternifolia)* for oral candidiasis of AIDS patients showed that 60% of patients responded positively to this treatment.[11]

Homeopathy
One hundred HIV-positive individuals were randomised to receive either individualised homeopathic remedies or placebo for 15–30 days.[12] There were positive effects on CD4 cell counts only in the homeopathically treated group.

Massage
Twenty-eight neonates born to HIV-positive mothers were randomised to receive either 15-minute massages daily for 10 days or no intervention.[13] The clinical score to evaluate the infants' development showed better outcomes for the neonates treated with massage. An RCT with 42 HIV-positive subjects suggested that regular massage therapy has no effect on immune function but, combined with stress management, improves quality of life.[14] Another RCT with 24 HIV-positive adolescents showed that regular massage is superior to progressive muscle relaxation in reducing anxiety and low mood.[15]

Ozone therapy
In an RCT regular ex vivo ozone treatment of peripheral blood followed by re-injection was carried out for 8 weeks. Compared with placebo treatment, no positive effects on immunological markers were observed.[16]

Spiritual healing
A double-blind RCT of distant healing versus no intervention including 40 patients suffering from advanced AIDS showed better outcomes in the experimental compared with the control group.[17] In another CCT,[18] 20 HIV-infected children were randomised to receive either therapeutic touch or 'mimic therapeutic touch'. The results show that active therapy reduced anxiety while the sham intervention did not.

Stress management
Several forms of stress management may offer useful adjunctive options in caring for AIDS patients. The cumulative evidence from these clinical trials is encouraging (Table 2.3), although no study controlled for placebo effects.[19–25]

Supplements
Short-term **arginine** supplementation may increase killer cell function in AIDS patients.[26] Similarly, vitamin deficiencies of AIDS patients will improve with adequate supplementation.

Topical **capsaicin** as a treatment for neuropathic pain was tested against placebo in an RCT.[27] After one week's treatment,

Table 2.3 **RCTs of stress management for AIDS/HIV infection**

Reference	Sample size	Interventions [regimen]	Result	Comment
Coates[19]	64 asymptomatic individuals	A) Stress management training [8 w] B) No intervention	Number of sexual partners decreased, no effect on immune system	No control of placebo-effects
Taylor[20]	10 asymptomatic individuals	A) Behavioural stress management [10 w] B) No intervention	Positive changes for anxiety, self-esteem and T cell count	Small sample size, no control of placebo-effects
McCain[21]	45 AIDS patients and HIV-positive individuals	A) Stress management programme [6 w] B) No intervention	Lowering of stress score	No control of placebo-effects, no effects on immune function
Lutgendorf[22]	40 male AIDS patients	A) Cognitive–behavioural stress management [10 w] B) No intervention	Reduction of dysphoria, anxiety and HSV1–2 titre	Some indication for dose–effect relationship
Fukunishi[23]	19 HIV-positive individuals	A) Relaxation therapy [3 mo] B) Psychotherapy C) No intervention	Anger reduced most by relaxation therapy	Very small sample, no control for placebo-effects
McCain[24]	148 HIV-positive individuals	A) Relaxation training and social support B) No intervention	Well-being and quality of life improved more with A	No control for placebo effects
Lechner[25]	330 women with AIDS	A) Individual stress management [10 w] B) Group therapy plus individual stress management [10 w]	Quality of life improved more in B than in A	

patients treated with capsaicin cream reported more pain than controls.

Malnutrition of AIDS patients often results in deficiencies of L-carnitine or glutathione. **Carnitine** supplementation, in turn, might ameliorate zidovudine-induced myopathies and normalise lymphocyte function.[28]

Cystein-supplementation normalises glutathione levels in HIV-positive patients[29] and enhances immune function.[30]

Advanced stages of AIDS are usually associated with malnutrition which, in turn, might impair immune function. RCTs of **glutamine** supplementation[31] or L-glutamine plus antioxidants[32] or omega-3 fatty acid[33] produced encouraging results in terms of preservation of body weight and nelfinavir-induced diarrhoea.[34]

Multivitamin supplementation of breastfeeding HIV-positive mothers reduced child mortality and HIV transmission,[35] and increased mean CD4+ cell count in children.[36] When given to HIV-positive adults, multivitamin supplements may enhance survival[37] and delay progression of HIV-disease.[38]

An RCT of **probiotics** failed to show an effect on diarrhoea or gastrointestinal symptoms.[39]

Supplementation with **selenium** has been shown to reduce anxiety[40] and reduce hospitalisation rates[41] of HIV-infected individuals.

Vitamin A supplements have been shown to improve growth of infants[42,43] and may prevent the deterioration in gut integrity of HIV-infected infants.[44] It is, however, unlikely to affect genital shedding of virus[45,46] and could even increase the risk of HIV transmission.

Other therapies

A CCT[47] evaluated the outcome of a complex CAM programme including diet, physical activity, smoking cessation, herbal remedies, stress reduction and emotional support in asymptomatic HIV-positive individuals. The results were compared with those in patients who had not received these interventions. After 30 months there were some encouraging differences in terms of CD4 and CD8 counts. These findings require independent replication.

Overall recommendation

None of the numerous 'AIDS cures' which regularly emerge only to vanish months later can be recommended. CAM interventions used in palliative and supportive care may prove to be useful; this applies in particular to regular aerobic exercise, stress management programmes of various types and massage therapy. Vitamins and other supplements show some promise.

Table 2.4
Summary of clinical evidence for AIDS/HIV infection

Treatment	Weight of Evidence	Direction of evidence	Serious safety concerns
Acupuncture (symptomatic)	O	⬊	Yes (see p 294)
Exercise (symptomatic)	OOO	⬆	Yes (see p 5)
Guided imagery (palliative)	O	⇨	No (see p 359)
Herbal medicine			
Boxwood	O	⬈	Yes (see p 476)
Chinese herbal mixture	O	⬊	Yes (see p 5)
St John's wort	O	⬇	Yes (see p 463)
Tea tree oil (candidiasis)	O	⬈	Yes (see p 466)
Homeopathy	O	⬈	No (see p 327)

Treatment	Weight of evidence	Direction of evidence	Serious safety concerns
Massage (palliative)	OO	⬀	No (see p 334)
Ozone therapy	O	⬇	Yes (see p 360)
Spiritual healing (palliative)	O	⬀	No (see p 351)
Stress management (palliative)	OOO	⬆	No (see p 361)
Supplements			
Arginine	O	⬀	No (see p 482)
Capsaicin cream (symptomatic)	O	⬇	Yes (see p 5)
Carnitine	O	⬀	No (see p 482)
Cystein	O	⬀	No (see p 5)
Glutamine	O	⬀	No (see p 483)
Multivitamin	OO	⬆	No (see p 5)
Probiotics	O	⬇	No (see p 5)
Selenium	O	⬀	Yes (see p 484)
Vitamin A	OO	⬄	Yes (see p 5)

REFERENCES

1 Ernst E. Complementary AIDS therapies: the good, the bad and the ugly. Int J STD AIDS 1997;8:281–285

2 Gore-Felton C, Vosvick M, Power R, Koopman C, Ashton E, Bachmann M H, Israelski D, Spiegel D. Alternative therapies: a common practice among men and women living with HIV. J Assoc Nurses AIDS Care 2003;14:17–27

3 Shlay J C, Chaloner K, Max M B, Flaws B, Reichelderfer P, Wentworth D, Hillman S, Brizz B, Cohn D L. Acupuncture and amitriptyline for pain due to HIV-related peripheral neuropathy: a randomized controlled trial. Terry Beirn Community Programs for Clinical Research on AIDS. JAMA 1998;280:1590–1595

4 Beal M W, Nield-Anderson L. Acupuncture for symptom relief in HIV-positive adults: lessons learned from a pilot study. Altern Ther Health Med 2000;6:33–42

5 Nixon S, O'Brien K, Glazier R, Tynan A. Aerobic exercise interventions for adults living with HIV/AIDS. The Cochrane Database of Systematic Reviews 2005, Issue 2. Art. No.: CD001796

6 Eller L S. Effects of cognitive–behavioral interventions on quality of life in persons with HIV. Int J Nurs Stud 1999;36:223–233

7 Durant J, Chantre P, Gonzalez G, Vandermander J, Halfon P, Rousse B, Guedon D, Rahelinirina V, Chamaret S, Montagnier L, Dellamonica P. Efficacy and safety of Buxus sempervirens L. preparations (SPV$_{30}$) in HIV-infected asymptomatic patients: a multicentre, randomized, double-blind, placebo-controlled trial. Phytomedicine 1998;5:1–10

8 Burack J H, Cohen M R, Hahn J A, Abrams D I. Pilot randomized controlled trial of Chinese herbal treatment for HIV-associated symptoms. J Acquir Immun Defic Syndr Hum Retrovirol 1996;12:386–393

9 Weber R, Christen L, Loy M, Schaller S, Christen S, Joyce C R, Ledermann U, Ledergerber B, Cone R, Luthy R, Cohen M R. Randomized, placebo-controlled trial of Chinese herb therapy for HIV-1-infected individuals. J AIDS 1999;22:56–64

10 Gulick R M. Phase I studies of hypericin, the active compound in St John's wort, as an antiretroviral agent in HIV-infected adults: AIDS clinical trials group protocols 150 and 258. Ann Intern Med 1999; 130:510–514

11 Vazquez J A, Zawawi A A. Efficacy of alcohol-based and alcohol-free melaleuca oral solution for the treatment of fluconazole-refractory

oropharyngeal candidiasis in patients with AIDS. HIV Clin Trials 2002;3:379–385

12　Rastogi D P, Singh V P, Singh V, Dey S K, Rao K. Homeopathy in HIV infection: a trial report of double-blind placebo controlled study. Br Homeopath J 1999;88:49–57

13　Scafidi F, Field T. Massage therapy improves behavior in neonates born to HIV-positive mothers. J Pediatr Psychol 1996;21:889–897

14　Birk T J, McGrady A, MacArthur R D, Khuder S. The effects of massage therapy alone and in combination with other complementary therapies on immune system measures and quality of life in human immunodeficiency virus. J Altern Complement Med 2000;6:405–414

15　Diego M A, Field T, Hernandez-Reif M, Shaw K, Friedman L, Ironson G. HIV adolescents show improved immune function following massage therapy. Int J Neurosci 2001;106:35–45

16　Garber G E, Cameron D W, Hawley-Foss N, Greenway D, Shannon-M E. The use of ozone-treated blood in the therapy of HIV infection and immune disease: a pilot study of safety and efficacy. AIDS 1991;5:981–984

17　Sicher F, Targ E, Moore D, Smith H S. A randomized double-blind study of the effect of distant healing in a population with advanced AIDS. Report of a small scale study. West J Med 1998;169:356–363

18　Ireland M. Therapeutic touch with HIV-infected children: a pilot study. J Assoc Nurses AIDS Care 1998;9:68–77

19　Coates T J, McKusick L, Kuno R, Stites D P. Stress reduction training changed number of sexual partners but not immune function in men with HIV. Am J Pub Health 1989;79:885–887

20　Taylor D N. Effects of a behavioral stress-management program on anxiety, mood, self-esteem, and T-cell count in HIV positive men. Psychol Rep 1995;76:451–457

21　McCain N L, Zeller J M, Cella D F, Urbanzki P A, Novak R M. The influence of stress management training in HIV disease. Nurse Res 1996;45:246–253

22　Lutgendorf S K, Antoni M H, Ironson G, Klimas N, Starr K, Schneiderman N, McCabe P, Kumar M, Cleven K, Fletcher M A. Cognitive behavioral stress management intervention decreases dysphoria and herpes simplex virus-Type 2 antibody titers in symptomatic HIV seropositive gay men. J Consulting Clin Psychol 1997;65:31–43

23　Fukunishi I, Hosaka T, Matsumoto T, Hayashi M, Negishi M, Moriya H. Liaison psychiatry and HIV (II): application of relaxation in HIV positive patients. Psychiat Clin Neurosci 1997;51:5–8

24　McCain N L, Munjas B A, Munro C L, Elswick R K, Robins J L, Ferreira-Gonzalez A, Baliko B, Kaplowitz L G, Fisher E J, Garrett C T, Brigle K E, Kendall L C, Lucas V, Cochran K L. Effects of stress management on PNI-based outcomes in persons with HIV disease. Res Nurs Health 2003;26:102–117

25　Lechner S C, Antoni M H, Lydston D, LaPerriere A, Ishii M, Devieux J, Stanley H, Ironson G, Schneiderman N, Brondolo E, Tobin J N, Weiss S. Cognitive–behavioral interventions improve quality of life in women with AIDS. J Psychosom Res 2003;54:253–261

26　Swanson B, Keithley J K, Zeller J M, Sha B E. A pilot study of the safety and efficacy of supplemental arginine to enhance immune function in persons with HIV/AIDS. Nutrition 2002;18:688–690

27　Paice J A, Ferrams C E V, Lashley F R. Topical capsaicin in the management of HIV-associated peripheral neuropathy. J Pain Sympt Manage 2000;19:45–52

28　Mintz M. Carnitine in human immunodeficiency virus type 1 infection/acquired immune deficiency syndrome. J Child Neurol 1995;10:Suppl 2:40–44

29　Micke P, Beeh K M, Schlaak J F, Buhl R. Oral supplementation with whey proteins increases plasma glutathione levels of HIV-infected patients. Eur J Clin Invest 2001;31:171–178

30　Breitkreutz R, Pittack N, Nebe C T, Schuster D, Brust J, Beichert M, Hack V, Daniel V, Edler L, Droge W. Improvement of immune functions in HIV infection by sulfur supplementation: two randomized trials. J Mol Med 2000;78:55–62

31　Wilmore D W. Glutamine-antioxidant supplementation increases body cell mass in AIDS patients with weight loss: a randomized, double-blind controlled trial. Nutrition 1999;15:860–864

32　Shabert J K, Winslow C, Lacey J M, Wilmore D W. Glutamine-antioxidant supplementation increases body cell mass in AIDS patients with weight loss: a randomized, double-blind controlled trial. Nutrition 1999;15:860–864

33　de Luis Roman D A, Bachiller P, Izaola O, Romero E, Martin J, Arranz M, Eiros Bouza J M, Aller R. Nutritional treatment for acquired immunodeficiency virus infection using an enterotropic peptide-based formula enriched with n-3 fatty acids: a randomized prospective trial. Eur J Clin Nutr 2001;55:1048–1052

34　Huffman F G, Walgren M E. L-glutamine supplementation improves nelfinavir-associated diarrhea in HIV-infected individuals. HIV Clin Trials 2003;4:324–329

35 Fawzi W W, Msamanga G I, Hunter D, Renjifo B, Antelman G, Bang H, Manji K, Kapiga S, Mwakagile D, Essex M, Spiegelman D. Randomized trial of vitamin supplements in relation to transmission of HIV-1 through breastfeeding and early child mortality. AIDS 2002;16:1935–1944

36 Fawzi W W, Msamanga G I, Wei R, Spiegelman D, Antelman G, Villamor E, Manji K, Hunter D. Effect of providing vitamin supplements to human immunodeficiency virus-infected, lactating mothers on the child's morbidity and CD4+ cell counts. Clin Infect Dis 2003;36:1053–1062

37 Jiamton S, Pepin J, Suttent R, Filteau S, Mahakkanukrauh B, Hanshaoworakul W, Chaisilwattana P, Suthipinittharm P, Shetty P, Jaffar S. A randomized trial of the impact of multiple micronutrient supplementation on mortality among HIV-infected individuals living in Bangkok. AIDS 2003;17:2461–2469

38 Fawzi W W, Msamanga G I, Spiegelman D, Wei R, Kapiga S, Villamor E, Mwakagile D, Mugusi F, Hertzmark E, Essex M, Hunter D J. A randomized trial of multivitamin supplements and HIV disease progression and mortality. N Engl J Med 2004;351:23–32

39 Salminen M K, Tynkkynen S, Rautelin H, Poussa T, Saxelin M, Ristola M, Valtonen V, Jarvinen A. The efficacy and safety of probiotic Lactobacillus rhamnosus GG on prolonged, non-infectious diarrhea in HIV patients on antiretroviral therapy: a randomized, placebo-controlled, crossover study. HIV Clin Trials 2004;5:183–191

40 Shor-Posner G, Lecusay R, Miguez M J, Moreno-Black G, Zhang G, Rodriguez N, Burbano X, Baum M, Wilkie F. Psychological burden in the era of HAART: impact of selenium therapy. Int J Psychiatry Med 2003;33:55–69

41 Burbano X, Miguez-Burbano M J, McCollister K, Zhang G, Rodriguez A, Ruiz P, Lecusay R, Shor-Posner G. Impact of a selenium chemoprevention clinical trial on hospital admissions of HIV-infected participants. HIV Clin Trials 2002;3:483–491

42 Villamor E, Mbise R, Spiegelman D, Hertzmark E, Fataki M, Peterson K E, Ndossi G, Fawzi W W. Vitamin A supplements ameliorate the adverse effect of HIV-1, malaria, and diarrheal infections on child growth. Pediatrics 2002;109:E6

43 Kennedy-Oji C, Coutsoudis A, Kuhn L, Pillay K, Mburu A, Stein Z, Coovadia H. Effects of vitamin A supplementation during pregnancy and early lactation on body weight of South African HIV-infected women. J Health Popul Nutr 2001;19:167–176

44 Filteau S M, Rollins N C, Coutsoudis A, Sullivan K R, Willumsen J F, Tomkins A M. The effect of antenatal vitamin A and beta-carotene supplementation on gut integrity of infants of HIV-infected South African women. J Pediatr Gastroenterol Nutr 2001;32:464–470

45 Baeten J M, McClelland R S, Corey L, Overbaugh J, Lavreys L, Richardson B A, Wald A, Mandaliya K, Bwayo J J, Kreiss J K. Vitamin A supplementation and genital shedding of herpes simplex virus among HIV-1-infected women: a randomized clinical trial. J Infect Dis 2004;189:1466–1471

46 Baeten J M, McClelland R S, Overbaugh J, Richardson B A, Emery S, Lavreys L, Mandaliya K, Bankson D D, Ndinya-Achola J O, Bwayo J J, Kreiss J K. Vitamin A supplementation and human immunodeficiency virus type 1 shedding in women: results of a randomized clinical trial. J Infect Dis 2002;185:1187–1191

47 Kaiser J D, Donegan E. Complementary therapies in HIV disease. Alt Ther Health Med 1996;2:42–46

ALZHEIMER'S DISEASE

**Synonyms/
Subcategories**

Alzheimer's dementia, presenile dementia, primary neuronal degeneration.

Definition

Dementia is characterised by chronic, global, non-reversible impairment in cerebral function. It usually results in loss of memory (initially of recent events), loss of executive function (such as the ability to make decisions or sequence complex tasks), and changes in personality. Alzheimer's disease is a type of dementia characterised by an insidious onset and slow deterioration, and involves speech, motor, personality, and executive function impairment. It should be diagnosed after other systemic, psychiatric, and neurological causes of dementia have been excluded clinically and by laboratory investigation.

**Related
conditions**

Other forms of (senile) dementia, e.g. vascular dementia, Lewy body dementia.

CAM usage

Herbal treatments and other dietary supplements are often advocated and used. Several complementary therapies (e.g. massage, reflexology, music therapy), which are aimed at improving quality of life, are used in palliative care of Alzheimer's patients.

**Clinical
evidence**

In many clinical studies of CAM the participants were not diagnosed according to accepted criteria. Thus, mixed or ill-defined populations of dementia patients have often been studied. Even though this discussion is on Alzheimer's disease, such studies have also been included.

Acupuncture
Several uncontrolled studies from China suggest that acupuncture can be beneficial for dementia patients (e.g.[1,2]). As these studies lack scientific rigour and are open to bias, conclusions regarding the efficacy of acupuncture for Alzheimer's disease cannot be drawn.

Aromatherapy
Several small uncontrolled studies of aromatherapy report some benefit in terms of well-being, (e.g.[3]), but the data are far from compelling. One controlled trial reported no difference between *Lavendula officinalis*, *Citrus aurantium* and *Malaleuca alternifolia* compared with no aroma for patients with dementia.[4]

Electrostimulation
An RCT assessed the effects of low-frequency cranial electrostimulation on rest–activity rhythm and salivary cortisol in patients with Alzheimer's disease.[5] There were no beneficial effects.

Herbal medicine

The Kampo mixture **Choto-san** has been tested in an RCT with 139 patients suffering from vascular dementias.[6] Choto-san was superior to placebo in terms of global improvement and several other outcome measures.

A Cochrane review of all double-blind RCTs included 33 trials which tested the effects of **ginkgo** (*Ginkgo biloba*) for treating cognitive impairment and dementia.[7] It concluded that there is encouraging evidence of improvement in cognition and function associated with ginkgo. There is no subgroup analysis of patients with Alzheimer's disease. These findings are supported by the results of a subsequent double-blind RCT.[8] No beneficial effects were reported by another double-blind RCT.[9] A meta-analysis concluded that ginkgo improved cognitive function in Alzheimer's disease (Box 2.1).[10] Another systematic review identified three RCTs including 493 patients and concluded that the efficacy of ginkgo as a treatment for Alzheimer's disease appears to be less than that of donepezil, metrifonate and rivastigmine.[11]

Box 2.1
Meta-analysis
Ginkgo for Alzheimer's disease
Oken[10]

- Included were placebo-controlled, double-blind RCTs, testing standardised ginkgo extracts and using objective assessments of cognitive function
- Four studies were included (n = 424)
- Their methodological quality was, on average, good
- Overall effect size was 0.40 which translated into a 3% difference in the Alzheimer's disease Assessment Scale – cognitive subtest
- Conclusion: there is a small effect of 3–6-month treatment with 120–240 mg of ginkgo extract

Ginseng (*Panax ginseng*) is often advocated for improving mental performance and might therefore have some potential in Alzheimer's disease. One Norwegian study with geriatric patients found no benefit in terms of activities of daily living, cognition, somatic symptoms, depression or anxiety.[12]

Huperzine A, an alkaloid isolated from the Chinese herb *Huperzia serrata,* is a reversible, selective acetylcholinesterase inhibitor. CCTs from China suggest that it improves memory deficiencies in patients with various forms of dementia.[13]

One RCT reported that patients treated with **lemon balm** *(Melissa officinalis)* for four months experienced better cognitive function than those treated with placebo.[14]

One RCT reported that patients treated with **sage** (*Salvia officinalis*) for four months experienced better cognitive function than those treated with placebo.[15]

Massage
The evidence from clinical trials suggesting that massage therapy can reduce anxiety or alter behaviour in Alzheimer's patients is encouraging but far from compelling at present.[16]

Music therapy
An RCT including 18 patients implied that exposure to soothing music can reduce aggressive behaviour in Alzheimer's disease.[17] Other studies confirm positive behavioural changes[18,19] but the evidence is so far not convincing.

Supplements
A Cochrane review assessed the evidence of **alpha-tocopherol** for Alzheimer's disease.[20] It identified one double-blind RCT (n = 341) and concluded that there is insufficient evidence of efficacy for vitamin E in the treatment of Alzheimer's disease. Numerous other nutritional supplements are being advocated for Alzheimer's. In most cases the evidence from clinical trials is absent or unconvincing. Some encouraging, albeit preliminary trial evidence exists for **acetyl-l-carnitine, dimethylaminoethanol, lecithin**, and **phosphatidylserine**.[21] Unfortunately, the size of the effect is usually small and therefore of questionable clinical relevance.

Therapeutic touch
Fifty-seven residents, aged 67 to 93 years, exhibiting behavioural symptoms of dementia, were randomised to either therapeutic touch, a placebo group and a group receiving usual care.[22] Therapeutic touch was given twice daily for 5–7 minutes for three days. The results indicated a difference in overall behavioural symptoms of dementia when the experimental group was compared with the placebo and control groups.

Table 2.5
Summary of clinical evidence for Alzheimer's disease

Treatment	Weight of evidence	Direction of evidence	Serious safety concerns
Acupuncture	O	⇨	Yes (see p 294)
Aromatherapy	O	⇨	Yes (see p 301)
Electrostimulation	O	⇩	Yes (see p 5)
Herbal medicine			
Choto-san	O	⇧	Yes (see p 5)
Ginkgo	OOO	⇧	Yes (see p 404)
Huperzia serrata	O	⬀	Yes (see p 477)
Lemon balm	O	⇧	Yes (see pp 5, 479)
Panax ginseng	O	⇩	Yes (see p 407)
Sage	O	⇧	Yes (see p 481)
Massage	O	⬀	No (see p 334)

Treatment	Weight of evidence	Direction of evidence	Serious safety concerns
Music therapy	O	↗	No (see p 360)
Supplements			
Acetyl-l-carnitine	O	↗	No (see p 482)
Alpha-tocopherol	O	⇨	No (see p 5)
Dimethylamino-ethanol	O	↗	Yes (see p 5)
Lecithin	O	↗	Yes (see p 5)
Phosphatidylserine	O	↗	Yes (see p 5)
Therapeutic touch	O	↗	No (see p 351)

Overall recommendation

Much of the evidence regarding CAM for Alzheimer's disease is too preliminary for strong recommendations. The only exception is ginkgo, which has a modest effect and is reasonably safe. As there is little evidence from comparative trials of ginkgo and conventional drugs for Alzheimer's disease, its therapeutic value relative to conventional therapies is uncertain.

REFERENCES

1   Xudong G. The influence of acupuncture modalities on the treatment of senile dementia: a brief review. Am J Acup 1996;24:105–109

2   Geng J. Treatment of 50 cases of senile dementia by acupuncture combined with inhalation of herbal drugs and oxygen. J Trad Chin Med 1999;19:287–289

3   Brooker D J, Snape M, Johnson E, Ward D, Payne M. Single case evaluation of the effects of aromatherapy and massage on disturbed behavior in severe dementia. Br J Clin Psychol 1997;36:287–296

4   Gray S G, Clair A A. Influence of aromatherapy on medication administration to residential-care residents with dementia and behavioral challenges. Am J Alzheimers Dis Other Demen 2002;17:169–174

5   Scherder E, Knol D, van Someren E, Deijen J B, Binnekade R, Tilders F, Sergeant J. Effects of low-frequency cranial electrostimulation on the rest-activity rhythm and salivary cortisol in Alzheimer's disease. Neurorehabil Neural Repair 2003;17:101–108

6   Terasawa K, Shimada Y, Kita T et al. Choto-san in the treatment of vascular dementia: a double-blind, placebo controlled study. Phytomedicine 1997;4:15–22

7   Birks J, Grimley Evans J. Ginkgo biloba for cognitive impairment and dementia. The Cochrane Database of Systematic Reviews 2002, Issue 4. Art. No.: CD003120

8   Kanowski S, Hoerr R. Ginkgo biloba extract EGb 761 in dementia: intent-to-treat analyses of a 24-week, multi-center, double-blind, placebo-controlled, randomized trial. Pharmacopsychiatry 2003;36:297–303

9   van Dongen M, van Rossum E, Kessels A, Sielhorst H, Knipschild P. Ginkgo for elderly people with dementia and age-associated memory impairment: a randomized clinical trial. J Clin Epidemiol 2003;56:367–376

10 Oken B S, Storzbach D M, Kaye J A. The efficacy of Ginkgo biloba on cognitive function in Alzheimer disease. Arch Neurol 1998;55:1409–1415

11 Wolfson C, Moride Y, Perrault A, Momoli F, Demers L, Oremus M. Drug treatments for Alzheimers's disease: 1. A comparative analysis of clinical trials 2000: 1–124. Ottawa, ON, Canada: Canadian Coordinating Office for Health Technology Assessment (CCOHTA)

12 Thommassen B, Laake K. Ginseng – no identifiable effect in geriatric rehabilitation. Tidsskr Nor Laegeforen 1997;117:3839–3841

CONDITIONS

13 Tang X C, Han Y F. Pharmacological profile of huperzine A, a novel acetylcholinesterase inhibitor from Chinese herb. CNS Drug Rev 1999;5:281–300

14 Akhondzadeh S, Noroozian M, Mohammadi M, Ohadinia S, Jamshidi A H, Khani M. Melissa officinalis extract in the treatment of patients with mild to moderate Alzheimer's disease: a double blind, randomised, placebo controlled trial. J Neurol Neurosurg Psychiatry 2003;74:863–866

15 Akhondzadeh S, Noroozian M, Mohammadi M, Ohadinia S, Jamshidi A H, Khani M. Salvia officinalis extract in the treatment of patients with mild to moderate Alzheimer's disease: a double blind, randomized and placebo-controlled trial. J Clin Pharm Ther 2003;28:53–59

16 Opie J, Rosewarne R, O'Connor D W. The efficacy of psychosocial approaches to behavior disorders in dementia: a systematic literature review. Aust NZ J Psych 1999;33:789–799

17 Clark M E, Lipe A W, Bilbrey M. Use of music to decrease aggressive behaviors in people with dementia. J Gerontol Nurs 1998;24:10–17

18 Ott B R, Owens N J. Complementary and alternative medicines for Alzheimer's disease. J Geriatr Psychiatr Neurol 1998;11:163–173

19 Gerdner L A. Effects of individualized versus classical 'relaxation' music on the frequency of agitation in elderly persons with Alzheimer's disease and related disorders. Int Psychogeriatr 2000;12:49–65

20 Tabet N, Birks J, Grimley Evans J, Orrel M, Spector A. Vitamin E for Alzheimer's disease. The Cochrane Database of Systematic Reviews 2000, Issue 4. Art. No.: CD002854

21 Wettstein V A. Cholinesterase inhibitors and Ginkgo extracts: are they comparable in the treatment of dementia? Fortschritte der Medizin 1999;1(suppl 1):11–18

22 Woods D L, Craven R F, Whitney J. The effect of therapeutic touch on behavioral symptoms of persons with dementia. Altern Ther Health Med 2005;11:66–74

ANXIETY

Synonyms/ subcategories

State anxiety, trait anxiety. International Classification of Disease (ICD-10) categories: phobic anxiety disorder (agoraphobia, social phobia, specific phobias); other anxiety disorders (panic disorder, generalised anxiety disorder, mixed anxiety and depression disorder); obsessive-compulsive disorder. Reaction to severe stress and adjustment disorders (acute stress reaction, posttraumatic stress disorder, adjustment reaction); dissociative (conversion) disorders; other neurotic disorders (including neurasthenia and depersonalisation or derealisation).

Definition

Excessive fearfulness and tensions accompanied by an increased motor tension (restlessness, muscle tension, trembling, fatigability), autonomic hyperactivity (tachycardia, shortness of breath, dry mouth, cold hands) and increased vigilance and scanning (feeling keyed up, impaired concentration) unattached to a clearly identifiable stimulus.

CAM usage

Forty-three percent of people who suffer from anxiety attacks have used CAM in the last 12 months.[1] The therapies most commonly used include relaxation, exercise, herbs, art/music therapy and megavitamins.[2] In addition, hypnosis, meditation and yoga are widely adopted for the treatment of stress. A recent review included 108 different CAM interventions for anxiety.[3]

**Clinical
evidence**

Acupuncture

In two RCTs with patients suffering from minor depression or anxiety disorder (n = 56 and 36), needle acupuncture was acutely followed by a more pronounced relaxation response than sham-acupuncture.[4,5] An RCT (n = 55) comparing the effects on state anxiety of ear-acupuncture and sham-acupuncture suggested anxiolytic effects of acupuncture in healthy volunteers.[6] Similar results were generated in pre-hospital transport and pre-operative settings,[7,8] as well as in mental stress.[9] Acupressure has been shown to reduce verbal stress scores in a small RCT (n = 25) with healthy volunteers.[10]

Aromatherapy

A systematic review[11] (Box 2.2) concluded that, although there are anxiolytic effects, these are short term and probably too modest to have clinical relevance. A Cochrane review found limited evidence that aromatherapy massage reduces anxiety in cancer patients.[12] More recent studies have generated both negative[13–15] and positive[16] results of various types of aromatherapy for stress or anxiety reduction.

Box 2.2
Systematic review
**Aromatherapy for
anxiety**
Cooke[11]

- Thirteen RCTs, of which six related to treatment of anxiety (452 patients)

- Quality of all studies was poor

- Five showed short-term superiority of aromatherapy

- Conclusion: modest, short-term effect which is unlikely to be clinically relevant

Autogenic training

A systematic review[17] (Box 2.3) found six CCTs of forms of 'autogenic training' that often only included part of the classic technique. Only two studies involved patient groups, but both had positive outcomes for anxiety. Subsequent trials have confirmed

Box 2.3
Systematic review
**Autogenic training
for anxiety**
Ernst[17]

- Eight CCTs, 245 participants

- Six trials on induced anxiety in volunteers; two on patient groups

- Majority of trials methodologically flawed

- Positive results, in at least some subgroups, in all studies. No decrease in panic attacks

- Conclusion: lack of uniform training procedures and poor methodological quality prevent firm conclusions

CONDITIONS

the anxiolytic activity of autogenic training in children with behavioural problems[18] and patients after angioplasty.[19]

Biofeedback

Among 45 individuals with generalised anxiety disorder included in an RCT, eight sessions of EMG and EEG biofeedback were both superior to pseudomeditation control at reducing trait anxiety.[20] Combined alpha-wave EEG and EMG biofeedback training (ten weekly sessions) improved test anxiety in a controlled trial with 163 students with examination phobia, compared with no training (quoted in[21]). Regular EEG biofeedback sessions on 5 days a week for combat-related posttraumatic stress disorder resulted in improvements in several clinical psychology scales compared with standard medication treatments (quoted in[21]) Only three out of 15 biofeedback patients had relapsed at 30 months, compared with all 14 traditionally treated patients. Other CCTs demonstrate that various forms of biofeedback can reduce the response to a cardiovascular stressor[22] and alleviate social stress in socially anxious people.[23] However, there are also negative RCTs, such as one involving 66 psychiatric patients where EEG biofeedback showed no difference from placebo biofeedback or untreated controls.[24]

Electrostimulation

A meta-analysis[25] (Box 2.4) found evidence in favour of the effectiveness of electrostimulation although not conclusively so, because of the small size of studies and problems with blinding.

Box 2.4
Meta-analysis
**Electrostimulation
for anxiety**
Klawansky[25]

- Eight subject-blind RCTs with 249 patients

- Either primary anxiety or alcohol- or drug-related anxiety

- Quality issues limit the findings

- Pooled effect size 0.59 (CI 0.23 to 0.95)

- Cautiously positive conclusion

Exercise

Exercise can reduce anxiety acutely, as shown in an RCT with 85 volunteers randomised to aerobic exercise, relaxation or no treatment control.[26] Both interventions diminished induced anxiety more than the control. In an RCT including 46 patients with panic disorder and agoraphobia, 10 weeks of walking (4 miles three times/week) was less effective than clomipramine, but both were superior to placebo.[27]

Flower remedies

A systematic review including two rigorous RCTs found no evidence that (Bach) Flower Remedies reduce exam stress.[28]

Herbal medicine

A large RCT (n = 264) showed that a combination of *Crataegus oxyacantha, Eschscholzia californica* and magnesium is more effective than placebo in reducing anxiety in patients with generalised anxiety disorder.[29]

There is poor-quality evidence for the efficacy of **German chamomile** (*Matricaria recutita*), in the treatment of anxiety.[30]

A systematic review[31] (Box 2.5) concluded that **kava** (*Piper methysticum*) was relatively safe and effective for the treatment of anxiety symptoms.

Box 2.5
Systematic review
Kava for anxiety
Pittler[31]

- Eleven RCTs involving 645 participants

- Kava extract from 300 to 800 mg/day in divided doses

- Quality was varied but good in some studies

- All studies showed positive effects of kava

- Meta-analysis of six studies showed weighted mean difference of 5.0 (CI 1.1 to 8.8) points on Hamilton Anxiety Scale

- No serious adverse effects were reported

- Conclusion: kava extract appears to be an effective symptomatic treatment option for anxiety

Short-term anxiolytic effects were also seen after administration of **lemon balm** (*Melissa officinalis*) in healthy volunteers.[32]

Passion flower (*Passiflora incarnata*) has been tested in an RCT with 36 patients suffering from generalised anxiety disorder.[33] The herbal medicine generated similarly positive results as oxazepam.

No anxiolytic effects of **valerian** (*Valeriana officinalis*) extract were noted in an RCT with 66 patients suffering from generalised anxiety disorder.[34]

Homeopathy

The evidence on the value of homeopathy for this indication is inconsistent. One controlled trial suggested that homeopathy may have an effect in reducing agitation in children after surgery.[35] Two RCTs found homeopathy not superior to placebo in 72 adults with anxiety.[36,37]

Hypnotherapy

Hypnosis is widely offered for dental phobia and in one controlled trial there was no difference between the effect of hypnosis, group therapy and individual desensitisation, though all were superior to no treatment.[38] A long-term follow-up concluded that hypnosis can help patients with dental anxiety.[39] For the management of agoraphobia, hypnosis may be offered as part of desensitisation management, at the time of exposure to the anxiety-provoking situation. However, one crossover study in 64 patients found that, although patients preferred it, hypnosis did not make any observable difference to the patients' behaviour at the time of the exposure.[40] Anxiety was reduced more effectively by hypnosis when given to children before painful and stressful procedures (bone marrow aspiration, lumbar puncture) than by a non-hypnotic behavioural technique.[41]

Imagery

A systematic review of six RCTs of imagery as an adjuvant therapy found some evidence that this approach alleviates anxiety in cancer patients.[42]

Massage

An overview of ten studies showed that massage therapy decreases anxiety in a variety of settings.[43] Massage therapy given to depressed pregnant adolescents twice a week for 5 weeks was shown to be superior to relaxation therapy in an RCT involving 26 women.[44] The anxiolytic effect of massage was confirmed in small CCTs of healthy pregnant women,[45] women undergoing amniocentesis,[46] women during childbirth,[47] women with breast cancer,[48] chronic pain patients,[49] and patients during cataract surgery.[50] In a further RCT of 21 elderly institutionalised patients, massage was shown to reduce anxiety to a greater extent than no intervention, though it was not different from attention control (conversation).[51] An RCT (n = 69) showed that massage was not more effective than a relaxation audio-tape in reducing stress.[52]

Meditation

There is evidence that meditation can reduce anxiety levels and neuroendocrine responses to stress more effectively than situation control in volunteers placed in stressful conditions[53] and uncontrolled studies have suggested benefits in patients with anxiety. In one RCT, 28 individuals receiving an 8-week stress reduction programme based on mindfulness meditation evidenced greater reductions in overall psychological symptoms, improvements in sense of control and measure of spiritual experiences compared with non-intervention control.[54] A systematic review which included observational studies as well as controlled trials on relaxation techniques for trait anxiety (Box 2.6) found the effect size for meditation to be 0.70 (SD 0.40) compared with progressive muscle relaxation (0.38, SD 0.40).[55] A meta-analysis of controlled and uncontrolled studies of mindfulness-based stress reduction suggested anxiolytic effects of this approach,[56] while another review pointed out that the primary data are methodologically weak and concluded that 'the available evidence does not support a strong endorsement of this approach'.[57]

Box 2.6
Systematic review
Relaxation techniques for anxiety
Eppley[55]

- Included were all observational and controlled trials in which the outcome was trait anxiety

- Relaxation studies involving psychiatric patients were excluded

- Progressive muscle relaxation 22 studies, meditation 70 studies, biofeedback 17 studies (subject numbers not stated)

- Overall effect sizes: progressive muscle relaxation 0.38 (SD 0.40); other forms of relaxation (largely biofeedback) 0.40 (0.35); meditation 0.70 (0.40)

- Effect size related to duration and hours of use of technique

- Conclusion: certain relaxation techniques may reduce trait anxiety

Music therapy

An RCT involving 56 patients admitted to a coronary care unit compared two or three sessions of either listening to light classical music or following relaxation instructions for 30 minutes. Neither therapy had any effect on anxiety and subjects had no benefit compared with untreated controls.[58] A systematic review of 29 RCTs showed that music therapy reduces anxiety in hospitalised patients,[59] a notion subsequently confirmed by recent studies in a large variety of settings.[60–68]

Relaxation

Studies of several forms of anxiety were systematically reviewed[55] (Box 2.6). For panic disorder specifically, relaxation was shown to be less effective than cognitive therapy in an RCT of 64 subjects but both were superior to minimal contact control.[69] These results are supported by other good-quality RCTs. For management of agoraphobia, relaxation training was as effective as exposure and cognitive treatment and all were more effective than weekly individual therapy sessions in an RCT.[70] There were few differences between the active treatments and the results were maintained at one year. A comparative trial suggested that applied relaxation and cognitive therapy are similarly effective in generalised anxiety disorder.[71] Other studies have confirmed the anxiolytic effects of various relaxation programmes in healthy, stressed volunteers.[72]

Relaxation has been used to manage the anxiety associated with medical conditions. In patients with newly diagnosed cancer, relaxation with or without imagery improved anxiety as well as other aspects of mood.[73] In a similar population, there was a reduction in state anxiety after relaxation compared with untreated controls but there was no effect on trait anxiety.[74] In a small RCT dyspnoea, anxiety and airway obstruction were reduced in the relaxation group while the control group receiving standard management remained the same or became worse.[75] Positive results were also generated for night eating syndrome[76] and dental anxiety.[77] A specific relaxation technique, progressive muscle relaxation, has been shown to improve quality of life in patients with colon cancer.[78]

Relaxation training has been used to reduce the anxiety associated with a variety of medical and surgical procedures and to improve some aspects of healing.[79] For minor surgery there is considerable evidence of patient benefit and one study found relaxation to be superior to attention control in facilitating the ease of general anaesthesia in day-case surgery.[80] Audiotapes with relaxation instructions were superior to music tapes or blank tapes at reducing both anxiety and pain (assessed both subjectively and objectively) during femoral angiography.[81] A relaxation procedure before magnetic resonance imaging scan reduced the anxiety associated with the scan more than no intervention in an RCT involving 149 subjects.[82] In an RCT of 53 women undergoing radiation therapy for early-stage breast cancer, relaxation with guided imagery was an effective intervention for reducing anxiety and enhancing comfort, compared with no intervention.[83]

Spinal manipulation

Although there are no studies on anxiety as the presenting complaint, in one RCT state anxiety in hypertensive patients was measured after **chiropractic**, placebo chiropractic or no treatment control in 21 hypertensive patients.[84] There was no difference between the groups though chiropractic was associated with a fall in blood pressure.

Spiritual healing

Positive findings for **therapeutic touch** in the treatment of anxiety have been suggested in RCTs compared with no treatment in 40 healthy professional caregivers/students[85] and compared with sham therapeutic touch in 20 HIV-infected children[86] and 99 hospitalised burn patients.[87] Compared with a placebo, **Reiki** healing was more effective in 46 stressed patients in reducing anxiety.[88]

Other therapies

Breathing exercises showed considerable promise in a large (n = 272) RCT of adults suffering from dental anxiety.[89]

A small CCT (n = 23) suggested that **reflexology** reduces anxiety in cancer patients.[90]

Rolfing (structural integration) was superior to no intervention in reducing state anxiety in an RCT of 48 persons.[91]

An RCT found **tai chi** to be as effective as moderate walking exercise (and both better than reading control) in alleviating

induced anxiety in 96 practitioners of tai chi.[92] A recent RCT
confirmed the anxiolytic activity of regular tai chi.[93]

Two small CCTs (n = 50 and 54) suggested that **yoga** reduces
exam stress.[94,95]

**Overall
recommendation**

For generalised anxiety disorder, drug management is fraught
with problems. Kava is currently banned in some countries due
to safety concerns but may yet prove to be a useful short-term
alternative when used under close individual observation.
Psychological interventions are as successful as medications for
anxiety and often more acceptable. For patients who are willing
to undertake a mind–body approach, guided imagery, meditation,

Table 2.6
Summary of
clinical evidence
for anxiety

Treatment	Weight of evidence	Direction of evidence	Serious safety concerns
Acupuncture	OO	⬈	Yes (see p 294)
Aromatherapy	OO	⬈	Yes (see p 301)
Autogenic training	OO	⬈	Yes (see p 305)
Biofeedback	OO	⬈	No (see p 310)
Electrostimulation	OO	⬈	Yes (see p 5)
Exercise	O	⬆	Yes (see p 5)
Flower remedies	OO	⬇	No (see p 307)
Guided imagery	OOO	⬈	No (see p 359)
Herbal medicine			
German chamomile	O	⬈	Yes (see p 376)
Kava	OOO	⬆	Yes (see p 427)
Lemon balm	O	⬈	Yes (see pp 5, 479)
Passionflower	O	⬈	Yes (see p 446)
Valerian	O	⬇	Yes (see p 469)
Homeopathy	OO	⬂	No (see p 327)
Hypnotherapy	OO	⬈	Yes (see p 331)
Massage	OOO	⬆	No (see p 334)
Meditation	OOO	⬈	Yes (see p 338)
Music therapy	OOO	⬆	No (see p 360)
Relaxation	OOO	⬆	No (see p 348)
Spinal manipulation			
Chiropractic	O	⬇	Yes (see p 316)
Spiritual healing			
Reiki	O	⬆	No (see p 360)
Therapeutic touch	OO	⬈	No (see p 351)

CONDITIONS

CONDITIONS

autogenic training or relaxation can be encouraged as the evidence is in favour. Electrostimulation may also be recommended. Relaxation massage and music therapy can also be useful in reducing anxiety in a range of settings.

For panic disorder and the various forms of phobia, conventional therapies should be used in the first instance. Hypnotherapy may have specific use in some circumstances (e.g. dental phobia).

REFERENCES

1 Eisenberg D M, Davis R, Ettner S L, Appel S, Wilkey S, Van Rompay M, Kessler R C. Trends in alternative medicine use in the United States, 1990–1997: Results of a Follow-up National Survey. JAMA 1998;280:1569–1575

2 Astin J A. Why patients use alternative medicine. JAMA 1998;279:1548–1553

3 Jorm A F, Christensen H, Griffiths K M, Parslow R A, Rodgers B, Blewitt K A. Effectiveness of complementary and self-help treatments for anxiety disorders. Med J Aust 2004;181:S29–46

4 Eich H, Agelink M W, Lehmann E, Lemmer W, Klieser E. Acupuncture in patients with minor depressive episodes and generalized anxiety. Results of an experimental study. [Article in German] Fortschr Neurol Psychiatr 2000;68:137–144

5 Agelink M W, Sanner D, Eich H, Pach J, Bertling R, Lemmer W, Klieser E, Lehmann E. Does acupuncture influence the cardiac autonomic nervous system in patients with minor depression or anxiety disorders? [Article in German] Fortsch Neurol Psychiatr 2003; 71:141–149

6 Wang S M, Kain Z N. Auricular acupuncture: a potential treatment for anxiety. Anesth Analg 2001;92:548–553

7 Kober A, Scheck T, Schubert B, Strasser H, Gustorff B, Bertalanffy P, Wang S M, Kain Z N, Hoerauf K. Auricular acupuncture as a treatment for anxiety in prehospital transport settings. Anesthesiology 2003;98: 1328–1332

8 Wang S M, Peloquin C, Kain Z N. The use of auricular acupuncture to reduce preoperative anxiety. Anesth Analg 2001;93:1178–1180

9 Middlekauff H R, Hui K, Yu J L, Hamilton M A, Fonarow G C, Moriguchi J, Maclellan W R, Hage A. Acupuncture inhibits sympathetic activation during mental stress in advanced heart failure patients. J Card Fail 2002;8:399–406

10 Fassoulaki A, Paraskeva A, Patris K, Pourgiezi T, Kostopanagiotou G. Pressure applied on extra 1 acupuncture point reduces bispectral index values and stress in volunteers. Anesth Analg 2003;96:885–890

11 Cooke B, Ernst E. Aromatherapy: a systematic review. Br J Gen Pract 2000;50:493–496

12 Fellowes D, Barnes K, Wilkinson S. Aromatherapy and massage for symptom relief in patients with cancer. The Cochrane Database of Systematic Reviews 2004 Issue 3. Art. No.: CD002287

13 Soden K, Vincent K, Craske S, Lucas C, Ashley S. A randomized controlled trial of aromatherapy massage in a hospice setting. Palliat Med 2004;18:87–92

14 Graham P H, Browne L, Cox H, Graham J. Inhalation aromatherapy during radiotherapy: results of a placebo-controlled double-blind randomized trial. J Clin Oncol 2003;21:2372–2376

15 Wiebe E. A randomized trial of aromatherapy to reduce anxiety before abortion. Eff Clin Pract 2000;3:166–169

16 Motomura M, Sakurai A, Yotsuya Y. Reduction of mental stress with lavender odorant. Percept Mot Skills 2001;93:713–718

17 Ernst E, Kanji N. Autogenic training for stress and anxiety: a systematic review. Complement Ther Med 2000;8:106–110

18 Goldbeck L, Schmid K. Effectiveness of autogenic relaxation training on children and adolescents with behavioral and emotional problems. J Am Acad Child Adolesc Psychiatry 2003;42:1046–1054

19 Kanji N, White A R, Ernst E. Autogenic training reduces anxiety after coronary angioplasty: a randomized clinical trial. Am Heart J 2004;147:E10

20 Rice K M, Blanchard E B, Purcell M. Biofeedback treatments of generalized anxiety disorder: preliminary results. Biofeedback Self Reg 1993;18:93–105

21 Moore N C. A review of EEG biofeedback treatment of anxiety disorders. Clin Electroencephalogr 2000;31:1–6

22 Goodie J L, Larkin K T. Changes in hemodynamic response to mental stress with heart rate feedback training. Appl Psychophysiol Biofeedback 2001;26:293–309

23 Harve A G, Clark D M, Ehlers A, Rapee R M. Social anxiety and self-impression: cognitive preparation enhances the beneficial effects of video feedback following a stressful social task. Behav Res Ther 2000;38:1183–1192

24 Watson C G, Herder J. Effectiveness of alpha biofeedback therapy: negative results. J Clin Psychol 1980;36:508–513

25 Klawansky S, Yeung A, Berkey C, Shah N, Phan H, Chalmers T C. Meta-analysis of randomized controlled trials of cranial electrotherapy stimulation: efficacy in treating selected psychological and physiological conditions. J Nerv Ment Dis 1996; 183:478–485

26 Crocker P R, Grozelle C. Reducing induced state anxiety: effects of acute aerobic exercise and autogenic relaxation. J Sports Med Phys Fitness 1991;31:277–282

27 Broocks A, Bandelow B, Pekrun G, George A, Meyer T, Bartmann U, Hillmer-Vogel U, Rüther E. Comparison of aerobic exercise, clomipramine and placebo in the treatment of panic disorder. Am J Psychiatr 1998;155:603–609

28 Ernst E. 'Flower remedies': a systematic review of the clinical evidence. Wien Klin Wochenschr 2002;114:963–966

29 Hanus M, Lafon J, Mathieu M. Double-blind, randomised, placebo-controlled study to evaluate the efficacy and safety of fixed combination containing two plant extracts (Crataegus oxyacantha and Eschscholtzia californica) and magnesium in mild-to-moderate anxiety disorders. Curr Med Res Opin 2004;20.63–71

30 Wong A H C, Smith M, Boon H S. Herbal remedies in psychiatric practice. Arch Gen Psychiatr 1998;55:1033–1044

31 Pittler M H, Ernst E. Kava extract for treating anxiety. The Cochrane Database of Systematic Reviews 2003, Issue 1. Art. No.: CD003383

32 Kennedy D O, Little W, Scholey A B. Attenuation of laboratory-induced stress in humans after acute administration of Melissa officinalis (Lemon Balm). Psychosom Med 2004;66:607–613

33 Akhondzadeh S, Naghavi H R, Vazirian M, Shayeganpour A, Rashidi H, Khani M. Passionflower in the treatment of generalized anxiety: a pilot double-blind randomized controlled trial with oxazepam. J Clin Pharm Ther 2001;26:363–367

34 Adreatini R, Sartori V A, Seabra M L, Leiter J R. Effect of valepotriates (valerian extract) in generalized anxiety disorder: a randomized placebo-controlled pilot study. Phytother Res 2002;16:650–654

35 Alibou J P, Jobert J. Aconit en dilution homéopathique et agitation postopératoire de l'enfant. Pédiatrie 1990;45:465–466

36 McCutcheon L E. Treatment of anxiety with a homoeopathy remedy. J Appl Nutr 1996; 48:2–6

37 Bonne O, Shemer Y, Gorali Y, Katz M, Shalev A Y. A randomized, double-blind, placebo-controlled study of classical homeopathy in generalized anxiety disorder. J Clin Psychiatry 2003;64:282–287

38 Moore R, Abrahamsen R, Brodsgaard I. Hypnosis compared with group therapy and individual desensitization for dental anxiety. Eur J Oral Sci 1996;104:612–618

39 Moore R, Brodsgaard I, Abrahamsen R. A 3-year comparison of dental anxiety treatment outcomes: hypnosis, group therapy and individual desensitization vs. no specialist treatment. Eur J Oral Sci 2002;110:287–295

40 Van Dyck R, Spinhoven P. Does preference for type of treatment matter? A study of exposure in vivo with or without hypnosis in the treatment of panic disorder with agoraphobia. Behav Modif 1997;21:172–186

41 Zeltzer L, LeBaron S. Hypnosis and non-hypnotic techniques for reduction of pain and anxiety during painful procedures in children and adolescents with cancer. J Pediatr 1982;101:1032–1035

42 Roffe L, Schmidt K, Ernst E. A systematic review of guided imagery as an adjuvant cancer therapy. Psychooncology 2005;14:607–617

43 Richards K C, Gibson R, Overton-McCoy A L. Effects of massage in acute and critical care. AACN Clin Issues 2000,11.77–96

44 Field T, Grizzle N, Scafidi F, Schanberg S. Massage and relaxation therapies' effects on depressed adolescent mothers. Adolescence 1996;31:903–911

45 Field T, Hernandez-Reif M, Hart S, Theakston H, Schanberg S, Kuhn C. Pregnant women benefit from massage therapy. J Psychosom Obstet Gynaecol 1999;20:31–38

46 Fischer R L, Bianculli K W, Sehdev H, Hediger M L. Does light pressure effleurage reduce pain and anxiety associated with genetic amniocentesis? A randomized clinical trial. J Matern Fetal Med 2000;9:294–297

47 Chang M Y, Wang S Y, Chen C H. Effects of massage on pain and anxiety during labour: a randomized controlled trial in Taiwan. J Adv Nurs 2002;38:68–73

48 Hernandez-Reif M, Ironson G, Field T, Hurley J, Katz G, Diego M, Weiss S, Fletcher M A, Schanberg S, Kuhn C, Burman I. Breast cancer patients have improved immune and

CONDITIONS

neuroendocrine functions following massage therapy. J Psychosom Res 2004;57:45–52

49 Walach H, Güthlin C, Konig M. Efficacy of massage therapy in chronic pain: a pragmatic randomized trial. J Altern Complement Med 2003;9:837–846

50 Kim M S, Cho K S, Woo H, Kim J H. Effects of hand massage on anxiety in cataract surgery using local anesthesia. Cataract Refract Surg 2001;27;884–890

51 Fraser J, Kerr J R. Psychophysiological effects of back massage on elderly institutionalized patients. J Adv Nurs 1993;18:238–245

52 Hanley J, Stirling P, Brown C. Randomised controlled trial of therapeutic massage in the management of stress. Br J Gen Pract 2003;53:20–25

53 MacLean C R K, Walton K G, Wenneberg S R, Levitsky D K, Mandarino J V, Waziri R, Schneider R H. Altered response of cortisol, GH, TSH and testosterone to acute stress after four months' practice of transcendental meditation (TM). Ann NY Acad Sci 1994;746:381–384

54 Astin J A. Stress reduction through mindfulness meditation. Effects on psychological symptomatology, sense of control and spiritual experiences. Psychother Psychosom 1997;66:97–106

55 Eppley K R, Abrams A I, Shear J. Differential effects of relaxation techniques on trait anxiety: a meta-analysis. J Clin Psychol 1989;45:957–974

56 Grossman P, Niemann L, Schmidt S, Walach H. Mindfulness-based stress reduction and health benefits. A meta-analysis. J Psychosom Res 2004;57:35–43

57 Bishop S R. What do we really know about mindfulness-based stress reduction? Psychosom Med 2002;64:71–83

58 Elliott D. The effects of music and muscle relaxation on patient anxiety in a coronary care unit. Heart Lung 1994;23:27–35

59 Evans D. The effectiveness of music as an intervention for hospital patients: a systematic review. J Adv Nurs 2002;37:8–18

60 Ferguson S L, Voll K V. Burn pain and anxiety: the use of music relaxation during rehabilitation. J Burn Care Rehabil 2004;25:8–14

61 Kain Z N, Caldwell-Andrews A A, Krivutza D M, Weinberg M E, Gaal D, Wang S M, Mayes L C. Interactive music therapy as a treatment for preoperative anxiety in children: a randomized controlled trial. Anesth Analg 2004;98:1260–1266

62 Smith J C, Joyce C A. Mozart versus new age music: relaxation states, stress, and ABC

relaxation theory. J Music Theor 2004;41:215–234

63 Irarte Roteta A. Music therapy effectiveness to decrease anxiety in mechanically ventilated patients. [Article in Spanish] Enferm Intesiva 2003;14:43–48

64 Chan Y M, Lee P W, Ng T Y, Ngan H Y, Wong L C. The use of music to reduce anxiety for patients undergoing colposcopy: a randomized trial. Gynecol Oncol 2003;91:213–217

65 Hayes A, Buffum M, Lanier E, Rodahl E, Sasso C. Gastroenterol Nurs 2003;26:145–149

66 Kwekkeboom K L. Music versus distraction for procedural pain and anxiety in patients with cancer. Oncol Nurs Forum 2003;30:433–440

67 Smolen D, Topp R, Singer L. The effect of self-selected music during colonoscopy on anxiety, heart rate, and blood pressure. Appl Nurs Res 2002;15:126–136

68 Taylor-Piliae R E, Chair S Y. The effect of nursing interventions utilizing music therapy or sensory information on Chinese patients' anxiety prior to cardiac catheterization: a pilot study. Eur J Cardiovasc Nurs 2002;1:203–211

69 Beck J G, Stanley M A, Baldwin L E, Deagle E A 3rd, Averill P M. Comparison of cognitive therapy and relaxation training for panic disorder. J Consult Clin Psychol 1994;62:818–826

70 Ost L G, Westling B E, Hellstrom K. Applied relaxation, exposure in vivo and cognitive methods in the treatment of panic disorder with agoraphobia. Behav Res Ther 1993;31:383–394

71 Arntz A. Cognitive therapy versus applied relaxation as treatment of generalized anxiety disorder. Behav Res Ther 2003;41:633–646

72 Deckro G R, Ballinger K M, Hoyt M, Wilcher M, Dusek J, Myers P, Greenberg B, Rosenthal D S, Benson H. The evaluation of a mind/body intervention to reduce psychological distress and perceived stress in college students. J Am Coll Health 2002;50:281–287

73 Bindemann S, Soukop M, Kaye S B. Randomised controlled study of relaxation training. Eur J Cancer 1991;27:170–174

74 Bridge L R, Benson P, Pietroni P C, Priest R G. Relaxation and imagery in the treatment of breast cancer. BMJ 1988;297:1169–1172

75 Gift A G, Moore T, Soeken K. Relaxation to reduce dyspnea and anxiety in COPD patients. Nurs Res 1992;41:242–246

76 Pawlow L A, O'Neil P M, Malcolm R J. Night eating syndrome: effects of brief relaxation training on stress, mood, hunger, and eating

patterns. Int J Obes Relat Metab Disord 2003; 27:970–978

77 Willumsen T, Vassend O. Effects of cognitive therapy, applied relaxation and nitrous oxide sedation. A five-year follow-up study of patients treated for dental fear. Acta Odontol Scand 2003;61:93–99

78 Cheung Y L, Molassiotis A, Chang A M. The effect of progressive muscle relaxation training on anxiety and quality of life after stoma surgery in colorectal cancer patients. Psychoncology 2003;12:254–266

79 Holden-Lund C. Effects of relaxation with guided imagery on surgical stress and wound healing. Res Nurs Health 1988;11:235–244

80 Markland D, Hardy L. Anxiety, relaxation and anaesthesia for day-case surgery. Br J Clin Psychol 1993;32:493–504

81 Mandle C L, Domar A D, Harrington D P, Leserman J, Bozadjian E M, Friedman R, Benson H. Relaxation response in femoral angiography. Radiology 1990,174:737–739

82 Lukins R, Davan I G, Drummond P D. A cognitive behavioural approach to preventing anxiety during magnetic resonance imaging. J Behav Ther Exp Psychiatr 1997; 28:97–104

83 Kolcaba K, Fox C. The effects of guided imagery on comfort of women with early stage breast cancer undergoing radiation therapy. Oncol Nurs Forum 1999;26:67–72

84 Yates R G, Lamping D L, Abram N L, Wright C. Effects of chiropractic treatment on blood pressure and anxiety: a randomized, controlled trial. J Manip Physiol Ther 1998; 11.484–488

85 Olson M, Sneed N. Anxiety and therapeutic touch. Issues Mental Health Nurs 1995; 16:97–108

86 Ireland M. Therapeutic touch with HIV-infected children: a pilot study. J Assoc Nurses AIDS Care 1998;9:68–77

87 Turner J G, Clark A J, Gauthier D K, Williams M. The effect of therapeutic touch on pain and anxiety in burn patients. J Adv Nurs 1998;28:10–20

88 Shore A G. Long-term effects of energetic healing on symptoms of psychological depression and self-perceived stress. Altern Ther Health Med 2004;10:42–48

89 Biggs Q M, Kelly K S, Toney J D. The effects of deep diaphragmatic breathing and focused attention on dental anxiety in a private practice setting. J Dent Hyg 2003;77:105–113

90 Stephenson N L, Weinrich S P, Tavakoli A S. The effects of foot reflexology on anxiety and pain in patients with breast and lung cancer. Oncol Nurs Forum 2000;27:67–72

91 Weinberg R S, Hunt V V. Effects of structural integration on state-trait anxiety. J Clin Psychol 1979;35:319–322

92 Jin P. Efficacy of Tai Chi, brisk walking, meditation, and reading in reducing mental and emotional stress. J Psychosom Res 1992;36: 361–370

93 Tsai J C, Wang W H, Chan P, Lin L J, Wang C H, Tomlinson B, Hsieh M H, Yang H Y, Liu J C. The beneficial effects of Tai Chi Chuan on blood pressure and lipid profile and anxiety status in a randomized controlled trial. J Altern Complement Med 2003;9:747–754

94 Malathi A, Damodaran A. Stress due to exams in medical students – role of yoga. Indian J Physiol Pharmacol 1999;43:218–224

95 Ray U S, Mukhopadhyaya S, Purkayastha S S, Asnani V, Tomer O S, Prashad R, Thakur L, Selvamurthy W. Effect of yogic exercises on physical and mental health of young fellowship course trainees. Indian J Physiol Pharmacol 2001;45:37–53

ASTHMA

Synonyms/ subcategories	Atopic asthma, bronchial asthma, extrinsic asthma, intrinsic asthma, nervous asthma, reflex asthma.
Definition	Asthma is characterised by variable airflow obstruction and airway hyper-responsiveness. Symptoms include dyspnoea, cough, chest tightness, and wheezing.
CAM usage	Surveys of patients with asthma have reported usage in up to 70% of adults[1] and 55% of children.[2,3] Breathing techniques, relaxation, homeopathy, herbal medicine and yoga are commonly used.

CONDITIONS

Clinical evidence

Acupuncture

The data on acupuncture are highly inconsistent and systematic reviews[4,5] of RCTs (Box 2.7) agree that the evidence is insufficient. This conclusion also ties in with subsequent RCTs which have generated both positive[6] and negative findings.[7-10]

Box 2.7
Systematic review
Acupuncture for asthma
McCarney[4]

- Eleven placebo-controlled RCTs involving 324 patients

- Quality was moderate overall

- Effects are no different from sham acupuncture

- Meta-analysis (two RCTs) for lung function: standard mean difference: 0.12 (95% CI −0.31 to 0.55)

- Conclusion: there is not enough evidence to make recommendations

Alexander technique

A Cochrane review[11] found no clinical trials of this modality as a treatment of asthma.

Autogenic training

An RCT comparing autogenic training with supportive psychotherapy in 24 adults with moderate or severe asthma showed clinically relevant improvement in lung function with autogenic training compared with controls.[12] Two other RCTs were less promising; a study with 38 adults found improvement of anxiety but no changes in lung function[13] and another in 31 adults detected no changes in symptoms or airway resistance, although the use of sympathomimetics decreased.[14]

Biofeedback

The evidence for biofeedback is encouraging. There were improvements in lung function and symptom scores in 33 children given biofeedback over 5 months, whereas those randomised to placebo biofeedback showed improvement in symptom scores only.[15] Another RCT with 20 adolescents showed improvement of symptoms (superior to an untreated control group) but no change in lung function.[16] A high quality RCT tested heart rate variability biofeedback against placebo in 94 adult asthmatics.[17] The results demonstrated a reduction in need for medication in patients receiving biofeedback.

Breathing techniques

Breathing techniques have repeatedly been systematically reviewed[18-20] (Box 2.8). Although yoga and physiotherapy exercises are encouraging,[18] particularly in terms of quality of life,[19] there is insufficient evidence to conclude that they are effective.

Box 2.8
Systematic review
**Breathing exer-
cises for asthma**
Ernst[18]

- Five RCTs with 150 adults with chronic asthma; one RCT in 38 children with acute asthma

- Interventions included breathing exercises as part of yoga and physiotherapy

- Quality: most studies flawed

- Conclusion: breathing exercises appear promising but insufficient evidence to make firm judgements

The Buteyko breathing technique (BBT) which involves learning to make breathing shallow and slow was tested in an RCT involving 39 patients with asthma. Those who were trained in BBT showed greater reduction in asthma medication use and improvement in quality of life than controls who received asthma education alone.[21] An RCT (n = 36) shows an improvement in quality of life and a reduction in medication compared with placebo.[22] The Buteyko technique was compared with Pranayama yoga in another RCT (n = 90).[23] The results demonstrated positive effects of Buteyko on symptoms but not on lung function.

Diet

Rigorous tests with randomised, double-blind, placebo-controlled challenge demonstrate that between 2% and 6% of asthmatic patients are hypersensitive to foods.[24] Apart from avoidance of known food allergens, particularly peanuts, in this group of patients, no recommendations can be made for any particular diet on the basis of current evidence. There is some evidence suggesting that reduced dietary intake of vitamins A, C and E as well as selenium and magnesium is associated with brittle asthma in children.[25]

Herbal medicine

A systematic review[26] (Box 2.9) found some encouraging evidence in single studies with *Picrorrizia kurroa, Solanum* spp, *Boswellia serrata,* Saibuko-to, cannabis (*Cannabis sativa*) and dried ivy (*Hedera helix*) extract, but insufficient to make firm judgements. Another systematic review focused specifically on

Box 2.9
Systematic review
**Herbal medicine
for asthma**
Huntley[26]

- Seventeen RCTs included

- Overall quality poor

- Six studies of traditional Chinese herbs (494 patients), eight using traditional Indian herbs (805 patients) and three with Kampo herbs (146 patients)

- Conclusion: some promising data but no fully convincing evidence for any of the herbal preparations ivy leaf extract for asthmatic children.[27] Five RCTs were included and an overall positive effect on respiratory function was noted. Further RCTs or CCTs found encouraging symptomatic effects of the Ayurvedic herbal mixture 'Amrita Bindu',[28] butterbur (*Petasites hybridus*),[29] a range of Chinese herbal mixtures,[30–33] and a Kampo medicine (TJ-96).[34]

Homeopathy

One version of homeopathy is 'isopathy' which employs high dilutions of a preparation of the allergen(s) to which the individual is sensitive. Isopathic treatment was superior to placebo in improving symptom scores of 28 adults over 21 days in one rigorous study,[35] though the clinical implications of this were far from certain in view of the short duration, small sample and small effect on lung function. The overall evidence from a systematic review of any type of homeopathy (Box 2.10) is insufficient to draw conclusions.[36] A further RCT with 96 asthmatic children tested individualised homeopathy against placebo and found no evidence for efficacy.[37]

Box 2.10
Systematic review
Homeopathy for asthma
McCarney[36]

- Six placebo-controlled RCTs involving 556 patients

- Quality was variable

- No trial reported a difference on validated symptom scales

- There were conflicting results in terms of lung function

- Conclusion: not enough evidence to reliably assess the possible role of homeopathy in asthma

Hypnotherapy

The evidence from three published RCTs (Table 2.7) is encouraging but not convincing.[38–40] Patients may become less aware of their degree of bronchoconstriction and therefore risk undertreating acute attacks of asthma.

Massage

In one RCT of 32 children, parents either massaged their children each evening or instructed them in relaxation.[41] There were improvements in lung function in younger children (aged 6–8 years) after massage for 30 days, compared with relaxation controls, but not in older children aged 9–11. The parents also noted a beneficial effect on themselves.

Meditation

One study attempted to compare transcendental meditation with reading relaxing literature in a crossover study, but was confounded by those who learned to meditate first and then contin-

Table 2.7 **RCTs of hypnotherapy for asthma**

Reference	Sample size	Interventions [regimen]	Result	Comment
Maher-Loughman[38]	62	A) Hypnosis [30 min/d] B) Standard medication	Symptomatic improvement greater with A	No statistical analysis
Anon[39]	252	A) Hypnosis [15 min/d] B) Relaxation & breathing exercises	Both groups improved similarly, lung function more with A	Functional changes not clinically relevant
Ewer[40]	44	A) Hypnosis [6 wkly sessions] B) Attention control (clinic visits)	Benefit in some lung functions in hypnosis-responsive subjects	Stratified by responsiveness

ued to practise after they were crossed over.[42] In the first period, those who meditated experienced a decrease in airway resistance.

Reflexology
An RCT in 30 patients given reflexology showed this treatment to have no benefit over an attention control.[43] A rigorous RCT (n = 40) compared reflexology with sham-reflexology and found no between-group differences relating to lung function, bronchial activity, medication use, symptoms, or quality of life.[44]

Relaxation
In view of the association between acute asthma and stress, regular relaxation would seem a promising approach to treatment. A systematic review identified 15 clinical trials (Box 2.11).[45] The methodological quality of these studies was often poor. There was some evidence that muscular relaxation improves lung function but for other relaxation techniques the evidence was unconvincing.[46–48]

Box 2.11
Systematic review
Relaxation for asthma
Huntley[45]

- Nine RCTs were included, five of progressive muscle/mental relaxation, two of hypnosis/self-hypnosis, two of biofeedback

- Methodological quality was unusually poor

- Conclusion: for no approach was the evidence conclusively positive

Spinal manipulation
A Cochrane review found no convincing evidence to show that spinal manipulation is effective.[49]

Supplements

A Cochrane review of nine RCTs of **fish oil** (omega-3 fatty-acid) supplements concluded that the evidence is insufficient.[50]

A small placebo-controlled RCT of **propolis** suggested a reduction in asthma attacks after taking this supplement.[51]

A Cochrane review with only one small trial found encouraging evidence that **selenium** supplementation may be a useful adjunctive therapy for chronic asthma.[52] Another Cochrane review of four **Vitamin C** trials concluded that the evidence is insufficient.[53] An RCT of **Vitamin E** supplementation found no benefit.[54]

Yoga

Compared with the matched controls, patients using long-term yoga showed a reduction in asthma medication use and number of asthma attacks and an increase in peak flow rate.[55] Two RCTs failed to find any effect on lung function, although mental improvements were noted.[56,57] An RCT (n = 30) of Sahaja yoga found limited beneficial effects on subjective and objective outcome measures.[58]

Other therapies

Encouraging results have been reported in CCTs of **humor therapy**,[59] **imagery**,[60,61] and **pulsatic electromagnetic therapy**.[62]

Table 2.8
Summary of clinical evidence for asthma

Treatment	Weight of evidence	Direction of evidence	Serious safety concerns
Acupuncture	OOO	⇨	Yes (see p 294)
Alexander technique	O	⇨	No (see p 299)
Autogenic training	OO	⇨	Yes (see p 305)
Biofeedback	OO	⬈	No (see p 310)
Breathing exercises	OO	⬈	No (see p 5)
Buteyko breathing	OO	⇧	No (see p 358)
Diet (allergy avoidance)	O	⇧	No (see p 5)
Herbal medicine			
Amrita Bindu	O	⬈	Yes (see p 5)
Boswellia serrata	O	⬈	Yes (see p 479)
Butterbur	O	⬈	Yes (see p 477)
Cannabis	O	⬈	Yes (see p 5)
Chinese herbal mixtures	O	⬈	Yes (see p 5)
Ivy	O	⬈	Yes (see p 479)
Picrorrizia kurroa	O	⬈	Yes (see p 5)

Treatment	Weight of evidence	Direction of evidence	Serious safety concerns
Saibuko-to	O	↗	Yes (see p 5)
Solanum	O	↗	Yes (see p 5)
TJ96 Kampo medicine	O	↗	Yes (see p 5)
Homeopathy	OO	↘	No (see p 327)
Hypnotherapy	OO	↗	Yes (see p 331)
Massage	O	↗	No (see p 334)
Meditation	O	↗	Yes (see p 338)
Reflexology	OO	↘	No (see p 345)
Relaxation	OO	⇒	No (see p 348)
Spinal manipulation			
Chiropractic	OO	↘	Yes (see p 316)
Supplements			
Fish oil	OO	↘	Yes (see p 483)
Propolis	O	↗	Yes (see p 454)
Selenium	OO	↘	Yes (see p 484)
Vitamin C	OO	⇒	Yes (see p 5)
Vitamin E	OO	↘	Yes (see p 5)
Yoga	OO	⇒	Yes (see p 356)

Overall recommendation

In comparison with conventional drugs with known risk/benefit profiles, no CAM therapy can be recommended as a sole treatment for asthma. However, some therapies may turn out to be useful adjuncts, e.g. Buteyko and other breathing exercises, exclusion diets, some herbal medicines, and massage.

REFERENCES

1 Ernst E. Complementary therapies for asthma: what patients use. J Asthma 1998;35:667–671
2 Ernst E. Use of complementary therapies in childhood asthma. Pediatr Asthma Allergy Immunol 1998;21:29–32
3 Andrews L, Lokuge S, Sawyer M, Lillywhite L, Kennedy D, Martin J. The use of alternative therapies by children with asthma: a brief report. J Paediatr Child Health 1998;34:131–134
4 McCarney R W, Brinkhaus B, Lasserson T J, Linde K. Acupuncture for chronic asthma. The Cochrane Database of Systematic Reviews 2003, Issue 3. Art No.: CD000008
5 Martin J, Donaldson A N, Villarroel R, Parmar M K, Ernst E, Higginson I J. Efficacy of acupuncture in asthma: systematic review and meta-analysis of published data from 11 randomised controlled trials. Eur Respir J 2002;20:846–852
6 Maa S H, Sun M F, Hsu K H, Hung T J, Chen H C, Yu C T, Wang C H, Lin H C. Effect of acupuncture or acupressure on quality of life of patients with chronic obstructive asthma: a pilot study. J Altern Complement Med 2003;9:659–670
7 Shapira M Y, Berkman N, Ben-David G, Avital A, Bardach E, Breuer R. Short-term acupuncture therapy is of no benefit in patients with moderate persistent asthma. Chest 2002;121:1396–1400
8 Gruber W, Eber E, Malle-Scheid D, Pfleger A, Weinhandl E, Dorfer L, Zach M S. Laser acupuncture in children and adolescents with exercise induced asthma. Thorax 2002;57:222–225

9 Malmstrom M, Ahlner J, Carlsson C, Schmekel B. No effect of Chinese acupuncture on isocapnic hyperventilation with cold air in asthmatics, measured with impulse oscillometry. Acupunct Med 2002;20:66–73

10 Medici T C, Grebski E, Wu J, Hinz G, Wuthrich B. Acupuncture and bronchial asthma: a long-term randomized study of the effects of real versus sham acupuncture compared to controls in patients with bronchial asthma. J Altern Complement Med 2002;8:737–750

11 Dennis J, Cates C. Alexander technique for chronic asthma. The Cochrane Database of Systematic Reviews 2000, Issue 2. Art No.: CD000995

12 Henry M, De Rivera J L G, Gonzalez-Martin I J, Abreu J. Improvement of respiratory function in chronic asthmatic patients with autogenic therapy. J Psychosom Res 1993;17:265–270

13 Spiess K, Sachs G, Buchinger C, Roggla G, Schnack C, Haber P. Zur Auswirkung von Informations-und Entspannungsgruppen auf die Lungenfunktion und psychophysische Befindlichkeit bei Asthmapatienten. Prax Klin Pneumol 1988;42:641–644

14 Deter H C, Allert G. Group therapy for asthma patients: a concept for the psychosomatic treatment of patients in a medical clinic – a controlled study. Psychother Psychosom 1983;40:95–105

15 Kotses H, Harver A, Segreto J, Glaus K D, Creer T L, Young G A. Long-term effects of biofeedback-induced facial relaxation on measures of asthma severity in children. Biofeedback Self Regul 1991;16:1–21

16 Coen B L, Conran P B, McGrady A, Nelson L. Effects of biofeedback-assisted relaxation on asthma severity and immune function. Pediatr Asthma Allergy Immunol 1996;10:71–78

17 Lehrer P M, Vaschillo E, Vaschillo B, Lu S E, Scardella A, Siddique M, Habib R H. Biofeedback treatment for asthma. Chest 2004;126:352–361

18 Ernst E. Breathing techniques – adjunctive treatment modalities for asthma? A systematic review. Eur Resp J 2000;15:969–972

19 Holloway E, Ram F S. Breathing exercises for asthma. The Cochrane Database of Systematic Reviews 2004, Issue 1. Art No.: CD001277.

20 Ram F S, Holloway E A, Jones P W. Breathing retraining for asthma. Respir Med 2003;97:501–507

21 Bowler S D, Green A, Mitchell C A. Buteyko breathing techniques in asthma: a blinded randomised controlled trial. Med J Aust 1998; 169:575–578

22 Opag A J, Cohen M M, Bailey M J, Abramson M J. A clinical trial of Buteyko breathing technique in asthma as taught by a video. J Asthma 2000;37:557–564

23 Cooper S, Oborne J, Newton S, Harrison V, Thompson-Coon J, Lewis S, Tattersfield A. Effect of two breathing exercises (Buteyko and Pranayama) in asthma: a randomised controlled trial. Thorax 2003;58:674–679

24 Monteleone C A, Sherman A R. Nutrition and asthma. Arch Intern Med 1997;157:23–34

25 Baker J C, Tunnicliffe W S, Duncanson R C, Ayres J G. Reduced dietary intakes of magnesium, selenium and vitamins A, C and E in patients with brittle asthma. Thorax 1995;50 (suppl 2):A75

26 Huntley A, Ernst E. Herbal medicines for asthma: a systematic review. Thorax 2000;55:925–929

27 Hofmann D, Hecker M, Volp A. Efficacy of dry extract of ivy leaves in children with bronchial asthma – a review of randomized controlled trials. Phytomedicine 2003;10:213–220

28 Kumar S S, Shanmugasundaram K R. Amrita Bindu – an antioxidant inducer therapy in asthma children. Ethnopharmacol 2004;90: 105–114

29 Lee D K, Haggart K, Robb F M, Lipworth B J. Butterbur, a herbal remedy, confers complementary anti-inflammatory activity in asthmatic patients receiving inhaled corticosteroids. Clin Exp Allergy 2004;34:110–114

30 Zhang J. TCM treatment of bronchial asthma. J Tradit Chin Med 2000;20:101–103

31 Hong G, Zhang Y, Huang J. Clinical and experimental study on treatment of asthma with juanxiao tablet. [Article in Chinese] Zhongguo Zhong Xi Yi Jie He Za Zhi 1999;19:93–95

32 Xu L, Hua Q, Wang L. Clinical and experimental study on effect of Chanbei Kechuanping in treating bronchial asthma. [Article in Chinese] Zhongguo Zhong Xi Yi Jie He Za Zhi 2000;20:649–652

33 Kong L F, Gua L H, Zheng XY. Effect of yiqi bushen huoxue herbs in treating children asthma and on levels of nitric oxide, endothelin-1 and serum endothelial cells. [Article in Chinese] Zhongguo Zhong Xi Yi Jie He Za Zhi 2001;21:667–669

34 Urata Y, Yoshida S, Irie Y, Tanigawa T, Amayasu H, Nakabayashi M, Akahori K. Treatment of asthma patients with herbal medicine TJ-96: a randomized controlled trial. Respir Med 2002;96:469–474

35 Reilly D, Taylor M A, Beattie N G, Campbell J H, McSharry C, Aitchison T C, Carter R, Stevenson R D. Is evidence for homoeopathy reproducible? Lancet 1994;344:1601–1606

36 McCarney R W, Linde K, Lasserson T J. Homeopathy for chronic asthma. The Cochrane Database of Systematic Reviews 2003, Issue 4. Art No.: CD000353

37 White A, Slade P, Hunt C, Hart A, Ernst E. Individualized homeopathy as an adjunct in the treatment of childhood asthma: a randomized placebo controlled trial. Thorax 2003;58:317–321

38 Maher-Loughnan G P, Macdonald N, Mason A A, Fry L. Controlled trial of hypnosis in the symptomatic treatment of asthma. BMJ 1962;2:371–376

39 Anon. Hypnosis for asthma: a controlled trial. BMJ 1968;4:71–76

40 Ewer T C, Stewart D E. Improvement in bronchial hyper-responsiveness in patients with moderate asthma after treatment with a hypnotic technique: a randomised controlled trial. BMJ 1986;293:1129–1132

41 Field T, Henteleff T, Hernandez-Reif M, Martinez E, Mavunda K, Kuhn C, Schanberg S. Children with asthma have improved pulmonary functions after massage therapy. J Pediatr 1998;132:854–858

42 Wilson A F, Honsberger R, Chiu J T, Novey H S. Transcendental meditation and asthma. Respiration 1975;32:74–80

43 Peterson L N, Faurschou P, Olsen O T, Svendsen U G. Reflexology and bronchial asthma. Ugeskr Laeger 1992;154: 2065–2068

44 Brygge T, Heinig J H, Collins P, Ronborg S, Gehrchen P M, Hilden J, Heegaard S, Poulsen L K. Reflexology and bronchial asthma. Respir Med 2001;95:173–179

45 Huntley A, White A R, Ernst E. Relaxation therapies for asthma: a systematic review. Thorax 2002;57:127–131

46 Alexander A B, Miklich D R, Hershkoff H. The immediate effects of systematic relaxation training on peak expiratory flow rates in asthmatic children. Psychosom Med 1972; 34:388–394

47 Erskine J, Schonell M. Relaxation therapy in bronchial asthma. J Psychosom Res 1979; 23:131–139

48 Hock R A, Bramble J, Kennard D W. A comparison between relaxation and assertive training with asthmatic male children. Bio Psych 1977;12:593–596

49 Hondras M A, Linde K, Jones A P. Manual therapy for asthma. The Cochrane Database of Systematic Reviews 2001, Issue 1. Art No.: CD001002

50 Thien F C K, Woods R, De Lucas S, Abramson M J. Dietary marine fatty acids (fish oil) for asthma in adults and children. The Cochrane Database of Systematic Reviews 2002, Issue 2. Art No.: CD001283

51 Khayyal M T, el-Ghazaly M A, el-Khatib A S, Hatem A M, de Vries P J, el-Shafei S, Khattab M M. A clinical pharmacological study of the potential beneficial effects of a propolis food product as an adjuvant in asthmatic patients. Fundamen Clin Pharmacol 2003; 17:93–102

52 Allam M F, Lucena R A. Selenium supplementation for asthma. The Cochrane Database of Systematic Reviews 2001, Issue 4. Art. No.: CD003538

53 Ram F S, Rowe B H, Kaur B. Vitamin C supplementation for asthma. The Cochrane Database of Systematic Reviews 2004, Issue 3. Art No.: CD000993

54 Pearson P J, Lewis S A, Britton J, Fogarty A. Vitamin E supplements in asthma: a parallel group randomised placebo controlled trial. Thorax 2004;59:652–656

55 Nagarathna R, Nagendra H R. Yoga for bronchial asthma: a controlled study. BMJ 1985;291:1077–1079

56 Fluge T, Richter J, Fabel H, Zysno E, Weller E, Wagner T O. Long-term effects of breathing exercises and yoga in patients with bronchial asthma. Pneumologie 1994;48:484–490

57 Vedanthan P K, Kesavalu L N, Murthy K C, Duvall K, Hall M J, Baker S, Nagarathna S. Clinical study of yoga techniques in university students with asthma: a controlled study. Allergy Asthma Proc 1998;19:3–9

58 Manocha R, Marks G B, Kenchington P, Peters D, Salome C M. Sahaja yoga in the management of moderate to severe asthma: a randomised controlled trial. Thorax 2002;57:110–115

59 Kimata H. Effect of viewing humorous vs. non-humerous film on bronchial responsiveness in patients with bronchial asthma. Physiol Behav 2004;81:681–684

60 Epstein G N, Halper J P, Barrett E A, Birdsall C, McGee M, Baron K P, Lowenstein S. A pilot study of mind-body changes in adults with asthma who practice mental imagery. Altern Ther Health Med 2004;10:66–71

61 Freeman L W, Welton D. Effects of imagery, critical thinking, and asthma education on symptoms and mood state in adult asthma patients: a pilot study. J Altern Complement Med 2005;11:57–68

62 Sadlonova J, Korpas J, Salat D, Miko L, Kudlicka J. The effect of the pulsatile electromagnetic field in children suffering from bronchial asthma. Acta Physiol Hung 2003;90:327–334

ATOPIC ECZEMA

Synonyms/ subcategories

Atopic dermatitis, infantile eczema.

Definition

Atopic eczema (atopic dermatitis) is an inflammatory skin disease characterised by an itchy erythematous poorly demarcated skin eruption with a predilection for skin creases.

CAM usage

A survey of German eczema patients reported homeopathy, acupuncture, dietary therapy, autogenic training and relaxation as the most frequently used forms of CAM.[1]

Clinical evidence

Autogenic training

An RCT (n = 113) compared autogenic training (once weekly for 12 weeks) with cognitive–behavioural therapy, a dermatological education programme and standard medical care.[2] Results at one year follow-up indicated that autogenic training was as effective as the psychotherapy and superior to the educational programme and usual care in terms of skin condition and use of topical steroids.

Diet

Several RCTs[3–6] have investigated egg and cow's milk exclusion diets, with two of them showing positive results,[3,6] including one on the effect of maternal antigen avoidance on breast-fed infants.[6] RCTs of prevention of eczema in high-risk infants by maternal antigen avoidance during pregnancy and lactation[7] have been systematically reviewed. Based on only three trials each, it was concluded that the risk of the child developing eczema was likely to be reduced by exclusion diets during lactation, but not during pregnancy.

A Cochrane review of five studies found no convincing evidence that feeding infants without clinical allergy/intolerance on an adapted soy milk formula instead of human milk would be of benefit in the prevention of atopic eczema.[8]

Herbal medicine

Three RCTs of **borage** (*Borago officinalis*) seed oil involving mostly adult patients have produced conflicting results (Table 2.9).[9–11] A smaller crossover trial in children using gamma-linolenic acid from borage seeds reported a strong placebo response and no difference between the interventions.[12] Collectively these data fail to demonstrate the effectiveness of borage oil.

Encouraging but not fully convincing were data also published for **black seed** (*Nigella sativa*) oil.[13]

A meta-analysis of nine placebo-controlled trials of oil of **evening primrose** (*Oenothera biennis*) demonstrated a positive effect.[14] However, the results of subsequent RCTs do not tend to support this result (Table 2.10).[15–18]

Table 2.9 **Double-blind RCTs of borage oil for atopic eczema**

Reference	Sample size	Interventions [dosage]	Result	Comment
Baslau[9]	50	A) Borage oil [2 × 1000 mg/d for 12 w] B) Placebo (palm oil)	A superior to B on severity index	Placebo response of 43%
Henz[10]	160	A) Borage oil [3 × 500 mg/d for 24 w] B) Placebo (miglyol)	A no different from B on Costa score	Non-compliance seemed likely from plasma lipid measurements
Takwale[11]	151	A) Borage oil [2–4 × 920 mg/d for 12 w] B) Placebo	A no different from B on SASSAD score	No difference in response of children or adults; medication well tolerated

Table 2.10 **Double-blind RCTs of evening primrose oil for atopic eczema**

Reference	Sample size	Interventions [dosage]	Result	Comment
Berth-Jones[15]	123	A) Evening primrose oil [6 g/d for 16 w] B) Evening primrose & fish oil [5 g & 1.3 g] C) Placebo	A or B no different from C on severity scores	Children and adults included but no differential effects
Biagi[16]	51	A) Evening primrose oil [500 mg kg/d for 8 w] B) Evening primrose oil [250 mg kg/d] C) Placebo	A superior to C on severity scores; B no different from C	Infants all, 8 years; very high doses used; significant difference was borderline
Whitaker[17]	39	A) Evening primrose oil [600 mg/d for 16 w] B) Placebo	A no different from B on symptom scores	Patients with chronic hand dermatitis
Hederos[18]	60	A) Evening primrose oil [500 mg/d for 16 w] B) Placebo	A no different from B on symptom scores	Patients aged 1–16 years

A non-randomised trial (n = 161) of a topical preparation containing **German chamomile** (*Matricaria recutita*) suggested it may be as useful as hydrocortisone, but no statistical analysis was carried out.[19] A subsequent RCT reported slight superiority over hydrocortisone but little difference with placebo.[20]

Topical preparations of **liquorice** (*Glycyrrhiza glabra*)[21] and **St John's wort** (*Hypericum perforatum*)[22] have also generated encouraging findings which require independent replication.

A systematic review of the Chinese herbal mixture **Zemaphyte**,[23] included only two RCTs from the same researchers who reported positive results for a herbal combination in both

CONDITIONS

adults and children. A subsequent independent crossover RCT of the same preparation found it to be no different from placebo.[24] A Cochrane review of these three RCTs and an open label study concluded that this approach 'may be effective'.[25]

A mixture of *Eleutherococcus*, *Achillea millefolium* and *Lamium album* did not generate any benefit over placebo in a small (n = 49) RCT with a 2-week treatment period.[26]

Hypnotherapy

An RCT including children (n = 31) compared the effects of hypnotherapy (four sessions over 8 weeks) with biofeedback (skin conductance) and an attention control condition where children discussed their eczema and kept a symptom diary.[27] After 5 months the hypnotherapy and biofeedback groups had improved more than the control group on severity of eczema, but not area of coverage.

Supplements

A substantial body of evidence from RCTs suggests that **probiotics** are effective in the prevention and treatment of atopic eczema in infants and children.[28-33]

A double-blind RCT of supplementation with **selenium** (alone and combined with Vitamin E) found no difference in severity of eczema compared with placebo.[34] More recently, an open, uncontrolled study found levels reduced in children with atopic eczema and suggested that selenium-supplementation generated positive clinical effects.[35]

Zinc has been investigated in a double-blind RCT with children.[36] It was not superior to placebo in any outcome measure.

Other therapies

A small sham-controlled RCT of **autologous blood therapy** showed a mild but positive effect on a symptom score in adults with atopic eczema.[37]

Table 2.11 **Summary of clinical evidence for atopic eczema**

Treatment	Weight of evidence	Direction of evidence	Serious safety concerns
Autogenic training	O	⇧	Yes (see p 305)
Biofeedback	O	⬈	No (see p 310)
Diet			
Exclusion in children/adults	OO	⬈	No (see p 5)
Exclusion during pregnancy	O	⇩	No (see p 5)
Exclusion during lactation	O	⬈	No (see p 5)
Herbal medicine			
Borage oil	OO	⇨	Yes (see p 476)
Black seed oil	O	⬈	Yes (see p 476)

Treatment	Weight of evidence	Direction of evidence	Serious safety concerns
Evening primrose oil	OOO	↘	Yes (see p 393)
German chamomile	O	↗	Yes (see p 376)
Liquorice	O	↗	Yes (see p 479)
St John's wort	O	↗	Yes (see p 462)
Zemaphyte	OO	↗	Yes (see p 5)
Hypnotherapy	O	↗	Yes (see p 331)
Supplements			
Probiotics	OO	↗	No (see p 5)
Selenium	O	↗	Yes (see p 484)
Zinc	O	↗	Yes (see p 5)

A crossover trial with eight children receiving either **massage** with essential oils (aromatherapy) or massage alone found no difference in clinical signs of atopic eczema.[38]

Overall recommendation

There is no convincing evidence for the effectiveness of any complementary therapy in treating or preventing eczema. The therapies with the most encouraging evidence are autogenic training, biofeedback, hypnotherapy, some dietary approaches, and some supplements. They are considered relatively risk-free and may be worth considering as an adjunct to effective conventional treatments.

REFERENCES

1 Augustin M, Zschocke I, Buhrke U. Attitudes and prior experience with respect to alternative medicine among dermatological patients: the Freiburg questionnaire on attitudes to naturopathy (FAN). Forsch Komplementärmed 1999;6:26–29

2 Ehlers A, Stangier U, Gieler U. Treatment of atopic dermatitis: a comparison of psychological and dermatological approaches to relapse prevention. J Consult Clin Psychol 1995;63:624–635

3 Lever R, MacDonald C, Waugh P, Aitchison T. Randomised controlled trial of advice on an egg exclusion diet in young children with atopic eczema and sensitivity to eggs. Pediatr Allergy Immunol 1998;9:13–19

4 Atherton D J, Sewall M, Soothill J F, Wells R S, Chilvers C E D. A double-blind controlled cross-over trial of an antigen-avoidance diet in atopic eczema. Lancet 1978;25:401–403

5 Neild V S, Marsden R A, Bailes J A, Bland J M. Egg and milk exclusion diets in atopic eczema. Br J Dermatol 1986;114:117–123

6 Cant A J, Bailes J A, Marsden R A, Hewitt D. Effect of maternal dietary exclusion on breast fed infants with eczema: two controlled studies. BMJ Clin Res Ed 1986;293:231–233

7 Kramer M S, Kakuma R. Maternal dietary antigen avoidance during pregnancy and/or lactation for preventing or treating atopic disease in the child. The Cochrane Database of Systematic Reviews 2003, Issue 4. Art. No.: CD000133

8 Osborn D A, Sinn J. Soy formula for prevention of allergy and food intolerance in infants. The Cochrane Database of Systematic Reviews 2004, Issue 3. Art. No.: CD003741

9 Baslau M, Thaci D. Atopic dermatitis: borage oil for systemic therapy. Zeitschr Dermatol 1996;182:131–136

10 Henz B M, Jablonska S, van de Kerkhof P C M, Stingl G, Blaszczyk M, Vandervalk P G, Veenhuizen R, Muggli R, Raederstorff D. Double-blind, multicentre analysis of the efficacy of borage oil in patients with atopic eczema. Br J Dermatol 1999;140:685–688

11 Takwale A, Tan E, Agarwal S, Barclay G, Ahmed I, Hotchkiss K, Thompson J R, Chapman T, Berth-Jones J. Efficacy and tolerability of borage oil in adults and children with atopic eczema: randomised, double-blind, placebo controlled, parallel group trial. BMJ 2003;327:1385

12 Borreck S, Hildebrandt A, Forster J. Borage seed oil and atopic dermatitis. Klinische Pädiatrie 1997;209:100–104

13 Kalus U, Pruss A, Bystron J, Jurecka M, Smekalova A, Lichius J J, Kiesewetter H. Effect of Nigella sativa (black seed) on subjective feeling in patients with allergic diseases. Phytother Res 2003;17:1209–1214

14 Morse P F, Horrobin D F, Manku M S. Meta-analysis of placebo-controlled studies of the efficacy of Epogam in the treatment of atopic eczema. Relationship between plasma essential fatty acid changes and clinical response. Br J Dermatol 1989;121:75–90

15 Berth-Jones J, Graham-Brown R A. Placebo-controlled trial of essential fatty acid supplementation in atopic dermatitis. Lancet 1993;341:1557–1560. Erratum in: Lancet 1993;342:564.

16 Biagi P L, Bordoni A, Hrelia S, Celadon M, Ricci G P, Cannella V, Patrizi A, Specchia F, Masi M. The effect of gamma-linolenic acid on clinical status, red cell fatty acid composition and membrane microviscosity in infants with atopic dermatitis. Drugs Exp Clin Res 1994;20:77–84

17 Whitaker D K, Cilliers J, de Beer C. Evening primrose oil (Epogam) in the treatment of chronic hand dermatitis: disappointing therapeutic results. Dermatology 1996;193:115–120

18 Hederos C A, Berg A. Epogam evening primrose oil treatment in atopic dermatitis and asthma. Arch Dis Child 1996;75: 494–497

19 Aertgeerts P, Albring M, Klaschka F, Nasemann T, Patzelt-Wenczler R, Rauhut K, Weigl B. Comparative testing of Kamillosan cream and steroidal (0.25% hydrocortisone, 0.75% fluocortin butyl ester) and non-steroidal (5% bufexamac) dermatologic agents in maintenance therapy of eczematous diseases. Zeitschr für Hautkrankheiten 1985;60:270–277

20 Patzelt-Wenczler R, Ponce-Pöschl E. Proof of efficacy of Kamillosan cream in atopic eczema. Eur J Med Res 2000;5:171–175

21 Saeedi M, Morteza-Semnani K, Ghoreishi M R. The treatment of atopic dermatitis with licorice gel. J Dermatolog Treat 2003;14:153–157

22 Schempp C M, Windeck T, Hezel S, Simon J C. Topical treatment of atopic dermatitis with St John's wort cream – a randomized, placebo controlled, double blind half-side comparison. Phytomedicine 2003;10:31–37

23 Armstrong N C, Ernst E. The treatment of eczema with Chinese herbs: a systematic review of randomised clinical trials. Br J Clin Pharmacol 1999;48:262–264

24 Fung A Y, Look P C, Chong L Y, But P P, Wong E. A controlled trial of traditional Chinese herbal medicine in Chinese patients with recalcitrant atopic dermatitis. Int J Dermatol 1999;38:387–392

25 Zhang W, Leonard T, Bath-Hexall F, Chambers C A, Lee C, Humphreys R, Williams H C. Chinese herbal medicine for atopic eczema. The Cochrane Database of Systematic Reviews 2005, Issue 2. Art. No.: CD002291

26 Shapira M Y, Raphaelovich Y, Gilad L, Or R, Dumb A J, Ingber A. Treatment of atopic dermatitis with herbal combination of Eleutherococcus, Achillea millefolium and Lamium album has no advantage over placebo: a double blind, placebo-controlled, randomized trial. J Am Acad Dermatol 2005;52:691–693

27 Sokel B, Christie D, Kent A, Lansdown R, Atherton D. A comparison of hypnotherapy and biofeedback in the treatment of childhood atopic eczema. Contemp Hypnosis 1993;10:145–154

28 Kalliomaki M, Salminen S, Arvilommi H, Kero P, Kiskinen P, Isolauri E. Probiotics in primary prevention of atopic disease: a randomized placebo-controlled trial. Lancet 2001;357:1076–1079

29 Isolauri E, Arvola T, Sutas Y, Moilanen E, Salminen S. Probiotics in the management of atopic eczema. Clin Exp Allergy 2000;30: 1604–1610

30 Rautava S, Kalliomaki M, Isolauri E. Probiotics during pregnancy and breast-feeding might confer immunomodulatory protection against atopic disease in the infant. J Allergy Clin Immunol 2002;109:119–121

31 Kirjavainen P V, Arvola T, Salminen S J, Isolauri E. Aberrant composition of gut microbiota of allergic infants: a target of

bifidobacterial therapy at weaning? Gut 2002;51:51–55

32 Kirjavainen P V, Salminen S J, Isolauri E. Probiotic bacteria in the management of atopic disease: underscoring the importance of viability. J Pediatr Gastroenterol Nutr 2003;36:223–227

33 Rosenfeldt V, Benfeldt E, Nielsen S D, Michaelsen K F, Jeppesen D L, Valerius N H, Paerregaard A. Effect of probiotic Lactobacillus strains in children with atopic dermatitis. J Allergy Clin Immunol 2003;111:389–395

34 Fairris G M, Perkins P J, Lloyd B, Hinks L, Clayton B E. The effect on atopic dermatitis of supplementation with selenium and vitamin E. Acta Derm Venereol 1989;69:359–362

35 Ranjbar A, Pizzulli A. Selen und atopische Dermatitis. Erfahrungsheilkd 2002;10:665–674

36 Ewing C I, Gibbs A C, Ashcroft C, David T J. Failure of oral zinc supplementation in atopic eczema. Eur J Clin Nutr 1991;45:507–510

37 Pittler M H, Armstrong N C, Cox A, Collier P M, Hart A, Ernst E. Randomized, double-blind, placebo-controlled trial of autologous blood therapy for atopic dermatitis. Br J Dermatol 2003;148:307–313

38 Anderson C, Lis-Balchin M, Kirk-Smith M. Evaluation of massage with essential oils on childhood atopic eczema. Phytother Res 2000;14:452–456

CONDITIONS

BACK PAIN

Synonyms/ subcategories	Mechanical back pain, idiopathic back pain, non-specific back pain, low back pain, back ache, lumbago.
Definition	Pain, muscle tension or stiffness below the costal margin with many (often undefined) causes. Acute means less than 12 weeks.
Related conditions	Back pain with specific causes, i.e. specific back pain (e.g. due to ankylosing spondylitis, vertebral canal stenosis, etc.) can be differentiated from non-specific back pain where no cause can be identified. The latter type is much more common.
CAM usage	Back pain is the most frequent indication for which patients try CAM (e.g.[1]). The most commonly employed CAM treatments include acupuncture, herbal remedies, massage therapy and spinal manipulation (chiropractic or osteopathy). In our survey of CAM organisations (see p 4) the following treatments were recommended for back pain: Bowen technique, chiropractic, magnet therapy, massage, reflexology and yoga.
Clinical evidence	*Acupuncture* Systematic reviews have generated contradictory conclusions. Two new meta-analyses generated overall positive results (Box 2.12).[2,3]
	Alexander technique A systematic review[4] included one CCT with back pain sufferers and showed encouraging results for this approach.
	Exercise Systematic reviews of therapeutic exercise have drawn positive conclusions (Box 2.13).[5,6] It seems important that the treatment

Box 2.12
Meta-analysis
Acupuncture for back pain
Manheimer[2]

- Thirty-three RCTs were included, of which 22 were meta-analysed
- The methodological quality was variable but for some studies it was good
- For short-term pain relief of chronic pain the standardised mean difference was 0.54 (95% CI 0.35 to 0.73) compared with sham treatment
- For acute pain, the data were inconclusive
- Conclusions: acupuncture is effective for chronic low back pain

Box 2.13
Systematic review
Exercise for chronic back pain
Hayden[6]

- Forty-three RCTs were included
- Methodological quality was variable
- Overall results were positive
- High-dose exercise programmes were superior to low dose
- Conclusion: exercise may improve pain and function in chronic back pain

is individually designed, includes stretching and strengthening, and is supervised.[7]

Herbal medicine
Several herbal remedies have shown promising results in alleviating musculoskeletal pain.[8] The only one that has been investigated specifically for back pain is **devil's claw** (*Harpagophytum procumbens*). A systematic review (Box 2.14) of devil's claw included four RCTs on back pain and concluded that this remedy is an effective symptomatic treatment.[9]

Box 2.14
Systematic review
Harpagophytum procumbens for low back pain
Gagnier[9]

- Four RCTs were included
- Methodological quality was good on average
- There is moderate evidence that 100 mg harpagoside/day is effective for back pain
- Conclusion: this remedy is an effective symptomatic treatment for low back pain

Massage

A Cochrane review (Box 2.15) included eight RCTs and arrived at a cautiously positive conclusion.[10]

Box 2.15
Systematic review
Massage for back pain
Furlan[10]

- Eight RCTs were included
- Five RCTs were of high methodological quality
- Various comparator interventions were used
- Results were not uniform
- Conclusion: massage might be beneficial

Spinal manipulation

A Cochrane review of all types of manipulation and mobilisation failed to show that these approaches are superior to other treatment options (Box 2.16).[11] A systematic review of osteopathic manipulative treatment for low back pain found greater pain reductions with osteopathy compared to active control treatment, placebo or no treatment.[11a]

Box 2.16
Meta-analysis
Spinal manipulation/mobilisation for low-back pain
Assendelft[11]

- Thirty-nine RCTs were included
- Methodological quality was variable
- Acute low-back pain: spinal manipulation therapy was superior only to sham, ineffective or harmful interventions, but not to GP care, analgesics, physical therapy, exercise or back school
- For chronic low-back pain results were similar
- Conclusion: there is no evidence that spinal manipulation therapy is superior to other treatments

Water injections

Sterile water injections have been used for a number of pain syndromes. The theory is that such injections stimulate skin nociceptors and thus close the 'gate' for peripheral pain perception. Two placebo-controlled RCTs suggested that they are effective in alleviating back pain of various causes.[12,13]

Other therapies

A combination of **back school, relaxation** and **qi gong** yielded promising preliminary results[14] and there are some encouraging data related to **hypnotherapy**[15] and **yoga**.[16,17]

Overall recommendation

The most promising CAM treatments for back pain are exercise, acupuncture, devil's claw, massage, and sterile water injections. Perhaps with the exception of therapeutic exercise, none of these

CONDITIONS

therapies are completely risk free, but serious complications are rare. The effect sizes of CAM modalities for low back pain are invariably small to moderate, yet this also applies to all conventional treatments of back pain.[18] The bottom line therefore is that the above options, particularly exercise, are worthy of consideration. The most important advice to back pain sufferers is to keep up normal activity as much as possible and to realise that having back problems is not a disease but entirely normal.

Table 2.12
Summary of clinical evidence for back pain

Treatment	Weight of evidence	Direction of evidence	Serious safety concerns
Acupuncture	OOO	↗	Yes (see p 294)
Alexander technique	O	↗	No (see p 299)
Exercise	OOO	↗	Yes (see p 5)
Herbal medicine			
Devil's claw	OOO	↗	Yes (see p 389)
Massage	OO	↗	No (see p 334)
Spinal manipulation			
(chronic pain)	OOO	↗	Yes (see pp 316, 343)
(acute pain)	OOO	↗	Yes (see pp 316, 343)
Water injections	O	↗	Yes (see p 5)

REFERENCES

1 Eisenberg D M, David R B, Ettner S L, Appel S, Wilkey S, Van Rompay M, Kessler R C. Trends in alternative medicine use in the United States, 1990–1997. JAMA 1998;280:1569–1575

2 Manheimer E, White A, Berman B, Forys K, Ernst E. Meta-analysis: acupuncture for low back pain. Ann Intern Med 2005;142:651–663

3 Furlan A D, van Tulder M, Cherkin D, Tsukayama H, Lao L, Koes B, Berman B. Acupuncture and dry-needling for low back pain: an updated systematic review within the framework of the Cochrane collaboration. Spine 2005;30:944–963

4 Ernst E, Canter P H. The Alexander technique: a systematic review of controlled clinical trials. Forsch Komplementarmed Klass Naturheilkd 2003;10:325–329

5 Brox J I, Hagen K B, Juel N G, Storheim K. Is exercise therapy and manipulation effective in low back pain? [Article in Norwegian] Tidsskr Nor Laegeforen 1999;119:2042–2050

6 Hayden J A, van Tulder M W, Tomlinson G. Systematic review: strategies for using exercise therapy to improve outcomes in chronic low back pain. Ann Intern Med 2005;142:776–785

7 Hayden J A, van Tulder M W, Malmivaara A V, Koes B W. Meta-analysis: exercise

therapy for non-specific low back pain. Ann Intern Med 2005;142:765–775

8 Ernst E, Chrubasik S. Phyto-antiinflammatories. A systematic review of randomized, placebo-controlled, double-blind trials. Rheum Dis Clin North Am 2000;26:13–27

9 Gagnier J J, Chrubasik S, Manheimer E. Harpagophytum procumbens for osteoarthritis and low back pain: a systematic review. BMC Complement Altern Med 2004;4:13

10 Furlan A D, Brosseau L, Imamura M, Irvin E. Massage for low-back pain: a systematic review within the framework of the Cochrane Collaboration Back Review Group. Spine 2002;27:1896–1910

11 Assendelft W J J, Morton S C, Yu Emily I, Suttorp M J, Shekelle P G. Spinal manipulative therapy for low back pain. The Cochrane Database of Systematic Reviews 2004, Issue 1. Art No: CD000447

11a Licciardone J C, Brimhall A K, King L N. Osteopathic manipulative treatment for low back pain: a systematic review and meta analysis of randomized controlled trials. BMC Musculoskelet Disord 2005;6:43

12 Labrecque M, Nouwen A, Bergeron M, Rancourt J. A randomized controlled trial of

non-pharmacologic approaches for relief of low back pain during labor. J Fam Pract 1999;48:259–263

13 Trolle B, Moller M, Kronborg H, Thomsen S. The effect of sterile water blocks on low back labor pain. Am J Obstet Gynecol 1991;164:1277–1281

14 Berman B M, Sing B B. Chronic low back pain: an outcome analysis of a mind–body intervention. Complement Ther Med 1997;5:29–35

15 McCauley J D, Thelen M H, Frank R G, Willard R R, Callen K E. Hypnosis compared to relaxation in the outpatient management of chronic low back pain. Arch Phys Med Rehab 1983;64:548–552

16 Nespor K. Psychosomatics of back pain and the use of yoga. Int J Psychosom 1989;36:72–78

17 Williams K A, Petronis J, Smith D, Goodrich D, Wu J, Ravi N, Doyle Jr E J, Gregory Juckett R, Munoz Kolar M, Gross R, Steinberg L. Effect of Iyengar yoga therapy for chronic low back pain. Pain 2005;115:107–117

18 Van Tulder M W, Koes B W, Bouter L M. Conservative treatment of acute and chronic non-specific low back pain: a systematic review of the most common interventions. Spine 1997;22.2128–2156

BENIGN PROSTATIC HYPERPLASIA

Synonyms   Benign prostatic hypertrophy, nodular hyperplasia of the prostate.

Definition   Glandular and stromal hyperplasia occurring very commonly in the middle and lateral lobes of the prostate gland of older men, forming nodules that may increasingly obstruct the urethra. Clinically, it is characterised by lower urinary tract symptoms (urinary frequency, urgency, a weak and intermittent stream, needing to strain, a sense of incomplete emptying, and nocturia) and can lead to complications, including acute urinary retention.

CAM usage   Herbal medicine is the option most commonly used to treat this condition.

Clinical evidence

Herbal medicine

The evidence for African plum (*Pygeum africanum*) extract has been assessed in a meta-analysis (Box 2.17).[1] Some concerns relate to the short duration of studies and the heterogeneity in

Box 2.17
Meta-analysis
***Pygeum africanum*
for benign prosta-
tic hyperplasia**
Wilt[1]

- Eighteen RCTs including 1562 patients; 17 double-blind RCTs

- Improvement in the combined outcome of urologic symptoms and flow measures (effect size −0.8 SD, CI −1.4 to −0.3)

- Improvement in overall symptoms (risk ratio 2.1, CI 1.40 to 3.1)

- Adverse events were mild and similar to placebo

- Conclusion: The overall standardised effect size and the summary improvement in global symptoms, nocturia, peak urine flow and residual urine volume suggests that *Pygeum africanum* is effective in men with symptomatic benign prostatic hyperplasia. This benefit is of modest size and appears to be clinically significant

CONDITIONS

the study design, the use of phytotherapeutic preparations and the types of reported outcomes. However, the available data from this meta-analysis suggests that African plum modestly improves urologic symptoms and flow measures.

Several RCTs have assessed the effectiveness of **nettle** (*Urtica dioica*) root extract (Table 2.13).[2-6] These largely report beneficial effects of nettle root extract compared with placebo. The results of the largest trial on the subject corroborate these findings suggesting beneficial effects. Additional positive evidence relates to combination preparations with saw palmetto (*Serenoa repens*) extract[7] or African plum (*Pygeum africanum*) extract.[8]

A systematic review[9] identified one RCT that evaluated the efficacy of **pumpkin** (*Cucurbita pepo*) seed extract. This RCT was conducted double-blind and assessed a combination preparation of 80 mg pumpkin seed extract and 80 mg saw palmetto extract per tablet. It reports an improvement of urinary flow, frequency and time spent urinating after 3 months of treatment with two tablets three times daily, compared with placebo. Beneficial effects are also suggested by an uncontrolled study.[10] These encouraging findings require confirmation in independent trials.

The evidence for **rye grass pollen** (*Secale cereale*) extract has been assessed in a meta-analysis (Box 2.18).[11] Concerns relate to the short duration of the trials, limited number of patients, omissions in reported outcomes and the unknown quality of the preparations used. The comparative trials had no confirmed active control. Further independent confirmation in large RCTs is required.

Table 2.13 **Double-blind RCTs of nettle root extract for benign prostatic hyperplasia**

Reference	Sample size	Interventions [dosage]	Result	Comment
Vontabel[2]	50	A) Nettle [600 mg/d for 9 w] B) Placebo	A superior to B in micturition volume	No difference in subjective complaints
Dathe[3]	79	A) Nettle [600 mg/d for 4–6 w] B) Placebo	A improvement of mean and maximal urinary flow B No improvement	Intergroup differences not reported
Fischer[4]	40	A) Nettle [1.2 g/d for 6 mo] B) Placebo	A superior to B in symptom score	Long treament period
Engelmann[5]	41	A) Nettle [6 ml/d for 3 mo] B) Placebo	A superior to B in International Prostate Symptom Score (IPSS)	No difference in micturition volume and maximal urinary flow
Schneider[6]	246	A) Nettle [459 mg/d for 1 y] B) Placebo	A superior to B in IPSS	Large trial over long treatment period

Box 2.18
Meta-analysis
Rye grass pollen for benign prostatic hyperplasia
Wilt[11]

- Four RCTs of Cernilton; two placebo-controlled, two comparative (Tadenan) including a total of 444 patients; three double-blind

- Self-rated improvement of urinary symptoms versus placebo (risk ratio 2.40, CI 1.21 to 4.75), versus tadenan (risk ratio 1.42, CI 1.21 to 4.75)

- Reduction in nocturia versus placebo (risk ratio 2.05, CI 1.41 to 3.0)

- Adverse events were rare and mild

- Conclusion: The trials were limited by short duration, limited number of enrollees, gaps in reported outcomes, and unknown quality of the preparations utilised. The available evidence suggests Cernilton is well tolerated and modestly improves overall urologic symptoms including nocturia

The evidence for saw palmetto (*Serenoa repens*) extract has been assessed in a meta-analysis (Box 2.19),[12] Despite the low quality of some RCTs, the relatively large body of data provides convincing evidence that saw palmetto improves urinary tract symptoms and peak urine flow. These results are largely corroborated by another meta-analysis[13] of a single standardised extract and by double-blind RCTs[14–18] published since these meta-analyses (Table 2.14).

Box 2.19
Meta-analysis
Saw palmetto for benign prostatic hyperplasia
Wilt[12]

- Twenty-one RCTs including 3139 patients; 18 double-blind RCTs

- Improvement in self-rating of urinary tract symptoms compared with placebo (risk ratio 1.76, CI 1.21 to 2.54)

- Improvement in peak urine flow compared with placebo (weighted mean difference 1.86 ml/s, CI 0.60 to 3.12)

- Reduction in nocturia compared with placebo (weighted mean difference −0.76 per evening, CI −1.22 to −0.32)

- Similar improvements in urinary tract symptom scores and peak urine flow compared with finasteride

- Adverse effects were mild and infrequent

- Conclusion: Saw palmetto provides mild to moderate improvement in urinary symptoms and flow measures. It produced similar improvement in urinary symptoms and flow compared with finasteride and is associated with fewer adverse events

Table 2.14 **Double-blind RCTs of saw palmetto for benign prostatic hyperplasia**

Reference	Sample size	Interventions [dosage]	Result	Comment
Debruyne[14]	124	A) Saw palmetto [320 mg/d for 1y] B) Tamsulosin [0.4 mg/d for 1 y]	No difference in IPSS	Patients with severe BPH (IPSS > 19)
Willets[15]	100	A) Saw palmetto [320 mg/d for 12 w] B) Placebo	No difference in IPSS	Short treatment period
Debruyne[16]	542	A) Saw palmetto [320 mg/d for 1 y] B) Tamsulosin [0.4 mg/d for 1 y]	Equivalence in IPSS	Prostate specific antigen remained stable
Glemain[17]	329	A) Tamsulosin + saw palmetto [0.4 + 320 mg/d for 1 y] B) Tamsulosin + placebo [0.4 mg/d for 1 y]	No difference in IPSS	No difference in max. urine flow
Giannakopoulos[18]	100	A) Saw palmetto [320 mg/d for 1y] B) Saw palmetto [480 mg/d for 1 y]	Reductions from baseline for IPSS, no difference between groups	No adverse events occurred

Overall recommendation

The evidence for the short- and medium-term effectiveness of saw palmetto extract is convincing. Saw palmetto seems to improve urinary tract symptom scores and peak urine flow to a similar degree as conventional oral medication with finasteride or tamsulosin. Given the nature and frequency of adverse events, saw palmetto extract can be recommended as an oral treatment for benign prostatic hyperplasia. However, compelling long-term data are not yet available. Short-term data for African plum extract indicate that it is effective for improving overall and urologic symptoms. Similarly for rye grass pollen, there is some evidence available to suggest that it improves urinary symptoms and nocturia. For nettle extract the evidence is encouraging but not compelling.

Table 2.15 **Summary of clinical evidence for benign prostatic hyperplasia**

Treatment	Weight of evidence	Direction of evidence	Serious safety concerns
Herbal medicine			
African plum	OOO	⇧	Yes (see p 476)
Nettle	OO	⇧	Yes (see p 444)
Pumpkin seed	O	⬈	Yes (see pp 5, 480)
Rye grass pollen	OO	⬈	Yes (see pp 5, 480)
Saw palmetto	OOO	⇧	Yes (see p 458)

REFERENCES

1 Wilt T, Ishani A, MacDonald R, Rutks I, Stark G. Pygeum africanum for benign prostatic hyperplasia. The Cochrane Database of Systematic Reviews 1998, Issue 1. Art. No.: CD001044

2 Vontobel HP, Herzog R, Rutishauser G, Kres H. Results of a double-blind study on the effectiveness of ERU (extractum radicis Urticae) capsules in conservative treatment of benign prostatic hyperplasia. Urologe A 1985;24:49–51

3 Dathe G, Schmid H. Phytotherapie der benignen Prostatahyperplasie. Urologe B 1987;27: 223–226

4 Fischer M, Wilpert. Wirkprüfung eines Phytopharmakons zur Behandlung der benignen Prostatahyperplasie. In: Rutishauser G (ed). Benigne Prostata-hyperplasie III. Zuckerschwerdt, München 1992, p 79–84

5 Engelmann U, Boos G, Kres H. Therapie der benignen Prostatahyperplasie mit Bazoton Liquidum. Urologe B 1996;36:287–291

6 Schneider T, Rubben H. Stinging nettle root extract (Bazoton-uno) in long term treatment of benign prostatic syndrome (BPS). Results of a randomized, double-blind, placebo controlled multicenter study after 12 months. Urologe A 2004;43:302–306

7 Bondarenko B, Walther C, Funk P, Schläfke S, Engelmann U. Long-term efficacy and safety of PRO 160/120 (a combination of sabal and urtica extract) in patients with lower urinary tract symptoms (LUTS). Phytomedicine 2003;10;Suppl 4:53–55

8 Krzeski T, Kazon M, Borkowski A, Witeska A, Kuczera J. Combined extract of Urtica dioica and Pygeum africanum in the treatment of benign prostatic hyperplasia: double-blind comparison of two doses. Clin Therapeut 1993;15:1011–1020

9 Wilt TJ, Ishani A, Rutks I, MacDonald R. Phytotherapy for benign prostatic hyperplasia. Public Health Nutr 2000;3:459–472

10 Schiebel-Schlosser G, Friedrich M. Phytotherapy of BPH with pumpkin seeds – a multicentric clinical trial. Zeitschr für Phytotherapie 1998;19:71–76

11 Wilt T, MacDonald R, Ishani A, Rutks I, Stark G. Cernilton for benign prostatic hyperplasia. The Cochrane Database of Systematic Reviews 2000, Issue 2. Art. No.: CD001042

12 Wilt T, Ishani A, MacDonald R. Serenoa repens for benign prostatic hyperplasia. The Cochrane Database of Systematic Reviews 2002, Issue 3. Art. No.: CD001423

13 Boyle P, Robertson C, Lowe F, Roehrborn C. Meta-analysis of clinical trials of permixon in the treatment of symptomatic benign prostatic hyperplasia. Urology 2000;55:533–539

14 Debruyne F, Boyle P, Calais Da Silva F, Gillenwater JG, Hamdy FC, Perrin P, Teillac P, Vela-Navarrete R, Raynaud JP, Schulman CC. Evaluation of the clinical benefit of permixon and tamsulosin in severe BPH patients-PERMAL study subset analysis. Eur Urol 2004;45:773–779; discussion 779–780

15 Willetts KE, Clements MS, Champion S, Ehsman S, Eden JA. Serenoa repens extract for benign prostate hyperplasia: a randomized controlled trial. BJU Int 2003;92:267–270

16 Debruyne F, Koch G, Boyle P, Da Silva FC, Gillenwater JG, Hamdy FC, Perrin P, Teillac P, Vela-Navarrete R, Raynaud JP. Comparison of a phytotherapeutic agent (Permixon) with an alpha-blocker (Tamsulosin) in the treatment of benign prostatic hyperplasia: a 1-year randomized international study. Eur Urol 2002;41:497–506; discussion 506–507

17 Glemain P, Coulange C, Billebaud T, Gattegno B, Muszynski R, Loeb G. Groupe de l'essai OCOS. Tamsulosin with or without Serenoa repens in benign prostatic hyperplasia: the OCOS trial. Prog Urol 2002;12:395–403; discussion 404

18 Giannakopoulos X, Baltogiannis D, Giannakis D, Tasos A, Sofikitis N, Charalabopoulos K, Evangelou A. The lipidosterolic extract of Serenoa repens in the treatment of benign prostatic hyperplasia: a comparison of two dosage regimens. Adv Ther 2002;19:285–296

CONDITIONS

CANCER

Synonyms/ subcategories	Malignant tumours or neoplasms.
Definition	General term used to describe any type of malignant neoplasm, most of which invade surrounding tissues, may metastasise and can recur after treatment.
Related conditions	Precancerous conditions.
CAM usage	Cancer patients are understandably desperate to try any treatment that offers hope; therefore, many cancer patients use CAM. A systematic review of 26 surveys from 13 countries found an average prevalence of CAM use of 31%.[1]
	Each decade seems to have had its own cancer 'cure' that achieved some prominence, only to fade away as new therapies emerged. The following treatments are popular at present: co-enzyme Q10, diets, herbal remedies, homeopathy, hypnotherapy, meditation, relaxation, reflexology, shark cartilage, spiritual healing/therapeutic touch, visualisation.[1] Some of these therapies are promoted as 'cures', some are used for palliative care and some are promoted for cancer prevention.
Clinical evidence	Even though there can be considerable overlap, the clinical evidence is divided into three parts: cancer prevention, cancer 'cures' and palliative/supportive care.
Cancer prevention	*Diet*
	Many measures to prevent cancer relate to the dietary intake of plant-derived compounds. Some of those often promoted by proponents of CAM are discussed below.

Several lines of evidence suggest that the regular consumption of **Allium** vegetables, such as onion or garlic, is tumour protective. A systematic review[2] summarised 20 epidemiological studies in this area. With one exception, they all suggest that *Allium* vegetables convey some protection against cancers, particularly those of the gastrointestinal tract. A meta-analysis of 18 epidemiological studies found a relative risk estimate of colorectal cancer for dietary garlic consumption of 0.69 (95% CI 0.55 to 0.89). For stomach cancer it was 0.53 (95% CI 0.31 to 0.92).[3]

A meta-analysis of five RCTs with a total of 4349 individuals found no evidence to suggest that increasing **dietary fibre** intake will reduce the incidence or recurrence of adenomatous polyps and carcinomas within a 2–4 year period.[4]

The polyphenols in **green tea** (*Camellia sinensis*) exhibit protective effects against cancer. Epidemiological studies suggest that the regular consumption of green tea conveys a moderate reduction of cancer risk, particularly cancers of the upper digestive tract. A systematic review of the data cautiously concluded that: 'There is some evidence that green tea may prevent the occurrence of some cancers'.[5] More recently, encouraging epidemiological evidence has been summarised specifically for gastrointestinal cancers.[6]

Indirect (e.g. epidemiological) evidence suggests that the regular consumption of **phytoestrogens** lowers the risk of some forms of malignancy, for instance, prostate cancer.[7]

A systematic review included 27 mostly epidemiological studies suggesting that regular consumption of **tomato** or tomato products which are rich in lycopene, reduces the risk of various malignancies, particularly prostate cancer.[8] Oral leukoplakia, a pre-cancerous lesion can be reduced through oral administration of a lycopene supplement.[9]

Vegetarianism is often claimed to protect against cancer. In a prospective study from the UK, 6000 non meat eaters and 5000 meat eaters were followed for 12 years.[10] All-cause and cancer mortality in the former population were approximately half of that of the control group. However, a meta-analysis of this and four similar studies including a total sample of 76 172 men and women found no difference in mortality between vegetarians and non-vegetarians from stomach, colorectal, lung or breast cancer.[11] However, high intake of plant foods has been shown to have a preventive influence in individuals at high risk for lung cancer.[12]

Exercise
A large body of evidence suggests that regular **exercise** reduces the risk of colon and breast cancer.[13]

Herbal medicine
Basic research implies that ginseng (*Panax ginseng*) is tumour protective through its effects on the immune system. An epidemiological study carried out in a ginseng-growing region in Korea[14] included 4634 individuals who were assessed by questionnaire on ginseng intake. During the 5 years of follow-up, those individuals who regularly consumed fresh ginseng had a dramatically reduced cancer risk.

Supplements
Antioxidants such as beta-carotene, vitamins A, C and E and selenium are often promoted for cancer prevention. A meta-analysis of 14 RCTs including 170 525 individuals suggested that such supplements increased mortality of gastrointestinal cancers.[15] Specifically, beta-carotene plus vitamin A or E increased mortality. An in-depth review concluded that it is uncertain whether vitamin C supplementation beyond normal dietary intake has any preventative effects.[16] A large RCT (n = 738) showed that long-term vitamin E supplementation does not

prevent cancer.[17] For selenium, the data seem to vary according to cancer type: a protective effect may exist for prostate cancer,[18] no effect for basal cell carcinoma and an increased risk of both squamous cell carcinoma and non-melanoma skin cancer;[19] a protective effect may exist for all cancers in males.[20]

A systematic review of two RCTs including a total of 1346 subjects found that **calcium** supplementation (1200–2000 mg/ day) for 3–4 years conveys a modest risk reduction of colorectal cancer.[21]

One case-control study (n = 797) supports evidence from in vitro studies to suggest that regular intake of **fish oil** reduces the risk of prostate cancer.[22]

Table 2.16
Summary of clinical evidence of cancer prevention

Treatment	Weight of evidence	Direction of evidence	Serious safety concerns
Diet			
Allium vegetables	OOO	⇧	No (see p 5)
Green tea	OOO	⇧	No (see p 417)
Phytoestrogens	OO	⬈	Yes (see p 450)
Dietary fibre	O	⬈	No (see p 5)
Tomato (lycopene)	OOO	⇧	No (see p 5)
Vegetarianism	OO	⇨	Yes for vegan diet (see p 5)
Exercise	OOO	⇧	Yes (see p 5)
Herbal medicine			
Ginseng, Panax	O	⇧	Yes (see p 407)
Supplements			
Antioxidants	OOO	⇨	No (see p 5)
Calcium	O	⬈	No (see p 5)
Fish oil	O	⇧	No (see p 483)

Cancer 'cures'

Claims to cure cancer, lower the tumour burden or prolong the life of cancer patients are rife within CAM.

Di Bella therapy

The 'Di Bella therapy' consists of melatonin, bromocriptine, either somatostatin or octreotide, and retinoid solution (as well as cyclophosphamide and hydroxyurea in some cases). Eleven independent, multicentre, uncontrolled phase II studies including 386 patients with advanced cancer were initiated in Italy.[23] None of the patients showed complete remission and only three patients had a partial remission. A retrospective comparison of 314 patients versus matched patients from Italian cancer registers showed a shorter average survival time for Di Bella's patients.[24]

Diet

Proponents of 'alternative' diets claim that their approach can prolong the life of cancer patients. A review of the evidence found no convincing data in support of this hypothesis.[25] In particular, retrospective data suggesting a six-fold increase in 5-year survival rates of melanoma patients treated with the **Gerson diet**[26] are unconvincing due to seriously flawed methodology.

Similar claims for a **macrobiotic diet** are also not supported by evidence from rigorous clinical trials. One third of cancer patients on a macrobiotic diet have been shown to experience problems due to weight loss, the restrictive and unpalatable nature of the regimen and the expense and inaccessibility of some ingredients used in this diet.[27]

Herbal medicine

Numerous herbal medicines have been tried for cancer and a comprehensive systematic review[28] is available.

Fifty patients with advanced solid malignant tumours for whom no effective standard anticancer therapy existed were treated in a CCT, either with melatonin (20 mg/day) or with melatonin and *Aloe vera* tincture (1 ml twice daily).[29] No response was seen in the former group while two partial responses were observed in the group treated with *Aloe vera*.

Essiac is a herbal mixture which is popular in North America and consists of *Arctium lappa, Rheum palmatum, Rumex acetosella* and *Ulmus fulva*. Two systematic reviews did not find a single published clinical trial.[28,30] Several unpublished investigations were identified and there was some indirect evidence for anticancer activity of several of the constituent herbs. Essiac has also been associated with considerable risks.[28]

Three independent systematic reviews of RCTs of **mistletoe** (*Viscum album*)[31–33] are available. They fail to demonstrate that mistletoe extracts are beneficial either for improving quality of life or prolonging survival time (Box 2.20).

CONDITIONS

Box 2.20
Systematic review
Mistletoe for cancer
Ernst[33]

- Ten trials involving 2470 participants were included

- Most of the studies had considerable weaknesses in terms of study design, reporting or both

- Some of the weaker studies implied benefits of mistletoe extracts, particularly in terms of quality of life. None of the methodologically stronger trials exhibited efficacy in terms of quality of life, survival or other outcome measures

- Conclusion: rigorous trials of mistletoe extracts fail to demonstrate efficacy of this therapy

The herbal formula **PC–SPES** contains *Chrysanthemum morifolium, Ganoderma lucidium, Glycyrrhiza glabra, Isatis indigotica, Panax pseudoginseng, Robdosia rubesceus, Scutellaria baicalensis* and *Serenoa repens*. The mixture was shown to lower prostate-specific antigen in patients with prostate cancer and to inhibit the growth of prostate cancer cells in vitro.[34] The preparation has been withdrawn because of adulteration with prescription drugs.

A systematic review[28] located one CCT (n = 48) of **Reishi** (*Ganoderma lucidum*) for various advanced cancers. Three grams of extract were given for 30 days. Compared with placebo patients, those treated with Reishi experienced an improvement in immune function and symptoms.

A plethora of clinical trials of **Chinese** and other **Asian herbal mixtures** are available (Table 2.17).[35–44] All of them report posi-

Table 2.17   **Controlled clinical trials of Asian herbal mixtures as cancer treatments**

Reference	Sample size	Treatment	Indication	Result
Li[35]	48	Chang'ai Kangfu	Large intestinal cancer	Improved immune function and clinical recovery
Xu[36]	188	Destagnation	Nasopharyngal cancer	Improved survival rate compared with radiotherapy
Guo[37]	38	Fuzheng Yiai	Intestinal cancer	Prolonged survival compared with chemotherapy
Liu[38]	100	Individualised herbal mixtures	Lung cancer	Prolonged survival compared with chemotherapy
Liu[39]	76	Individualised herbal mixtures	Lung cancer	Prolonged survival compared with chemotherapy
Lan[40]	47	Individualised herbal mixtures	Lung cancer	Prolonged survival compared with radiotherapy
Wang[41]	58	Individualised herbal mixtures	Pancreatic cancer	Prolonged survival compared with radio-therapy
Zhou[42]	120	Shenqui Fuzheng	Gastric cancer	Higher remission rate compared with chemotherapy
Oka[43]	260	Sho saiko-to	Liver cancer	Prolonged survival compared with chemotherapy
Wang[44]	62	Yiqu Huoxue	Oesophageal cancer	Prolonged survival compared with chemo- and radiotherapy

tive findings but their methodological rigour is sometimes unclear. A Cochrane review had a focus on Chinese herbal mixtures for oesophageal cancer and confirmed that the data are positive but, due to methodological limitations, weak.[45]

Supplements

The (partly) herbal mixture **714-X** contains camphor, ammonium chloride and nitrate, sodium chloride, ethyl alcohol and water. It is being promoted in North America and Europe, particularly for prostate cancers. A systematic review found several animal studies but no clinical trials that supported its benefit.[46] The conclusion was that 'Side-effects appear to be minimal, but evidence of its effectiveness is limited'.

Beta-glucan extracts from mushrooms (e.g. *Coriolus versiculor* or *schizophyllum commune*) have been studied in several CCTs. Encouraging results emerged for gastrointestinal cancers and negative ones for other malignancies.[47]

A systematic review[48] of all clinical trials of **hydrazine sulfate** included three RCTs from the USA. Many studies were methodologically weak. None of the RCTs suggested positive effects. Therefore it was concluded that 'The value of hydrazine sulfate as an antitumour agent – specifically its capacity to stabilise tumour size, cause tumour regression and improve survival – remains uncertain'.[48]

Laetrile has been tested in clinical trials (e.g.[49]). No clinically relevant benefit was found, either in terms of cure, survival or stabilisation of cancer growth or improvement of symptoms.

Several studies have tested the efficacy of **melatonin** supplementation for slowing tumour progression.[50] One RCT, for instance, suggested that patients with brain metastases treated with melatonin experienced a longer survival time compared with patients who received supportive care only.[51]

Shark cartilage is claimed to have anti-angiogenesis effects that might inhibit malignant growth. Preclinical investigations supported this hypothesis.[52] One RCT (n = 83) found no difference in overall survival or quality of life between patients receiving standard care plus a shark cartilage product versus standard care plus placebo.[53] This confirms the results of a previous uncontrolled pilot study of shark cartilage as the sole anticancer therapy.[54]

Preclinical studies have demonstrated that bovine **thymus extracts** restore lymphocyte function, improve immunological variables, activate natural killer cells, increase cytotoxic activity as well as mitogen-induced interferon levels in human lymphocytes and inhibit tumour growth in animals. A systematic review of all RCTs[55] did not, however, arrive at positive conclusions (Box 2.21). Injectable thymus preparations can cause severe allergic reactions and have the potential of transmitting serious infections.

Ukrain is a semi-synthetic compound derived from *Chelidonium majus* marketed as a cancer therapy. A systematic review (Box 2.22) found no conclusive evidence for its efficacy.[56]

Box 2.21
Systematic review
Thymus extracts for cancer
Ernst[55]

- Thirteen RCTs were included with a total of 802 patients suffering from various cancers
- Methodological quality was, on average, poor
- Five studies suggested benefits of thymus therapy
- Conclusion: 'no compelling evidence exists for the clinical efficacy of thymus therapy in human cancers'

Box 2.22
Systematic review
Ukrain for cancer
Ernst[56]

- Seven CCTs were found including a diverse range of cancers
- Methodological quality was poor
- All trials were positive
- Conclusion: no compelling evidence

Support group therapy

While there is little doubt that support groups can help cancer patients in numerous ways, it is uncertain whether this approach also prolongs their life. A meta-analysis of support group therapies of cancer patients found no convincing evidence for such an effect (Box 2.23).[57]

Box 2.23
Systematic review
Group therapies for prolonging survival of cancer patients
Smedslund[57]

- 14 CCTs included 2626 patients
- Methodological quality was variable
- The eight RCTs showed no overall treatment effect
- There was some indication that individual treatments might be superior
- Conclusion: data are not compelling

Other therapies

The Bristol Cancer Help Centre Study is a tragic example of the profound confusion that may result from seriously flawed research.[58] The trial apparently demonstrated that the survival rate of those breast cancer patients treated by an adjunctive **package of CAM modalities** was poorer than for controls. Yet the study was not randomised and thus baseline differences are a probable cause for the finding.

A matched-pair comparison was conducted of survival of cancer patients receiving standard care with those receiving a package of CAM (autogenous immune-enhancing vaccine, bacille Calmette-Guérin, vegetarian diets and coffee enemas) in addition.[59] There were no differences in survival times but patients in the experimental group reported poorer quality of life.

Table 2.18
Summary of clinical evidence of cancer 'cures'

Treatment	Weight of evidence	Direction of evidence	Serious safety concerns
Di Bella therapy	OO	⇩	Yes (see p 5)
Diets			
Gerson	O	⬀	Yes (see p 5)
Macrobiotic	O	⬂	Yes (see p 5)
Herbal medicine			
Aloe vera	O	⬀	Yes (see p 364)
Essiac	O	⇨	Yes (see p 5)
Mistletoe	OOO	⇨	Yes (see p 441)
PC-SPES	O	⬀	Yes (see p 5)
Reishi	O	⬀	Yes (see p 480)
Asian mixtures	OOO	⇨	Yes (see p 5)
Supplements			
'714-X'	O	⬂	Yes (see p 5)
Beta glucan	OO	⇨	Yes (see p 482)
Hydrazine sulfate	O	⇨	Yes (see p 483)
Laetrile	OO	⇩	Yes (see p 483)
Melatonin	O	⬀	Yes (see p 435)
Shark cartilage	O	⇩	Yes (see p 461)
Thymus extracts	OO	⇩	Yes (see p 484)
Ukrain	OO	⬀	Yes (see p 5)
Support group therapy	OOO	⇩	No (see p 5)

Palliative/ supportive care

Many CAM modalities have the potential to increase well-being, e.g. by alleviating the symptoms of the disease or reducing the adverse effects of conventional treatments. Thus they are often used in addition to conventional treatments in palliative and supportive care for cancer patients.

Acupuncture

Systematic reviews suggest that acupuncture[60] and acupressure[61] reduce chemotherapy-induced nausea. This conclusion is also supported by recent RCTs.[62,63] However, an RCT (n = 80) with adequate control for placebo-effects found no difference between real and sham acupuncture.[64] A systematic review of six clinical trials testing the effectiveness of acupuncture to control cancer pain found no compelling evidence for this indication (Box 2.24).[65]

Encouraging data suggest that acupuncture alleviates radiation-induced xerostomia.[66] Lastly, acupuncture may reduce vasomotor symptoms in men receiving hormone therapy for prostate cancer.[67]

Box 2.24
Systematic review
Acupuncture for cancer pain
Lee[65]

- Two RCTs and four uncontrolled clinical trials
- Methodological quality was, on average, poor
- Best studies fail to show positive effects
- Conclusion: effectiveness not proven

Aromatherapy and massage

A Cochrane review[68] found that aromatherapy and/or massage have positive short-term effects on the well-being of cancer patients. The question of whether essential oils are important for this effect remains unanswered (Box 2.25).

Box 2.25
Systematic review
Aromatherapy/ massage for cancer
Fellowes[68]

- Eight RCTs including 357 patients
- Methodological quality was variable
- Most consistent effect was short-term anxiolytic effect
- Conclusion: short-term benefits on psychological well-being

Exercise

A substantial body of evidence suggests that regular physical **exercise** will reduce the severity of treatment-related symptoms such as fatigue and nausea.[69]

Herbal medicine

Aloe vera gel was tested against placebo in an RCT (n = 58) for control of radiation-induced mucositis.[70] The results failed to demonstrate any beneficial effects. In a similar RCT of *Aloe vera*, no decrease in skin reaction was noted at low dose radiotherapy.[71] But with high dose radiotherapy (> 2700 cGy) skin reactions occurred on average 2 weeks later compared with placebo.

Black cohosh (*Actaea racemosa*), administered for 60 days, was not superior to placebo in controlling hot flushes after conventional therapy for breast cancer in an RCT (n = 85).[72] In another RCT for tamoxifen-induced hot flushes, black cohosh was administered for 1 year.[73] The results show a reduction in the number and severity of hot flushes.

Cranberry (*Vaccinium macrocarpon*) juice was submitted to an RCT including 112 men with prostate cancer to determine whether it affects the urinary symptoms after radiation therapy.[74] No beneficial effects compared with placebo were noted.

Calendula officinalis cream was compared with trolamine cream in an RCT (n = 254) testing their usefulness in preventing radiation-induced dermatitis in breast cancer patients.[75] The occurrence of grade 2 dermatitis was 41% with calendula and 63% with trolamine.

Ginseng (*Panax ginseng*) is, according to a small (n = 20) but controlled pilot study, effective in treating fatigue of cancer patients receiving chemotherapy.[76]

Ginkgo *(Ginkgo biloba)* reduced limb heaviness in an RCT including 48 patients with upper extremity lymphoedema after breast cancer treatment.[77]

A multitude of **Chinese and other herbal mixtures** has been submitted to CCTs (Table 2.19).[78–82] The results are invariably positive but the reliability of the data and their methodological rigour are sometimes doubtful. A Cochrane review of Chinese herbal mixtures for adverse effects after chemotherapy for colorectal cancer with four CCTs confirmed these methodological uncertainties associated with these studies but concluded that decoctions of Huang qi compounds may be effective.[83]

Table 2.19 **Controlled clinical trials of Asian herbal mixtures for supportive cancer care**

Reference	Sample size	Treatment	Indication	Result
Zou[78]	60	Astragalus	Lung cancer	Improvement of quality of life
Pan[79]	60	Fuzheng Yiliu	Gastrointestinal cancer	Reduction of adverse effects
Mori[80]	44	Hangeshashin-to	Lung cancer	Prevention of diarrhoea
Cai[81]	92	Individualised herbal mixtures	Lung cancer	Reduction of adverse effects of radiotherapy
Liu[82]	80	Shenmai	Breast cancer	Reduction of postoperative complications

Homeopathy

An RCT (n = 66) of Belladonna 7cH and X-ray 15cH tested whether this homeopathic mixture would prevent radiation-induced dermatitis.[84] There were no differences compared with placebo.

Hypnotherapy

Several RCTs have suggested the usefulness of hypnotherapy in palliative cancer care. It was effective in controlling pain and nausea/vomiting.[85,86] In children, hypnotherapy was more effective than attention control in reducing nausea.[87,88] However, there is insufficient evidence for hypnotherapy to control procedural pain in children with cancer [89] and one RCT suggested its ineffectiveness in reducing anxiety in cancer patients receiving radiotherapy.[90]

Music therapy

RCTs show that music therapy, compared with usual care, improves quality of life[91] or reduces mood disturbance in cancer patients.[92] Another RCT (n = 60) suggested that procedural pain and anxiety are not influenced by music therapy when compared with simple distraction.[93] Compared with no additional treatments, music therapy plus guided imagery improved mood and quality of life of cancer patients in a small (n = 8) RCT.[94]

Reflexology

A small, sham-controlled RCT (n = 12) generated no convincing evidence that reflexology improves quality of life of cancer patients.[95] A less rigorously controlled CCT with 23 breast and lung cancer patients suggested reflexology reduces anxiety and pain.[96]

Relaxation

The effectiveness of several relaxation therapies has been tested repeatedly. In one RCT the programme consisted of breathing exercises, muscle relaxation and imagery. This regimen was superior in controlling pain of cancer patients to no intervention.[97] A similar RCT with 35 cancer patients after stem cell transplantation found that a 6-week relaxation programme reduced fatigue in these patients.[98]

In another RCT, 96 women with advanced breast cancer were randomised to receive either regular relaxation training and imagery or standard care only. The experimental group experienced better quality of life than the control group.[99] Other relaxation therapies supported by similar data from RCTs or CCTs include a comprehensive coping strategy programme with guided imagery,[100] mindfulness meditation,[101–103] stress management training,[104] autogenic training,[105] and progressive muscle relaxation training.[106–109]

Spiritual healing

Several CCTs have tested the effectiveness of **therapeutic touch** to reduce anxiety[110] or increase well-being[111] in cancer patients. Due to weaknesses in study design, it is unclear whether the observed positive effects were due to a specific therapeutic or a non-specific (placebo) effect.

Supplements

A systematic review of cannabinoids in supportive cancer care found 20 RCTs. The authors concluded that **cannabinoids** are not superior to codeine in controlling cancer pain. As they cause central nervous depression their introduction into routine care is 'undesirable'.[112]

A systematic review found encouraging albeit not convincing evidence that **Co-enzyme Q10** reduces the toxicity of cancer therapies (Box 2.26).[113]

Box 2.26
Systematic review
**Co-enzyme Q10
for improving
tolerability of
cancer treatments**
Roffe[113]

- Six CCTs (three RCTs) were included

- Methodological quality was poor

- In five studies patients received anthracyclines

- Conclusion: evidence is not compelling

Oral mixtures of proteolytic **enzymes** (Wobe Mucos) are marketed in Germany with the controversial claim of benefiting the well-being of cancer patients. A systematic review included seven prospective clinical studies, including 692 patients in total.[114] The authors concluded: 'Enzyme therapy has generally been found to be a well-tolerated form of treatment for the relief of side-effects caused by other tumour therapies and for improving quality of life'. Due to methodological limitations of the primary data, this hypothesis still requires testing in rigorous RCTs.

Factor AF2 is an extract from liver and spleen of newborn lambs promoted for reducing adverse effects of chemotherapy. Four RCTs are available and there is some albeit not conclusive suggestion that this remedy might reduce myelotoxicity.[115]

Fish oil supplements are rich in omega-3 polyunsaturated fatty acids. One RCT (n = 60) failed to show that fish oil supplements influence appetite, tiredness, nausea, well-being, calorie intake, nutritional status or function of cachectic cancer patients.[116] Another RCT with 44 postoperative cancer patients suggested improvement of liver function and decrease of weight loss after fish oil supplements.[117] A small RCT (n = 24) of fish oil plus melatonin failed to show that this treatment has anticachetic effects.[118]

Phytoestrogens are, according to an RCT (n = 62), not effective in alleviating the hot flushes experienced by breast cancer patients.[119] Two RCTs (n = 113 and 177) yield the same results for **soy products**.[120,121]

**Overall
recommendation**

CAM has a role in palliative/supportive cancer care. This area clearly deserves more research; in particular, we need to know which treatments are in any way superior to conventional methods of palliative/supportive cancer care. Until more data are available some CAM therapies, e.g. acupressure, acupuncture, aromatherapy, calendula, hypnotherapy, massage, music therapy, relaxation therapies, can be cautiously recommended in this setting.

Some dietary regimens aimed at cancer prevention are supported by good epidemiological evidence; they can thus be recommended provided the principle of a balanced diet is not jeopardised. The evidence for antioxidant supplements is unconvincing. CAM should be used in conjunction but not instead of mainstream cancer prevention (e.g. smoking cessation).

Most CAM cancer 'cures' are burdened with important risks and offer little or no prospect of benefit; they should therefore not be recommended. Those CAM cancer 'cures' for which the evidence is encouraging invariably require further study before sound advice can be provided.

Table 2.20
Summary of clinical evidence of palliative care

Treatment	Weight of evidence	Direction of evidence	Serious safety concerns
Acupuncture or acupressure (nausea)	OO	↗	Yes (see p 294)
Acupuncture (pain)	OO	⇒	Yes (see p 294)
Acupuncture (xerostomia)	O	↗	Yes (see p 294)
Aromatherapy/ massage	OOO	⇑	Yes (see p 301)
Exercise	OOO	⇑	Yes (see p 5)
Herbal medicine			
Aloe vera gel	OO	⇒	Yes (see p 364)
Black cohosh	OO	⇒	Yes (see p 373)
Cranberry	O	⇓	Yes (see p 387)
Calendula	O	⇑	Yes (see p 477)
Ginkgo	O	↗	Yes (see p 404)
Ginseng, Panax	O	↗	Yes (see p 407)
Asian mixtures	OOO	⇒	Yes (see p 5)
Homeopathy	O	⇓	No (see p 327)
Hypnotherapy	O	↗	Yes (see p 331)
Music therapy	OO	↗	No (see p 360)
Reflexology	OO	↘	No (see p 345)
Relaxation	OO	⇑	No (see p 348)
Spiritual healing	OO	↗	No (see p 351)
Supplements			
Cannabinoids	OOO	⇒	No (see p 5)
Co-enzyme Q10	OO	↗	No (see p 385)
Enzymes	OOO	↗	No (see p 5)
Factor AF2	OO	↗	Yes (see p 5)
Fish oil	OO	⇒	Yes (see p 483)
Phytoestrogens	O	⇓	Yes (see p 450)
Soy products	OO	⇓	Yes (see p 5)

REFERENCES

1 Ernst E, Cassileth B R. The prevalence of complementary/alternative medicine in cancer. A systematic review. Cancer 1998;83:777–782

2 Ernst E. Can allium vegetables prevent cancer? Phytomedicine 1997;4:79–83

3 Fleischauer A T, Poole C, Arab L. Garlic consumption and cancer prevention: meta-analyses of colorectal and stomach cancers. Am J Clin Nutr 2000;72:1047–1052

4 Asano T, McLeod R S. Dietary fiber for the prevention of colorectal adenomas and carcinomas. The Cochrane Database of Systematic Reviews 2002, Issue 2. Art No.:CD003430

5 Kaegi E. Unconventional therapies for cancer: 2 Green tea. Can Med Assoc J 1998;158:1621–1624

6 Borrelli F, Capasso R, Russo A, Ernst E. Systematic review: green tea and gastrointestinal cancer risk. Aliment Pharmacol Ther 2004;19:497 510

7 Storm S S, Yamamura Y, Duphorne C M. Phytoestrogen intake and prostate cancer: a case control study using a new database Nutr Cancer 1999;33:20–25

8 Boon H, Wong J. Botanical medicine and cancer: a review of the safety and efficacy. Expert Opin Pharmacother 2004;5:2485–2501

9 Singh M, Krishanappa R, Bagewadi A, Keluskar V. Efficacy of oral lycopene in the treatment of oral leukoplakia. Oral Oncology 2004;40:591–596

10 Thorogood M, Mann J, Appleby P, McPherson K. Risk of death from cancer and ischaemic heart disease in meat and non meat-eaters. BMJ 1994;108:1667 1671

11 Key T J, Fraser G E, Thorogood M. Mortality in vegetarians and non-vegetarians: detailed findings from a collaborative analysis of 5 prospective studies. Am J Clin Nutr 1999;70:5165–5245

12 Neuhouser M L, Patterson R E, Thornquist M D, Omenn G S, King I B, Goodman G E. Fruits and vegetables are associated with lower lung cancer risk only in the placebo arm of the beta-carotene and retinol efficacy trial (CARET). Cancer Epidemiol Biomarkers Prev 2003;12:350–358

13 Dimeo F. Welche Rolle spielt körperliche Aktivität in der Prävention, Therapie und Rehabilitation von neoplastischen Erkrankungen? Deutsche Zeitschr Sportmed 2004;55:177–182

14 Yun T-K, Choi S-Y. Non-organ specific cancer prevention of ginseng: a prospective study in Korea. Int J Epidemiol 1998;27:359–364

15 Bjelakovic G, Nikolova D, Simonetti R G, Gluud C. Antioxidant supplements for prevention of gastrointestinal cancers: a systematic review and meta-analysis. Lancet 2004;364:1219–1228

16 Lee K W, Lee II J, Surh Y-J, Lee C Y. Vitamin C and cancer chemoprevention: reappraisal. Am J Clin Nutr 2003;78:1074–1078

17 Lonn E, Bosch J, Yusuf S, Sheridan P, Pogue J, Arnold J M, Ross C, Arnold A, Sleight P, Probstfield J, Dagenais G R. HOPE and HOPE-TOO Trial Investigators. Effects of long-term vitamin E supplementation on cardiovascular events and cancer: a randomized controlled trial. JAMA 2005;293:1338–1347

18 Duffield-Lillico A J, Dalkin B L, Reid M E, Turnbull B W, Slate E H, Jacobs E T, Marshall J R, Clark L C. Nutritional Prevention of Cancer Study Group. Selenium supplementation, baseline plasma selenium status and incidence of prostate cancer: an analysis of the complete treatment period of the Nutritional Prevention of Cancer Trial. BJU Int 2003;91:608–612

19 Duffield-Lillico A J, Slate E H, Reid M E, Turnbull B W, Wilkins P A, Combs G F Jr, Park H K, Gross E G, Graham G F, Stratton M S, Marshall J R, Clark L C. Nutritional Prevention of Cancer Study Group. Selenium supplementation and secondary prevention of non-melanoma skin cancer in a randomized trial. J Natl Cancer Inst 2003;95:1477–1481

20 Duffield-Lillico A J, Reid M E, Turnbull B W, Combs G F Jr, Slate E H, Fischbach L A, Marshall J R, Clark L C. Baseline characteristics and the effect of selenium supplementation on cancer incidence in a randomized clinical trial: a summary report of the Nutritional Prevention of Cancer Trial. Cancer Epidemiol Biomarkers Prev 2002;11:630–639

21 Weingarten M A, Zalmanovici A, Yaphe J. Dietary calcium supplementation for preventing colorectal cancer and adenomatous polyps. The Cochrane Database of Systematic Reviews 2004, Issue 1. Art No.: CD003548

22 Norrish A E, Skeaff C M, Arribas G L, Sharpe S J, Jackson R T. Prostate cancer risk and consumption of fish oils: a dietary biomarker-based case-control study. Br J Cancer 1999;81.1238–1242

23 Italian Study Group for the Di Bella Multitherapy Trials. Evaluation of an unconventional cancer treatment (the Di Bella multitherapy): results of phase II trials in Italy. BMJ 1999;318:224–228

24 Buiatti A, Arniani S, Verdecchia A, Tomatis L and the Italian Cancer Registries. Results

from a historical survey of the survival of cancer patients given Di Bella multitherapy. Cancer 1999;86:2143–2149

25 Ernst E, Cassileth B. Cancer diets, fads and facts. Cancer Prevent Int 1996;2:181–187

26 Hildenbrand G. Five-year survival rates of melanoma patients treated by diet therapy after the manner of Gerson: a retrospective review. Alt Ther Health Med 1995;4:29–37

27 Downer S M, Cody M M, McCluskey P, Wilson P D, Arnott S J, Lister T A, Slevin M L. Pursuit and practice of complementary therapies by cancer patients receiving conventional treatment. BMJ 1994;309:86–89

28 Boon H, Wong J. Botanical medicine and cancer: a review of the safety and efficacy. Expert Opin Pharmacother 2004;5:2485–2501

29 Lissoni P, Giana L, Zerbini S, Trabattoni P, Rovelli F. Biotherapy with the pineal immunomodulating hormone melatonin versus melatonin plus aloe vera in untreatable advanced solid neoplasms. Natural Immunity 1998;16:27–33

30 Kaegi E. Unconventional therapies for cancer: 1 Essiac. Can Med Assoc J 1998;158:897–902

31 Kaegi E. Unconventional therapies for cancer: 3 Iscador. Can Med Assoc J 1998;158:1157–1159

32 Kleijnen J, Knipschild P. Mistletoe treatment for cancer: review of controlled trials in humans. Phytomedicine 1994;1:255–260

33 Ernst E, Schmidt K, Steuer-Vogt M K. Mistletoe for cancer? A systematic review of randomised clinical trials. Int J Cancer 2003;107:262–267

34 De La Taille A, Hayek O R, Buttyan R, Bagiella E, Burchardt M, Katz A E. Effects of a phytotherapeutic agent, PC-SPES, on prostate cancer: a preliminary investigation on human cell lines and patients. Br J Urol Int 1999;84:845–850

35 Li H, Li H, Tang Z. Effect of chang'ai kangfu decoction on immunity in postoperational patients with large intestine cancer [Chinese]. Zhongguo Zhong Xi Yi Jie He Za Zhi 2000;20:580–582

36 Xu G Z, Cai W M, Qin D X, Yan J H, Wu X L, Zhang H X, Hu Y H, Gu X Z. Chinese herb "destagnation" series I: Combination of radiation with destagnation in the treatment of nasopharyngeal carcinoma (NPC): a prospective randomized trial on 188 cases. Int J Rad Oncol Biol Phys 1989;16:297–300

37 Guo Z. Clinical observation on treatment of 38 cases of postoperational large intestinal cancer by fuzheng yiai decoction combined with chemotherapy [Chinese]. Zhongguo Zhong Xi Yi Jie He Za Zhi 1999;19:20–22

38 Liu X, Wang B, Fu X. Clinical study on treatment of advanced non-small cell lung cancer with Chinese herbal medicine combined with synchronous radio- and chemotherapy [Chinese]. Zhongguo Zhong Xi Yi Jie He Za Zhi 2000; 20:427–429

39 Liu C L, Wang Y D, Jin X J. Clinical observation on treatment of non-small cell lung cancer with Chinese herbal medicine combined with bronchial arterial infusion chemotherapy [Chinese]. Zhongguo Zhong Xi Yi Jie He Za Zhi 2001;21:579–581

40 Lan X, Jiang Y. The therapeutic effects of the radiotherapy plus TCM treatment observed in senile non-parvicellular lung cancer patients at the late stage. J Tradit Chin Med 2003;23:32–34

41 Wang B, Liu X, Wu Z. Effect of qi replenishing and blood circulation activating drugs in treatment of middle-advanced pancreatic cancer with radio- and chemotherapy [Chinese]. Zhongguo Zhong Xi Yi Jie He Za Zhi 2000;20:736–738

42 Zhou K, Wang J, Liu B. Clinical study on effect of shenqi fuzheng injection combined with chemotherapy in treating gastric cancer [Chinese]. Zhongguo Zhong Xi Yi Jie He Za Zhi 1999;19:11–13

43 Oka H, Yamamoto S, Kuroki T, Harihara S, Marumo T, Kim SR, Monna T, Kobayashi K, Tango T. Prospective study of chemoprevention of hepatocellular carcinoma with Sho-saiko- to (TJ-9). Cancer 1995;76:743–749

44 Wang B, Liu X, Fu X. Clinical observation on effect of yiqi huoxue decoction in comprehensive treatment on advanced stage of esophageal cancer [Chinese]. Zhongguo Zhong Xi Yi Jie He Za Zhi 1999;19:589–591

45 Chen Zhiyu, Wu Taixiang, Yang Xiaoyan, Wei Jiafu, Wang Qin, Liu Guanjian. Medicinal herbs for esophageal cancer. The Cochrane Database of Systematic Reviews 2003, Issue 4. Art. No.: CD004520

46 Kaegi E. Unconventional therapies for cancer: 714-X. Can Med Assoc J 1998;158:1327–1329

47 Vickers A. Botanical medicines for the treatment of cancer: rationale, overview of current data, and methodological considerations for phase I and II trials. Cancer Invest 2002;20:1069–1079

48 Kaegi E. Unconventional therapies for cancer: 4 Hydrazine sulfate. Can Med Assoc J 1998;158:897–902

49 Moertel C G, Fleming T R, Rubin J. A clinical trial of amygdalin (Laetrile) in the treatment of human cancer. New Engl J Med 1982;306:201–206

50 Jacobson J S, Workman S B, Kronenberg F. Research on complementary/alternative medicine for patients with breast cancer: a review of the biomedical literature. J Clin Oncol 2000;18:668–683

51 Lissoni P, Barni S, Ardizzoa A. A randomized study with pineal hormone melatonin versus supportive care alone in patients with brain metastases due to solid neoplasms. Cancer 1994;73:699–701

52 Ernst E. Antiangiogenic shark cartilage as a treatment for cancer? Perfusion 1998;11:49

53 Loprinzi C L, Levitt R, Barton D L; North Central Cancer Treatment Group. Evaluation of shark cartilage in patients with advanced cancer: a North Central Cancer Treatment Group trial. Cancer 2005;104:176–182

54 Miller D R, Anderson G T, Stark J J, Granick J L, Richardson D. Phase I/II trial of the safety and efficacy of shark cartilage in the treatment of advanced cancer. J Clin Oncol 1998;16:3649–3655

55 Ernst E. Thymus therapy for cancer? A criteria-based, systematic review. Eur J Cancer 1997;33:531–535

56 Ernst E, Schmidt K. Ukrain – a new cancer cure? A systematic review of randomised clinical trials. BMC Cancer 2005;5:69

57 Smedslund G, Ringdal G I. Meta-analysis of the effects of psychosocial interventions on survival time in cancer patients. J Psychosom Res 2004;57:123–131

58 Bagenal F S, Easton D F, Harris E, Chilvers C E D, McElwain T J. Survival of patients with breast cancer attending Bristol Cancer Help Centre. Lancet 1990;336:606–610

59 Cassileth B R, Lusk E J, Guerry D, Blake A D, Walsh W P, Kascius L, Schultz D J. Survival and quality of life among patients receiving unproven as compared with conventional cancer therapy. New Engl J Med 1991;324:1180–1185

60 Vickers A J. Can acupuncture have specific effects on health – a systematic review of acupuncture trials. J Roy Soc Med 1996;89:303–311

61 Klein J, Griffiths P. Acupressure for nausea and vomiting in cancer patients receiving chemotherapy. Br J Community Nurs 2004;9:383–388

62 Roscoe J A, Morrow G R, Hickok J T, Bushunow P, Pierce H I, Flynn P J, Kirshner J J, Moore D F, Atkins J N. The efficacy of acupressure and acustimulation wrist bands for the relief of chemotherapy-induced nauseas and vomiting. A University of Rochester Cancer Center Community Clinical Oncology Program multicenter study. J Pain Symptom Manage 2003;26:731–742

63 Shin Y H, Kim T I, Shin M S, Juon H S. Effect of acupressure on nausea and vomiting during chemotherapy cycle for Korean postoperative stomach cancer patients. Cancer Nurs 2004;27:267–274

64 Streitberger K, Friedrich-Rust M, Bardenheuer H, Unnebrink K, Windeler J, Goldschmidt H, Egerer G. Effect of acupuncture compared with placebo-acupuncture at P6 as additional antiemetic prophylaxis in high-dose chemotherapy and autologous peripheral blood stem cell transplantation: a randomized controlled single-blind trial. Clin Cancer Res 2003;9:2538–2544

65 Lee H, Schmidt K, Ernst E. Acupuncture for the relief of cancer-related pain – a systematic review. Eur J Pain 2005;9:437–444

66 Rydholm N, Strang P. Acupuncture for patients in hospital-based home care suffering from xerostomia. J Palliat Care 1999;15:20–23

67 Hammar M, Frisk J, Grimas O. Acupuncture treatment of vasomotor symptoms in men with prostatic carcinoma: a pilot study. J Urol 1999;161:853–857

68 Fellowes D, Barnes K, Wilkinson S. Aromatherapy and massage for symptom relief in patients with cancer. The Cochrane Database of Systematic Reviews 2004, Issue 3. Art No.: CD002287

69 Dimeo F. Welche Rolle spielt körperliche Aktivität in der Prävention, Therapie und Rehabilitation von neoplastischen Erkrankungen? Deutsche Zeitschr Sportmed 2004;55:177–182

70 Su C K, Mehta V, Ravikumar L, Shah R, Pinto H, Halpern J, Koong A, Goffinet D, Le Q T. Phase II double-blind randomized study comparing aloe vera versus placebo to prevent radiation-related mucositis in patients with head-and-neck neoplasms. Int J Radiat Oncol Biol Phys 2004;60:171–177

71 Olsen S L, Raub W Jr, Bradley C, Johnson M, Macias J L, Love V, Markoe A. The effect of aloe vera gel/mild soap versus mild soap alone in preventing skin reactions in patients undergoing radiation therapy. Oncol Nurs Forum 2001;28:543–547

CONDITIONS

72 Jacobson J S, Troxel A B, Evans J, Klaus L, Vahdat L, Kinne D, Lo K M, Moore A, Rosenman P J, Kaufman E L, Neugut A I, Grann V R. Randomized trial of black cohosh for the treatment of hot flashes among women with a history of breast cancer. J Clin Oncol 2001 19:2739–2745

73 Hernandez Munoz G, Pluchino S. Cimicifuga racemosa for the treatment of hot flushes in women surviving breast cancer. Maturitas 2003;44(Suppl1):S59–S65

74 Campbell G, Pickles T, D'yachkova Y. A randomised trial of cranberry versus apple juice in the management of urinary symptoms during external beam radiation therapy for prostate cancer. Clin Oncol (R Coll Radiol) 2003;15:322–328

75 Pommier P, Gomez F, Sunyach M P, D'Hombres A, Carrie C, Montbarbon X. Phase III randomized trial of Calendula officinalis compared with trolamine for the prevention of acute dermatitis during irradiation for breast cancer. J Clin Oncol 2004;22:1447–1453

76 Younus J, Collins A, Wang X. A double-blind, placebo-controlled pilot study to evaluate the effects of ginseng on quality of life in adult chemotherapy–naïve cancer patients. Proc Am Soc Clin Oncol 2003;22:733a

77 Cluzan R V, Pecking A P, Mathiex-Fortunet H, Leger Picherit E. Efficacy of BN165 (Ginkor Fort) in breast cancer related upper limb lymphedema: a preliminary study. Lymphology 2004;37:47–52

78 Zou Y H, Liu X M. Effect of astragalus injection combined with chemotherapy on quality of life in patients with advanced non-small cell lung cancer [Article in Chinese]. Zhongguo Zhong Xi Yi Jie He Za Zhi 2003;23:733–735

79 Pan B, Cheng T, Nan K J, Qiu G Q, Sun X C. Effect of Fuzheng Yiliu decoction combined with chemotherapy on patients with intermediate and late stage gastrointestinal cancer. World J Gastroenterol 2005;11:439–442

80 Mori K, Kondo T, Kamiyama Y, Kano Y, Tominaga K. Preventive effect of Kampo medicine (Hangeshashin-to) against irinotecan-induced diarrhea in advanced non-small-cell lung cancer. Cancer Chemother Pharmacol 2003;51:403–406

81 Cai H B, Dai F G, Min Q F, Shi M, Miao J X, Luo R C. Clinical study of the effects of radiotherapy in combination with traditional Chinese medicine on non-small cell lung cancer [Article in Chinese]. Di Yi Jun Yi Da Xue Xue Bao 2002;22:1112

82 Liu P, Cao Y, Qiao X. Clinical study on shenmai injection in promoting postoperative recovery in patients of breast cancer [Article in Chinese]. Zhongguo Zhong Xi Yi Jie He Za Zhi 2000;20:328–329

83 Taixiang W, Munro A J, Guanjian L. Chinese medical herbs for chemotherapy side effects in colorectal cancer patients. The Cochrane Database of Systematic Reviews 2005, Issue 1. Art. No.: CD004540

84 Balzarini A, Felisi E, Martini A, De Conno F. Efficacy of homeopathic treatment of skin reactions during radiotherapy for breast cancer: a randomised, double-blind clinical trial. Br Homeopath J 2000;89:8–12

85 Syrjala K L, Cummings C, Donaldson G W. Hypnosis or cognitive behavioral training for the reduction of pain and nausea during cancer treatment: a controlled clinical trial. Pain 1992;48:137–146

86 Elkins G, Cheung A, Marcus J, Palamara L, Rajab M H. Hypnosis to reduce pain in cancer survivors with advanced disease: a prospective study. J Cancer Integr Med 2004;2:167–172

87 Hawkins P J, Liossi C, Ewart W, Hatira P, Kosmidis V H, Varvutsi M. Hypnotherapy for control of anticipatory nausea and vomiting in children with cancer: preliminary findings. Psycho-Oncology 1995;4:101–106

88 Zeltzer L K, Dolgin M J, LeBaron S, LeBaron C. A randomized, controlled study of behavioral intervention for chemotherapy distress in children with cancer. Pediatrics 1991;88:34–42

89 Wild M R, Espie C. The efficacy of hypnosis in the reduction of procedural pain and distress in pediatric oncology: a systematic review. J Dev Behav Pediatr 2004;25:207–213

90 Stalpers L J, da Costa H C, Merbis M A, Fortuin A A, Muller M J, van Dam F S. Hypnotherapy in radiotherapy patients: a randomized trial. Int J Radiat Oncol Biol Phys 2005;61:499–506

91 Hilliard R E. The effects of music therapy on the quality and length of life of people diagnosed with terminal cancer. J Music Therap 2003;40:113–137

92 Cassileth B R, Vickers A J, Magill L A. Music therapy for mood disturbance during hospitalization for autologous stem cell transplantation. Cancer 2003;98:2723–2729

93 Kwekkeboom K L. Music versus distraction for procedural pain and anxiety in patients with cancer. Oncol Nurs Forum 2003;30:433–440

94 Burns D S. The effect of the bonny method of guided imagery and music on the mood and life quality of cancer patients. J Music Ther 2001;38:51–65

95 Hodgson H. Does reflexology impact on cancer patients' quality of life? Nurs Stand 2000;14:33–38

96 Stephenson N L, Weinrich S P, Tavakoli A S. The effects of foot reflexology on anxiety and pain in patients with breast and lung cancer. Oncol Nurs Forum 2000;27:67–72

97 Sloman R, Brown P, Aldana E, Chee E. The use of relaxation for the promotion of comfort and pain relief in persons with advanced cancer. Contemporary Nurse 1994;3:6–12

98 Kim S D, Kim H S. Effects of a relaxation breathing exercise on anxiety, depression, and leukocyte in hemopoietic stem cell transplantation patients. Cancer Nurs 2005;28:79–83

99 Walker L G, Walker M B, Ogston K, Heys S D, Ah-See A K, Miller I D, Hutcheon A W, Sarkar T K, Eremin O. Psychological, clinical and pathological effects of relaxation training and guided imagery during primary chemotherapy. Br J Cancer 1999;80:262–268

100 Gaston-Johansson F, Fall-Dickson J M, Nanda J, Ohly K V, Stillman S, Krumm S, Kennedy M J. The effectiveness of the comprehensive coping strategy program on clinical outcomes in breast cancer autologous bone marrow transplantation. Cancer Nurs 2000;23:277–285

101 Speca M, Carlson L E, Goodey E, Angen M. A randomized, wait-list controlled clinical trial: the effect of a mindfulness meditation-based stress reduction program on mood and symptoms of stress in cancer outpatients. Psychosom Med 2000;62:613–622

102 Carlson L E, Ursuliak Z, Goodey E, Angen M, Speca M. The effects of a mindfulness meditation-based stress reduction program on mood and symptoms of stress in cancer outpatients: 6-month follow-up. Support Care Cancer 2001;9:112–123

103 Shapiro S L, Bootzin R R, Figueredo A J, Lopez A M, Schwartz G E. The efficacy of mindfulness-based stress reduction in the treatment of sleep disturbance in women with breast cancer: an exploratory study. J Psychosom Res 2003;54:85–91

104 XJacobsen P B, Meade C D, Stein K D, Chirikos T N, Small B J, Ruckdeschel J C. Efficacy and costs of two forms of stress management training for cancer patients undergoing chemotherapy. J Clin Oncol 2002;20:2851–2862

105 Hidderley M, Holt M. A pilot randomized trial assessing the effects of autogenic training in early stage cancer patients in relation to psychological status and immune system responses. Eur J Oncol Nurs 2004;8:61–65

106 Baider L, Peretz T, Hadani P E, Koch U. Psychological intervention in cancer patients: a randomized study. Gen Hosp Psychiatry 2001;23:272–277

107 Molassiotis A, Yung H P, Yam B M, Chan F Y, Mok T S. The effectiveness of progressive muscle relaxation training in managing chemotherapy-induced nausea and vomiting in Chinese breast cancer patients: a randomised controlled trial. Support Care Cancer 2002;10:237–246

108 Sloman R. Relaxation and imagery for anxiety and depression control in community patients with advanced cancer. Cancer Nurs 2002;25:432–435

109 Cheung Y L, Molassiotis A, Chang A M. The effect of progressive muscle relaxation training on anxiety and quality of life after stoma surgery in colorectal cancer patients. Psychooncology 2003;12:254–266

110 Samarel N, Fawcett J, Davis M M, Ryan F M. Effects of dialogue and therapeutic touch on preoperative and postoperative experiences of breast cancer surgery: an exploratory study. Oncol Nurs Forum 1998;25:1369–1376

111 Giasson M, Bouchard L. Effect of therapeutic touch on the well-being of persons with terminal cancer. J Holistic Nurs 1998;16: 383–398

112 Campbell F A, Tramer M R, Carroll D, Reynolds D J, Moore R A, McQuay H J. Are cannabinoids an effective and safe treatment option in the management of pain? A qualitative systematic review. BMJ 2001;323:13–16

113 Roffe L, Schmidt K, Ernst E. Efficacy of Coenzyme Q10 for improved tolerability of cancer treatments: a systematic review. J Clin Oncol 2004;22:4418–4424

114 Leipner J, Saller R. Systematic enzyme therapy in oncology. Forsch Komplementärmed Klass Naturheilkd 2000;7:45

115 Philipp T, Rossion I. Factor AF2 as a complementary cancer therapy: an overview. Anticanc Res 2004;24:3393–3698

116 Bruera E, Strasser F, Palmer J L, Willey J, Calder K, Amyotte G, Baracos V. Effect of fish oil on appetite and other symptoms in patients with advanced cancer and anorexia/cachexia: a double-blind, placebo-controlled study. J Clin Oncol 2003;21:129–134

117 Heller A R, Rossel T, Gottschlich B, Tiebel O, Menschikowski M, Litz R J, Zimmermann T, Koch T. Omega-3 fatty acids improve liver and pancreas function in postoperative cancer patients. Int J Cancer 2004;111:611–616

118 Persson C, Glimelius B, Rönnelid J, Nygren P. Impact of fish oil and melatonin on

cachexia in patients with advanced gastrointestinal cancer: a randomized pilot study. Nutrition 2005;21:170–178

119 Nikander E, Kilkkinen A, Metsa-Heikkila M, Adlercreutz H, Pietinen P, Tiitinen A, Ylikorkala O. A randomized placebo controlled crossover trial with phytoestrogens in treatment of menopause I breast cancer patients. Obstet Gynecol 2003;101:1213–1220

120 Van Patten C L, Olivotto I A, Chambers G K, Gelmon K A, Hislop T G, Templeton E, Wattie A, Prior J C. Effect of soy phytoestrogens on hot flashes in postmenopausal women with breast cancer: a randomized, controlled clinical trial. J Clin Oncol 2002;20:1449–1455

121 Quella S K, Loprinzi C L, Barton D L, Knost J A, Sloan J A, LaVaseur B I, Swan D, Krupp K R, Miller K D, Novotny P J. Evaluation of soy phytoestrogens for the treatment of hot flashes in breast cancer survivors: a North Central Cancer Treatment Group Trial. J Clin Oncol 2000;18:1068–1074

CHRONIC FATIGUE SYNDROME

Synonyms/ subcategories

Akureyri disease, Iceland disease, neurasthenia, postviral fatigue syndrome, Royal Free disease, Tapanui flu, yuppie flu.

Definition

A condition of severe, disabling fatigue accompanied by symptoms such as musculoskeletal pain, sleep disturbances and impaired concentration and short-term memory, as well as headache.

CAM usage

According to a US survey,[1] massage and exercise were frequently employed for chronic fatigue syndrome (CFS). Acupuncture and kinesiology are also often used.[2]

Clinical evidence

Exercise
A Cochrane review[3] found encouraging evidence for exercise, but it was often associated with poor compliance (Box 2.27).

Box 2.27
Systematic review
Exercise for chronic fatigue
Edmonds[3]

- Five RCTs were included

- Methodological quality was variable but good in some instances

- Fatigue and physical functioning responded positively to exercise while for depression data were not conclusive

- Combining exercise with antidepressants or education generated best outcomes

- Conclusion: some patients may benefit from exercise

Herbal medicine
Conflicting results have been reported by two placebo-controlled RCTs of oil of **evening primrose** (*Oenothera biennis*) combined with fish oil (Table 2.21).[4,5] There were several key differences between these two trials, i.e. diagnosis, duration of illness and placebo, which may explain the discrepant results. **Siberian ginseng** (*Eleutherococcus senticosus*) was tested in an

Table 2.21 **Double-blind RCTs of evening primrose oil for chronic fatigue syndrome**

Reference	Sample size	Interventions [dosage]	Result	Comment
Behan[4]	63	A) Evening primrose and fish oil [4 g/d for 3 mo] B) Placebo (liquid paraffin)	A superior to B on symptom ratings	Diagnosis was postviral fatigue syndrome not CFS
Warren[5]	50	A) Evening primrose and fish oil [4 g/d for 3 mo] B) Placebo (sunflower oil)	A no different from B on symptom ratings	Neither group improved

RCT (n = 96).[6] Both the placebo and the ginseng group showed improvements but no differential effects were noted.

Homeopathy

A double-blind RCT (n = 61) of classical homeopathy reported improvements in 33% of the homeopathic group compared with 4% of the placebo group based on self-assessments.[7] However, no statistical analysis was reported. A further RCT (n = 103) tested a similar approach and found more improvement on a symptom score with individualised homeopathy compared with placebo.[8]

Supplements

In an uncontrolled trial of 3 months of specific **amino acid** supplementation, 15 of 20 patients reported over 50% improvement in symptoms.[9] Energy and mental function were the areas of greatest improvement.

A small (n = 14) double-blind, placebo-controlled, crossover RCT was conducted of an intravenous combination of folic acid, bovine liver extract and vitamin B_{12}.[10] A substantial placebo response was observed, but no difference between the interventions.

A large double-blind RCT (n = 326) of CFS patients investigated the effect of **isobutyryl-thiamine disulfide**.[11] No improvements were observed compared with placebo.

L-carnitine was compared with amantadine in a crossover RCT (n = 30) for 2 months.[12] Clinical improvements were reported for L-carnitine but not amantadine, while tolerability was far superior with L-carnitine.

In a double-blind, placebo-controlled RCT (n = 32), intravenous **magnesium** improved energy, pain and emotional symptoms.[13] However, subsequent open studies found no magnesium deficiency in CFS patients and no benefit from magnesium injections.[14,15]

When **melatonin** (5 mg per day) was compared in an RCT (n = 30) with phototherapy, neither intervention generated beneficial effects.[16]

CONDITIONS

Oral **nicotinamide adenine dinucleotide** (NADH) (10 mg daily for 4 weeks) produced modest improvements in symptoms in a small (n = 26) crossover placebo-controlled RCT.[17] No severe adverse events were reported. When NADH was compared with psychological therapy in a small RCT (n = 31), a slight superiority of NADH was noted.[18]

A **polynutrient** supplement with vitamins, minerals and co-enzymes generated encouraging results compared with placebo in an RCT with 53 CFS patients.[19]

Other therapies

A non-randomised trial (n = 58) reported superior results with **osteopathy** (20 sessions over 12 months) than no intervention.[20]

Relaxation was used in the control arm of an RCT.[21] It was a successful treatment in 19% of patients, which was less than cognitive–behaviour therapy.

Overall recommendation

Good evidence exists only for exercise treatment. Encouraging data have emerged for homeopathy and NADH. As none of these approaches are associated with major risks, they may well be worth trying in combination with cognitive–behavioural therapy, the only conventional therapy of demonstrable effectiveness.

Table 2.22
Summary of clinical evidence for chronic fatigue syndrome

Treatment	Weight of evidence	Direction of evidence	Serious safety concerns
Exercise	OOO	⇧	Yes (see p 5)
Herbal medicine			
Evening primrose oil	OO	⇨	Yes (see p 393)
Siberian ginseng	O	⬃	Yes (see p 409)
Homeopathy	OO	⇧	No (see p 327)
Supplements			
Amino acids	O	⬈	No (see p 5)
Folic acid	O	⇩	Yes (see p 5)
Isobutyryl-thiamine disulfide	O	⇩	No (see p 5)
L-carnitine	O	⬈	No (see p 482)
Magnesium	O	⬃	Yes (see p 5)
Melatonin	O	⇩	Yes (see p 435)
NADH	OO	⇧	No (see p 484)
Polynutrients	O	⇧	No (see p 5)

REFERENCES

1 Astin J A. Why patients use alternative medicine. JAMA 1998;279:1548–1553

2 Az S, Gregg V H, Jones D. Chronic fatigue syndrome: sufferers' evaluation of medical support. J Roy Soc Med 1997;90:250–254

3 Edmonds M, McGuire H, Price J. Exercise therapy for chronic fatigue syndrome. The Cochrane Database of Systematic Reviews 2004, Issue 3. Art No: CD003200

4 Behan P O, Behan W M, Horrobin D. Effect of high doses of essential fatty acids on the postviral fatigue syndrome. Acta Neurol Scand 1990;82:209–216

5 Warren G, McKendrick M, Peet M. The role of essential fatty acids in chronic fatigue syndrome. A case-controlled study of red-cell membrane essential fatty acids (EFA) and a placebo-controlled treatment study with high dose of EFA. Acta Neurol Scand 1999;99:112–116

6 Hartz A J, Bentler S, Noyes R, Hoehns J, Logemann C, Sinift S, Butani Y, Wang W, Brake K, Ernst M, Kautzman H. Randomized controlled trial of Siberian ginseng for chronic fatigue. Psychol Med 2004;34:51–61

7 Awdry R. Homeopathy may help ME. Int J Alt Compl Med 1996;14:12–16

8 Weatherley-Jones E, Nicholl J P, Thomas K J, Parry G J, McKendrick M W, Green S T, Stanley P J, Lynch S P. A randomised, controlled, triple-blind trial of the efficacy of homeopathic treatment for chronic fatigue syndrome. J Psychosom Res 2004;56:189–197

9 Bralley J A, Lord R S. Treatment of chronic fatigue syndrome with specific amino acid supplementation. J Appl Nutr 1994;46:74–78

10 Kaslow J E, Rucker L, Onishi R. Liver extract-folic acid–cyanocobalamin versus placebo for chronic fatigue syndrome. Arch Intern Med 1989;149:2501–2503

11 Tiev K P, Cabane J, Imbert J C. Treatment of chronic postinfectious fatigue: randomised double-blind study of two doses of sulbutiamine (400–600 mg/day) versus placebo. Revue de Médecine Interne 1999;20:912–918

12 Plioplys A V, Plioplys S. Amantadine and L-carnitine treatment of chronic fatigue syndrome. Neuropsychobiology 1997;35:16–23

13 Cox I M, Campbell M J, Dowson D. Red blood cell magnesium and chronic fatigue syndrome. Lancet 1991;337:757–760

14 Gantz N M. Magnesium and chronic fatigue. Lancet 1991;338:66

15 Clague J E, Edwards R H T, Jackson M J. Intravenous magnesium loading in chronic fatigue syndrome. Lancet 1992;340:124–125

16 Williams G, Waterhouse J, Mugarza J, Minors D, Hayden K. Therapy of circadian rhythm disorders in chronic fatigue syndrome: no symptomatic improvement with melatonin or phototherapy. Eur J Clin Invest 2002;32:831–837

17 Forsyth L M, Preuss H G, MacDowell A L, Chiazze L, Birkmayer G D, Bellanti J A. Therapeutic effects of oral NADH on the symptoms of patients with chronic fatigue syndrome. Ann Allergy Asthma Immunol 1999;82:185–191

18 Santaella M L, Font I, Disdier O M. Comparison of oral nicotinaminde adenine dinucleotide (NADH) versus conventional therapy for chronic fatigue syndrome. P R Health Sci J 2004;23:89–93

19 Brouwers F M, Van Der Werf S, Bleijenberg G, Van Der Zee L, Van Der Meer J W. The effect of polynutrient supplements on fatigue and physical activity of patients with chronic fatigue syndrome: a double-blind randomized controlled trial. QJM 2002;95:677–683

20 Perrin R N, Edwards J, Hartley P. An evaluation of the effectiveness of osteopathic treatment on symptoms associated with myalgic encephalomyelitis. A preliminary report. J Med Engineering Technol 1998;22:1–13

21 Deale A, Chalder T, Marks L, Wessely S. Cognitive behaviour therapy for chronic fatigue syndrome: a randomised controlled trial. Am J Psychiatr 1997;154:408–414

CONDITIONS

CHRONIC HEART FAILURE

Synonyms/ subcategories
Heart failure, cardiac failure, left ventricular failure, right ventricular failure.

Definition
Heart failure occurs when abnormality of cardiac function causes failure of the heart to pump blood at a rate sufficient for metabolic requirements under normal filling pressure. It can be caused by systolic or diastolic dysfunction and is associated with neurohormonal changes.

CAM usage
One classic conventional drug for chronic heart failure (CHF) of plant origin is digitalis. Another treatment that has been shown to be beneficial by reducing death rates and hospital admissions compared with usual care is graded physical exercise training. Neither option, however, can be considered CAM. The CAM treatment modalities that are most frequently recommended for CHF are herbal medicines and non-herbal dietary supplements. A survey suggests that garlic, ginger and parsley are most frequently used by CHF patients.[1]

Clinical evidence

Acupuncture
One small (n = 12) RCT suggested that auriculo-acupuncture might improve left ventricular function in patients with dilating cardiomyopathy and CHF.[2] This study requires replication in a more rigorous RCT.

Herbal medicine
The **Ayurvedic** herb *Terminalia arjuna* has been tested in a small (n = 12) crossover RCT with CHF patients in stage IV New York Heart Association.[3] The results show that there was an improvement of all relevant signs and symptoms of CHF in patients treated with *Terminalia arjuna*. After the trial, all patients received treatment for up to 28 months and the clinical improvement continued, including amelioration in quality of life. These findings require confirmation.

A number of traditional **Chinese medicines** have been tested in RCTs for this condition.[4–7] Only single RCTs are available for each of the tested medicines. For three of these, positive effects have been reported which require independent replication.[4–6] Injection of shengmai was reported to decrease the digoxin level compared with controls.[7]

Ginseng (*Panax ginseng*) was tested in a CCT (n = 45) with three parallel arms.[8] The first group was treated with digoxin, the second with ginseng and the third with a combination of both. Haemodynamic measurements suggested improvements in the two groups treated with ginseng compared with the digoxin only group.

A systematic review of **hawthorn** (*Crataegus*) extract of leaf with flower identified 13 double-blind RCTs.[9] The meta-analysis suggested that for maximal workload, hawthorn extract was more beneficial than placebo (Box 2.28). This conclusion is supported by the results of an independent analysis of trials using a single standardised preparation.[10] Double-blind RCTs that tested extract of crataegus berries also reported beneficial effects compared with placebo.[11,12] Several comparative clinical trials imply that it is as effective as conventional drugs.[9]

Two RCTs assessed the effects of **milk vetch** (Astragalus) injection and compared it with nitroglycerine added to an intravenous drip.[13,14] For left ventricular ejection fraction, both trials report an improvement compared with controls.

Box 2.28
Meta-analysis
Hawthorn extract for chronic heart failure
Pittler MH[9]

- Thirteen double-blind, placebo controlled RCTs met all inclusion criteria, eight of which were included in a meta-analysis

- For maximal workload the weighted mean difference was 7 Watt (CI 3 to 11 Watt, n = 310)

- For pressure-heart rate the weighted mean difference was −20 (CI −32 to −8, n = 264)

- Reported adverse events were mild, infrequent and transient and were nausea, dizziness, cardiac and gastrointestinal complaints

- Conclusion: the results suggest that adjunctive treatment with hawthorn extract is beneficial compared with placebo in patients with chronic heart failure

Supplements

Co-enzyme Q10 is being recommended for, amongst other conditions, hypertension, coronary heart disease and CHF. Several trials, most of which have methodological weaknesses, have suggested that it is effective for CHF.[15] Two rigorous RCTs demonstrated that co-enzyme Q10 supplementation does not improve left ventricular function or quality of life in CHF patients.[16,17]

Nitric oxide formed by the action of **L-arginine** increases blood flow and could therefore have positive effects in CHF. An RCT (n = 15) tested this hypothesis by treating CHF patients with an oral L-arginine-containing supplements or with placebo.[18] The results show the expected increase in blood flow and improvement of functional status by an increase in the 6-minute walking distance. Another double-blind RCT showed a prolongation of exercise duration compared with placebo.[19]

In chronic heart failure, the myocardium is depleted of carnitine, co-enzyme Q10 and taurine. **MyoVive**, a supplement which contains these agents was tested in a double-blind RCT.[20] The left ventricular end-diastolic volume decreased in the supplement group compared with placebo. It was concluded that, because the risk of death for surgical revascularisation is related to preoperative left ventricular end-diastolic volume, supplementation could improve outcomes.

An RCT assessing the effects of **vitamin** E supplementation included 2545 women and 6996 men.[21] Patients were treated with 400 IU of vitamin E for 4.5 years. A composite of myocardial infarction, stroke and death from cardiovascular causes was the primary outcome measure. It was concluded that in patients with high risk for cardiovascular events, treatment with vitamin E had no apparent effect on cardiovascular outcomes. An extension of this trial also concluded that vitamin E supplementation does not prevent major cardiovascular events and may even increase the risk for heart failure.[22]

Another RCT also reported that supplementation with vitamin E does not result in any improvements in prognostic or functional indices or in quality of life.[23]

Overall recommendation

There is conclusive evidence for extract of hawthorn leaves with flowers as a symptomatic therapy in mild to moderate CHF. For extract of hawthorn berries encouraging evidence is emerging. Other encouraging data relate to astragalus and L-arginine, but the weight of the evidence is not strong enough for a firm recommendation. The evidence regarding co-enzyme Q10 is ambiguous. These treatments are unlikely to be associated with serious risks when taken under medical supervision. Conventional treatments for CHF, which are well established and of proven effectiveness exist. Thus the above herbal and non-herbal dietary supplements should only be prescribed in cases where the patient insists on complementary medicine.

Table 2.23
Summary of clinical evidence for chronic heart failure

Treatment	Weight of evidence	Direction of evidence	Serious safety concerns
Acupuncture	O	⬀	Yes (see p 294)
Herbal medicine			
Ayurvedic medicines	O	⇧	Yes (see p 5)
Chinese medicines	O	⬀	Yes (see p 5)
Ginseng	O	⬀	Yes (see p 407)
Hawthorn	OOO	⇧	Yes (see p 422)
Milk vetch	OO	⇧	Yes (see pp 5, 479)
Supplements			
Co-enzyme Q10	OO	⇨	Yes (see p 385)
L-arginine	OO	⇧	No (see p 482)
MyoVive	O	⬀	Yes (see p 5)
Vitamin E	OOO	⇩	Yes (see p 5)

REFERENCES

1 Ackman M L, Campbell J B, Buzak K A. Use of non-prescription medications by patients with congestive heart failure. Ann Pharmacother 1999;33:674–679

2 Zhou J R. Effect of auriculo-acupuncture plus needle embedding in heart point on left cardiac, humoral and endocrine function. Chung Kuo Chung Hsi I Chieh Ho Tsa Chih K 1993;13:153–154

3 Bharani A, Ganguly A, Bhargava K D. Salutary effect of Terminalia arjuna in patients with severe refractory heart failure. Int J Cardiol 1995;49:191–199

4 An H Y, Huang L J, Jin J S. Preliminary exploration on effect of yiqi wenyang huoxue lishui treatment on neuroendocrine system in patients with congestive heart failure. Zhongguo Zhong Xi Yi Jie He Za Zhi 2002;22:349–352

5 Li L, Zhang J, Xu F. Clinical study on lixin pill in treating congestive heart failure. Zhongguo Zhong Xi Yi Jie He Za Zhi 2000;20:341–343

6 Li G, Qi W, Xiong K. Clinical observation on 51 patients of acute myocardial infarction treated with thrombolytic therapy combined with Chinese herbal medicine. Zhongguo Zhong Xi Yi Jie He Za Zhi 1999;19:461–462

7 Mao J Y, Xu W R, Wang H H. Clinical study on effect of shengmai injection on serum concentration and pharmacokinetic parameters of digoxin in patients with congestive heart failure. Zhongguo Zhong Xi Yi Jie He Za Zhi 2003;23:347–350

8 Ding D Z, Shen T K, Cui Y Z. The effects of red ginseng on the congestive heart failure and its mechanism. Chung Kuo Ching Hsi I Chieh Ho Tsa Chih 1995;15:325–327

9 Pittler M H, Schmidt K, Ernst E. Hawthorn extract for treating chronic heart failure: Meta-analysis of randomized trials. Am J Med 2003;114:665–674

10 Eichstädt H, Störk T, Funk P, Köhler S. Coronary heart disease treated with Crataegus extract WS 1442 – a comparison of four randomized clinical studies. Perfusion 2003;16:217–223

11 Rietbrock N, Hamel M, Hempel B, Mitrovic V, Schmidt T, Wolf G K. Actions of standardized extract of crataegus berries on exercise tolerance and quality of life in patients with congestive heart failure. Arzneimittelforschung 2001;51:793–798

12 Degenring F H, Suter A, Weber M, Saller R. A randomized double blind placebo controlled clinical trial of a standardized extract of fresh cratagues berries (crataegisan) in the treatment of patients with congestive heart failure NYHA II. Phytomedicine 2003;10:363–369

13 Zhou Z L, Yu P, Lin D. Study on effect of astragalus injection in treating congestive heart failure. Zhongguo Zhong Xi Yi Jie He Za Zhi 2001;21:747–749

14 Liu Z G, Xiong Z M, Yu X Y. Effect of astragalus injection on immune function in patients with congestive heart failure. Zhongguo Zhong Xi Yi Jie He Za Zhi 2003;23:351–353

15 Ernst E. The cardiovascular 'miracle drug' ubiquinone. Herz Kreislauf 1999;31:79–81

16 Watson P S, Scalia G M, Galbraith A, Burstow D J, Bett N. Coenzyme Q did not affect severe heart failure or quality of life. J Am Coll Cardiol 1999;33:1549–1552

17 Khatta M, Alexander B S, Krichten C M, Fisher M L, Freudenberger R, Robinson S W, Gottlieb S S. The effect of Coenzyme Q10 in patients with congestive heart failure. Ann Intern Med 2000;132:636–640

18 Rector R S, Bank A J, Mullen K A, Tscumperlin L K, Sih R, Pillai K, Kubo S H. Randomized, double-blind, placebo-controlled study of supplemental oral L-arginine in patients with heart failure. Circulation 1996;93:2135–2141

19 Bednarz B, Jaxa-Chamicc T, Gebalska J, Herbaczynska-Cedro K, Ceremuzynski L. L-arginine supplementation prolongs exercise capacity in congestive heart failure. Kardiol Pol 2004;60:348–353

20 Jeejeebhoy F, Keith M, Freeman M, Barr A, McCall M, Kurian R, Mazer D, Errett L. Nutritional supplementation with MyoVive repletes essential cardiac myocyte nutrients and reduces left ventricular size in patients with left ventricular dysfunction. Am Heart J 2002;143:1092–1100

21 Yusuf S, Dagenais G, Pogue J, Bosch J, Sleight P. Vitamin E supplementation and cardiovascular events in high-risk patients. The heart outcomes prevention evaluation study investigators. N Engl J Med 2000;342:154–160

22 Lonn E, Bosch J, Yusuf S, Sheridan P, Pogue J, Arnold J M, Ross C, Arnold A, Sleight P, Probstfield J, Dagenais G R. HOPE and HOPE-TOO Trial Investigators. Effects of long-term vitamin E supplementation on cardiovascular events and cancer: a randomized controlled trial. JAMA 2005;293:1338–1347

23 Keith M E, Jeejeebhoy K N, Langer A, Kurian R, Barr A, O'Kelly B, Sole M J. A controlled clinical trial of vitamin E supplementation in patients with congestive heart failure. Am J Clin Nutr 2001;73:219–224

CHRONIC VENOUS INSUFFICIENCY

Synonyms   Post-thrombotic syndrome, post-thrombophlebitic syndrome.

Definition   Chronic venous insufficiency (CVI) is caused by poorly functioning valves within the lumen of the veins. Blood flows from the
deep to the superficial venous systems through these incompetent valves, causing persistent superficial venous hypertension,
which leads to varicosity of the superficial veins. Common sites
of valvular incompetence include the saphenofemoral and
saphenopopliteal junctions and perforating veins connecting the
deep and superficial venous systems along the length of the leg.
Symptoms of varicose veins include distress about cosmetic
appearance, pain, itch, limb heaviness, and cramps.

CAM usage   Herbal medicine and hydrotherapy are popular complementary
therapies for this condition, particularly in some European
countries.

Clinical   ***Herbal medicine***
evidence   A double-blind RCT investigating the effects of **buckwheat**
(*Fagopyrum esculentum*) tea in 67 patients[1] reported some beneficial effects for lower leg volume and symptom scores, which
were, however, not different from placebo.

The clinical evidence on **butcher's broom** (*Ruscus aculeatus*)
is mostly based on RCTs using combination preparations (e.g.[2-4]).
These studies report beneficial effects such as a reduction of
venous capacity as well as an improvement of symptoms. A
meta-analysis included 20 placebo-controlled RCTs, which tested
the effectiveness of Cyclo 3 fort, a combination preparation
containing *Ruscus aculeatus*, hesperidine methychalcone and
ascorbic acid.[5] It concluded that the preparation reduces the
severity of the symptoms associated with CVI more than placebo.
A double-blind RCT of a monopreparation reported positive
effects for leg volume, ankle and leg circumferences.[6]

A review assessing the evidence for **French maritime pine**
(***Pinus pinaster***) bark extract suggested effectiveness for treating
CVI.[7] This is, however, based on a small number of RCTs and fur-
ther study is required.

One double-blind RCT investigated the effects of a combination preparation containing **ginkgo** (*Ginkgo biloba*) extract, trox-
erutin and heptaminol.[8] Patients (n = 48) received either 625 mg
of the preparation or placebo daily for 4 weeks. Clinical symptom
scores were not different between treatment and control groups.

In a placebo-controlled double-blind RCT (n = 87) patients
were given either 30 or 60 mg **gotu kola** (*Centella asiatica*) extract
twice daily for 60 days.[9] The results suggest an improvement of
microcirculatory parameters such as transcutaneous PO_2 compared with baseline. In a placebo-controlled double-blind RCT, 94
outpatients received either 120 mg or 60 mg titrated extract of

Centella asiatica daily for 2 months.[10] Beneficial effects are reported for the symptoms of heaviness in the lower limbs and oedema compared with placebo. These findings are corroborated by another double-blind RCT, reporting an improvement of night cramps, pruritus and oedema after the administration of 60 mg gotu kola extract for 30 days compared with placebo.[11]

A systematic review found compelling evidence for the effectiveness of oral **horse chestnut** (*Aesculus hippocastanum*) seed extract (Box 2.29).[12] The reviewed studies assessed patients with mild to moderate forms of CVI. Leg oedema and symptoms such as pain, tenseness and fatigue were reduced compared with placebo. This is corroborated by independent reviews and meta-analyses.[13,14]

Box 2.29
Systematic review
Horse chestnut seed extract for chronic venous insufficiency
Pittler[12]

- Sixteen RCTs testing monopreparations were included

- Leg pain was assessed in seven placebo-controlled trials (n = 595)

- Six studies (n = 543) reported a reduction of leg pain on various measurement scales compared with placebo

- Oedema was assessed in six placebo-controlled trials (n = 567). Four trials (n = 461) reported a reduction compared with placebo

- Conclusion: The evidence implies that horse chestnut seed extract is an efficacious and safe short-term treatment

A large double-blind RCT (n = 260) compared 360 and 720 mg of **red vine** (*Vitis vinifera*) leaf extract daily with placebo in patients with mild to moderate forms of CVI.[15] This study reports a reduction of lower leg volume and calf circumference compared with placebo and an improvement of CVI symptoms after a treatment period of 12 weeks. Another double-blind RCT reports a reduction of leg circumference at calf and ankle levels and an increase in microvascular blood flow and oxygen tension.[16]

Hydrotherapy

The results of two RCTs[17,18] which applied cold water stimuli alone or in combination with warm water application suggest beneficial effects for this condition (Table 2.24). The effects of mineral thermal water containing carbon dioxide have been assessed in another RCT.[19] It is reported that venous function was markedly improved after 20 minutes of bathing compared with baseline. A large (n = 2504) observational study reported that the occurrence of acute venous episodes, working days missed, number and duration of hospital admissions, consumption of drugs and physical therapies were reduced in the year after two cycles of thermal hydrotherapy.[20]

CONDITIONS

Table 2.24 **Parallel-armed RCTs of hydrotherapy for chronic venous insufficiency**

Reference	Sample size	Interventions [regimen]	Result	Comment
Ernst E[17]	61	A) Cold water applications [5 × w for 24 d] B) No treatment	A superior to B for symptoms of cramps and pain	Beneficial effects also on ankle and calf circumference
Saradeth T[18]	122	A) Cold (12–18°C) and warm (35–38°C) water applications [10 min/d for 24 d] B) No treatment	A superior to B for symptoms of cramps, pain and pruritus	Beneficial effects also on foot volume, ankle and calf circumference

Supplements

An RCT tested a combination of **alpha-tocopherol**, rutin, *Melilotus officinalis* and *Centella asiatica* in CVI patients without compression stockings.[21] Symptoms such as cramps and leg swelling were reduced at the end of the 4-week treatment period.

Overall recommendation

The evidence for the effectiveness of horse chestnut seed extract is convincing. Given the low frequency of adverse effects and suggestions that it may be as effective as conventional compression therapy, it seems worthy of consideration. The evidence for butcher's broom looks encouraging. Other therapies where encouraging evidence emerges are French maritime pine, gotu kola, red vine leaf and hydrotherapy. Further studies are needed to assess the effectiveness of these treatments. For other complementary therapies for this condition the evidence is unconvincing.

Table 2.25
Summary of clinical evidence for chronic venous insufficiency

Treatment	Weight of evidence	Direction of evidence	Serious safety concerns
Herbal medicine			
Buck wheat	O	⬀	Yes (see p 476)
Butcher's broom	OOO	⬀	Yes (see p 476)
French maritime pine	OO	⬀	Yes (see p 478)
Ginkgo	O	⬂	Yes (see p 404)
Gotu kola	OO	⇧	Yes (see p 478)
Horse chestnut	OOO	⇧	Yes (see p 427)
Red vine leaf	OO	⬀	Yes (see p 414)
Hydrotherapy	OO	⇧	Yes (see p 358)
Supplements			
Alpha-tocopherol	O	⬀	Yes (see p 5)

REFERENCES

1   Ihme N, Kiesewetter H, Jung F, Hoffmann K H, Birk A, Müller A, Grützner K I. Leg edema protection from a buckwheat herb tea in patients with chronic venous insufficiency: a single blind, randomised, placebo-controlled clinical trial. Eur J Clin Pharmacol 1996;50:443–447

2   Rudofsky G, Diehm C, Grua J-D, Hartmann M, Schultz-Ehrenburg H-K, Bisler H. Chronisch venöse Insuffizienz. Münch Med Wochenschr 1990;132:205–210

3   Weindorf N, Schultz-Ehrenburg U. Kontrollierte Studie zur oralen Venentonisierung der primären Varikosis mit Ruscus aculeatus und Trimethy-lherperidinchalkon. Z Hautkr 1987;62:28–38

4   Cappelli R, Nicora M, Di Perri T. Use of extract of ruscus aculeatus in venous disease in the lower limbs. Drugs Exp Clin Res 1988;14:277–283

5   Boyle P, Diehm C, Robertson C. Meta-analysis of clinical trials of Cyclo 3 Fort in the treatment of chronic venous insufficiency. Int Angiol 2003;22:250–262

6   Vanscheidt W, Jost V, Wolna P, Lucker P W, Müller A, Theurer C, Patz B, Grutzner K I. Efficacy and safety of a Butcher's broom preparation (Ruscus aculeatus L. extract) compared to placebo in patients suffering from chronic venous insufficiency. Arzneimittelforschung 2002;52:243–250

7   Rohdewald P. A review of the French maritime pine bark extract (Pycnogenol), a herbal medication with a diverse clinical pharmacology. Int J Clin Pharmacol Ther 2002;40:158–168

8   Janssens D, Michiels C, Guillaume G, Cuisinier B, Louagie Y, Remacle J. Increase in circulating endothelial cells in patients with primary chronic venous insufficiency: protective effect of Ginkgor Fort in a randomized double-blind, placebo-controlled clinical trial. J Cardiovasc Pharmacol 1999;33:7–11

9   Cesarone M R, Laurora G, De Sanctis M T, Incandela L, Grimaldi R, Marelli C, Belcaro G. The microcirculatory activity of Centella asiatica in venous insufficiency. A double-blind study. Minerva Cardioangiologica 1994;42:299–304

10 Pointel J P, Boccalon H, Cloarec M, Ledevehat C, Joubert M. Titrated extract of Centella asiatica (TECA) in the treatment of venous insufficiency of the lower limbs. Angiology 1987;38:46–50

11 Allegra C, Pollari G, Criscuolo A, Bonifacio M, Tabassi D. L'estratto di Centella asiatica nelle flebopatie degli arti inferiori. Clin Ther 1981;99:507–513

12 Pittler M H, Ernst E. Horse chestnut seed extract for chronic venous insufficiency. The Cochrane Database of Systematic Reviews 2004, Issue 2. Art. No.: CD003230

13 Siebert U, Brach M, Sroczynski G, Berla K. Efficacy, routine effectiveness, and safety of horse chestnut seed extract in the treatment of chronic venous insufficiency. A meta-analysis of randomized controlled trials and large observational studies. Int Angiol 2002;21:305–315

14 Tiffany N, Boon H, Ulbricht C, Basch E, Bent S, Barrette E P, Smith M, Sollars D, Dennehy C E, Szapary P. Horse chestnut: a multidisciplinary clinical review. J Herb Pharmacother 2002;2:71–85

15 Kiesewetter H, Koscielny J, Kalus U, Vix J M, Peil H, Petrini O, van Toor B S, de Mey C. Efficacy of orally administered extract of red vine leaf AS 195 (folia vitis viniferae) in chronic venous insufficiency (stages I–II). A randomized, double-blind, placebo-controlled trial. Arzneimittelforschung 2000;50:109–117

16 Kalus U, Koscielny J, Grigorov A, Schaefer F, Peil H, Kiesewetter H. Improvement of cutaneous microcirculation and oxygen supply in patients with chronic venous insufficiency by orally administered extract of red vine leaves AS 195: a randomised, double-blind, placebo-controlled, crossover study. Drugs R D 2004;5:63–71

17 Ernst E, Saradeth T, Resch K L. A single blind randomized, controlled trial of hydrotherapy for varicose veins. Vasa 1991;20:147–152

18 Saradeth T, Ernst E, Resch K L. Hydrotherapy for varicose veins – a randomized controlled trial. Eur J Phys Med 1993;3:123–124

19 Hartmann B, Drews B, Bassenge E. Effects of bathing in CO_2-containing thermal water on the venous hemodynamics of healthy persons with venous diseases. Phys Med Rehabil Kurortmed 1993;3:153–157

20 Coccheri S, Nappi G, Valenti M, Di Orio F, Altobelli E, De Luca S; Naiade Study Group. Changes in the use of health resources by patients with chronic phlebopathies after thermal hydrotherapy. Report from the Naiade project, a nation-wide survey on thermal therapies in Italy. Int Angiol 2002;21:196–200

21 Cataldi A, Gasbarro V, Viaggi R, Soverini R, Gresta E, Mascoli F. Effectiveness of the combination of alpha tocopherol, rutin, melilotus, and centella asiatica in the treatment of patients with chronic venous insufficiency. Minerva Cardioangiol 2001;49:159–163

CONDITIONS

CONSTIPATION

Synonyms   Obstipation, costiveness.

Definition   Bowel actions twice a week or less, for two consecutive weeks, especially in the presence of features such as straining at stool, abdominal discomfort, and sensation of incomplete evacuation. The Rome II criteria diagnoses chronic constipation on the basis of two or more of the following symptoms for at least 12 weeks in the preceding year: straining at defecation on at least a quarter of occasions; stools that are lumpy/hard on at least a quarter of occasions; sensation of incomplete evacuation on at least a quarter of occasions; and three or fewer bowel movements a week.

CAM usage   Herbal medicine is an option frequently used to treat constipation.

Clinical evidence

Acupuncture
A systematic review stated that there is little data on the efficacy of acupuncture in patients with constipation.[1] It identified two controlled trials. In one study including 17 children with chronic constipation, acupuncture gradually increased the frequency of bowel movement during a 10-week treatment period. In adult patients, acupuncture was administered using needles that were electrically stimulated at 10 Hz. There were no differences between treatment and control periods in stool frequency and colonic transit time.

Biofeedback
A systematic review[2] of both the paediatric and adult research included ten studies using a parallel treatment design; seven of which were RCTs. It concluded that although most studies report positive results using biofeedback to treat constipation, quality research is lacking. This is supported by another independent systematic review which concluded that the evidence is insufficient to support the efficacy of biofeedback for gastrointestinal conditions.[3]

Herbal medicine
A herbal combination preparation containing *Aloe vera* was tested in a double-blind RCT (n = 35).[4] There was an increase in bowel movements in the treatment group compared with baseline, which was not different from placebo. Overall, more patients in the treatment group considered themselves improved compared with those in the placebo group.

An RCT (n = 50) assessed the effects of a liquid **Ayurvedic** herbal preparation (Misrakasneham) including *Clitoria ternatea*, *Curcuma longa* and *Vitis vinifera* as well as castor oil in the management of opioid-induced constipation.[5] There were no differences compared with controls who received senna.

Patients with constipation-predominant irritable bowel syndrome were included in a double-blind RCT testing the combination preparation **Padma Lax.**[6] Improvement was demonstrated in the Padma Lax group compared with placebo in constipation, severity of abdominal pain, and its effect on daily activities, incomplete evacuation, abdominal distension and flatulence.

A systematic review identified seven RCTs, which assessed the effectiveness of **psyllium** (*Plantago ovata*) (Box 2.30).[7] It concluded that there is evidence to support its use for chronic constipation. Another double-blind RCT[8] assessed 20 patients, of whom ten had associated irritable bowel syndrome. Stools per week and fecal weight increased in the treatment group compared with baseline, while there were no such changes in the placebo group.

Box 2.30
Systematic review
Psyllium for chronic constipation
Ramkumar[7]

- Only RCTs published in English and conducted on adult subjects were reviewed

- Moderate evidence (Grade B according to the United States Preventive Services Task Force guidelines) was found to support the use of psyllium

- There was a paucity of quality data regarding many commonly used agents including milk of magnesia, senna, bisacodyl, and stool softeners

- Conclusion: There is evidence to support the use of psyllium in chronic constipation

Massage

The evidence for abdominal massage has been assessed in a systematic review (Box 2.31).[9] Concerns relate to the heterogeneity of the studies in terms of trial design, patient samples and type of massage used. The review cautiously concludes that abdominal massage could be a potentially effective treatment option for this condition.

Box 2.31
Systematic review
Abdominal massage for constipation
Ernst[9]

- One RCT and three CCTs including 101 patients

- Trial quality was low

- Two CCTs report an improvement in stool frequency and stool consistency while this is not corroborated by data from an RCT

- Conclusion is limited due to the small number and low quality of available trials

Reflexology

One hundred and thirty postoperative women were randomised to receive one 15-minute session daily for 5 days of either reflexology, leg and foot massage or talking.[10] There were no intergroup differences in stool frequency after the treatment period and after 4 days of follow-up. This is supported by the findings of another single-blind CCT.[11]

Supplements

A systematic review of RCTs concluded that the benefits of treatment with **fibre** are marginal for irritable bowel syndrome-related constipation.[12] A Cochrane review for constipation in pregnancy identified two RCTs (Box 2.32).[13] Fibre supplements increased the frequency of defecation, and led to softer stools.

Box 2.32
Systematic review
**Interventions for
constipation in
pregnancy**
Jewell[13]

- RCTs testing any treatment were included

- Two RCTs were identified

- Fibre supplements increased the frequency of defecation (OR 0.18, CI 0.05 to 0.67)

- Stimulant laxatives are more effective than bulk-forming laxatives (OR 0.30, CI 0.14 to 0.61)

- Conclusion: Fibre in the form of bran or wheat fibre are likely to help women experiencing constipation in pregnancy. If the problem fails to resolve, stimulant laxatives are likely to prove more effective

A **probiotic** beverage containing *Lactobacillus casei* Shirota was tested in a double-blind, placebo-controlled RCT.[14] The consumption of the beverage resulted in an improvement in self-reported severity of constipation and stool consistency. The occurrence and degree of flatulence or bloating sensation did not change. In a double-blind RCT (n = 84) children received lactulose plus colony-forming units of Lactobacillus GG or a placebo.[15] Treatment success was assessed as spontaneous bowel movements and was similar in the control and experimental groups, which led to the conclusion that Lactobacillus GG was not an effective adjunct to lactulose in treating constipation in children.

Other therapies

Two RCTs investigating **electrical stimulation therapy**[16] or relaxation response **meditation**[17] report encouraging data, but require independent replication for any firm recommendation. Another CCT investigated the acute effects of **mineral water** containing sulfate (2754 mg/l) on bowel movements and stool consistency.[18] Beneficial effects are reported for the time to bowel movement and stool consistency in favour of mineral water compared with tap water.

Overall recommendation

The evidence for the short-term effectiveness of biofeedback training is encouraging but more quality research is warranted. Given its relative safety and the risks of long-term conventional treatments, it is a reasonable option for constipated patients. In adult patients there is no concrete evidence for its long-term effectiveness, while conventional treatment is also often limited to short-term relief. In paediatric patients the evidence suggests some benefit from adding biofeedback to conventional treatment, but there seems to be little long-term benefit. Evidence supports the use of psyllium in chronic constipation. Encouraging data exist for fibre supplements in pregnancy-related constipation and constipation in irritable bowel syndrome patients. Abdominal massage may also be beneficial for some patients.

Table 2.26
Summary of clinical evidence for constipation

Treatment	Weight of evidence	Direction of evidence	Serious safety concerns
Acupuncture	OO	⇨	Yes (see p 294)
Biofeedback	OOO	⇗	No (see p 310)
Herbal medicine			
Aloe vera	O	⇗	Yes (see p 364)
Ayurveda	O	⇗	Yes (see p 5)
Padma Lax	O	⇑	Yes (see p 5)
Psyllium	OOO	⇑	Yes (see p 480)
Massage	OO	⇗	No (see p 334)
Reflexology	O	⇩	No (see p 345)
Supplements			
Fibre	OOO	⇗	Yes (see p 5)
Probiotics	OO	⇨	Yes (see p 5)

REFERENCES

1 Ouyang H, Chen J D. Review article: therapeutic roles of acupuncture in functional gastrointestinal disorders. Aliment Pharmacol Ther 2004;20:831–841

2 Heymen S, Jones K R, Scarlett Y, Whitehead W E. Biofeedback treatment of constipation: a critical review. Dis Colon Rectum 2003;46:1208–1217

3 Coulter I D, Favreau J T, Hardy M L, Morton S C, Roth E A, Shekelle P. Biofeedback interventions for gastrointestinal conditions: a systematic review. Altern Ther Health Med 2002;8:76–83

4 Odes H S, Madar Z. A double-blind trial of a celandin, aloe vera and psyllium laxative preparation in adult patients with constipation. Digestion 1991;49:65–71

5 Ramaesh P R, Kumar K S, Rajagopal M R, Balachandran P, Warrier P K. Managing morphine-induced constipation: a controlled

CONDITIONS

comparison of an Ayurvedic formulation and senna. J Pain Symptom Manage 1998;16:240–244

6 Sallon S, Ben-Arye E, Davidson R, Shapiro H, Ginsberg G, Ligumsky M. A novel treatment for constipation-predominant irritable bowel syndrome using Padma Lax, a Tibetan herbal formula. Digestion 2002;65:161–171

7 Ramkumar D, Rao S S. Efficacy and safety of traditional medical therapies for chronic constipation: systematic review. Am J Gastroenterol 2005;100:936–971

8 Tomás-Ridocci M, Añón R, Minguez M, Zaragoza A, Ballester J, y Benages A. Eficacia del Plantago ovaata como regulador del tránsito intestinal. Estudio doble ciego comparativo frente a placebo. Rev Esp Enf Digest 1992;82:17–22

9 Ernst E. Abdominal massage therapy for chronic constipation: A systematic review of controlled clinical trials. Forsch Komplementarmed 1999;6:149–151

10 Kesselring A, Spichiger E, Müller M. Fussre-flexzonenmassage. Pflege 1998;11:213–218

11 Tovey P. A single-blind trial of reflexology for irritable bowel syndrome. Br J Gen Pract 2002;52:19–23

12 Bijkerk C J, Muris J W, Knottnerus J A, Hoes A W, de Wit N J. Systematic review: the role of different types of fiber in the treatment of irritable bowel syndrome. Aliment Pharmacol Ther 2004;19:245–251

13 Jewell D J, Young G. Interventions for treating constipation in pregnancy. Cochrane Database Systc Rev 2001, Issue 2. Art. No.: CD001142

14 Koebnick C, Wagner I, Leitzmann P, Stern U, Zunft HJ. Probiotic beverage containing Lactobacillus casei Shirota improves gastrointestinal symptoms in patients with chronic constipation. Can J Gastroenterol 2003;17:655–659

15 Banaszkiewicz A, Szajewska H. Ineffectiveness of Lactobacillus GG as an adjunct to lactulose for the treatment of constipation in children: a double-blind, placebo-controlled randomized trial. J Pediatr 2005;146:364–369

16 Chang H S, Myung S J, Yang S K, Jung H Y, Kim T H, Yoon I J, Kwon O R, Hong W S, Kim J H, Min Y I. Effect of electrical stimulation in constipated patients with impaired rectal sensation. Int J Colorectal Dis 2003;18:433–438

17 Keefer L, Blanchard E B. The effects of relaxation response meditation on the symptoms of irritable bowel syndrome: results of a controlled treatment study. Behav Res Ther 2001;39:801–811

18 Gutenbrunner C, Gundermann G. Kontrollierte Studie über die abführende Wirkung eines Heilwassers. Z Allg Med 1998;74:648–651

CROHN'S DISEASE

Synonyms	Morbus Crohn, inflammatory bowel disease.
Related conditions	Ulcerative colitis.
Definition	Crohn's disease causes inflammation, deep ulcers and scarring to the wall of the intestine and often occurs in patches. It can affect the gastrointestinal system anywhere from the mouth to the anus but most commonly affects the small intestine and/or colon.
CAM usage	Herbal and non-herbal dietary supplements such as ginseng, *Aloe vera*, and vitamins as well as chiropractic therapy, reflexology and homeopathy are frequently used.[1-3]
Clinical evidence	*Acupuncture* A systematic review identified no prospective clinical studies on acupuncture for inflammatory bowel disease including Crohn's

disease.[4] A subsequent RCT aimed to assess the change in the Crohn's disease activity index (CDAI) and quality of life.[5] Fifty-one patients with mild to moderately active Crohn's disease received acupuncture or sham-acupuncture for ten sessions over a period of 4 weeks. The CDAI decreased compared with placebo, whereas quality of life improved in both groups. No other evidence from prospective clinical trials exist.

Biofeedback

A systematic review assessed the evidence of biofeedback for gastrointestinal conditions.[6] It identified no controlled trials in Crohn's disease.

Herbal medicine

A double-blind RCT tested the effects of *Boswellia serrata* extract H15 in 102 patients.[7] Compared with mesalazine there was no difference in CDAI, whereas comparison with baseline showed a reduction of CDAI in both groups.

Relaxation

Relaxation and short-term psychodynamic therapy in addition to standardised glucocorticoid therapy was tested on the somatic course of disease and on psychosocial status.[8] After one year of treatment and another year of follow-up it was concluded that, although a tendency toward fewer surgical interventions, fewer relapses and a reduction of depression was noted, the results failed to demonstrate effectiveness.

Supplements

A non-systematic review assessed the effectiveness of **fish oil** for inflammatory bowel disease.[9] It identified eight placebo controlled trials of which at least three were RCTs including patients with Crohn's disease. Patients received n-3 fatty acids from fish oil for up to 24 months. It was concluded that the data indicate potential effectiveness in the treatment of Crohn's disease. This conclusion is supported by another double-blind RCT published since the review.[10]

A small (n = 14) double-blind RCT investigated whether oral **glutamine** supplements in addition to routine treatment are able to restore increased intestinal permeability in patients with Crohn's disease.[11] It was concluded that glutamine does not seem to restore impaired intestinal permeability.

Two placebo-controlled RCTs assessed the effects of **probiotics** using *Lactobacillus* GG.[12,13] The trials found that *Lactobacillus* GG did neither prevent endoscopic recurrence nor reduce the severity of recurrent lesion and that there was no benefit in maintaining medically induced remission.

Supplementation with **vitamin E and C** resulted in a reduction in indices of oxidative stress such as breath pentanc and ethane output.[14] The authors concluded that patients with inactive or mildly active disease can be oxidatively stressed and have increased requirements for antioxidant vitamins.

A double-blind placebo controlled RCT tested an adjunctive **yeast** preparation containing *Saccharomyces boulardii* and assessed its effects on diarrhoea in Crohn's patients.[15] A reduction in bowel movements compared with baseline was noted which did not occur in the placebo group. *Saccharomyces boulardii* was also tested in addition to treatment with mesalamine in an RCT.[16] Treatment with the yeast preparation and mesalamine resulted in a reduction of clinical relapses, which did not occur to the same extent when treated with mesalamine alone.

Overall recommendation

The evidence is not sufficiently compelling to recommend any CAM therapy for treating Crohn's disease. The evidence is encouraging for fish oil and a yeast preparation containing *Saccharomyces boulardii* but further trials are required for firm recommendations.

Table 2.27
Summary of clinical evidence for Crohn's disease

Treatment	Weight of evidence	Direction of evidence	Serious safety concerns
Acupuncture	O	↗	Yes (see p 294)
Biofeedback	O	⇨	No (see p 310)
Herbal medicine			
Boswellia serrata	O	↗	Yes (see p 479)
Relaxation	O	↘	No (see p 348)
Supplements			
Fish oil	OO	↗	Yes (see p 483)
Glutamine	O	↘	Yes (see p 483)
Probiotics	OO	⇩	Yes (see p 5)
Vitamins	O	↗	Yes (see p 5)
Yeast	OO	↗	Yes (see p 5)

REFERENCES

1 Hilsden R J, Meddings J B, Verhoef M J. Complementary and alternative medicine use by patients with inflammatory bowel disease: An Internet survey. Can J Gastroenterol 1999;13:327–332

2 Hilsden R J, Scott C M, Verhoef M J. Complementary medicine use by patients with inflammatory bowel disease. Am J Gastroenterol 1998;93:697–701

3 Verhoef M J, Scott C M, Hilsden R J. A multimethod research study on the use of complementary therapies among patients with inflammatory bowel disease. Altern Ther Health Med 1998;4:68–71

4 Diehl D L. Acupuncture for gastrointestinal and hepatobiliary disorders. J Altern Complement Med 1999;5:27–45

5   Joos S, Brinkhaus B, Maluche C, Maupai N, Kohnen R, Kraehmer N, Hahn E G, Schuppan D. Acupuncture and moxibustion in the treatment of active Crohn's disease: a randomized controlled study. Digestion 2004;69:131–139

6   Coulter I D, Favreau J T, Hardy M L, Morton S C, Roth E A, Shekelle P. Biofeedback interventions for gastrointestinal conditions: a systematic review. Altern Ther Health Med 2002;8:76–83

7   Gerhardt H, Seifert F, Buvari P, Vogelsang H, Repges R. Therapy of active Crohn disease with Boswellia serrata extract H 15. Z Gastroenterol 2001;39:11–17

8   Keller W, Pritsch M, Von Wietersheim J, Scheib P, Osborn W, Balck F, Dilg R, Schmelz-Schumacher E, Doppl W, Jantschek G, Deter H C; The German Study Group on Psychosocial Intervention in Crohn's Disease. Effect of psychotherapy and relaxation on the psychosocial and somatic course of Crohn's disease: main results of the German Prospective Multicenter Psychotherapy Treatment study on Crohn's Disease. J Psychosom Res 2004;56:687–696

9   Belluzzi A, Boschi S, Brignola C, Munarini A, Cariani G, Miglio F. Polyunsaturated fatty acids and inflammatory bowel disease. Am J Clin Nutr 2000;71 (Suppl):339S–342S

10 Geerling B J, Badart-Smook A, Van Deursen C, Van Houwelingen A C, Russel M G, Stockbrugger R W, Brummer R J. Nutritional supplementation with n-3 fatty acids and antioxidants in patients with Crohn's disease

in remission: effects on antioxidant status and fatty acid profile. Inflamm Bowel Dis 2000;6:77–84

11 Den Hond E, Hiele M, Peeters M, Ghoos Y, Rutgeerts P. Effect of long-term oral glutamine supplements on small intestinal permeability in patients with Crohn's disease. J Parenter Enteral Nutr 1999;23:7–11

12 Prantera C, Scribano M L, Falasco G, Andreoli A, Luzi C. Ineffectiveness of probiotics in preventing recurrence after curative resection for Crohn's disease: a randomized controlled trial with Lactobacillus GG. Gut 2002;51:405–409

13 Schultz M, Timmer A, Herfarth H H, Sartor R B, Vanderhoof J A, Rath H C. Lactobacillus G G in inducing and maintaining remission of Crohn's disease. BMC Gastroenterol 2004;4:5

14 Aghdassi E, Wendland B E, Steinhart A H, Wolman S L, Jeejeebhoy K, Allard J P. Antioxidant vitamin supplementation in Crohn's disease decreases oxidative stress: a randomized controlled trial. Am J Gastroenterol 2003;98:348–353

15 Plein K, Hotz J. Therapeutic effects of Saccharomyces boulardii on mild residual symptoms in a stable phase of Crohn's disease with special respect to chronic diarrhea – a pilot study. Z Gastroenterol 1993;31:129–134

16 Guslandi M, Mezzi G, Sorghi M, Testoni P A. Saccharomyces boulardii in maintenance treatment of Crohn's disease. Dig Dis Sci 2000;45:1462–1464

DEPRESSION

Synonyms/ subcategories	Depressive disorder, depressive illness, dysthymic disorder, neurotic depression, psychotic depression.
Definition	Persistent low mood, loss of interest and enjoyment and reduced energy. Mild to moderate depression is characterised by depressive symptoms and some functional impairment. Severe depression is characterised by additional agitation or psychomotor retardation with marked somatic symptoms.

Depressed mood as a result of other conditions, e.g. multiple sclerosis or cancer, is excluded from this discussion.

CAM usage

Depression is one of the most common reasons for using CAM. The most popular therapies include exercise, herbal medicine, relaxation and spiritual healing.[1,2]

Clinical evidence

Acupuncture

A systematic review[3] of six RCTs demonstrated that the evidence for acupuncture was inconclusive (Box 2.33).

Box 2.33
Systematic review
Acupuncture for depression
Mukaino[3]

- Six RCTs were found with a total of 509 patients

- Only three of these were of good methodological quality

- The results were inconsistent

- Conclusion: the evidence from RCTs is insufficient for firm recommendations

Autogenic training

A systematic review of all clinical trials of autogenic training (for any condition) found encouraging evidence for its effectiveness in depression.[4]

Exercise

A large body of positive evidence exists for the antidepressant effects of exercise. The majority of studies are not of high quality, but over a dozen RCTs collectively provide convincing evidence of efficacy in clinically depressed patients. Two meta-analyses have found effects after pooling the data. One included 80 studies of any design with all types of participants.[5] The other was restricted to controlled trials with clinically depressed patients (Box 2.34).[6] Both aerobic and non-aerobic forms of exercise were effective. Three RCTs have suggested that aerobic exercise may be as effective as psychological or pharmacological treatment (Table 2.28).[7-9] Whether the antidepressant effects demonstrated are specific to the exercise itself or are due to associated variables is unclear. A further RCT suggested beneficial effects of combining exercise with light exposure.[10]

Guided imagery

A review of 46 studies of guided imagery (regardless of indication) found 'preliminary evidence for the effectiveness of guided imagery in the management of depression'.[11]

Box 2.34
Meta-analysis
Exercise for depression
Craft[6]

- Thirty controlled trials including 2158 patients
- Depression as primary disorder or secondary to other psychiatric disorder
- Comparison groups were mainly waiting lists or psychotherapy
- Trial quality ranged from good to poor
- Significant effect of exercise (mean effect size −0.72; SE 0.10)
- Conclusion: all types of exercise appear to have similar effects

Table 2.28 **RCTs of exercise compared with psychiatric treatment for depression**

Reference	Sample size	Interventions [regimen]	Result	Comment
Klein[7]	74	A) Running [2 × 45 min/w for 12 w] B) Meditation/relaxation C) Group psychotherapy	A no different from B or C	Improvements maintained at 9 mo
Freemont[8]	49	A) Running [3 × 20 min/w for 10 w] B) Cognitive therapy C) Combination of A & B	A no different from B or C	Improvements maintained at 4 mo
Blumenthal[9]	156	A) Walking/jogging [3 × 45 min/w for 16 w] B) Sertraline [200 mg/d] C) Combination of A & B	A no different from B or C; less relapse in A after 6 mo	Patients were all ≥ 50 years

Herbal medicine

Ginkgo (*Ginkgo biloba*) was tested against placebo in a small RCT with 27 patients suffering from 'winter depression'.[12] The results failed to demonstrate effectiveness.

Lavender (*Lavandula angustifolia*) was compared with imipramine in a small RCT with 45 moderately depressed patients.[13] Depressive symptoms improved similarly in both groups, and the authors concluded that lavender 'may be of therapeutic benefit'.

Saffron (*Crocus sativus*) generated similar improvements as imipramine in a small RCT with 30 patients suffering from mild to moderate depression.[14]

There is compelling evidence for the efficacy of St John's wort (*Hypericum perforatum*) in mild to moderate depression from numerous meta-analyses A recent meta-analysis (Box 2.35), which includes also the more recent negative RCTs,[15] comes to a positive conclusion for mild to moderate depression. This overall encouraging finding was modified[16] and it was noted that the

Box 2.35
Meta-analysis
St John's wort for depression
Roder[15]

- Thirty RCTs were included

- Mainly but not exclusively mild–moderate depression

- Trial quality generally good

- Placebo-controlled trials with a total of 2129 patients favoured St John's wort (RR = 0.66, 95% CI 0.57 to 78, NNT = 42)

- Five compared with other antidepressants (n = 2231, RR = 0.96, 95% CI 0.85 to 1.08)

- Favourable side effects profile

- Conclusion: St John's wort is effective for mild–moderate depression

effect size was inversely related to the sample size in placebo controlled RCTs. Newer RCTs and those originating from countries other than Germany tended to generate smaller response rates.

Magnet therapy

An RCT tested exposure to a magnetic field (15 micro T) against sham-therapy in 24 patients on antidepressants. The results suggest that magnetic therapy has a positive additional symptomatic effect.[17]

Massage

Massage was more effective in improving symptoms of depression and anxiety, night time sleep and cortisol levels than watching relaxing videos in an RCT (n = 72) involving children and adolescent inpatients with depression and adjustment disorder.[18] A further recent RCT confirmed these positive findings[19] and a meta-analysis of all RCTs of massage therapy (regardless of indication) concluded that 'reduction of depression were massage therapy's largest effects'.[20]

Mindfulness-based stress reduction

A systematic review of all clinical studies of this approach (regardless of indication) found encouraging evidence that mindfulness-based stress reduction reduces depression.[21]

Music therapy

An RCT of depressed elderly patients (n = 30) found superior results with a music-based intervention than no treatment.[22] The intervention involved various therapeutic modalities. Other RCTs with depressed adolescent females who listened to rock music while control groups received massage[23] or simply relaxed[24] reported changes to physiological and biochemical parameters but not mood or behaviour.

Relaxation

Three small RCTs have suggested that relaxation training is superior to no treatment and potentially similar to cognitive–behavioural therapy (Table 2.29).[25-27] Clearly, non-specific effects are difficult to control for with this therapy. Nonetheless, the evidence can be considered encouraging.

Table 2.29 **RCTs of relaxation therapy for depression**

Reference	Sample size	Interventions [regimen]	Result	Comment
Reynolds[25]	30	A) Relaxation training [10 × 50 min over 5 w] B) Cognitive–behavioural therapy C) Waiting list	A no different from B; both superior to C	Patients were adolescents; improvements maintained at 5 w follow-up
Broota[26]	30	A) Progressive muscle relaxation [1 × 20 min/d for 3 d] B) Yoga and autosuggestion C) Discussion	A no different from B; both superior to C	Patients all on medication
Murphy[27]	37	A) Relaxation training [1–2 × 50 min/w for 12 w] B) Cognitive–behavioural therapy C) Desipramine [150–300 mg]	A no different from B; both superior to C	Substantial non-compliance in medication group

Supplements

Fish oil (omega-3 fatty acids) has been tested in an RCT with 36 depressed patients.[28] The response rates with docosahexaenoic acid (2 g/day) were similar to those of placebo. Another RCT tested a much larger dose (6.6 g/day) in 28 patients with major depression and found that this treatment alleviated depression more than placebo.[29]

Encouraging evidence was found in a systematic review for S-adenosylmethionine.[30]

Zinc was tested against placebo in an RCT with 14 severely depressed and medically treated patients.[31] The results suggest that 12 weeks of zinc supplementation (25 mg/day) has beneficial effects on the symptoms of depression.

Yoga

Four RCTs have tested the effectiveness of yoga for depression (Table 2.30).[32-35] The totality of this evidence suggests, but does not prove, that yoga reduces depressive symptoms.

CONDITIONS

Table 2.30 **RCTs of yoga for depression**

Reference	Sample size	Interventions [regimen]	Result	Comment
Broota[32]	30	A) Special technique developed from yoga (breathing, exercise, meditation) B) Progressive muscle relaxation C) Attention control (each 20 min on 3 consecutive days)	Reduction of symptoms favoured yoga	Author's own treatment technique
Khumar[33]	50	A) Shavasana yoga (breathing technique) B) No such intervention (30 min/day for 30 days)	Reduction of symptoms favoured yoga	No attempt to control for non-specific effects
Janakiramaiah[34]	45	A) Sundarshan Kriya yoga (breathing exercises) B) Electroconvulsive therapy C) Imipramine 150 mg/day (for 4 weeks)	Similar improvements in all 3 groups	Sample size far too small for equivalence trial
Rohini[35]	30	A) Sudarshan Kriya yoga B) Modified Sudarshan Kriya yoga (once/day for 4 weeks)	Similar improvements in all 3 groups	Were both treatments effective or ineffective?

Other therapies

In a small non-randomised trial (n = 20) with male inpatients, adjunctive **aromatherapy** enabled reductions to be made in the dose of antidepressants compared with patients under usual care.[36]

Single sessions of **dance and movement therapy** produced promising results in two small trials with inpatients when compared with no intervention.[37,38]

Reiki was compared with distant Reiki healing and with no treatment at all in an RCT with 46 patients.[39] The results suggest that both Reiki interventions reduced depressive symptoms.

Overall recommendation

No complementary treatment is more effective than conventional pharmacological or psychological interventions. Exercise and St John's wort, however, seem to be equivalent to conventional treatment and have fewer adverse effects. Other approaches for which research is encouraging include autogenic training, massage, relaxation and yoga. As these options are considered relatively safe and given the sizeable placebo response in depression, they may benefit some individuals.

Table 2.31
Summary of clinical evidence for depression

Treatment	Weight of evidence	Direction of evidence	Serious safety concerns
Acupuncture	OO	⇨	Yes (see p 294)
Autogenic training	OO	⬈	Yes (see p 305)
Exercise	OOO	⇧	Yes (see p 5)
Guided imagery	O	⇧	No (see p 359)
Herbal medicine			
Ginkgo	O	⇩	Yes (see p 404)
Lavender	O	⬈	Yes (see p 432)
Saffron	O	⬈	Yes (see p 481)
St John's wort	OOO	⇧	Yes (see p 463)
Magnetic therapy	O	⬈	No (see p 359)
Massage	OO	⇧	No (see p 334)
Mindfulness-based stress reduction	O	⬃	No (see p 360)
Music therapy	OO	⬈	No (see p 360)
Relaxation	OO	⇧	No (see p 348)
Supplements			
Fish oil	OO	⬈	Yes (see p 483)
S-adenosylmethionine	O	⬈	No (see p 484)
Zinc	O	⇧	No (see p 5)
Yoga	OO	⬈	Yes (see p 356)

CONDITIONS

REFERENCES

1 Astin J A. Why patients use alternative medicine. JAMA 1998;279:1548–1553

2 Eisenberg D M, Davis R B, Ettner S L, Appel S, Wilkey S, Rompay M V, Kessler R C. Trends in alternative medicine use in the United States, 1990–1997. JAMA 1998;280:1569–1575

3 Mukaino Y, Park J, White A, Ernst E. Effectiveness of acupuncture for depression: a systematic review of randomised controlled trials. Acupunct Med 2005;23:70–76

4 Stetter F, Kupper S. Autogenic training: a meta-analysis of clinical outcome studies. Appl Psychophysiol Biofeedback 2002;27:45–98

5 North T C, McCullagh P, Vu Tran Z. Effect of exercise on depression. Ex Sport Sci Rev 1990;18:379–415

6 Craft L L, Landers D M. The effect of exercise on clinical depression and depression resulting from mental illness: A meta-analysis. J Sport and Exercise Psychol 1998;20:339–357

7 Klein M H, Greist J H, Gurman A S, Neimeyer R A, Lesser D P, Bushnell N J, Smith, R E. A comparative outcome study of group psychotherapy vs exercise treatments for depression. Int J Ment Health 1985;13:148–177

8 Freemont J, Craighead L W. Aerobic exercise and cognitive therapy in the treatment of dysphoric moods. Cognitive Therapy and Research 1987;11:241–251

9 Blumenthal J A, Babyak M A, Moore K A, Craighead W E, Herman S, Khatri P, Waugh R, Napolitano M A, Forman L M, Appelbaum M, Doraiswamy P M, Krishnan K R. Effects of exercise training on older patients with major depression. Arch Intern Med 1999;159:2349–2356

10 Leppamaki S, Haukka J, Lonnqvist J, Partonen T. Drop-out and mood improvement: a randomized controlled trial with light exposure and physical exercise. BMC Psychiatry 2004;4:22

11 Eller L S. Guided imagery interventions for symptom management. Ann Rev Nurs Res 1999;17:57–84

12 Lingaerde O, Foreland A R, Magnusson A. Can winter depression be prevented by

Ginkgo biloba extract? A placebo-controlled trial. Acta Psychiatr Scand 1999;100:62–66

13 Akhondzadeh S, Kashani L, Fotouhi A, Jarvandi S, Mobaseri M, Moin M, Khani M, Jamshidi A H, Baghalian K, Taghizadeh M. Comparison of Lavandula angustifolia Mill. Tincture and imipramine in the treatment of mild to moderate depression: a double-blind, randomized trial. Prog Neuropsychopharmacol Biol Psychiatry 2003;27:123–127

14 Akhondzadeh S, Fallah-Pour H, Afkham K, Jamshidi A H, Khalighi-Cigaroudi F. Comparison of Crocus sativus L. and imipramine in the treatment of mild to moderate depression: a double-blind randomized trial. BMC Complement Altern Med 2004;4:12

15 Roder C, Schaefer M, Leucht S. Meta-analysis of effectiveness and tolerability of treatment of mild to moderate depression with St John's wort. [Article in German] Fortschr Neurol Psychiatr 2004;72:330–343

16 Linde K, Mulrow C, Berner M, Egger M. St John's Wort for depression. The Cochrane Database of Systematic Reviews 2005, Issue 2. Art No.: CD000448

17 Sieron A, Hese R T, Sobis J, Ciesla G. Estimation of therapeutical efficacy of weak variable magnetic fields with low value of induction in patients with depression. [Article in Polish] Psychiatr Pol 2004;38:217–225

18 Field T, Morrow C, Valdeon C, Larson S, Kuhn C, Schanberg S. Massage reduces anxiety in child and adolescent psychiatric patients. J Am Acad Child Adolesc Psychiatr 1992;31:125–131

19 Muller-Oerlinghausen B, Berg C, Scherer P, Mackert A, Moestl H P, Wolf J. Effects of slow-stroke massage as complementary treatment of depressed hospitalized patients. [Article in German] Dtsch Med Wochenschr 2004;129:1363–1368

20 Moyer C A, Rounds J, Hannum J W. A meta-analysis of massage therapy research. Psychol Bull 2004;130:3–18

21 Grossman P, Niemann L, Schmidt S, Walach H. Mindfulness-based stress reduction and health benefits. A meta-analysis. J Psychosom Res 2004;57:35–43

22 Hanser S B. Thompson L W. Effects of music therapy strategy on depressed older adults. J Gerontol 1994;49:265–269

23 Jones N A, Field T. Massage and music therapies attenuate frontal EEG asymmetry in depressed adolescents. Adolescence 1999;34:529–534

24 Field T, Martinez A, Nawrocki T, Pickens J, Fox N A, Schanberg S. Music shifts frontal EEG in depressed adolescents. Adolescence 1998;33:109–116

25 Reynolds W M, Coats K I. A comparison of cognitive–behavioral therapy and relaxation training for the treatment of depression in adolescents. J Consult Clin Psychol 1986;54:653–660

26 Broota A, Dhir R. Efficacy of two relaxation techniques in depression. J Pers Clin Stud 1990;6:83–90

27 Murphy G E, Carney R M, Knesevich M A, Wetzel R D, Whitworth P. Cognitive behavior therapy, relaxation training, and tricyclic antidepressant medication in the treatment of depression. Psychol Rep 1995;77:403–420

28 Marangell L B, Martinez J M, Zboyan H A, Kertz B, Kim H F, Puryear L J. A double-blind, placebo-controlled study of the omega-3 fatty acid docosahexaenoic acid in the treatment of major depression. Am J Psychiatry 2003;160:996–998

29 Su K P, Huang S Y, Chiu C C, Shen W W. Omega-3 fatty acids in major depressive disorder. A preliminary double-blind, placebo-controlled trial. Eur Neuropsychopharmacol 2003;13:267–271

30 Jorm A F, Christensen H, Griffiths K M, Rodgers B. Effectiveness of complementary and self-help treatments for depression. Med J Aust 2002;176:S84–S96

31 Nowak G, Siwek M, Dudek D, Zieba A, Pilc A. Effect of zinc supplementation on antidepressant therapy in unipolar depression: a preliminary placebo-controlled study. Pol J Pharmacol 2003;55:1143–1147

32 Broota A, Dhir R. Efficacy of two relaxation techniques in depression. J Pers Clin Stud 1990;6:83–90

33 Khumar S S, Kaur P, Kaur S. Effectiveness of Shavasana on depression among university students. Ind J Clin Psychol 1993;20:82–87

34 Janakiramaiah N, Gangadhar B N, Naga Venkatesha Murthy P J, Harish M G, Subbakrishna D K, Vedamurthachar A. Antidepressant efficacy of Sudarshan Kriya Yoga in melancholia: a randomized comparison with electroconvulsive therapy and imipramine. J Affect Dis 2000;57:255–259

35 Rohini V, Pandey R S, Janakiramaiah N, Gangadhar B N, Vedamurthachar A. A comparative study of full and partial Sudarshan Kriya Yoga (SKY) in major depressive disorder. NIMHANS J 2000;18:53–57

36 Komori T, Fujiwara R, Tanida M, Nomura J, Yokoyama M M. Effects of citrus fragrance on immune function and depressive states. Neuroimmunomodulation 1995;2:174–180

37 Brooks D, Stark A. The effect of dance/
    movement therapy on affect: a pilot study.
    Am J Dance Ther 1989;11:101–112
38 Stewart N J, McMullen L M, Rubin L D.
    Movement therapy with depressed
    inpatients: a randomized multiple single-

    case design. Arch Psychiatr Nurs
    1994;8:22–29
39 Shore A G. Long-term effects of energetic
    healing on symptoms of psychological
    depression and self-perceived stress. Altern
    Ther Health Med 2004;10:42–48

DIABETES

Synonyms   Sugar disease, sugar sickness

Definition   Diabetes mellitus is a group of disorders characterised by hypergly-caemia (definitions vary slightly: fasting plasma glucose = 7.0 mmol/l or = 11.1 mmol/l, 2 h after a 75 g oral glucose load, on two or more occasions). Intensive treatment is designed to achieve blood glucose values as close to the non-diabetic range as possible. The components of such treatment are education, counselling, monitoring, self management, and pharmacological treatment.

Related conditions / subcategories   Type 1 diabetes or insulin-dependent diabetes mellitus (IDDM), type 2 diabetes or non-insulin dependent diabetes mellitus (NIDDM), gestational diabetes.

CAM usage   A national US survey on CAM reported that 95 of 2055 respondents reported having diabetes, of whom 57% reported CAM use in the past year; fewer respondents (35%) reported use specifically for diabetes.[1] Therapies used for diabetes included solitary prayer/spiritual practices (28%), herbal remedies (7%), commercial diets (6%), and folk remedies (3%). Excluding solitary prayer, only 20% of respondents used CAM to treat diabetes. The prevalence of CAM therapy use among patients with diabetes is similar to that among the general population.

Clinical evidence   A systematic review assessed the effectiveness and safety of all herbal treatments, vitamin and mineral supplements for glucose control in patients with diabetes (Box 2.36).[2] The review concluded that there is insufficient evidence to draw definitive conclusions about the effectiveness of individual herbs and supplements. The best evidence from adequately designed RCTs is available for *Coccinia indica* and American ginseng (*Panax quinquefolius*). Chromium has been the most widely studied non-herbal supplement. Other supplements with encouraging preliminary results include *Gymnema sylvestre*, *Aloe vera*, vanadium, *Momordica charantia*, and *Opuntia streptacantha*.

Herbal medicine

A systematic review assessed the effectiveness of **Ayurvedic interventions** for diabetes mellitus (Box 2.37).[3] Holy basil, fenugreek and the herbal formulas Ayush-82 and D-400 may have a glucose-lowering effect and deserve further study. For *Coccinia indica* and

CONDITIONS

Box 2.36
Systematic review
Herbs and dietary supplements for diabetes
Yeh[2]

- 108 trials examining 36 herbs and nine vitamin and/or mineral supplements (n = 4565) patients with diabetes or impaired glucose tolerance were analysed

- Forty-two RCTs and 16 non-randomised controlled trials were identified

- Of these 58 trials, the direction of the evidence for improved glucose control was positive in 76% (44 of 58).

- Very few adverse events were reported

- Conclusion: there is still insufficient evidence to draw definitive conclusions about the efficacy of individual herbs and supplements for diabetes

Gymnema sylvestre this review supports the findings of the above study.[2] Evidence of effectiveness of several other herbs is less extensive such as *C. tamala, Eugenia jambolana*, and *Momordica charantia*. An additional double-blind, placebo-controlled RCT

Box 2.37
Systematic review
Ayurvedic interventions for type 2 diabetes mellitus
Hardy[3]

- Herbal therapy was the most commonly studied treatment. Fifty-four identified articles contained the results of 62 studies

- Seven RCTs, ten CCTs, 38 case series (the most frequently used clinical design) and seven cohort studies were identified

- There is evidence to suggest that the single herbs *Coccinia indica*, holy basil, fenugreek, and *Gymnema sylvestre* and the herbal formulas Ayush-82 and D-400 have glucose-lowering effects

- Methodological shortcomings were observed

- Conclusion: no strong conclusions can be drawn

tested Pancreas Tonic, a mixture of Indian Ayurvedic herbs in type 2 diabetic patients.[4] Concurrent oral agents were unchanged and treatment for 3 months improved glucose control in patients with HbA$_{1c}$ levels between 10.0% to 12.0% compared with baseline.

Twenty patients with type 2 diabetes who took hyperglycaemic drugs as prescribed were assessed in an RCT and consumed 1.5 l oolong tea made of *Camellia sinensis* or water for 30 days.[5] Oolong tea lowered concentrations of plasma glucose levels whereas the water control group had not changed compared with baseline. Another trial assessing herbal tea failed to show an effect in type 2 diabetic patients.[6]

A Cochrane review assessed the effects of **Chinese herbal medicines** (Box 2.38).[7] It concluded that some herbal medicines have

CONDITIONS

Box 2.38
Systematic review
**Chinese herbal
medicines for type
2 diabetes mellitus**
Liu[7]

- Sixty-six RCTs, involving 8302 participants, met the inclusion criteria

- Methodological quality was generally low

- Sixty-nine different herbal medicines were tested

- Control groups received either placebo, hypoglycaemic drugs, or herbal medicines plus hypoglycaemic drugs

- Conclusion: it is not possible to recommend any of the examined herbs for clinical routine use

beneficial effects on blood glucose control in type 2 diabetes mellitus. However, it is not possible to recommend any of the examined herbs for clinical routine use, since the majority of the trials had low methodological quality and the benefit has not been confirmed by high-quality, large trials. Three additional RCTs report beneficial effects for three different Chinese herbal medicines.[8 10]

An RCT included 60 patients with type 2 diabetes to determine whether **cinnamon** (*Cinnamomum zeylanicum*) improves blood glucose, triglyceride, total cholesterol, HDL cholesterol, and LDL cholesterol levels.[11] Intake of 1, 3, or 6 g of cinnamon daily reduced serum glucose, triglyceride, LDL cholesterol, and total cholesterol.

Two RCTs testing **fenugreek** (*Trigonella foenum-graecum*) reported beneficial effects on blood glucose levels and triglycerides levels compared with baseline[12] and placebo.[13]

A systematic review identified one RCT which tested **ginseng** and reported improvement of fasting blood glucose levels and HbA_{1c} compared with baseline.[14] Additional RCTs of American ginseng (*Panax quinquefolius*) reported some positive results.[15,16]

A systematic review included 18 RCTs which tested soluble fibre from **guar gum** (*Cyamopsis tetragonolobus*). Eight of these tested guar gum in patients with diabetes mellitus (Box 2.39).[17] Overall, intergroup differences are reported for total and LDL cholesterol in favour of guar gum. These findings are supported by an RCT comparing a moderate fibre group, given predominately insoluble fibre, with a high fibre group of equal amounts of soluble and insoluble fibre.[18] It concluded that high intake of dietary fibre, particularly of the soluble type improves glycaemic control, decreases hyperinsulinaemia, and lowers plasma lipid concentrations in patients with type 2 diabetes.

Ipomoea batatas (Caiapo), an extract of white sweet potatoes was evaluated in two RCTs.[19,20] Caiapo decreased 2 hour glucose levels after a 75 g oral glucose tolerance test and total cholesterol more than placebo and thus supported the findings of the earlier pilot study in type 2 diabetes.[20]

An RCT (n = 60) reported that the herbal product **Inolter** achieved better hypoglycaemic effects than placebo and

Box 2.39
Meta-analysis
Guar gum for reducing cholesterol in diabetic patients
Brown[17]

- Eighteen RCTs (n = 356) of 66 days duration on average were reviewed

- Eight were conducted in patients with diabetes mellitus

- Guar gum lowers total cholesterol by 0.03 mmol/l/g, CI −0.04 to −0.02 mmol/l/g, lowers LDL cholesterol by 0.03 mmol/l/g, CI −0.05 to −0.02 mmol/l/g

- Conclusion: The lipid lowering effect of guar gum is small within the practical range of intake

lowered serum lipids more than placebo in type 2 diabetic patients.[21]

Mulberry (*Morus indica*) leaves are reported to have hypoglycaemic and hypolipidaemic effects in pre–post assessments (n = 24).[22]

A systematic review included 12 RCTs which tested soluble fibre from **psyllium** (*Plantago ovata*) in hyperlipidaemic patients and suggested overall positive effects.[17] In men with type 2 diabetes and hypercholesterolaemia psyllium showed improvements in glucose and lipid values compared with placebo.[23] Serum total and LDL-cholesterol concentrations were lower in the psyllium group compared with the placebo group. This extends earlier findings in diabetic patients.[24,25]

A double-blind RCT (n = 77) was performed to investigate anti-diabetic effects of the French maritime pine (*Pinus pinaster*) bark extract, **Pycnogenol**.[26] Supplementation with Pycnogenol for 12 weeks, during which a standard anti-diabetic treatment was continued, lowered plasma glucose levels as compared with placebo.

Dietary supplementation with isoflavones from **red clover** (*Trifolium pratense*) was tested in postmenopausal type 2 diabetics (n = 16) in a double-blind RCT.[27] Mean daytime systolic and diastolic blood pressures were lowered during isoflavone therapy compared with placebo.

Two single RCTs, which tested *Tinospora crispa* powder[28] and **xioke tea**[29] reported no beneficial effects.

Supplements

A systematic review and meta-analysis identified 20 RCTs assessing the effect of **chromium** on glucose, insulin, or glycated haemoglobin HbA_{1c}.[30] It summarises data on 15 trials (n = 618) including 193 patients with type 2 diabetes and 425 healthy participants who had impaired glucose tolerance. It concluded that the data for patients with diabetes are inconclusive and that there is no effect on glucose or insulin concentrations in non-diabetic subjects. A placebo-controlled trial suggested that chromium supplementation was an effective treatment strategy to minimise increased oxidative stress in patients whose HbA_{1c} level was > 8.5%.[31]

Coenzyme Q10 was tested in a double-blind RCT (n = 77) in subjects with uncomplicated type 2 diabetes and dyslipidaemia. The main effect of Coenzyme Q10 was to decrease systolic and diastolic blood pressure and HbA$_{1c}$ compared with baseline.[32]

A Cochrane review aimed to determine the effects of **fish oil** supplementation on cardiovascular outcomes, cholesterol levels and glycaemic control in patients with type 2 diabetes mellitus (Box 2.40).[33] It concluded that it has no effect on glycaemic control. It lowers triglycerides and may raise LDL cholesterol, especially in hypertriglyceridaemic patients on higher doses of fish oil. A small (n = 11) double-blind RCT found no differences in weight, fasting glucose, and insulin levels, HbA$_{1c}$, total, LDL, and HDL cholesterol levels, but was associated with reductions in triglyceride levels.[34] Two RCTs found that fish oil leads to an increase in oxidative stress parameters,[35,36] whereas another RCT observed beneficial changes.[37] The results of a double-blind RCT suggested that fish oils alter vascular reactivity.[38]

Box 2.40
Systematic review
Fish oil for type 2 diabetes mellitus
Farmer[33]

- Eighteen RCTs (n – 823) of 12 weeks duration on average were included

- Doses of fish oil used ranged from 3 to 18 g/day

- Fish oil lowers triglycerides by 0.56 mmol/l, CI –0.71 to –0.40 mmol/l and raises LDL cholesterol by 0.21 mmol/l, CI 0.02 to 0.41 mmol/l in diabetic patients

- No adverse effects of the intervention were reported

- Conclusion: Fish oil lowers triglycerides, may raise LDL cholesterol and has no effect on glycaemic control

A placebo-controlled, double-blind RCT set out to evaluate possible effects of **glucosamine** supplementation on glycaemic control in patients with type 2 diabetes mellitus.[39] Mean HbA$_{1c}$ concentrations were not different between groups prior to glucosamine therapy. Posttreatment HbA$_{1c}$ concentrations were not different between groups, nor were there any differences within groups before and after treatment.

Three independent double-blind RCTs (n = 195) assessed the effects of **magnesium** for glycaemic control and reported no beneficial effects in type 2 diabetes.[40–42]

Two RCTs assessed the effects of dietary supplementation with **soy** protein in type 2 diabetes and report beneficial effects on fasting insulin, insulin resistance, total and LDL cholesterol compared with placebo and animal protein.[43,44] This is supported to a degree by a trial that assessed soybean-derived Touchi extract, a traditional Chinese food.[45]

The effects of **vitamin** E were assessed in patients with type 1 diabetes by three RCTs.[46–48] Improvements are reported in one of each trial for flow-mediated vasodilation, for retinal blood flow and in vitro peroxidisability of LDL and VLDL. In type 2 diabetes patients with peripheral sensorimotor polyneuropathy the data suggested improved nerve conduction velocity in median motor nerve fibres and tibial motor nerve latency.[49] Vitamin E also seems to increase the resistance of LDL to oxidation and decreases plasma levels of C-reactive protein.[50] Zinc, magnesium and vitamin C in addition to vitamin E increased HDL-c and apolipoprotein A1 levels,[51] whereas it reduced systolic and diastolic blood pressure compared with baseline.[52]

Zinc alone and in combination with chromium did not alter HbA_{1c} nor glucose homeostasis.[53,54] Potentially beneficial antioxidant effects are reported.

Other therapies

Single RCTs which report some positive effects tested **Qi-gong**[55] and **reflexology**[56] in type 2 diabetic patients.

Overall recommendation

There is evidence to suggest that guar gum is effective for lowering lipid levels in patients with type 2 diabetes. There are also some suggestions that it improves glycaemic control. Some Ayurvedic and Chinese herbal medicines have beneficial effects on blood glucose control. However, it is not possible to recommend any of the examined herbs for clinical routine use. Other medicines with encouraging data, which require further study, are fenugreek, *Ipomoea batatas*, psyllium and soy.

Table 2.32
Summary of clinical evidence for diabetes

Treatment	Weight of evidence	Direction of evidence	Serious safety concerns
Herbal medicine			
Ayurveda	OOO	⤴	Yes (see p 5)
Camellia sinensis	O	⇨	Yes (see p 417)
Chinese herbal medicines	OOO	⤴	Yes (see p 5)
Cinnamon	O	⤴	Yes (see p 477)
Fenugreek	OO	⇧	Yes (see p 478)
Ginseng	OO	⤴	Yes (see p 407)
Guar gum	OOO	⇧	Yes (see p 419)
Ipomoea batatas	OO	⇧	Yes (see p 477)
Inolter	O	⇧	Yes (see p 5)
Mulberry	O	⤴	Yes (see p 5)
Psyllium	OOO	⇧	Yes (see p 480)

Treatment	Weight of evidence	Direction of evidence	Serious safety concerns
Pycnogenol	◑	⇅	Yes (see p 4/8)
Red clover	○	⇧	Yes (see p 456)
Tinospora crispa	○	⇩	Yes (see p 5)
Xioke tea	○	⇩	Yes (see p 5)
Supplements			
Chromium	○○○	⇨	Yes (see p 482)
Coenzyme Q10	○	⬈	Yes (see p 385)
Fish oil	○○○	⬂	Yes (see p 483)
Glucosamine	○	⇩	Yes (see p 412)
Magnesium	○○	⇩	Yes (see p 5)
Soy	○○	⇧	Yes (see p 450)
Vitamin E	○○	⬃	Yes (see p 5)
Zinc	○○	⇨	Yes (see p 5)

CONDITIONS

REFERENCES

1   Yeh G Y, Eisenberg D M, Davis R B, Phillips R S. Use of complementary and alternative medicine among persons with diabetes mellitus: results of a national survey. Am J Public Health 2002;92:1648–1652

2   Yeh G Y, Eisenberg D M, Kaptchuk T J, Phillips R S. Systematic review of herbs and dietary supplements for glycemic control in diabetes. Diabetes Care 2003;26:1277–1294

3   Hardy M I., Coulter I, Venuturupalli S, Roth F A, Favreau J, Morton S C, Shekelle P, Ayurvedic interventions for diabetes mellitus: a systematic review. Evid Rep Technol Assess (Summ) 2001;41:2p

4   Hsia S H, Bazargan M, Davidson M B. Effect of Pancreas Tonic (an ayurvedic herbal supplement) in type 2 diabetes mellitus. Metabolism 2004;53:1166–1173

5   Hosoda K, Wang M F, Liao M L, Chuang C K, Iha M, Clevidence B, Yamamoto S. Antihyperglycemic effect of oolong tea in type 2 diabetes. Diabetes Care 2003;26:1714–1718

6   Ryan E A, Imes S, Wallace C, Jones S. Herbal tea in the treatment of diabetes mellitus. Clin Invest Med 2000;23:311–317

7   Liu J P, Zhang M, Wang W Y, Grimsgaard S. Chinese herbal medicines for type 2 diabetes mellitus. Cochrane Database Syst Rev 2002, Issue 3. Art. No.: CD003642

8   Gao S R, Bu J H, Zhu L Z. Preliminary exploration on effect of qilian decoction in intervention treatment of diabetes mellitus type 2 with insulin resistance and its influence on related inflammatory cytokines. Zhongguo Zhong Xi Yi Jie He Za Zhi 2004;24:593–595

9   Chen P, Zhu Z Z, Lang J M, Wei A, Chen F. Clinical observation on effect of Yiqi Yangyin Huoxue Tongfu principle in treating diabetes mellitus type 2 of secondary failure to sulfonylurea agents. Zhongguo Zhong Xi Yi Jie He Za Zhi 2004;24:585–588

10 Zhu L Q, Liu Y H, Huang M, Wei H, Liu Z. Study on improvement of islet beta cell function in patients with latent autoimmune diabetes mellitus in adults by integrative Chinese and Western medicine. Zhongguo Zhong Xi Yi Jie He Za Zhi 2004;24:581–584

11 Khan A, Safdar M, Ali Khan M M, Khattak K N, Anderson R A. Cinnamon improves glucose and lipids of people with type 2 diabetes. Diabetes Care 2003;26:3215–3218

12 Sharma R D, Raghuram T C, Rao N S. Effect of fenugreek seeds on blood glucose and serum lipids in type I diabetes. Eur J Clin Nutr 1990;44:301–306

13 Gupta A, Gupta R, Lal B. Effect of Trigonella foenum-graecum (fenugreek) seeds on glycaemic control and insulin resistance in type 2 diabetes mellitus: a double blind placebo controlled study. J Assoc Physicians India 2001;49:1057–1061

14 Vogler B K, Pittler M H, Ernst E. The efficacy of ginseng. A systematic review of

randomised clinical trials. Eur J Clin Pharmacol 1999;55:567–575

15   Vuksan V, Stavro M P, Sievenpiper J L, Beljan-Zdravkovic U, Leiter L A, Josse R G, Xu Z. Similar postprandial glycemic reductions with escalation of dose and administration time of American ginseng in type 2 diabetes. Diabetes Care 2000;23:1221–1226

16   Vuksan V, Sievenpiper J L, Koo V Y, Francis T, Beljan-Zdravkovic U, Xu Z, Vidgen E. American ginseng (Panax quinquefolius L) reduces postprandial glycemia in non-diabetic subjects and subjects with type 2 diabetes mellitus. Arch Intern Med 2000;160:1009–1013

17   Brown L, Rosner B, Willett W W, Sacks F M. Cholesterol-lowering effects of dietary fiber: a meta-analysis. Am J Clin Nutr 1999;69:30–42

18   Chandalia M, Garg A, Lutjohann D, von Bergmann K, Grundy S M, Brinkley L J. Beneficial effects of high dietary fiber intake in patients with type 2 diabetes mellitus. N Engl J Med 2000;342:1392–1398

19   Ludvik B, Neuffer B, Pacini G. Efficacy of Ipomoea batatas (Caiapo) on diabetes control in type 2 diabetic subjects treated with diet. Diabetes Care 2004;27:436–440

20   Ludvik B H, Mahdjoobian K, Waldhaeusl W, Hofer A, Prager R, Kautzky-Willer A, Pacini G. The effect of Ipomoea batatas (Caiapo) on glucose metabolism and serum cholesterol in patients with type 2 diabetes: a randomized study. Diabetes Care 2002;25:239–240

21   Agrawal R P, Sharma A, Dua A S, Chandershekhar Y C, Kochar D K, Kothari R P. A randomized placebo controlled trial of Inolter (herbal product) in the treatment of type 2 diabetes. J Assoc Physicians India 2002;50:391–393

22   Andallu B, Suryakantham V, Lakshmi Srikanthi B, Reddy G K. Effect of mulberry (Morus indica L.) therapy on plasma and erythrocyte membrane lipids in patients with type 2 diabetes. Clin Chim Acta 2001;314:47–53

23   Anderson J W, Allgood L D, Turner J, Oeltgen P R, Daggy B P. Effects of psyllium on glucose and serum lipid responses in men with type 2 diabetes and hypercholesterolemia. Am J Clin Nutr 1999;70:466–473

24   Uribe M, Dibildox M, Malpica S, Guillermo E, Villallobos A, Nieto L, Vargas F, Garcia Ramos G. Beneficial effect of vegetable protein diet supplemented with psyllium plantago in patients with hepatic encephalopathy and diabetes mellitus. Gastroenterology 1985;88:901–907

25   Pastors J G, Blaisdell P W, Balm T K, Asplin C M, Pohl S L. Psyllium fiber reduces rise in postprandial glucose and insulin concentrations in patients with non-insulin-dependent diabetes. Am J Clin Nutr 1991;53:1431–1435

26   Liu X, Wei J, Tan F, Zhou S, Wurthwein G, Rohdewald P. Antidiabetic effect of Pycnogenol French maritime pine bark extract in patients with diabetes type II. Life Sci 2004;75:2505–2513

27   Howes J B, Tran D, Brillante D, Howes L G. Effects of dietary supplementation with isoflavones from red clover on ambulatory blood pressure and endothelial function in postmenopausal type 2 diabetes. Diabetes Obes Metab 2003;5:325–332

28   Sangsuwan C, Udompanthurak S, Vannasaeng S, Thamlikitkul V. Randomized controlled trial of Tinospora crispa for additional therapy in patients with type 2 diabetes mellitus. J Med Assoc Thai 2004;87:543–546

29   Hale P J, Horrocks P M, Wright A D, Fitzgerald M G, Nattrass M, Bailey C J. Xiaoke tea, a Chinese herbal treatment for diabetes mellitus. Diabet Med 1989;6:675–676

30   Althuis M D, Jordan N E, Ludington E A, Wittes J T. Glucose and insulin responses to dietary chromium supplements: a meta-analysis. Am J Clin Nutr 2002;76:148–155

31   Cheng H H, Lai M H, Hou W C, Huang C L. Antioxidant effects of chromium supplementation with type 2 diabetes mellitus and euglycemic subjects. J Agric Food Chem 2004;52:1385–1389

32   Hodgson J M, Watts G F, Playford D A, Burke V, Croft K D. Coenzyme Q10 improves blood pressure and glycaemic control: a controlled trial in subjects with type 2 diabetes. Eur J Clin Nutr 2002;56:1137–1142

33   Farmer A, Montori V, Dinneen S, Clar C. Fish oil in people with type 2 diabetes mellitus. Cochrane Database Syst Rev 2001, Issue 3. Art. No.: CD003205

34   McManus R M, Jumpson J, Finegood D T, Clandinin M T, Ryan E A. A comparison of the effects of n-3 fatty acids from linseed oil and fish oil in well-controlled type II diabetes. Diabetes Care 1996;19:463–467

35   McGrath L T, Brennan G M, Donnelly J P, Johnston G D, Hayes J R, McVeigh G E. Effect of dietary fish oil supplementation on peroxidation of serum lipids in patients with non-insulin dependent diabetes mellitus. Atherosclerosis 1996;121:275–283

36   Pedersen H, Petersen M, Major-Pedersen A, Jensen T, Nielsen N S, Lauridsen S T, Marckmann P. Influence of fish oil supplementation on in vivo and in vitro oxidation resistance of low-density lipoprotein in type 2 diabetes. Eur J Clin Nutr 2003;57:713–720

37 Jain S, Gaiha M, Bhattacharjee J, Anuradha S. Effects of low-dose omega-3 fatty acid substitution in type-2 diabetes mellitus with special reference to oxidative stress a prospective preliminary study. J Assoc Physicians India 2002;50:1028–1033

38 McVeigh G E, Brennan G M, Cohn J N, Finkelstein S M, Hayes R J, Johnston G D. Fish oil improves arterial compliance in non-insulin-dependent diabetes mellitus. Arteriocler Thromb 1994;14:1425–1429

39 Scroggie D A, Albright A, Harris M D. The effect of glucosamine-chondroitin supplementation on glycosylated hemoglobin levels in patients with type 2 diabetes mellitus: a placebo-controlled, double-blinded, randomized clinical trial. Arch Intern Med 2003;163:1587–1590

40 Eriksson J, Kohvakka A. Magnesium and ascorbic acid supplementation in diabetes mellitus. Ann Nutr Metab 1995;39:217–223

41 Lima Mde L, Cruz T, Pousada J C, Rodrigues L E, Barbosa K, Cangucu V. The effect of magnesium supplementation in increasing doses on the control of type 2 diabetes. Diabetes Care 1998;21:682–686

42 Johnsen S P, Husted S E, Ravn H B, Stodkilde-Jorgensen H, Peltz-Andresen E, Christensen C K. Magnesium supplementation to patients with type II diabetes. Ugeskr Laeger 1999;161:945–948

43 Jayagopal V, Albertazzi P, Kilpatrick E S, Howarth E M, Jennings P E, Hepburn D A, Atkin SL. Beneficial effects of soy phytoestrogen intake in postmenopausal women with type 2 diabetes. Diabetes Care 2002;25:1709–1714

44 Azadbakht L, Shakerhosseini R, Atabak S, Jamshidian M, Mehrabi Y, Esmaill-Zadeh A. Beneficiary effect of dietary soy protein on lowering plasma levels of lipid and improving kidney function in type II diabetes with nephropathy. Eur J Clin Nutr 2003;57:1292–1294

45 Fujita H, Yamagami T, Ohshima K. Long-term ingestion of a fermented soybean-derived Touchi-extract with alpha-glucosidase inhibitory activity is safe and effective in humans with borderline and mild type-2 diabetes. Nutr 2001;131:2105–2108

46 Bursell S E, Clermont A C, Aiello L P, Aiello L M, Schlossman D K, Feener E P, Laffel L, King G L. High-dose vitamin E supplementation normalizes retinal blood flow and creatinine clearance in patients with type 1 diabetes. Diabetes Care 1999;22:1245–1251

47 Skyrme-Jones R A, O'Brien R C, Berry K L, Meredith I T. Vitamin E supplementation improves endothelial function in type I diabetes mellitus: a randomized, placebo-controlled study. J Am Coll Cardiol 2000;36:94–102

48 Engelen W, Keenoy BM, Vertommen J, De Leeuw I. Effects of long-term supplementation with moderate pharmacologic doses of vitamin E are saturable and reversible in patients with type 1 diabetes. Am J Clin Nutr 2000;72:1142–1149

49 Tutuncu NB, Bayraktar M, Varli K. Reversal of defective nerve conduction with vitamin E supplementation in type 2 diabetes: a preliminary study. Diabetes Care 1998;21:1915–1918

50 Upritchard JE, Sutherland WH, Mann JI. Effect of supplementation with tomato juice, vitamin E, and vitamin C on LDL oxidation and products of inflammatory activity in type 2 diabetes. Diabetes Care 2000;23:733–738.

51 Farvid MS, Siassi F, Jalali M, Hosseini M, Saadat N. The impact of vitamin and/or mineral supplementation on lipid profiles in type 2 diabetes. Diabetes Res Clin Pract 2004;65:21–28

52 Farvid MS, Jalali M, Siassi F, Saadat N, Hosseini M. The impact of vitamins and/or mineral supplementation on blood pressure in type 2 diabetes. J Am Coll Nutr 2004;23:272–279

53 Roussel AM, Kerkeni A, Zouari N, Mahjoub S, Matheau JM, Anderson RA. Antioxidant effects of zinc supplementation in Tunisians with type 2 diabetes mellitus. J Am Coll Nutr 2003;22:316–321

54 Anderson RA, Roussel AM, Zouari N, Mahjoub S, Matheau JM, Kerkeni A. Potential antioxidant effects of zinc and chromium supplementation in people with type 2 diabetes mellitus. J Am Coll Nutr 2001;20:212–218

55 Tsujiuchi T, Kumano H, Yoshiuchi K, He D, Tsujiuchi Y, Kuboki T, Suematsu H, Hirao K. The effect of Qi-gong relaxation exercise on the control of type 2 diabetes mellitus: a randomized controlled trial. Diabetes Care 2002;25:241–242

56 Wang XM. Treating type II diabetes mellitus with foot reflexotherapy. Zhongguo Zhong Xi Yi Jie He Za Zhi 1993;13:536–538, 517

CONDITIONS

DRUG/ALCOHOL DEPENDENCE

Synonyms/ subcategories
Chemical dependence (dependency), cocaine/opiate dependence, substance abuse, substance misuse.

Definition
Continued or increasing use of a chemical substance, to the extent of having negative consequences upon a person's life, in order to avoid physical or psychological withdrawal symptoms.

CAM usage
Acupuncture and hypnotherapy have been used with the aim of inducing changes in motivation among drug misusers. These therapies as well as others such as reflexology are used in a supportive way with the aim of reducing symptoms and stress during withdrawal. Courses of acupuncture treatment are mandated for this purpose by the state legislature in some areas of the USA. Acupuncture and biofeedback are sometimes used as adjuncts in relapse prevention.

Clinical evidence

Acupuncture
For alcohol dependence, some early RCTs reported positive effects on recidivist alcoholics.[1,2] The evidence since has been mixed (Table 2.33) with two trials reporting positive findings[3,4] and five suggesting that acupuncture has no great value in achieving or maintaining abstinence.[5-9]

In cocaine and opiate treatment programmes, uncontrolled analyses of acupuncture as an adjunct (e.g.[10]) have been promising. Findings from a systematic review (Box 2.41), however, do not support the use of acupuncture for the treatment of cocaine dependency.[11] This confirms the findings of a review of auricular acupuncture in the treatment of cocaine and crack abuse.[12] An RCT suggested that acupuncture reduced the severity of withdrawal symptoms associated with rapid opiate detoxification.[13] For heroin addicts, the evidence is conflicting. For example, in one RCT involving 60 subjects entering a methadone maintenance programme, cravings were greater in the group that had real acupuncture compared with those given placebo acupuncture.[14] In another RCT involving 100 subjects with heroin dependence, acupuncture increased the rate of continuation in treatment, although only six subjects remained in the study at 21 days.[15] One RCT (n = 181, thereof 121 in the acupuncture group) reported improvement in withdrawal symptoms after treatment with Han's Acupoint Nerve Stimulator.[16]

Biofeedback
Biofeedback training with relaxation increased the internal locus of control compared with no intervention in an RCT in young alcohol-dependent persons, a change that is associated with improved control over drinking habits.[17] Another RCT found lower relapse rates with EEG biofeedback in chronic alcohol

Table 2.33 **RCTs of acupuncture for alcohol dependence**

Reference	Sample size	Interventions [regimen]	Result	Comment
Toteva[3]	118	A) Acupuncture [12–15 sessions] B) Standard care	A better than B	Subjects already withdrawn from alcohol
Karst[4]	34	A) Acupuncture [ten sessions over 2 w] B) Placebo acupuncture	A better than B in withdrawal symptoms	In addition to standard medication
Worner[5]	56	A) Acupuncture [five sessions/w initially, total 39] B) Placebo acupuncture	A no different from B	
Rampes[6]	59	A) Acupuncture [weekly for 6 w] B) Placebo acupuncture C) Standard care	A no different from B or C	
Sapir Weise[7]	72	A) Acupuncture [five sessions/w initially, total 30] B) Placebo acupuncture	A no different from B	
Trümpler[8]	48	A) Laser acupuncture [daily session of 30–45 min until end of withdrawal] B) Needle acupuncture C) Sham laser stimulation	A no different from B or C	Inpatients undergoing alcohol withdrawal
Bullock[9]	503	A) Specific acupuncture B) Non-specific acupuncture C) Symptom-based acupuncture D) Conventional treatment	A no different from B, C or D	Improvement from baseline in all groups but no intergroup differences

Box 2.41
Meta-analysis
Acupuncture for cocaine dependence
Mills[11]

- Nine RCTs involving 1747 patients

- Large loss to follow-up, on average 50% (0 to 63%)

- Pooled OR estimating the effect of acupuncture on cocaine abstinence was 0.76 (95% CI, 0.45 to 1.27, p = 0.30, I2 = 30%, heterogeneity p = 0.19)

- Conclusion: the use of acupuncture for the treatment of cocaine dependence cannot be supported.

dependency compared with the standard Alcoholic Anonymous 12-step programme, as well as reductions in psycho-pathology.[18] Two RCTs comparing biofeedback with other treatments and with standard care alone in patients with severe alcohol dependence reached inconsistent conclusions. One RCT found it to improve retention in the project but not abstinence at 9 months,[19] another reported more non-drinking days over 18 months.[20]

CONDITIONS

CONDITIONS

Electrostimulation

Various forms of cranial electrostimulation have been applied to alleviate withdrawal symptoms. The RCTs available up to 1990 were reviewed[21] but because of the variety of electrical parameters and treatment regimens used and methodological problems no meaningful conclusions could be drawn. Since that time, more rigorous, double-blind RCTs with negative results have been published in cocaine/opiate dependence.[22,23]

Herbal medicine

Some withdrawal programmes in China involve colonic irrigation with **Chinese herbs** as a method of detoxification, but the only RCT located used inappropriate outcome measures and no conclusion can be drawn.[24] Modified **Banxia Houpu** decoction administered at the beginning of detoxification showed better improvement of protracted heroin abstinence syndrome than the mixture administered at the end of detoxification or placebo.[25] **Kudzu** (*Pueraria lobata*) is a long-established Chinese herbal remedy which has been used for treatment of alcohol dependence, but a small RCT in 38 persons found no effect on craving or sobriety scores compared with placebo.[26] **WeiniCom,** a Chinese herbal compound was reported to be more effective in alleviating withdrawal symptoms and craving in patients with acute opioid withdrawal symptoms than control standard treatment.[27]

Ginkgo *(Ginkgo biloba)* was compared with piracetam and placebo in a double-blind RCT of 44 cocaine-dependent subjects.[28] Ginkgo was not superior to placebo and piracetam aggravated symptoms.

A double-blind RCT tested **passion flower** (*Passiflora incarnata*) in addition to opiate detoxification with clonidine against clonidine administered alone.[29] Both treatments were equally effective in treating physical symptoms yet mental symptoms improved more with passionflower.

Hypnotherapy

For alcohol dependence, a review found that the rigorous evidence about hypnotherapy was restricted to one RCT, the negative outcome of which was weakened by the failure to stratify according to hypnotic susceptibility.[30] There have been no rigorous investigations published since the review in 1981.

Relaxation

Relaxation has been used alone as the control method in several controlled trials and found to be of little benefit in drug withdrawal (though it may not have been applied optimally).[31,32] One small (n = 20) RCT found a beneficial effect on sleep patterns in institutionalised chronic alcoholic men, compared with no additional treatment.[33] Relaxation can promote restoration of normal sleep patterns in patients who are withdrawing from long-term hypnotic medication, as compared with no relaxation, but it makes little difference to the temporary disturbance during the actual drug withdrawal, according to an RCT in only 20 subjects.[34]

Supplements

Supplements during withdrawal and recovery may be necessary because appetite and quality of nutritional intake are often poor in all drug dependence, and metabolic disturbance may also be severe with excessive alcohol abuse.[35]

In addition, **amino acid** supplements have been used with the aim of restoring brain neurotransmitter concentrations: in alcohol dependency, three patients showed improved retention, stress reduction and ease of detoxification compared with 19 controls with standard treatment alone.[36]

In another double-blind controlled trial in 23 patients, **gamma-hydroxybutyric acid** reduced symptoms of alcohol withdrawal more effectively than placebo control.[37] These studies are still exploratory and require independent replication.

Other therapies

Regular, aerobic exercise was superior at reducing craving in a group of 90 alcohol-dependent patients compared with standard treatment in a controlled trial.[38]

Intercessory **prayer** was found to be of no benefit for alcohol dependency in an RCT of 40 subjects in which it was compared with no additional treatment.[39]

Qigong therapy for detoxification of heroin addicts was compared with standard medication and no treatment in an RCT (n = 86).[40] Withdrawal symptoms reduced more rapidly in the qigong group and anxiety scores were lower than in the other groups.

Therapeutic touch was associated with lower anxiety scores in an RCT of 54 pregnant women with chemical dependency when compared with shared activity with a nurse or standard ward care.[41]

Yoga was not superior to dynamic group psychotherapy in an RCT of 61 patients undergoing methadone maintenance therapy, as assessed by a range of psychological, sociological and biological measures.[42]

Overall recommendation

For the management of chemical dependence, the major areas of action are in motivating changes in behaviour, bringing patients into detoxification and therapy and maintaining abstinence. In alcohol dependent patients biofeedback with relaxation may have a role in the first two areas; its role in treating withdrawal symptoms, however, remains uncertain. Maintenance of abstinence is best attempted with multiple interventions including support and teaching of coping strategies and substitute behaviours. CAM appears to have little to offer in comparison with current methods such as Alcoholics or Narcotics Anonymous or cognitive–behavioural therapy. For dependence on prescribed hypnotic drugs, relaxation may help restore normal sleep patterns.

Table 2.34
Summary of clinical evidence for drug/alcohol dependence

Treatment	Weight of evidence	Direction of evidence	Serious safety concerns
Acupuncture			
(alcohol)	OO	⇒	Yes (see p 294)
(cocaine & opiates)	OOO	↘	Yes (see p 294)
Biofeedback	OO	↗	No (see p 310)
Electrostimulation	OO	↘	Yes (see p 5)
Herbal medicine			
Banxi	O	↗	Yes (see p 476)
Chinese herbs (rectally)	O	⇒	Yes (see p 5)
Ginkgo	O	⇓	Yes (see p 404)
Kudzu	O	⇓	Yes (see p 479)
Passionflower	O	↗	Yes (see p 446)
WeiniCom	O	↗	Yes (see p 5)
Hypnotherapy			
(alcohol)	O	⇓	Yes (see p 331)
Relaxation	OO	⇒	No (see p 348)
Supplements			
Amino acids	O	↗	Yes (see p 5)
Gamma-hydroxybutyric acid	O	↗	Yes (see p 483)

REFERENCES

1 Bullock M L, Umen A J, Culliton P D, Olander R T. Acupuncture treatment of alcohol recidivism: a pilot study. Alcohol Clin Exp Res 1987;11:292–295

2 Bullock M L, Culliton P D, Olander R T. Controlled trial of acupuncture for severe recidivist alcoholism. Lancet 1989;333:1435–1439

3 Toteva S, Milanov I. The use of body acupuncture for treatment of alcohol dependence and withdrawal syndrome: a controlled study. Am J Acup 1996;24:19–25

4 Karst M, Passie T, Friedrich S, Wiese B, Schneider U. Acupuncture in the treatment of alcohol withdrawal symptoms: a randomized, placebo-controlled inpatient study. Addict Biol 2002;7:415–419

5 Worner T M, Zeller B, Schwarz H, Zwas F, Lyon D. Acupuncture fails to improve treatment outcome in alcoholics. Drug Alcohol Depend 1992;30:169–173

6 Rampes H, Periera S, Mortimer A, Manoharan S, Knowles M. Does electroacupuncture reduce craving for alcohol? A randomized study. Complement Ther Med 1997;5:19–26

7 Sapir-Weise R, Berglund M, Frank A, Kristenson H. Acupuncture in alcoholism treatment: a randomized out-patient study. Alcohol and Alcoholism 1999;34:629–635

8 Trümpler F, Oez S, Stahli P, Brenner H D, Juni P. Acupuncture for alcohol withdrawal: a randomized controlled trial. Alcohol Alcohol 2003;38:369–375

9 Bullock M L, Kiresuk T J, Sherman R E, Lenz S K, Culliton P D, Boucher T A, Nolan C J. A large randomized placebo controlled study of auricular acupuncture for alcohol dependence. J Subst Abuse Treat 2002;22:71–77

10 Shwartz M, Saitz R, Mulvey K, Brannigan P. The value of acupuncture detoxification programs in a substance abuse treatment system. J Subst Abuse Treat 1999;17:305–312

11 Mills E J, Wu P, Gagnier J, Ebbert J O. Efficacy of acupuncture for cocaine dependence: a systematic review and meta-analysis. Harm Reduct J 2005;2:4

12 D'Alberto A. Auricular acupuncture in the treatment of cocaine/crack abuse: a review of the efficacy, the use of the National Acupuncture Detoxification Association protocol, and the selection of sham points. J Altern Complement Med 2004;10:985–1000

13 Montazeri K, Farahnakian M, Saghaei M. The effect of acupuncture on the acute withdrawal symptoms from rapid opiate detoxification. Acta Anaesthesiol Sin 2002;40:173–177

14 Wells E A, Jackson R, Dias O R et al. Acupuncture as an adjunct to methadone treatment services. Am J Addict 1995;4:169–214

15 Washburn A M, Fullilove R E, Fullilove M T, Keenan P A, McGee B, Morris K A, Sorensen J L, Clark W W. Acupuncture heroin detoxification: a single-blind clinical trial. J Subst Abuse Treat 1993;10:345–351

16 Zhang B, Luo F, Liu C. [Treatment of 121 heroin addicts with Han's acupoint nerve stimulator] Zhongguo Zhong Xi Yi Jie He Za Zhi 2000;20:593–595 Chinese.

17 Sharp C, Hurford D P, Allison J, Sparks R, Cameron B P. Facilitation of internal locus of control in adolescent alcoholics through a brief biofeedback-assisted autogenic relaxation training procedure. J Subst Abuse Treat 1997;14:55–60

18 Peniston E G, Kulkosky P J. Alpha-theta brainwave training and beta-endorphin levels in alcoholics. Alcohol Clin Exp Res 1989;13:271–279

19 Richard A J, Montoya I D, Nelson R, Spence R T. Effectiveness of adjunct therapies in crack cocaine treatment. J Subst Abuse Treat 1995;12:401–413.

20 Tuab E, Steiner S S, Weingarten E, Walton K G. Effectiveness of broad spectrum approaches to relapse prevention in severe alcoholism: a long-term, randomized, controlled trial of transcendental meditation, EMG biofeedback and electronic neurotherapy. Alcohol Treat Quart 1994;11:187–220

21 Alling F A, Johnson B D, Eldoghazy E. Cranial electrostimulation (CES) use in the detoxification of opiate-dependent patients. J Subst Abuse Treat 1990;7:173–180

22 Gariti P, Auriacombe M, Incmikoski R, McLellan A T, Patterson L, Dhopesh V, Mezochow J, Patterson M, O'Brien C. A randomized double-blind study of neuroelectric therapy in opiate and cocaine detoxification. J Subst Abuse 1992;4:299–308

23 Patterson M A, Patterson L, Flood N V et al. Electrostimulation in drug and alcohol detoxification: significance of stimulation criteria in clinical success. Addict Res 1993;1:130–144

24 Sha L J, Zhang Z X, Cheng L X. [Colonic dialysis therapy of Chinese herbal medicine in abstinence of heroin addicts – report of 75 cases] [Chinese]. Chung-Kuo Chung Hsi i Chieh Ho Tsa Chih 1997;17:76–78

25 Huang D B, Yu Z F, Fu L. [Clinical observation on effect of modified banxia houpu decoction in treating patients with protracted heroin abstinence syndrome] Zhongguo Zhong Xi Yi Jie He Za Zhi 2004;24:216–219 Chinese.

26 Hao W, Zhao M. A comparative clinical study of the effect of WeiniCom, a Chinese herbal compound, on alleviation of withdrawal symptoms and craving for heroin in detoxification treatment. J Psychoactive Drugs 2000;32:277–284

27 Shebek J, Rindone J P. A pilot study exploring the effect of kudzu root on the drinking habits of patients with chronic alcoholism. J Alt Compl Med 2000;6:45–48

28 Kampman K, Majewska M D, Tourian K, Dackis C, Cornish J, Poole S, O'Brien C. A pilot trial of piracetam and ginkgo biloba for the treatment of cocaine dependence. Addict Behav 2003;28:437–448

29 Akhondzadeh S, Kashani L, Mobaseri M, Hosseini S H, Nikzad S, Khani M. Passionflower in the treatment of opiates withdrawal: a double-blind randomized controlled trial. J Clin Pharm Ther 2001;26:369–373

30 Wadden T A, Penrod J H. Hypnosis in the treatment of alcoholism: a review and appraisal. Am J Clin Hypnosis 1981;24:41–47

31 Brown R A, Evans D M, Miller I W, Burgess E S, Müller T I. Cognitive–behavioral treatment for depression in alcoholism. J Consult Clin Psychol 1997;65:715–726

32 Rohsenow D J, Monti P M, Martin R A, Michalec E, Abrams D B. Brief coping skills treatment for cocaine abuse: 12-month substance use outcomes. J Consult Clin Psychol 2000;68:515–520

33 Greeff A P, Conradie W S. Use of progressive relaxation training for chronic alcoholics with insomnia. Psychol Reports 1998;82:407–412

34 Lichstein K L, Peterson B A, Riedel B W, Means M K, Epperson M T, Aguillard R N. Relaxation to assist sleep medication withdrawal. Behav Modification 1999;23:379–402

35 Beckley-Barrett L M, Mutch P B. Position of the American Dietetic Association: nutrition intervention in treatment and recovery from chemical dependence. ADA Reports 1990;90:1274–1277

36 Blum K, Trachtenberg M C, Ramsay J C. Improvement of inpatient treatment of the

alcoholic as a function of neurotransmitter restoration: a pilot study. Int J Addict 1988;23:991–998

37 Gallimberti L, Canton G, Gentile N, Ferri M, Cibin M, Ferrara S D, Fadda F, Gessa G L. Gamma-hydroxybutyric acid for treatment of alcohol withdrawal syndrome. Lancet 1989;334:787–789

38 Ermalinski R, Hanson P G, Lubin B, Thornby J I, Nahormek P A. Impact of a body-mind treatment component on alcoholic inpatients. J Psychosoc Nurs Ment Health Serv 1997;35:39–45

39 Walker S R, Tonigan J S, Miller W R, Corner S, Kahlich L. Intercessory prayer in the

treatment of alcohol abuse and dependence: a pilot investigation. Alt Ther Health Med 1997;3:79–86

40 Li M, Chen K, Mo Z. Use of qigong therapy in the detoxification of heroin addicts. Altern Ther Health Med 2002;8:50–54, 56–59

41 Larden C N, Palmer M L, Janssen P. Efficacy of therapeutic touch in treating pregnant inpatients who have a chemical dependency. J Holist Nurs 2004;22:320–332

42 Shaffer H J, Lasalvia T A. Comparing Hatha yoga with dynamic group psychotherapy for enhancing methadone maintenance treatment: a randomized clinical trial. Alt Ther Health Med 1997;3:57–66

ERECTILE DYSFUNCTION

Synonyms/ subcategories
Impotence, male erectile dysfunction.

Definition
Erectile dysfunction (ED) is defined as the persistent inability to obtain or maintain sufficient rigidity of the penis to allow satisfactory sexual performance.

CAM usage
Acupuncture, herbal medicine and hypnotherapy are frequently used.

Clinical evidence

Acupuncture
One RCT (n = 15) evaluated acupuncture as a treatment for patients with non-organic ED.[1] Improvements in sexual function were reported in the treatment group, which were not different from the control group. Another RCT (n = 22) administered acupuncture specific against ED or acupuncture specific against headache and allowed non-responders to cross over from the control group to the treatment group.[2] A satisfactory response was achieved in 68% of the treatment group and in 9% of the control group.

Biofeedback
A systematic review evaluated the effectiveness of biofeedback in general and identified one systematic review for ED.[3] Based on the data from clinical trials, the evidence is inconclusive for this condition.

Herbal medicine
A double-blind RCT tested the effects of the crude preparation of *Butea superba* on ED in Thai males.[4] The sexual record indicated that 82.4% of the patients exhibited noticeable improvement. Safety parameters were unaffected. It was concluded that the

plant preparation appears to improve erectile function in ED without apparent toxicity.

An uncontrolled pilot study (n = 60) assessed the effects of **ginkgo** (*Ginkgo biloba*) extract in antidepressant-induced sexual dysfunction.[5] Patients were treated with up to 240 mg daily with positive effects being reported on all four phases of the sexual response cycle, including penile erection.

Ginseng (*Panax* spp, *Eleutherococcus senticosus*) is widely believed to have aphrodisiac effects for patients with sexual dysfunction. A systematic review of ginseng for any indication, however, found no double-blind RCTs despite extensive searches.[6] In one placebo-controlled RCT (n = 90), patients were treated with either Korean red ginseng (*Panax ginseng*) or trazodone. The results suggested superiority of ginseng for penile rigidity, girth, libido and patient satisfaction.[7] Another double-blind trial (n = 45) tested Korean red ginseng and found a beneficial difference on the International Index of Erectile Function compared with placebo.[8] It concluded that Korean red ginseng can be an effective alternative for patients with ED.

Hypnotherapy

Two RCTs assessed the effects of hypnotic suggestions on sexual function.[1,9] Both studies originate from the same research group and included patients with no detectable organic cause. Both studies found improvements in sexual function and report that hypnotic suggestion is more effective than the administration of oral placebo. Independent replication of these findings is warranted.

Pelvic floor exercise

One RCT compared a pelvic floor exercise programme with surgery.[10] One hundred and fifty patients with erectile dysfunction and proven vascular leakage were included and 78 randomised to the training programme, which was given five times in weekly sessions and supervised by a trained physiotherapist. It was concluded that, although in cases of severe venous leakage surgery is superior to a pelvic floor exercise programme, in mild forms pelvic floor exercise is an alternative to surgery.

Supplements

A double-blind RCT (n = 50) tested 5 g daily of **L-arginine**.[11] It found no difference in sexual function compared with placebo. Another double-blind RCT (n = 45) compared a combination preparation of L-arginine glutamate and yohimbine hydrochloride with yohimbine hydrochloride alone and placebo.[12] The on-demand oral administration of the 6 g L-arginine glutamate and 6 mg yohimbine combination preparation is effective in improving mild to moderate ED.

CONDITIONS

The effects of **yohimbine**, the main active constituent of yohimbe bark (*Pausinystalia yohimbe*), have been assessed in a meta-analysis (Box 2.42).[13] Its results suggest that yohimbine is effective for this condition. An independent review confirmed these findings.[14] There is no trial that compared yohimbine with sildenafil.

Box 2.42
Meta-analysis
Yohimbine for erectile dysfunction
Ernst[13]

- Seven double-blind RCTs including 419 patients

- Trial quality generally good

- Erectile dysfunction due to organic or non-organic etiologies

- Superior to placebo in response rate (odds ratio 3.85, CI 2.22 to 6.67)

- Adverse events were reversible and infrequent

Overall recommendation

There is convincing evidence for the effectiveness of yohimbine for erectile dysfunction from organic or non-organic causes. Its risk–benefit ratio is favourable, which renders it an option worthy of consideration. Comparative studies with conventional oral medication such as sildenafil are not available. For other therapies such as acupuncture and Korean red ginseng, the evidence is encouraging but not compelling. Given the possibility of a large placebo response, hypnotherapy may also be beneficial for some patients.

Table 2.35
Summary of clinical evidence for erectile dysfunction

Treatment	Weight of evidence	Direction of evidence	Serious safety concerns
Acupuncture	OO	↗	Yes (see p 294)
Biofeedback	OO	⇨	No (see p 310)
Herbal medicine			
Butea superba	O	↗	Yes (see p 5)
Ginkgo	O	↗	Yes (see p 404)
Ginseng	OO	⇧	Yes (see p 407)
Hypnotherapy	O	⇧	Yes (see p 331)
Pelvic floor exercise	O	↗	No (see p 5)
Supplements			
L-arginine	OO	⇨	Yes (see p 482)
Yohimbine	OOO	⇧	Yes (see p 474)

REFERENCES

1 Aydin S, Ercan M, Caskurlu T, Tasci A I, Karaman I, Odabas O, Yilmaz Y, Agargun M Y, Kara H, Sevin G. Acupuncture and hypnotic suggestions in the treatment of non-organic male dysfunction. Scand J Urol Nephrol 1997;31:271–274

2 Engelhardt P F, Daha L K, Zils T, Simak R, Konig K, Pfluger H. Acupuncture in the treatment of

psychogenic erectile dysfunction: first results of a prospective randomized placebo-controlled study. Int J Impot Res 2003;15:343–346

3   Ernst E. Systematic reviews of biofeedback. Phys Med Rehab Kuror 2003;13:321–324

4   Cherdshewasart W, Nimsakul N. Clinical trial of Butea superba, an alternative herbal treatment for erectile dysfunction. Asian J Androl 2003;5:243–246

5   Cohen A J, Bartlik B. Ginkgo biloba for anti-depressant-induced sexual dysfunction. J Sex Marital Ther 1998;24:139–413

6   Vogler B K, Pittler M H, Ernst E. The efficacy of ginseng. A systematic review of randomised clinical trials. Eur J Clin Pharmacol 1999;55:567–575

7   Choi H K, Seong D H, Rha K H. Clinical efficacy of Korean red ginseng for erectile dysfunction. Int J Impot Res 1995;7:181–186

8   Hong B, Ji Y H, Hong J H, Nam K Y, Ahn T Y. A double-blind crossover study evaluating the efficacy of Korean red ginseng in patients with erectile dysfunction: a preliminary report. J Urol 2002;168:2070–2073

9   Aydın S, Odabas O, Ercan M, Kara H, Agargun M Y. Efficacy of testosterone,

trazodone, and hypnotic suggestion in the treatment of non-organic male sexual dysfunction. Br J Urol 1996;77:256–260

10 Claes H, Baert L. Pelvic floor exercise versus surgery in the treatment of impotence. Br J Urol 1993;71:52–57

11 Chen J, Wollman Y, Chernichovsky T, Iaina A, Sofer M, Matzkin H. Effect of oral administration of high-dose nitric oxide donor L-arginine in men with organic erectile dysfunction: results of a double-blind, randomized, placebo-controlled study. BJU Int 1999;83:269–273

12 Lebret T, Herve J M, Gorny P, Worcel M, Botto H. Efficacy and safety of a novel combination of L arginine glutamate and yohimbine hydrochloride: a new oral therapy for erectile dysfunction. Eur Urol 2002;41:608–613

13 Ernst E, Pittler M H. Yohimbine for erectile dysfunction: a systematic review and meta-analysis of randomized clinical trials. J Urol 1998;159:433–436

14 Tam S W, Worcel M, Wyllie M. Yohimbine: a clinical review. Pharmacol Ther 2001;91:215–243

FIBROMYALGIA

Synonyms   Fibromyalgia syndrome, tension myalgia.

Definition   A painful disorder, more common in women, in which diffuse pain, stiffness, fatigue, functional impairment and disrupted sleep are associated with the presence of bilateral tender points.

CAM usage   Sufferers of fibromyalgia commonly use CAM. One survey found that 91% had used CAM.[1] CAM therapies frequently used include massage, dietary therapies, vitamins and herbs, relaxation and imagery, spirituality/prayer, acupressure, acupuncture, biofeedback and meditation.[2]

Clinical evidence   One systematic review of CCTs of all types of CAM treatments[3] and one of various non-pharmacological approaches[4] are available.

Acupuncture

One good-quality RCT[5] in 70 subjects found that 25% of subjects improved markedly, 50% had satisfactory relief of symptoms and 25% had no benefit. This study was the principal evidence in a systematic review[6] (Box 2.43) which reached a positive overall conclusion. A recent study shows that acupuncture increases microcirculatory blood flow over tender points in fibromyalgia patients, thus reducing pain.[7] A further CCT compared acupuncture with connective tissue massage and found the former to be more effective than the latter.[8]

Box 2.43
Systematic review
Acupuncture for fibromyalgia
Berman[6]

- Three RCTs and four cohort studies involving 300 subjects
- Quality of studies highly variable
- A single high-quality RCT suggests that acupuncture is more effective than placebo for relieving pain and morning stiffness
- Other studies are inconclusive, but compatible with this result
- Long-term effects remain unknown
- Conclusion: based on a single high-quality study the evidence suggests that real acupuncture is more effective than sham acupuncture, further robust data on effectiveness are required

Biofeedback

Although several RCTs have suggested that fibromyalgia patients can benefit from various mind–body therapies, appropriate attention controls have rarely been used. In one controlled study, 12 patients received 15 sessions of either biofeedback or sham biofeedback over 5 weeks.[9] Persistent improvements in tender points, pain intensity and morning stiffness were found. In an RCT involving 119 subjects, biofeedback with relaxation was compared with exercise, a combination of biofeedback and exercise, and attention control.[10] Biofeedback was superior to the control group only in terms of tender points and enhanced self-efficacy of function.

Exercise

A Cochrane review[11] (Box 2.44) produced good evidence for aerobic exercise to increase physical capacity and alleviate symptoms of patients suffering from fibromyalgia.

Box 2.44
Systematic review
Exercise for treating fibromyalgia syndrome
Busch[11]

- Seventeen RCTs involving 724 patients
- Quality was variable but seven studies were rigorous
- All four high quality studies of aerobic exercise showed greater improvements compared with controls
- For other forms of exercise, the evidence is less conclusive
- Poor reporting was a common weakness of these studies
- Conclusion: aerobic exercise training has beneficial effects on physical capacity and symptoms

Herbal medicine

An open, uncontrolled study of **ginkgo** *(Ginkgo biloba)* combined with Co-enzyme Q10 (200 mg daily of each for 84 days) yielded encouraging results with 64% of patients noting improvement.[12]

Homeopathy

In one RCT, 30 patients receiving homeopathic *Rhus toxicoden-dron*[13] recorded greater reduction in tender points, pain and sleep disturbance, but global assessment was not different. An RCT (n = 62) also found good symptomatic improvements when comparing individualised homeopathy against placebo in a double-blind fashion.[14]

Massage

Connective tissue massage was compared with no treatment or attention control in an RCT involving 52 patients.[15] The treated group experienced greater relief of pain and depression and improvement in quality of life. A small (n = 37) CCT compared regular Swedish massage for 4 weeks with standard care and suggested modest symptomatic effects which, however, were not substantiated at 28-week follow-up.[16]

Mind–body therapies

A systematic review[17] found encouraging results for mind–body therapies such as meditation, hypnotherapy, relaxation, etc. (Box 2.45). A more recent RCT confirmed positive effects of imagery on pain[18] while a further RCT suggested mindfulness meditation plus Qigong to be more helpful than education plus support.[19]

Box 2.45
Systematic review
**Mind–body
therapies for
fibromyalgia**
Hadhazy[17]

- Thirteen CCTs involving 802 patients were included

- Quality was variable, but seven trials were rigorous

- Mind–body therapies improved self-efficacy (strong evidence), quality of life (limited evidence), and pain (limited evidence)

- Whether mind–body therapies are superior to physiotherapy, psychotherapy or education is not clear

- Conclusion: exercise is more effective than mind–body therapies

Supplements

Forty-five patients treated with topical **capsaicin** reported less tenderness and a significant increase in grip strength, but no difference in pain scores compared with placebo.[20]

Of four placebo-controlled RCTs of **s-adenosyl-L-methionine** (SAMe), three suggested positive effects on pain. The negative RCT, however, was the one rated to have the highest methodological quality.[3]

CONDITIONS

Other therapies

From one small study (n = 39), there is a suggestion that **balneotherapy** with plain fresh-water baths reduces pain and the addition of valerian to the water may improve other outcomes such as well-being and sleep.[21] Similarly encouraging results emerged from an RCT[22] and a CCT[23] of balneotherapy without the addition of herbal extracts.

A small (n = 19) RCT found that, although treatment with **chiropractic manipulation** and soft tissue massage was associated with improvements in many parameters such as spinal pain and mobility, the changes were not superior to no treatment in terms of the physical symptoms.[24] Outcome measures specific to fibromyalgia were not used.

Compared with an educational programme, regular **Feldenkrais** treatment was followed by only minor functional improvements which were not maintained over time.[25]

An RCT in which 40 patients with fibromyalgia were randomised to receive either **hypnotherapy** or physical therapy for 12 weeks found improvements in several measures including pain ratings, sleep disturbance and somatic and psychological discomfort scores, though not physicians' global assessments.[26]

Low-dose **laser therapy** was not found to provide any greater relief of pain than placebo laser in a crossover study involving 60 patients.[27]

Two RCTs suggested that, compared with placebo, **magnet therapy** may decrease pain in patients with fibromyalgia.[28,29]

A small, uncontrolled study of **melatonin** (3 mg per day at bedtime for 30 days) suggested a reduction in tender points and improvement of sleep.[30]

A single trial suggested that **music therapy** was associated with reduced pain and disability in chronic pain patients, including fibromyalgia, compared with untreated controls, but no change in anxiety or depression.[31]

A small (n = 24) RCT with four parallel groups suggested that **osteopathic spinal manipulation** effectively reduced pain of fibromyalgia.[32]

A small, uncontrolled study of **therapeutic touch** found encouraging effects on pain.[33]

An RCT comparing **vegetarian diet** with amitriptyline therapy suggested a modest pain relief after dieting which, however, was much smaller than that observed with drug treatment.[34]

Overall recommendation

It is unlikely that any complementary therapy alone can have greater impact on fibromyalgia symptoms than conventional approaches. However, combinations of therapies are often used for fibromyalgia and CAM has something to offer in this context. For example, the judicious use of oral medications to deal with pain and insomnia can be usefully combined with biofeedback or (supervised) exercise and perhaps acupuncture.

Table 2.36
Summary of clinical evidence for fibromyalgia

Treatment	Weight of evidence	Direction of evidence	Serious safety concerns
Acupuncture	OO	⇧	Yes (see p 294)
Biofeedback	O	⇧	No (see p 310)
Exercise	OO	⇧	Yes (see p 5)
Homeopathy	O	⬈	No (see p 327)
Massage	O	⇧	No (see p 334)
Mind–body therapy	OO	⬈	No (see p 5)
Supplements			
S-adenosyl-L-methionine	OO	⬈	No (see p 484)
Capsaicin	O	⬈	Yes (see p 5)

REFERENCES

1 Pioro-Boisset M, Esdaile J M, Fitzcharles M-A. Alternative medicine use in fibromyalgia syndrome. Arthritis Care Res 1996;9:13–17

2 Nicassio P M, Schuman C, Kim J, Cordova A, Weisman M H. Psychosocial factors associated with complementary treatment use in fibromyalgia. J Rheumatol 1997;24:2008–2013

3 Holdcraft L C, Assefi N, Buchwald D. Complementary and alternative medicine in fibromyalgia and related syndromes. Best Pract Res Clin Rheumatol 2003;17:667–683

4 Sim J, Adams N. Systematic review of randomized controlled trials of non-pharmacological interventions for fibromyalgia. Clin J Pain 2002;18:324–336

5 Deluze C, Bosia L, Zirbs A, Chantraine A, Vischer T L. Electroacupuncture in fibromyalgia: results of a controlled trial. BMJ 1992;305:1249–1252

6 Berman B M, Ezzo J, Hadhazy V, Swyers J P. Is acupuncture effective in the treatment of fibromyalgia? J Fam Pract 1999;48:213–218

7 Sprott H, Jeschonneck M, Grohmann G, Hein G. Änderung der Durchblutung über den tender points bei Fibromyalgie-Patienten nach einer Akupunkturtherapie (gemessen mit der Laser-Doppler-Flowmetrie). Wien Klin Wochenschr 2000;112:580–586

8 Uhlemann C, Schreiber T U, Smolenski U C, Loth D. Randomisierte Studie zur Akupunktur und Bindegewebmassage als Therapieoption bei Patienten mit Fibromyalgiesyndrom (FMS). Phys Med Rehab Kuror 2001;11:153

9 Ferraccioli G, Gherilli L, Scita F, Nolli M, Mozzani M, Fontana S, Scorsonelli M, Tridenti A, De Risio C. E MG-biofeedback training in fibromyalgia syndrome. J Rheumatol 1987;14:820–825

10 Buckelew S P, Conway R, Parker J, Deuser W E, Read J, Witty T E, Hewett J E, Minor M, Johnson J C, Van Male L, McIntosh M J, Nigh M, Kay D R. Biofeedback/relaxation training and exercise interventions for fibromyalgia: a prospective trial. Arthritis Care Res 1998;11:196–209

11 Busch A, Schachter CL, Peloso P M, Bombardier C. Exercise for treating fibromyalgia syndrome. The Cochrane Database of Systematic Reviews 2002, Issue 2 Art. No: CD003786

12 Lister R E. An open, pilot study to evaluate the potential benefits of coenzyme Q_{10} combined with Ginkgo biloba extract in fibromyalgia syndrome. J Int Med Res 2002;30:195–199

13 Fisher P, Greenwood A, Huskisson E C, Turner P, Belon P. Effect of homeopathic treatment on fibrositis (primary fibromyalgia). BMJ 1989;299:365–366

14 Bell I R, Lewis D A, Brooks A J, Schwartz G E, Lewis S E, Walsh B T, Baldwin C M. Improved clinical status in fibromyalgia patients treated with individualized homeopathic remedies versus placebo. Rheumatology (Oxford) 2004;43:577–582

15 Brattberg G. Connective tissue massage in the treatment of fibromyalgia. Eur J Pain 1999;3:235–245

16 Alnigenis M N Y, Bradly J D, Wallick J, Emsley C L. Massage therapy in the management of fibromyalgia: a pilot study. J Musculoskeletal Pain 2001;9:55–68

17 Hadhazy V A, Ezzo J, Creamer P, Berman B M. Mind–body therapies for the treatment of

fibromyalgia. A systematic review. J Rheumatol 2000;27:2911–2918

18 Fors E A, Sexton H, Gotestam K G. The effect of guided imagery and amitriptyline on daily fibromyalgia pain: a prospective, randomized, controlled trial. J Psychiatr Res 2002;36: 179–187

19 Astin J A, Berman B M, Bausell B, Lee W L, Hochberg M, Forys K L. The efficacy of mindfulness meditation plus Qigong movement therapy in the treatment of fibromyalgia: a randomized controlled trial. J Rheumatol 2003;30:2088–2089

20 McCarty D J, Csuka M, McCarthy G, Trotter D. Treatment of pain due to fibromyalgia with topical capsaicin: a pilot study. Semin Arthritis Rheum 1994;23(suppl 3):41–47

21 Ammer K, Melnizky P. Medicinal baths for treatment of generalized fibromyalgia [German]. Forsch Komplementärmed 1999;6:80–85

22 Neumann L, Sukenik S, Bolotin A, Abu-Shakra M, Amir M, Flusser D, Buskila D. The effect of balneotherapy at the Dead Sea on the quality of life of patients with fibromyalgia syndrome. Clin Rheumatol 2001;20:15–19

23 Evcik D, Kizilay B, Gokcen E. The effects of balneotherapy on fibromyalgia patients. Rheumatol Int 2002:22:56–59

24 Blunt K L, Rajwani M H, Guerriero R C. The effectiveness of chiropractic management of fibromyalgia patients: a pilot study. J Manip Physiol Ther 1997;20:389–399

25 Aspegren Kendall S, Ekselius L, Gerdle B, Sörén B, Bengtsson A. Feldenkrais intervention in fibromyalgia patients: a pilot study. J Musculoskelet Pain 2001;9:25–35

26 Haanen H C M, Hoenderdos H T W, Romunde L K J, Hop W C, Mallee C, Terwiel J P, Hekster G B. Controlled trial of hypnotherapy

in the treatment of refractory fibromyalgia. J Rheumatol 1991;18:72–75

27 Waylonis G W, Wilke S, O'Toole D, Waylonis D A, Waylonis D B. Chronic myofascial pain: management by low-output helium-neon laser therapy. Arch Phys Med Rehabil 1998;69:1017–1020

28 Alfano P, Taylor A G, Foresman P A, Dunkl P R, McConnell G G, Conaway M R, Gillies G T. Static magnetic fields for treatment of fibromyalgia: a randomized controlled trial. J Altern Complement Med 2001;7:53–64

29 Colbert A P, Markov M S, Banerji M, Pilla A. Magnetic mattress pad use in patients with fibromyalgia: a randomized, double-blind pilot study. J Back Musculoskel Rehab 1999; 13:19–31

30 Citera G, Arras M A, Maldonado-Cocco J A. The effect of melatonin in patients with fibromyalgia: a pilot study. Clin Rheumatol 2000;19:9–13

31 Müller-Busch H C, Hoffmann P. Aktive Musiktherapie bei chronischen Schmerzen. Schmerz 1997;11:91–100

32 Gamber R G, Shores J H, Russo D P, Jimenez C, Rubin B R. Osteopathic manipulative treatment in conjunction with medication relieves pain associated with fibromyalgia syndrome: results of a randomized clinical pilot project. J Am Osteopath Ass 2002;102:321–325

33 Denison B. Touch the pain away: new research on therapeutic touch and persons with fibromyalgia syndrome. Holist Nurs Pract 2004;18:142–151

34 Azad K A, Alam M N, Haq S A, Nahar S, Chowdury M A, Ali S M, Ullah A K. Vegetarian diet in the treatment of fibromyalgia. Bangladesh Med Res Counc Bull 2000;26:41–47

HANGOVER

Synonyms	Holdover.
Related conditions	Medication hangover.
Definition	Hangover describes a set of transient symptoms resulting from excessive consumption of alcohol and withdrawal of alcohol from the body. Symptoms vary from individual to individual. The most common complaints are headache, nausea, sluggishness, and irritability.

CAM usage   Data from websites suggest that herbal and non-herbal dietary supplements are popular for preventing and treating alcohol hangover.

Clinical evidence   To assess the clinical evidence for the effectiveness of any type of medical intervention for preventing or treating alcohol hangover, systematic searches were conducted to identify all RCTs (Box 2.46).[1] Four RCTs which assessed complementary treatments were included. The tested agents were borage (*Borago officinalis*), artichoke (*Cynara scolymus*), *Opuntia ficus-indica* and a **yeast**-containing preparation. All RCTs were conducted double-blind and placebo-controlled. Intergroup differences for overall symptom scores and individual symptoms were reported for borage and a yeast-containing combination preparation. Some beneficial effects are also reported for *Opuntia ficus-indica*. For all other reviewed interventions no differences are reported.[1]

Box 2.46
Systematic review
Interventions for alcohol hangover
Pittler[1]

- Four RCTs of complementary treatments and four RCTs of conventional treatments were included

- All were double-blind and placebo-controlled

- One RCT is available for each of: borage, artichoke, *Opuntia ficus-indica* and a yeast-containing preparation

- One RCT was published for each of the conventional agents propanolol, tropisetron, tolfenamic acid and fructose or glucose

- For borage and a yeast-containing combination preparation there were intergroup differences for overall symptom scores and individual symptoms

- Conclusion: There is not sufficient evidence to suggest that any complementary or indeed conventional intervention is effective for preventing or treating alcohol hangovers

Overall recommendation   The data do not provide sufficient evidence to suggest that any complementary therapy is effective for treating or preventing the alcohol hangover. Similarly, there is no effective conventional intervention for preventing or treating this condition. Therefore, the most effective way to avoid alcohol-induced hangover is by practising abstinence or enjoying alcohol only in moderation.

CONDITIONS

Table 2.37
Summary of clinical evidence for alcohol hangover

Treatment	Weight of evidence	Direction of evidence	Serious safety concerns
Herbal medicine			
Artichoke	O	⇘	Yes (see p 368)
Borage	O	⇗	Yes (see p 476)
Opuntia ficus-indica	O	⇗	Yes (see p 5)
Yeast	O	⇗	Yes (see p 5)

REFERENCE

1   Pittler MH, Verster JC, Ernst E. Interventions for preventing or treating alcohol hangover. Systematic review of randomised trials. BMJ 2005;331:1515–1518

HAY FEVER

Synonyms/ subcategories

Seasonal allergic rhinitis, pollenosis.

Definition

Type I immediate hypersensitivity reaction mediated by specific IgE antibody to a seasonal allergen, leading to mucosal inflammation characterised by sneezing, itching, rhinorrhoea, nasal blockage and conjunctivitis.

CAM usage

The best treatment for allergic rhinitis is, of course, to avoid allergens but this is not usually practical. Allergies are one of the main reasons for using complementary therapies, according to a US survey,[1] almost half of patients with allergies try a natural product with herbal medicine and relaxation used the most. A German survey found that hay fever was the allergy most commonly treated with CAM (62%) and that only four treatment modalities accounted for almost the entire usage: homeopathy, autologous blood injection, acupuncture and bioresonance.[2]

Clinical evidence

Acupuncture

Uncontrolled studies have previously suggested that acupuncture has value in the management of hay fever, but the evidence from RCTs (Table 2.38) is mixed and suggests that effects may be attributable to non-specific factors. Three RCTs found acupuncture to be superior in preventing[3] or treating[4,5] hay fever symptoms yet three found no difference between acupuncture and sham groups for either prevention[6] or treatment.[7,8]

Diet

One RCT assessed the effects of an antigen avoidance diet during infancy on later development of atopy.[9] Common allergens such as cow's milk, egg and peanuts were avoided during gestation

Table 2.38 **RCTs of acupuncture for hay fever**

Reference	Sample size	Interventions [regimen]	Result	Comment
Williamson[3]	30	A) Acupuncture [1 session/w for 3 w] B) Conventional medication	A superior to B for prevention	Conclusion unclear statistics uncertain
Xue[4]	26	A) Acupuncture [three sessions/w for 4 w] B) Sham acupuncture	A superior to B for treatment	Superior for subjective symptoms but not for relief medication scores
Ng[5]	72	A) Acupuncture [two sessions/w for 8 w] B) Sham acupuncture	A superior to B for treatment	Childhood persistent rhinitis
Wolkenstein[6]	24	A) Acupuncture [one session/w for 9 w] B) Sham acupuncture	A no different from B for prevention	Outcome was nasal allergen provocation
Williamson[7]	102	A) Acupuncture [3–4 sessions over 4 w] B) Sham acupuncture	A no different from B for treatment	Medication use and symptoms decreased in both groups
Magnusson[8]	40	A) Acupuncture [two sessions/w for 8 w] B) Sham acupuncture	A no different from B for treatment	For one allergen, mugwort, greater reduction in level of specific IgE and skin test reaction

and first 3 years of life (n = 165). Prevalence of hay fever or other allergies was no different from the control group at age 7 years.

Herbal medicine

Four out of five RCTs of **butterbur** (*Petasites hybridus*) (Table 2.39) report positive findings. Two found it to be more effective than placebo,[10,11] one superior to placebo and equally effective as fexofenadine,[12] and one equally effective as cetirizine.[13] One small RCT found it not to be clinically effective.[14]

One RCT of a **Chinese herbal formula** consisting of 18 herbs found it to be superior to acupuncture in relieving nasal and

Table 2.39 **Double-blind RCTs of butterbur for hay fever**

Reference	Sample size	Interventions [regimen]	Result	Comment
Schapowal[10]	186	A) High dose butterbur [three tablets/day for 2 w] B) Low dose butterbur [two tablets/day for 2 w] C) Placebo	A and B superior to C	Dose relationship between the two butterbur doses

table continues

CONDITIONS

Reference	Sample size	Interventions [regimen]	Result	Comment
Lee[11]	16	A) Butterbur [100 mg/day for 1w] B) Fexofenadine [180 mg/day for 1 w] C) Placebo	A and B superior to C	A and B equally effective double-blind
Lee[12]	22	A) Butterbur [100 mg/day for 2 w] B) Placebo	A superior to B	
Schapowal[13]	125	A) Butterbur [four tablets/day for 2 w] B) Cetirizine [one tablet/day for 2 w]	A and B equally effective	More adverse events in B double-blind
Gray[14]	35	A) Butterbur [100 mg/day for 2 w] B) Placebo	A not superior to B	Double-blind

non-nasal symptoms.[15] Two RCTs tested different formulas of Chinese herbal medicines administered in addition to acupuncture. One found it to be effective in relieving subjective symptoms of hay fever[16] while the other found no difference between active and placebo groups.[17]

A double-blind RCT of **grapeseed** extract generated no evidence supporting its efficacy in the treatment of seasonal allergic rhinitis.[18]

A double-blind RCT (n = 69) of **stinging nettle** (*Urtica dioica*) taken for one week reported higher global ratings of improvement than for placebo, but no statistical analysis was conducted.[19]

Tinospora cordifolia was reported to decrease all symptoms of allergic rhinitis in a double-blind, placebo-controlled RCT in patients with allergic rhinitis.[20]

Homeopathy

Seven placebo-controlled RCTs of *Galphimia glauca* from one research group were subjected to meta-analysis by the same researchers (Box 2.47).[21] Collectively the results suggested that the remedy is effective for both ocular and nasal symptoms. The success rate of 79% is comparable to conventional treatments, with minimal adverse events reported. Encouraging results were reported from a small pilot RCT (n = 36) of homeopathic grass pollens versus placebo.[22] The same research team conducted a larger (n = 144) double-blind placebo-controlled RCT testing homeopathic dilutions of specific antigens identified for each hay fever patient by skin tests.[23] Symptom scores and use of antihistamines were reduced more in the homeopathic group. A double-blind RCT compared a homeopathic nasal spray with a conventional one (cromolyn sodium) over 42 days in 146 hay fever sufferers.[24] Quality of life assessments indicated therapeutic equivalence of the two treatments. Findings of a placebo-controlled RCT (n = 40) of a homeopathic remedy prepared from common allergens specific to the Southwest region of the USA indicated benefits in reducing symptoms and improving quality of life in patients with seasonal allergic rhinitis in this area.[25]

Box 2.47
Meta-analysis
Homeopathic
Galphimia glauca
for hay fever
Lüdtke[21]

- Seven randomised double-blind placebo-controlled trials and four not placebo-controlled trials involving 1038 patients (752 in placebo-controlled trials)

- Overall rate of improved eye-symptoms is about 1.25 (CI 1.09 to 1.43) times higher in the verum than in the placebo group

- Verum success rate is estimated by 79.3% (CI 74.1% to 85.0%) comparable with those of conventional antihistaminics

- No side effects occurred

- Conclusion: a significant superiority of *Galphimia glauca* over placebo is demonstrated. However, as not all of the single studies were analysed by intention to treat analysis the results may be biased

Hypnotherapy
An RCT (n = 47) tested the effects of hypnotic suggestion on skin reactions to allergen prick tests in individuals with hay fever and asthma.[26] Hypnosis was associated with smaller weals, but specific suggestions had no influence. An RCT (n = 79) reported improvements of symptoms with self-hypnosis in patients with moderate to severe allergic rhinitis to grass or birch pollen.[27]

Supplements
Fish oil supplementation was investigated in a double-blind placebo-controlled RCT (n = 37) involving pollen-sensitive individuals with hay fever and asthma.[28] Various outcomes measured over a pollen season revealed no differences between the fish oil and placebo groups.

In a double-blind, placebo-controlled RCT (n = 112) **vitamin E** supplementation in addition to the regular antiallergic treatment reduced nasal symptom scores in hay fever patients but not ocular symptoms or relief medication scores.[29]

Overall recommendation
Encouraging evidence exists for a homeopathic preparation of *Galphimia glauca*. Whether it is as effective as conventional medication still needs to be directly investigated. Adverse events are rare with homeopathic remedies, so it might be an option for patients dissatisfied with their orthodox medication. The results for butterbur are also encouraging and it seems to be associated with fewer adverse events than conventional medication. There

is not convincing evidence from clinical trials for the effective-ness of any other complementary therapy in the prevention or treatment of hay fever.

Table 2.40
Summary of clinical evidence for hay fever

Treatment	Weight of evidence	Direction of evidence	Serious safety concerns
Acupuncture			
(prevention)	O	⇨	Yes (see p 294)
(treatment)	OOO	⇨	Yes (see p 294)
Diet (prevention)	O	⇩	No (see p 5)
Herbal medicine			
Butterbur	OO	⬈	Yes (see p 477)
Chinese herbal formula	OO	⬈	Yes (see p 5)
Grapeseed	O	⇩	Yes (see p 414)
Nettle	O	⬈	Yes (see p 444)
Tinaspora cordifolia	O	⇧	Yes (see p 5)
Homeopathy	OO	⇧	No (see p 327)
Hypnosis	OO	⬈	Yes (see p 331)
Supplements			
Fish oil	O	⇩	Yes (see p 483)
Vitamin E	O	⬈	Yes (see p 5)

REFERENCES

1 Zuckerman G B, Bielory L. Complementary and alternative medicine herbal therapies for atopic disorders. Am J Med 2002;113 suppl9A:47S–51S

2 Schafer T, Riehle A, Wichmann H E, Ring J. Alternative medicine in allergies – prevalence, patterns of use, and costs. Allergy 2002;57:694–700

3 Williamson L. Hay fever prophylaxis using single point acupuncture: a pilot study. Acup Med 1994;12:84–87

4 Xue C C, English R, Zhang J J, Da Costa C, Li C G. Effect of acupuncture in the treatment of seasonal allergic rhinitis: a randomized controlled clinical trial. Am J Chin Med 2002;30:1–11

5 Ng D K, Chow P Y, Ming S P, Hong S H, Lau S, Tse D, Kwong W K, Wong M F, Wong W H, Fu Y M, Kwok K L, Li H, Ho J C. A double-blind, randomized, placebo-controlled trial of acupuncture for the treatment of childhood persistent allergic rhinitis. Pediatrics 2004;114:1242–1247

6 Wolkenstein E, Horak F. [Protective effect of acupuncture on allergen provoked rhinitis] Wien Med Wochenschr 1998;148:450–453

7 Williamson L, Yudkin P, Livingstone R, Prasad K, Fuller A, Lawrence M. Hay fever treatment in general practice: a randomised controlled trial comparing standardised Western acupuncture with sham acupuncture. Acup Med 1996;14:6–10

8 Magnusson A L, Svensson R E, Leirvik C, Gunnarsson R K. The effect of acupuncture on allergic rhinitis: a randomized controlled clinical trial. Am J Chin Med 2004;32:105–115

9 Zeiger R S, Heller S. The development and prediction of atopy in high-risk children: follow up at age seven years in a prospective randomized study of combined maternal and infant food allergen avoidance. J Allergy Clin Immunol 1995;95:1179–1190

10 Schapowal A; Petasites Study Group. Butterbur Ze339 for the treatment of intermittent allergic rhinitis: dose-dependent efficacy in a

prospective, randomized, double-blind, placebo-controlled study. Arch Otolaryngol Head Neck Surg 2004;130:1381–1386

11 Lee D K, Carstairs I J, Haggart K, Jackson C M, Currie G P, Lipworth B J. Butterbur, a herbal remedy, attenuates adenosine monophosphate induced nasal responsiveness in seasonal allergic rhinitis. Clin Exp Allergy 2003;33:882–886

12 Lee D K, Gray R D, Robb F M, Fujihara S, Lipworth B J. A placebo-controlled evaluation of butterbur and fexofenadine on objective and subjective outcomes in perennial allergic rhinitis. Clin Exp Allergy 2004;34:646–649

13 Schapowal A; Petasites Study Group. Randomised controlled trial of butterbur and cetirizine for treating seasonal allergic rhinitis. BMJ 2002;324:144–146

14 Gray R D, Haggart K, Lee D K, Cull S, Lipworth B J. Effects of butterbur treatment in intermittent allergic rhinitis: a placebo controlled evaluation. Ann Allergy Asthma Immunol 2004;93:56–60

15 Xue C C, Thien F C, Zhang J J, Da Costa C, Li C G. Treatment for seasonal allergic rhinitis by Chinese herbal medicine: a randomized placebo controlled trial. Altern Ther Health Med 2003;9:80–87

16 Brinkhaus B, Hummelsberger J, Kohnen R, Seufert J, Hempen C H, Leonhardy H, Nogel R, Joos S, Hahn E, Schuppan D. Acupuncture and Chinese herbal medicine in the treatment of patients with seasonal allergic rhinitis: a randomized-controlled clinical trial. Allergy 2004;59:953–960

17 Xue C C, Thien F C, Zhang J J, Yang W, Da Costa C, Li C G. Effect of adding a Chinese herbal preparation to acupuncture for seasonal allergic rhinitis: randomised double-blind controlled trial. Hong Kong Med J 2003;9:427–434

18 Bernstein D I, Bernstein C K, Deng C, Murphy K J, Bernstein I L, Bernstein J A, Shukla R. Evaluation of the clinical efficacy and safety of grapeseed extract in the treatment of fall seasonal allergic rhinitis: a pilot study. Ann Allergy Asthma Immunol 2002;88:272–278

19 Mittman P. Randomized, double-blind study of freeze-dried *Urtica dioica* in the treatment of allergic rhinitis. Planta Med 1990;56:44–47

20 Badar V A, Thawani V R, Wakode P T, Shrivastava M P, Gharpure K J, Hingorani L L, Khiyani R M. Efficacy of *Tinospora cordifolia* in allergic rhinitis. J Ethnopharmacol 2005;96:445–449

21 Lüdtke R, Wiesenauer M. A meta-analysis of the homeopathic treatment of pollinosis with *Galphimia glauca*. Wien Med Wochenschr 1997;147:323–327

22 Reilly D T, Taylor M A. Potent placebo or potency? A proposed study model with initial findings using homoeopathically prepared pollens in hay fever. Br Homoeopath J 1985;74:65–74

23 Reilly D T, Taylor M A, McSharry C, Aitchison T. Is homoeopathy a placebo response? Controlled trial of homoeopathic potency, with pollen in hay fever as model. Lancet 1986;2:881–886

24 Weiser M, Gegenheimer L H, Klein P. A randomized equivalence trial comparing the efficacy and safety of Luffa comp-Heel nasal spray with cromolyn sodium spray in the treatment of seasonal allergic rhinitis. Forsch Komplementärmed 1999;6:142–148

25 Kim L S, Riedlinger J E, Baldwin C M, Hilli L, Khalsa S V, Messer S A, Waters R F. Treatment of seasonal allergic rhinitis using homeopathic preparation of common allergens in the southwest region of the US: a randomized, controlled clinical trial. Ann Pharmacother 2005;39:617–624

26 Fry L, Mason A A, Pearson R S. Effect of hypnosis on allergic skin responses in asthma and hay fever. BMJ 1964;1:1145–1148

27 Langewitz W, Izakovic J, Wyler J, Schindler C, Kiss A, Bircher A J. Effect of self hypnosis on hay fever symptoms – a randomised controlled intervention study. Psychother Psychosom 2005;74:165–172

28 Thien F C K, Mencia-Huerta J M, Lee T H. Dietary fish oil effects on seasonal hay fever and asthma in pollen-sensitive subjects. Am Rev Respir Dis 1993;147:1138–1143

29 Shahar E, Hassoun G, Pollack S. Effect of vitamin E supplementation on the regular treatment of seasonal allergic rhinitis. Ann Allergy Asthma Immunol 2004;92:654–658

HEADACHE

Synonyms/ sub-categories

Tension headache, chronic or episodic tension-type headache, cephalodynia, cephalalgia, cephalea, cerebralgia, encephalalgia, encephalodynia, cervicogenic headache (formerly muscle tension headache). For migraine see page 204.

Definition

The 1988 International Headache Society criteria for chronic tension-type headache are headaches on 15 or more days a month (180 days/year) for at least 6 months; pain that is bilateral, pressing, or tightening in quality, of mild or moderate intensity, which does not prohibit activities and is not aggravated by routine physical activity; presence of no more than one additional clinical feature (nausea, photophobia, or phonophobia) and no vomiting. Episodic tension-type headache can last for 30 minutes to 7 days and occurs for fewer than 180 days a year.

CAM usage

Thirty-two percent of Americans with headache have used CAM in the previous 12 months, most frequently relaxation and chiropractic.[1] Many other therapies are also used, especially herbal medicine, homeopathy, acupuncture and reflexology.

Clinical evidence

A Cochrane review[2] found encouraging evidence for spinal manipulation, therapeutic touch, electrotherapy, and transcutaneous electrical nerve stimulation (TENS) for treating tension-type headaches. It also noted that spinal manipulation and exercise are promising for cervicogenic headache.

Acupuncture

Three good-quality studies were included in a systematic review.[3] It concluded that acupuncture might have a role to play but the current evidence was not of sufficient quantity or quality to make firm recommendations. Since then, results of RCTs have been mixed. Three placebo-controlled RCTs (n = 69, n = 37 and n = 50) suggested positive effects on pain or quality of life.[4-6] Another pragmatic trial also generated positive results but the majority of patients suffered from migraine.[7] Three further RCTs (n = 39, n = 50, n = 30) showed no effects compared with sham acupuncture.[8-10]

Autogenic training

In one study, 146 patients with tension headache were randomised to autogenic training, hypnosis or waiting list control.[11] Autogenic training (but not hypnosis) was better than waiting list for symptom control.

Biofeedback

A systematic review[12] (Box 2.48) concluded that both relaxation and biofeedback (either on its own or in combination with relaxation) were superior to no treatment and to placebo therapy. Subsequent RCTs[13-15] (Table 2.41) have tested biofeedback in adolescents and adults, mainly in comparison with relaxation. The majority found biofeedback more effective. One study[16] demonstrated that the clinical improvements correlated with changes in self-efficacy but not in EMG or EEG activity. Another study[17] found that patients who have a preference for highly structured practice respond better when they are given explicit guidelines than when they are left to their own devices.

Box 2.48
Meta-analysis
Biofeedback and relaxation for headache
Bogaards[12]

- All prospective studies, including uncontrolled studies

- Seventy-eight studies with 175 groups were included in the review, involving 2866 patients

- Mean (SD) effect size from 29 studies of EMG biofeedback was 47% (26%)

- Mean (SD) effect size from 38 studies of relaxation was 36% (20%)

- For comparison, mean (SD) effect size from pharmacological treatment was 39% (23%) and for placebo treatment 20% (38%)

- Conclusion: biofeedback is likely to be an effective option for headache

Table 2.41   **Parallel-arm RCTs of biofeedback for headache**

Reference	Sample size	Interventions [regimen]	Result	Comment
Arena[13]	26	A) Frontal EMG biofeedback [12 sessions] B) Trapezius EMG biofeedback [12 sessions] C) Relaxation [7 sessions]	B better than A or C at 3 mo	
Bussone[14]	35	A) Biofeedback relaxation [10 sessions in 5 w] B) Relaxation placebo	A better than B at 1 y	Adolescents
Kroner-Herwig[15]	50	A) Biofeedback [12 30-min sessions in 6 w] B) Relaxation [6 1-h sessions in 6 w] C) Untreated control	No difference between A and B. Both better than C for some outcomes	Children; parental involvement had no influence

Herbal medicine
In an RCT involving 41 adults with a history of tension headache, 164 acute headache attacks were treated with either **peppermint** oil or placebo oil locally and either paracetamol (acetaminophen) or placebo tablet orally.[18] Peppermint oil was superior to placebo and not different from the analgesic drug in reducing headache.

The use of **tiger balm** was supported in one multicentre RCT in which 57 patients were given either tiger balm to apply locally, placebo balm or standard analgesic medication.[19] Tiger balm and medication were both more effective than placebo at reducing the headache intensity, though the success of subject blinding is questionable since tiger balm produces local warmth.

Homeopathy

One rigorous RCT with 98 subjects included patients with tension-type headache as well as those with migraine and found no benefit from 12 weeks of individualised homeopathy compared with placebo.[20] The results were similar after one year of follow-up.[21]

Hypnotherapy

Like other forms of therapy involving regular relaxation, self-hypnosis appears to be more effective than waiting list control (e.g.[22]). However, it is not clear whether it is superior to other forms of relaxation. Several trials have compared different combinations of therapies including hypnotherapy with various control interventions (e.g.[11,23]). Subjects who are highly hypnotisable tend to show a greater reduction of headaches than those who are less easily hypnotised.[11]

Relaxation

A systematic review[12] of biofeedback and relaxation (Box 2.48) concluded that relaxation is effective, with a mean effect size of 36%.

In children and adolescents, RCTs indicate that relaxation has a positive effect on tension headache, though the size of the effect is often modest. More than two-thirds of the children in one study (n = 26) recorded at least 50% improvement at follow-up after 6 months, compared with only a quarter of controls.[24] Follow-up over an average of 4 years found that continuing to practise relaxation maintained some of the improvements.[25] Most studies have compared relaxation with no treatment. One exception is a trial among 202 adolescents in which relaxation was compared with placebo relaxation (sitting quietly, thinking of an episode from their life) and no difference was found.[26] Relaxation techniques could therefore be of benefit predominantly through non-specific effects.

Spinal manipulation

The most recent and authoritative systematic review[27] of spinal manipulation found that, due to the small number and poor quality of the primary data, it is not possible to draw valid conclusions about the effectiveness of this approach (Box 2.49).

Other therapies

The role of **cranial electrotherapy**, which uses a stimulation apparatus to deliver a high-frequency, low-intensity current

Box 2.49
Systematic review
Spinal manipulation for tension-type headache
Lenssinck[27]

- Four RCTs were included
- Three studies were of chiropractic, one of osteopathic techniques
- Overall methodological quality was poor
- Best evidence synthesis was conducted
- Few adverse events were reported
- Conclusion: There is insufficient evidence

transcranially, is in treatment of acute headache rather than in prevention. It was found to be more effective than placebo in a multicentre RCT of 100 patients, reducing headache scores by 35% after 20 minutes compared with 18% in the placebo group.[28]

Guided imagery was used as an adjunct to standard medical treatment in an RCT of 260 adults with chronic tension headache with or without migraine.[29] The intervention group received a guided imagery tape to listen to every day for 1 month and controls received standard medical treatment alone. Guided imagery was superior in global assessment and some quality of life measures.

In one double-dummy RCT involving 32 patients, **reflexology** was compared with flunarizin. Improvements in headache were twice as great with reflexology, but the difference was not significant and methodological flaws prevent any firm conclusions.[30]

Non-contact **therapeutic touch** was more effective than mock therapeutic touch in the treatment of acute headache in an RCT of reasonable quality that involved 90 subjects, though the difference was no longer apparent after 4 hours.[31] Recent RCTs generated encouraging results for **percutaneous electrical nerve stimulation**,[32] **impulse magnetic-field therapy**,[33] and the **Trager approach**[34] as treatments for various types of headache.

Overall recommendation

The evidence is not convincing that any particular CAM therapy is more effective than placebo in preventing tension headaches. However, in the absence of genuinely safe and effective conventional treatments, patients may benefit from treatments involving relaxation. Relaxation in various forms, including muscular and mental relaxation, hypnotherapy and autogenic training, is simple, relatively safe and beneficial compared with no treatment. The addition of biofeedback may increase the benefit compared with simple relaxation alone. In the treatment of acute headache, preliminary evidence supports the use of tiger balm or peppermint oil locally, and possibly electrotherapy. It seems unlikely, however, that these options are superior to conventional drugs like amitriptyline.

Table 2.42
Summary of clinical evidence for headache

Treatment	Weight of evidence	Direction of evidence	Serious safety concerns
Acupuncture	OO	⇨	Yes (see p 294)
Autogenic training	O	⬈	Yes (see p 305)
Biofeedback	OOO	⬈	No (see p 310)
Herbal medicine			
Peppermint oil (local)	O	⇧	Yes (see p 448)
Tiger balm (local)	O	⬈	Yes (see p 5)
Homeopathy	O	⇩	No (see p 327)
Hypnotherapy	OO	⬈	Yes (see p 331)
Relaxation	OO	⬈	No (see p 348)
Spinal manipulation	OO	⇨	Yes (see p 316)

REFERENCES

1 Eisenberg D M, Davis R, Ettner S L, Appel S, Wilkey S, Rompay M V. Trends in alternative medicine use in the United States, 1990–1997. JAMA 1998;280:1569–1575

2 Bronfort G, Nilsson N, Haas M, Evans R, Goldsmith C H, Assendelft W J J, Bouter L M. Non-invasive treatments for chronic/recurrent headache. The Cochrane Database of Systematic Reviews 2004, Issue 3. Art No. CD001878

3 Melchart D, Linde K, Fischer P, Berman B, White A, Vickers A, Allais G. Acupuncture for idiopathic headache. The Cochrane Database of Systematic Reviews 2001, Issue 1. Art No. CD001218

4 Karst M, Reinhard M, Thum P, Wiese B, Rollnik J, Fink M. Needle acupuncture in tension-type headache: a randomized, placebo-controlled study. Cephalalgia 2001;21:637–642

5 Xue C C, Dong L, Polus B, English R A, Zheng Z, Da Costa C, Li C G, Story D F. Electroacupuncture for tension-type headache on distal acupoints only: a randomized, con- trolled, crossover trial. Headache 2004;44:333–341

6 Ebneshahidi N S, Heshmatipour M, Moghaddami A, Eghtesadi-Araghi P. The effects of laser acupuncture on chronic ten- sion headache – a randomised controlled trial. Acupunct Med 2005;23:13–18

7 Vickers A J, Rees R W, Zollman C E, McCarney R, Smith C M, Ellis N, Fisher P, Van Haselen R. Acupuncture for chronic headache in primary care: large, pragmatic, randomised trial. BMJ 2004;328:744

8 Karst M, Rollnik J D, Fink M, Reinhard M, Piepenbrock S. Pressure pain threshold and needle acupuncture in chronic tension-type headache – a double-blind placebo-controlled study. Pain 2000;88:199–203

9 White A R, Resch K L, Chan J C, Norris C D, Modi S K, Patel J N, Ernst E. Acupuncture for episodic tension-type headache: a multicentre randomized controlled trial. Cephalalgia 2000;20:632–637

10 Karakurum B, Karaalin O, Coskun O, Dora B, Ucler S, Inan L. The 'dry-needle technique': intramuscular stimulation in tension-type headache. Cephalalgia 2001;21:813–817

11 Ter Kuile M M, Spinhoven P, Linssen A C G, Zitman F G, Van Dyck R, Rooijmans H G M. Autogenic training and cognitive self-hypnosis for the treatment of recurrent headaches in three different subject groups. Pain 1994;58:331–340

12 Bogaards M C, ter Kuile M M. Treatment of recurrent tension headache: a meta-analytic review. Clin J Pain 1994;10:174–190

13 Arena J G, Bruno G M, Hannah S L, Meador K J. A comparison of frontal electromyographic biofeedback training, trapezius electromyo- graphic biofeedback training, and progressive muscle relaxation therapy in the treatment of tension headache. Headache 1995;35:411–419

14 Bussone G, Grazzi L, D'Amico D, Leone M, Andraski F. Biofeedback-assisted relaxation training for young adolescents with tension- type headache: a controlled study. Cephalalgia 1998;18:463–467

15 Kroner-Herwig B, Mohn U, Pothmann R. Comparison of biofeedback and relaxation in the treatment of pediatric headache and the influence of parent involvement on outcome. Appl Psychophysiol Biofeedback 1998;23:143–157

16 Rokicki L A, Holroyd K A, France C R, Lipchik G L, France J L, Kvaal S A. Change mechanisms associated with combined relaxation/E MG biofeedback training for chronic tension headache. Applied Psychophysiol Biofeedback 1997;22:21–41

17 Hart J D. Predicting differential response to EMG biofeedback and relaxation training: the role of cognitive structure. J Clin Psychol 1984;40:453–457

18 Gobel H, Fresenius J, Heinze A, Dworschak M, Soyka D. Effectiveness of Oleum menthae piperitae and paracetamol in therapy of headache of the tension type. Nervenarzt 1996;67:672–681

19 Schattner P, Randerson D. Tiger Balm as a treatment of tension headache. A clinical trial in general practice. Aust Fam Physician 1996;25:216,218,220 passim

20 Walach H, Haeusler W, Lower T, Mussbach D, Schamell U, Springer W, Stritzl G, Gaus W, Haag G. Classical homeopathic treatment of chronic headaches. Cephalalgia 1997;17:119–126

21 Walach H, Lowes T, Mussbach D, Schamell U, Springer W, Stritzl G, Haag G. The long-term effects of homeopathic treatment of chronic headaches: one year follow-up and single case time series analysis. Br Homeopath J 2001;90:61–62

22 Melis P M, Rooimans W, Spierings E L, Hoogduin C A. Treatment of chronic tension-type headache with hypnotherapy: a single-blind time controlled study. Headache 1991;31:686–689

23 Reich B A. Non-invasive treatment of vascular and muscle contraction headache: a comparative longitudinal clinical study. Headache 1989;29:34–41

24 Larsson B, Melin L. Chronic headaches in adolescents: treatment in a school setting with relaxation training as compared with information-contact and self-registration. Pain 1986;25:325–336

25 Engel J M, Rapoff M A, Pressman A R. Long-term follow-up of relaxation training for pediatric headache disorders. Headache 1992;32:152–156

26 Passchier J, Van Den Bree M B, Emmen H H, Osterhaus S O, Orlebeke J F, Verhage F. Relaxation training in school classes does not reduce headache complaints. Headache 1990;30:660–664

27 Lenssinck M L, Damen L, Verhagen A P, Berger M Y, Passchier J, Koes B W. The effectiveness of physiotherapy and manipulation in patients with tension-type headache: a systematic review. Pain 2004;112:381–388

28 Solomon S, Elkind A, Freitag F, Gallagher R M, Moore K, Swerdlow B, Malkin S. Safety and effectiveness of cranial electrotherapy in the treatment of tension headache. Headache 1989;29:445–450

29 Mannix L K, Chandurkar R S, Rybicki L A, Tusek D L, Solomon G D. Effect of guided imagery on quality of life for patients with chronic tension-type headache. Headache 1999;39:326–334

30 Lafuente A, Noguera M, Puy C, Molins A, Titus F, Sanz F. Effekt der Reflexzonenbehandlung am Fua bezüglich der prophylaktischen Behandlung mit Funarizin bei an Cephalea-Kopfschmerzen leidenden Patienten. Erfahrungsheilkunde 1990;39:713–715

31 Keller E, Bzdek V M. Effects of therapeutic touch on tension headache pain. Nurs Res 1986;35:101–106

32 Ahmed H E, White P F, Craig W F, Hamza M A, Ghoname E, Gajraj N M. Use of percutaneous electrical nerve stimulation (PENS) in the short-term management of headache. Headache 2000;40:311–315

33 Pelka R B, Jaenicke C, Gruenwald J. Impulse magnetic-field therapy for migraine and other headaches: a double-blind, placebo-controlled study. Adv Ther 2001;18:101–109

34 Foster K A, Liskin J, Cen S, Abbott A, Armisen V, Globe D, Knox L, Mitchell M, Shtir C, Azen S. The Trager approach in the treatment of chronic headache: a pilot study. Altern Ther Health Med 2004;10:40–46

CONDITIONS

HEPATITIS

Definition

Inflammation of the liver usually due to either viral infection or toxic agents.

Related conditions

Liver cirrhosis.

CAM usage

Several herbal medicines and some other food supplements are used for various forms of hepatitis.

Clinical evidence

A systematic review of complementary and alternative medicine in the treatment of chronic hepatitis C found 27 RCTs involving herbal products and supplements (Box 2.50).[1] No RCTs were identified for any other complementary therapy.

Box 2.50
Systematic review
Complementary and alternative medicine for hepatitis C
Thompson Coon[1]

- Twenty-seven RCTs involving herbal or other supplements were included

- Only 11 trials were of good methodological quality

- In 14 of the trials the supplement was administered in combination with interferon

- Greater clearance of the hepatitis C virus compared with control treatment was found for Bing Gan decoction, thymic extracts, zinc in combination with interferon and oxymatrine alone

- Normalisation of liver enzymes was greater during treatment with *Glycyrrhiza glabra*, CH-100, Yi Zhu decoction and Yi Er Gan Tang decoction than with control treatment

- Safety profiles at the doses studied look promising

- Conclusion: several promising complementary therapies were identified although extrapolation of the results is difficult due to methodological limitations

Herbal medicine

Two **Ayurvedic** herbal mixtures have been tested for hepatitis. Kamalahar, a mixture of six herbs was reported to improve clinical symptoms and liver enzymes in a placebo-controlled RCT with 52 patients suffering from acute viral hepatitis.[2] Preliminary data had suggested that the Ayurvedic herbal mixture LIV 52 might be effective for hepatitis[3] and liver cirrhosis.[4] However, a 2-year clinical trial including 188 patients with alcoholic liver cirrhosis revealed an increased mortality in the treatment compared with the placebo group and it should therefore be considered obsolete.[5]

A Cochrane review (Box 2.51) of **Chinese medicinal herbs** for chronic hepatitis B infections concluded that the evidence is too weak to make any recommendations for any of the ten single herbs or compounds included.[6] Another Cochrane review (Box 2.52) assessed whether Chinese medicinal herbs were effective in treating asymptomatic carriers of hepatitis B virus and found insufficient evidence for the three herbal medicines tested.[7]

CONDITIONS

Box 2.51
Systematic review
Chinese medicinal herbs for chronic hepatitis B
Liu[6]

- Nine trials of 936 patients with chronic hepatitis B were included

- Trials were randomised or quasi-randomised, blinded or unblinded

- Ten different Chinese medicines were tested

- Methodological quality was generally poor and considered adequate in only one trial

- Positive effects were found for Fuzheng Jiedu Tang and *Polyporus umbellatus* polysaccharide on the clearance of hepatitis B virus and on the diseased liver; no effects of the other examined herbs were found

- Chinese medicinal herbs may be associated with adverse effects

- Conclusion: the evidence is to weak to make any recommendations

Box 2.52
Systematic review
Chinese medicinal herbs for asymptomatic carriers of chronic hepatitis B infections
Liu[7]

- Three trials of 307 patients were included

- All were of poor methodological quality

- The herbal compound Jianpi Wenshen had significant effects on viral markers compared with interferon while *Phyllanthus amarus* and *Astragalus membranaceus* showed no antiviral effect compared with placebo

- Conclusion: due to the poor methodological quality and the small numbers there is insufficient evidence for these Chinese herbal medicines

Since these reviews, single trials of several Chinese herbal medicines have been published.

A decoction of *Astragalus polygonum* was more effective that jinshuibao capsules in treating liver fibrosis of chronic hepatitis B patients and in inhibiting hepatic inflammation.[8]

A small RCT reported **Da Ding Feng Zhu** to lower serum indexes of liver fibrosis due to chronic hepatitis B compared with colchicine.[9]

Fuzheng Huayu capsules were found to be effective in alleviating liver fibrosis in patients with hepatitis B in a double-blind RCT compared with Heluo Shugan capsules.[10]

Gaixan recipe combined with lamivudine was compared with Gaixan alone and lamivudine alone in an RCT of 122 patients with chronic hepatitis B.[11] The combined group showed positive results with regards to hepatic function.

Heije was found to improve T cell immune state in two RCTs of chronic hepatitis B patients.[12,13]

Jiedu yanggan gao, a Chinese herbal mixture containing 12 medicinal plants, was tested in a CCT with 96 patients suffering from chronic hepatitis B. It found greater normalisation of liver enzymes in the experimental compared with the control group.[14] The authors claim that eight patients in the treatment group were cured.

Kangxian baogan was reported to be more effective in treating liver fibrosis than conventional liver protecting treatment in an RCT of 81 patients with hepatitis B.[15]

A systematic review of *Sophora flavescens* root (Box 2.53) concluded that matrine, an alkaloid extracted from this traditional Chinese herb, may have antiviral activity and positive effects on liver biochemistry in chronic hepatitis B but that the evidence was not sufficient to recommend it for routine clinical use.[16] A subsequent RCT of 120 patients with hepatitis B found

Box 2.53
Meta-analysis
Sophora flavescens
**for chronic
hepatitis B**
Liu[16]

- Twenty-two RCTs included 2409 patients

- Methodological quality of the trials was generally low

- The combined results of the aqueous extract of *Sophora flavescens* (matrine) showed antiviral activity, positive liver biochemical effects, and improved symptoms

- The combination of aqueous extract of *Sophora flavescens* and interferon-alpha, thymosin, or basic treatment showed better effects on viral and liver biochemical responses

- No serious adverse events were reported

- Conclusion: the evidence is not sufficient to recommend matrine for routine clinical use due to the generally low methodological quality of the studies

matrine administered in addition to liver-protective drugs to be more effective in improving clinical symptoms, and recovery of liver functions than liver-protective drugs alone.[17]

Zhaoyangwan showed positive effects on chronic hepatitis B symptoms and posthepatic cirrhosis in an RCT of 50 patients with chronic hepatitis B.[18]

A systematic review of CAM for hepatitis C included seven RCTs.[1] Bing Gan in combination with interferon-alpha demonstrated greater clearance of the hepatitis C virus than control treatment. Normalisation of liver enzymes was reported to be greater during treatment with CH-100, Yi Zhu decoction and Yi Er Gan Tang decoction than with the control treatment. A subsequent RCT of a combination of Chinese medicinal herbs for symptomatic hepatitis C did not show any improvements in quality of life, liver chemistry results or viral load.[19]

The findings of four RCTs of **liquorice** (*Glycyrrhiza glabra*) included in a systematic review were inconclusive.[1]

A systematic review included four RCTs of **milk thistle** (*Silybum marianum*) for various forms of viral hepatitis.[20] The results were not uniformly positive, but overall showed an encouraging trend as well as a good safety profile. A Cochrane Review assessed the effects of milk thistle or its constituents in patients with alcoholic and/or hepatitis B or C virus liver diseases.[21] Its results question the beneficial effects of milk thistle for this indication. Silymarin extracted from the seeds of milk thistle for liver diseases has been evaluated in a systematic review.[22] Although the results for acute viral hepatitis were encouraging no firm conclusion were drawn.

Phyllanthus species have been shown to inhibit hepatitis virus DNA polymerase and surface antigen expression. A systematic review of 22 RCTs (Box 2.54) concluded that *Phyllanthus* species may have positive effects on antiviral activity and liver biochemistry in chronic hepatitis B viral infection and no serious adverse events occurred.[23] However, the evidence is not strong due to the generally low methodological quality and the variations of the herb. *Phyllanthus amarus* was considered equally effective as interferon alpha-1b in chronic viral hepatitis B recovery of liver function and inhibition of the replication of it.[24] *Phyllanthus urinaris* showed no demonstrable anti viral effect in chronic hepatitis B in a placebo-controlled double-blind RCT.[25]

Salvia miltiorrhiza and **Polyporus umbellatus** were tested alone or in combination in a three-armed RCT, including 90 patients with chronic hepatitis B. It reported high rates of liver enzyme normalisation and conversion of surface antigen in all these groups with results being consistently best for the combination therapy.[26] An RCT of three different doses (24, 16 and 8 ml) of *Salvia* injections administered in addition to Gexia Zhuyu decoction in patients with liver fibrosis caused by hepatitis B found that all doses improved clinical symptoms with the largest dose being the most effective.[27]

Sho-saiko-to, a mixture of skullcap, liquorice, bupleurum, ginseng, banxia, jujube and ginger, was tested in a CCT. It demonstrated that medication with sho-saiko-to normalises the cytokine production system in patients with hepatitis C.[28] An RCT showed better improvement of liver enzymes in the

Box 2.54
Systematic review
***Phyllantus* spp for
chronic hepatitis B**
Liu[23]

- Twenty-two RCTs including 1947 patients

- Methodological quality was good in five double-blind RCTs and low in the remaining 17 RCTs

- The combined results showed positive effects of *Phyllantus* on antiviral activity and liver biochemistry which was equally effective as interferon and better than non-specific treatment or other herbal medicines

- No serious adverse events were reported

- Conclusion: *Phyllantus* species may have positive effects; the evidence is not strong enough due the general low methodological quality and the variations of the herb

experimental group compared with the control group in 222 patients with chronic hepatitis.[29] The subgroup of patients with hepatitis B also showed a trend towards a decrease of viral antigen and an increase in antibodies. A further RCT including 260 patients with liver cirrhosis showed a trend towards longer survival after 5 years' treatment with sho-saiko-to.[30]

An RCT with 138 hepatitis B patients showed positive results for *Uncaria gambir* compared with placebo.[31] Unfortunately it is burdened with significant toxicity and should therefore be considered obsolete.

Supplements

Seven RCTs (n = 463) of antioxidants were included in a systematic review; six thereof in combination with interferon-alpha.[1] No differences in virological response were seen between treatment regimens in any of the trials. In a small RCT, high-dose vitamin E (800 IU twice daily) supplementation did not diminish ribavirin-associated haemolysis in hepatitis C treatment with combination standard alpha-interferon and ribavirin.[32]

Oral enzyme therapy was found to be equivalent to interferon-alpha, ribavarin or liver support therapy in one RCT; the study had however several methodological weaknesses.[1]

Epidemiological data from China suggested that **selenium** supplementation protects against hepatitis B infections and subsequent primary liver cancer. This was confirmed in a CCT with 226 hepatitis B surface antigen-positive patients.[33]

A systematic review identified five trials of **thymic extracts**.[1] In combination with interferon-alpha thymic extracts showed greater clearance of the hepatitis C virus than control but not when administered alone.

One RCT of **zinc** supplementation in combination with interferon-alpha found greater clearance of the hepatitis C virus than with interferon-alpha alone.[1]

Overall recommendation

Hepatitis can be both serious and difficult to treat. Conventional therapy (e.g. interferon) is by no means always successful. Encouraging evidence exists for *Phyllantus* spp and *Sophora flavescens* as well as for thymic extracts administered in combination with interferon as treatments for viral hepatitis, and for selenium as a means of prevention of liver cancer. The adverse events of thymic extracts require vigilance while *Phyllantus, S. flavescens* and selenium are associated with markedly fewer safety concerns. These options seem the most worthy of consideration in suitable cases. There is insufficient evidence for any other herbal or non-herbal supplements.

Table 2.43
Summary of clinical evidence for hepatitis

Treatment	Weight of evidence	Direction of evidence	Serious safety concerns
Herbal medicine			
Astragalus polygonum	O	↗	Yes (see pp 5, 479)
Bin gan	O	↗	Yes (see p 5)
CH-100	O	↗	Yes (see p 5)
Da Ding Feng Zhu	O	↗	Yes (see p 5)
Fuzheng Huayu	O	↗	Yes (see p 5)
Gaixan	O	↗	Yes (see p 5)
Heije	O	↗	Yes (see p 5)
Jiedu Yanggan Gao	O	↗	Yes (see p 5)
Kamalahar	O	↗	Yes (see p 5)
Kangxian Baogan	O	↗	Yes (see p 5)
Liquorice	OO	⇨	Yes (see p 479)
LIV 520	OO	⇩	Yes (see p 5)
Milk thistle	OO	↗	Yes (see p 439)
Phyllanthus spp	OOO	↗	Yes (see p 479)
Salvia miltiorrhiza & Polyporus umbellatus	O	↗	Yes (see p 478)
Sho-saiko-to	OO	↗	Yes (see p 476)
Sophora flavescens	OOO	↗	Yes (see p 5)
Uncaria gambir	O	⇩	Yes (see p 5)
Yi Zhu	O	↗	Yes (see p 5)
Yi Er Gan Tan	O	↗	Yes (see p 5)
Zhaoyangwan	O	↗	Yes (see p 5)

CONDITIONS

table continues

Treatment	Weight of evidence	Direction of evidence	Serious safety concerns
Supplements			
Antioxidants	OOO	⇓	Yes (see p 5)
Oral enzyme therapy	O	↗	Yes (see p 5)
Selenium	OO	↗	Yes (see p 484)
Thymus extracts	OO	↗	Yes (see p 484)
Zinc	O	↗	Yes (see p 5)

REFERENCES

1 Thompson Coon J, Ernst E. Complementary and alternative therapies in the treatment of chronic hepatitis C: a systematic review. J Hepatol 2004;40:491–500

2 Das D G. A double-blind clinical trial of Kamalahar, an indigenous compound preparation in acute viral hepatitis. Indian J Gastroenterol 1993;12:126–128

3 Desai V, Dudhia M, Ghandi V. A clinical study on infective hepatitis treated with LIV 52. Indian Paediatr 1997;3:197

4 Lotterer E, Etzel R. Pilotstudie einer kontrollierten klinischen Prüfung von Liv.52 bei Patienten mit alkoholischer Leberzirrhose. Forsch Komplementärmed 1995;2:12–14

5 Fleig W W, Morgan M Y, Holzer M A. The Ayurvedic drug LIV 52 in patients with alcoholic cirrhosis. Results of a prospective, double-blind, placebo-controlled clinical trial. J Hepatol 1997;26(suppl 1):127

6 Liu J P, McIntosh H, Lin H. Chinese medicinal herbs for chronic hepatitis B. Cochrane Database Syst Rev 2001; Issue 1. Art. No.: CD001940

7 Liu J P, McIntosh H, Lin H. Chinese medicinal herbs for asymptomatic carriers of hepatitis B virus infection. Cochrane Database Syst Rev 2001; Issue 2. Art. No.: CD002231

8 Chen H, Weng L. [Comparison on efficacy in treating liver fibrosis of chronic hepatitis B between Astragalus Polygonum anti-fibrosis decoction and jinshuibao capsule] Zhongguo Zhong Xi Yi Jie He Za Zhi 2000;20:255–257

9 Li W, Wang C, Zhang J. Effects of da ding feng zhu decoction in 30 cases of liver fibrosis. J Tradit Chin Med 2003;23:251–254

10 Liu P, Hu Y Y, Liu C, Xu L M, Liu C H, Sun K W, Hu D C, Yin Y K, Zhou X Q, Wan M B, Cai X, Zhang Z Q, Ye J, Tang B Z, He J. [Multicenter clinical study about the action of Fuzheng Huayu Capsule against liver fibrosis with chronic hepatitis B] Zhong Xi Yi Jie He Xue Bao 2003;1:89–102

11 Shen H, Alsatie M, Eckert G, Chalasani N, Lumeng L, Kwo P Y. Combination therapy with lamivudine and famciclovir for chronic hepatitis B infection. Clin Gastroenterol Hepatol 2004;2:330–336

12 Zhang S J, Chen Z X, Lao S X, Huang B J. Effect of Hejie decoction on T cell immune state of chronic hepatitis B patients. World J Gastroenterol 2004;10:1436–1439

13 Zhang S J, Chen Z X, Huang B J. [Effect of hejie decoction on T-cell receptor V beta 7 gene expression in patients of chronic hepatitis B] Zhongguo Zhong Xi Yi Jie He Za Zhi 2002;22:499–501

14 Chen Z. Clinical study of 96 cases with chronic hepatitis B treated with jiedu yang-gan gao by a double-blind method. Chin J Modern Develop Trad Med 1990;10:71–74

15 Liang T J, Zhang W, Zhang C Q. [Clinical study on treatment of liver fibrosis in patients of hepatitis B by kangxian baogan decoction] Zhongguo Zhong Xi Yi Jie He Za Zhi 2002;22:332–334

16 Liu J, Zhu M, Shi R, Yang M. Radix Sophorae flavescentis for chronic hepatitis B: a systematic review of randomized trials. Am J Chin Med 2003;31:337–354

17 Long Y, Lin X T, Zeng K L, Zhang L. Efficacy of intramuscular matrine in the treatment of chronic hepatitis B. Hepatobiliary Pancreat Dis Int 2004;3:69–72

18 Zhang C P, Tian Z B, Liu X S, Zhao Q X, Wu J, Liang Y X. Effects of Zhaoyangwan on chronic hepatitis B and posthepatic cirrhosis. World J Gastroenterol 2004;10:295–298

19 Jakkula M, Boucher T A, Beyendorff U, Conn S M, Johnson J E, Nolan C J, Peine C J,

Albrecht J H. A randomized trial of Chinese herbal medicines for the treatment of symptomatic hepatitis C. Arch Intern Med 2004;164:1341–1346

20 Mulrow C, Lawrence V, Jacobs B, Dennehy C, Sapp J, Ramirez G, Aguilar C, Montgomery K, Morbidoni L, Arterburn JM, Chiquette E, Harris M, Mullins D, Vickers A, Flora K. Report on milk thistle: effects on liver disease and cirrhosis and clinical adverse effects. Evidence Report/ Technology Assessment 2000 (unpublished)

21 Rambaldi A, Jacobs B P, Iaquinto G, Gluud C. Milk thistle for alcoholic and/or hepatitis B or C virus liver diseases. The Cochrane Database of Systematic Reviews 2005, Issue 2. Art. No.: CD003620

22 Saller R, Meier R, Brignoli R. The use of silymarin in the treatment of liver diseases. Drugs 2001;61:2035–2063

23 Liu J, Lin H, McIntosh H. Genus Phyllanthus for chronic hepatitis B virus infection: a systematic review. J Viral Hepat 2001;8:358–366

24 Xin-Hua W, Chang-Qing L, Xing-Bo G, Lin-Chun F. A comparative study of Phyllanthus amarus compound and interferon in the treatment of chronic viral hepatitis B. Southeast Asian J Trop Med Public Health 2001;32:140–142

25 Chan H L, Sung J J, Fong W F, Chim A M, Yung P P, Hui A Y, Fung K P, Leung P C. Double-blinded placebo-controlled study of Phyllanthus urinaris for the treatment of chronic hepatitis B. Aliment Pharmacol Ther 2003;18:339–345

26 Xiong L L. Therapeutic effect of combined therapy of Salvia miltiorrhiza and Polyporus umbellatus polysaccharide in the treatment of chronic hepatitis B. Chung Kuo Chung Hsi Chieh Ho Tsa Chih 1993;13:516–517, 533–535

27 She S F, Huang X Z, Tong G D. [Clinical study on treatment of liver fibrosis by different dosages of Salvia injection] Zhongguo Zhong Xi Yi Jie He Za Zhi 2004;24:17–20

28 Yamashiki M, Nishimura A, Suzuki H, Sakaguchi S, Kosaka Y. Effects of the Japanese herbal medicine 'Sho-Saiko-To' (TJ-9) on in vitro interleukin-10 production by peripheral blood monon-uclear cells of patients with chronic hepatitis C. Hepatology 1997;25:1390–1397

29 Hirayama C, Okumura M, Tanikawa K, Yano M, Mizuta M, Ogawa N. A multicenter randomized controlled clinical trial of Shosaiko- to in chronic active hepatitis. Gastroenterologia Japonica 1989;24:715–719

30 Oha H, Yamamoto S, Kuroki T. Prospective study of chemoprevention of hepatocellular carcinoma with Sho-saiko- to (TJ-9). Cancer 1995;76:743–749

31 Suzuki H, Yamamoto S, Hirayama C. Cianidanol therapy for HBe antigen positive chronic hepatitis. Liver 1986;6:35–44

32 Saeian K, Bajaj J S, Franco J, Knox J F, Daniel J, Peine C, McKee D, Varma R R, Ho S; Midwest Hepatitis Study Group. High-dose vitamin E supplementation does not diminish ribavirin-associated haemolysis in hepatitis C treatment with combination standard alpha-interferon and ribavirin. Aliment Pharmacol Ther 2004; 20:1189–1193

33 Yu S Y, Zhu Y J, Li W G. Protective role of Selenium against hepatitis B virus and primary liver cancer in Qidong. Biol Trace Element Res 1997;56:117–124

CONDITIONS

HERPES SIMPLEX

Synonyms/ subcategories Cold sores, herpes labialis, herpes genitalis.

Definition A variety of infections caused by herpes simplex virus types 1 and 2.

Related conditions Traumatic herpes, herpes gladiatorum.

CAM usage Herbal creams are commonly used for the treatment of acute lesions or prevention of recurrences.

Clinical evidence

Herbal medicine

A double-blind, placebo-controlled RCT (n = 50) of oral *Echinacea purpurea* extract found no benefit in the treatment of frequently recurrent genital herpes.[1]

Several studies have suggested that **lemon balm** (*Melissa officinalis*) speeds up the healing of herpes labialis lesions. A double-blind placebo-controlled RCT including 66 patients with acute herpes labialis demonstrated a commercial cream (Lomaherpan) to be effective in the treatment of herpes labialis symptoms.[2]

A double-blind RCT (n = 145) compared a topical preparation of **rhubarb and sage** extracts with a rhubarb monopreparation, and an aciclovir cream. It found the combined sage rhubarb preparation to be as effective as acyclovir cream in reducing the duration of symptoms and more effective than sage alone in reducing pain.[3]

A small RCT reported that the orally administered Chinese herbal preparation **Shenqi** reduced the recurrence rate of genital herpes to 26.5% compared with 72.4% in the control group.[4]

In a placebo-controlled RCT of **Siberian ginseng** (*Eleutherococcus senticosus*) root extract (4 g/day) including 93 individuals with recurrent herpes simplex infections, 75% in the experimental group reported improvements in severity duration or frequency of attacks while this figure was 34% in the placebo group.[5]

Topical application of **tea tree** (*Melaleuca alternifolia*) oil gel (6%) was not effective in the treatment of recurrent herpes labialis in a small placebo-controlled, investigator-blinded RCT.[6]

Supplements

A three-armed RCT testing the effectiveness of Canadian **propolis** against acyclovir or placebo administered on a tampon in 30 women with recurrent genital herpes reported faster average healing time and reduced incidence of superinfection in the propolis goup.[7]

A large RCT of **Vitamin A** in women coinfected with HIV-1 reported no decrease in herpes simplex virus shedding and infectivity.[8]

A double-blind, placebo-controlled RCT (n = 46) found **zinc oxide/glycine** cream to be effective in reducing the duration and severity of symptoms of facial and circumoral herpes infection.[9]

LongoVital, a preparation containing unspecified vitamins in daily recommended doses supplemented with dried and ground herbs from paprika, rosemary leaves, peppermint leaves, milfoil flowers, hawthorn leaves and flowers, and pumpkin seeds. The preparation was not superior to placebo in preventing recurrent herpes labialis but it was superior in reducing the number of recurrences after 2 months' intake.[10]

Overall recommendation

Herpes simplex infections are difficult to treat with conventional medications and recurrences are even more resistant to therapy. There is some encouraging evidence for some herbal and non-herbal supplements but the weight of the evidence is not sufficient for strong recommendations.

Table 2.44
Summary of clinical evidence for herpes simplex

Treatment	Weight of evidence	Direction of evidence	Serious safety concerns
Herbal medicine			
Echinacea purpurea (genital herpes)	O	⇩	Yes (see p 391)
Lemon balm (herpes labialis, treatment)	O	⇧	Yes (see pp 5, 479)
Rhubarb and sage combination (herpes labialis, treatment)	O	⇧	Yes (see p 5)
Shenqi (genital herpes, prevention)	O	⬀	Yes (see p 5)
Siberian ginseng (prevention)	O	⇧	Yes (see p 409)
Tea tree (herpes labialis, treatment)	O	⇩	Yes (see p 466)
Supplements			
Propolis (genital herpes)	O	⇧	Yes (see p 454)
Vitamin A (genital herpes)	O	⇩	Yes (see p 5)
Zinc oxide/glycine cream (genital herpes, treatment)	O	⇧	Yes (see p 5)
Longo Vital (herpes labialis, treatment)	O	⇩	Yes (see p 5)
(herpes labialis, prevention)	O	⬀	Yes (see p 5)

CONDITIONS

REFERENCES

1 Vonau B, Chard S, Mandalia S, Wilkinson D, Barton S E. Does the extract of the plant Echinacea purpurea influence the clinical course of recurrent genital herpes? Int J STD AIDS 2001;12:154–158

2 Koytchev R, Alken R G, Dundarov S. Balm mint extract (Lo-701) for topical treatment of recurring Herpes labialis. Phytomedicine 1999;6:225–230

3 Saller R, Buechi S, Meyrat R, Schmidhauser C. Combined herbal preparation for topical treatment of Herpes labialis. Forsch Komplementärmed Klass Naturheilkd 2001;8:373–382

4   Yu J B, Yin G W, He Q B. Immune modulatory and therapeutical effect of shenqi tablet accessory therapy in treating recurrent genital herpes [Chinese]. Zhongguo Zhong Xi Yi Jie He Za Zhi 2001;21:831–833

5   Williams M. Immuno-protection against herpes simplex type II infection by eleutherococcus root extract. Int J Alt Complement Med 1995;13:9–12

6   Carson C F, Ashton L, Dry L, Smith D W, Riley T V. Melaleuca alternifolia (tea tree) oil gel (6%) for the treatment of recurrent herpes labialis. J Antimicrob Chemother 2001;48:450–451

7   Vynograd N, Vynograd I, Sosnowski Z. A comparative multi-centre study of the efficacy of propolis, acyclovir and placebo in the treatment of genital herpes (HSV). Phytomedicine 2000;7:1–6

8   Baeten J M, McClelland R S, Corey L, Overbaugh J, Lavreys L, Richardson B A, Wald A, Mandaliya K, Bwayo J J, Kreiss J K. Vitamin A supplementation and genital shedding of herpes simplex virus among HIV-1-infected women: a randomized clinical trial. J Infect Dis 2004;189:1466–1471

9   Godfrey H R, Godfrey N J, Godfrey J C, Riley D. A randomized clinical trial on the treatment of oral herpes with topical zinc oxide/glycine. Altern Ther Health Med 2001;7:49–56

10 Pedersen A. LongoVital and herpes labialis: a randomised, double-blind, placebo-controlled study. Oral Dis 2001;7:221–225

HERPES ZOSTER

Synonyms   Shingles.

Definition   Herpes zoster is caused by activation of latent varicella zoster virus (human herpes virus 3) in people who have been rendered partially immune by a previous attack of chickenpox. Herpes zoster infects the sensory ganglia and their areas of innervation. It is characterised by pain along the distribution of the affected nerve, and crops of clustered vesicles over the area.

Related conditions   Postherpetic neuralgia.

CAM usage   Various CAM therapies are being advocated for the symptomatic treatment of postherpetic pain. Other treatments are claimed to enhance the healing process of the infection. Acupuncture is used both during infection and to treat neuralgia.

Clinical evidence   *Acupuncture*
Two RCTs of acupuncture for postherpetic pain have been published. Acupuncture was no more effective than mock TENS in one trial,[1] while a smaller trial suggested a short-term effect.[2] Thus there is no convincing evidence for its use in this condition.

Enzyme therapy
A commercial enzyme extract (Wobe-Mucos), consisting of trypsin, chymotrypsin, papainase and calf thymus hydrolysate, is promoted in Germany. Two RCTs have suggested that the intramuscular or oral administration of this preparation is equally effective as acyclovir in treating herpes zoster.[3,4] However, this evidence is weak due to methodological shortcomings in both studies.

Herbal medicine

A topical formulation of *Clinacanthus nutans* or placebo was applied five times daily to the affected area for 7–14 days in a CCT with 51 patients suffering from herpes zoster.[5] Compared with placebo, the experimental group exhibited faster healing of the skin lesions. Similarly encouraging results were reported from a subsequent larger RCT.[6]

One small double-blind RCT (n = 24) compared the effectiveness of different doses of topical **geranium** (*Pelargonium* spp) oil with capsaicin and placebo in the treatment of postherpetic neuralgia. Geranium oil treatment reduced spontaneous and evoked pain in a dose-dependent way and faster than capsaicin.[7]

Supplements

One systematic review including two double-blind, placebo-controlled RCTs (n = 175) of topical **capsaicin** (0.075%) cream for severe refractory postherpetic pain found it to be superior to placebo for symptomatic pain relief.[8] The effect size, however, was modest. A subsequent small RCT found no difference in pain between capsaicin and placebo.[9]

Other therapies

One small RCT of older patients who are at risk for shingles reported an increase in varicella-zoster virus specific cell-mediated immunity after 15 weeks of **tai chi chih**.[10]

Overall recommendation

Herpes zoster infection and its clinical sequelae are often difficult to control with conventional treatments. The evidence for some forms of CAM is encouraging but the weight of the evidence is mostly not sufficient for strong recommendations.

Table 2.45
Summary of clinical evidence for herpes zoster

Treatment	Weight of evidence	Direction of evidence	Serious safety concerns
Acupuncture	OO	⇨	Yes (see p 294)
Enzyme therapy	OO	⤴	Yes (see p 5)
Herbal medicine			
Clinacanthus nutans	O	⇧	Yes (see p 5)
Geranium oil	O	⇧	Yes (see p 478)
Supplements			
Capsaicin	OO	⤴	Yes (see p 480)

REFERENCES

1 Lewith G T, Field J, Machin D. Acupuncture compared with placebo in post-herpetic pain. Pain 1983;17:361–368

2 Rutgers M J, Van Romunde L K J, Osman P O. A small randomized comparative trial of

acupuncture versus transcutaneous electrical neurostimulation in postherpetic neuralgia. Pain Clin 1988;2:87–89.

3 Kleine M W, Stauder G M, Beese E W. The intestinal absorption of orally administered

hydrolytic enzymes and their effects in the treatment of acute herpes zoster as compared with those of oral acyclovir therapy. Phytomedicine 1995;2:7–15

4 Billigmann V P. Enzymtherapie – eine Alternative bei der Behandlung des Zoster. Fortschr Med 1995;113:39–44

5 Sangkitporn S, Chaiwat S, Balachandra K, Na-Ayudhaya T D, Bunjob M, Jayavasu C. Treatment of herpes zoster with Clinacanthus nutans (bi yaw yaw) extract. J Med Assoc Thailand 1995;78:624–627

6 Charuwichitratana S, Wongrattanapasson N, Timpatanapong P, Bunjob M. Herpes zoster: treatment with Clinacanthus nutans cream. Int J Dermatol 1996;35:665–666

7 Greenway F L, Frome B M, Engels T M 3rd, McLellan A. Temporary relief of postherpetic neuralgia pain with topical geranium oil. Am J Med 2003;115:586–587

8 Alper B S, Lewis P R. Treatment of postherpetic neuralgia: a systematic review of the literature. J Fam Pract 2002;51:121–128

9 Torre-Mollinedo F, Bárez E, Fernández-Landaluce A, Barreira R, Raposo F. Local capsaicine 0.025% in the management of postherpetic neuralgia. Rev Soc Esp Dolor 2001;8:468–475

10 Irwin M R, Pike J L, Cole J C, Oxman M N. Effects of a behavioral intervention, Tai Chi Chih, on varicella-zoster virus specific immunity and health functioning in older adults. Psychosom Med 2003;65:824–830

HYPERCHOLESTEROLAEMIA

Synonyms   Hypercholesteraemia, hypercholesterinaemia.

Definition   The presence of abnormally high levels of cholesterol in the plasma of the circulating blood.

Related conditions   Dyslipidaemia, hyperlipidaemia, hypertriglyceridaemia.

CAM usage   Total serum cholesterol levels can be lowered by dietary interventions, e.g. by reducing fat intake and by increasing regular physical exercise. Thus various lifestyle approaches can have an effect and are frequently promoted for hypercholesterolaemia. These approaches, however, are usually not specific to CAM. Several herbal and non-herbal dietary supplements are also used to lower cholesterol levels.

Clinical evidence

Herbal medicine

One placebo-controlled study assessed oral *Aloe vera* for hyperlipidaemia.[1] It reported no differences for total, LDL and HDL cholesterol, and serum triglyceride levels compared with placebo.

A Cochrane review (Box 2.55)[2] assessed the effects of artichoke (*Cynara scolymus*) in hypercholesterolaemic patients. Two RCTs were identified and both were conducted double-blind. Beneficial effects are reported, the evidence, however, is not compelling. This conclusion is supported by another systematic review, which assessed the evidence for all herbal medicines for reducing serum cholesterol levels.[3]

The Kampo medicine **Dai-saiko-to** was tested in a placebo-controlled RCT including 30 hypertensive patients.[4] Total cholesterol and triglyceride levels did not change but HDL cholesterol increased.

Box 2.55
Meta-analysis
Artichoke for hypercholestero-laemia
Pittler[2]

- Two RCTs were identified; both were double-blind and placebo-controlled

- One trial reported cholesterol reductions from 7.74 mmol/l to 6.31 mmol/l, which was different from placebo

- Another trial reported cholesterol reductions in a subgroup of patients with total cholesterol levels for more than 230 mg/dl

- Conclusion: beneficial effects are reported, the evidence, however, is not compelling

Fenugreek (*Trigonella foenum-graecum*) is often advocated for the purpose of normalising cardiovascular risk factors. Fenugreek seeds were tested in two RCTs and reduced total cholesterol, HDL and LDL cholesterol to a larger extent than placebo.[5,6]

Garlic (*Allium sativum*) is one of the best clinically investigated herbal remedies. Numerous RCTs have been published, some of high methodological quality.[7] An updated assessment is cautiously positive (Box 2.56).[8] Since then, two further double-blind placebo-controlled RCTs were published.[9,10] Both were negative. Consequently, the overall effect size is small, which casts doubt on the clinical relevance of the effect.

Box 2.56
Meta-analysis
Garlic for hyper-cholesterolaemia
Ernst[8]

- Sixteen double-blind, placebo-controlled RCTs were included (n = 971)

- The average quality of the studies was good

- On average, there was a reduction of 0.3 mmol/l (CI −0.6 to −0.2)

- Conclusion: garlic is superior to placebo but the effect is small and of debatable clinical relevance

Thirty-six patients with type II diabetes were randomised to receive either 100 mg or 200 mg **ginseng** (*Panax ginseng*) powder or placebo for 8 weeks.[11] Fasting glucose levels decreased but for the serum lipid profile there was no intergroup difference.

Theaflavin-enriched **green tea** (*Camellia sinensis*) extract was compared with placebo in a double-blind RCT (n = 240).[12] There were reductions compared with baseline for total and LDL cholesterol in the green tea group but not in the placebo group. It was concluded that this green tea extract is an effective adjunct for treating hypercholesterolaemia.

Guar gum is obtained from *Cyamopsis tetragonolobus* and has been shown to have total cholesterol lowering effects in hypercholesterolaemic patients.[13]

Four RCTs of **guggul** (*Commiphora mukul*), involving patients with hypercholesterolaemia, hyperlipidaemia or hyperlipoproteinaemia were included in a systematic review.[3] The results suggest reductions in total serum cholesterol compared with baseline.

Oat and other fibre products have repeatedly been shown to reduce total and LDL cholesterol.[14,15] For a meta-analysis raw data of all included trials were obtained and pooled (Box 2.57).[16] They indicate that the effect size of oat products for reducing total cholesterol levels is small. Another meta-analysis supported these results.[17]

Box 2.57
Meta-analysis
Oat fibre for hypercholesterol-aemia
Ripsin[16]

- Ten RCTs were included

- Methodological quality of the trials was, on average, good

- Total cholesterol fell by 0.13 mmol/l, CI −0.2 to −0.1

- Stronger effects were noted if initial cholesterol levels were high or dosage of oat fibre was large

- Conclusion: oat fibres cause a modest reduction in total cholesterol

Psyllium (*Plantago ovata*) is advocated as a bulk laxative and was evaluated in a meta-analysis of eight RCTs. It reported that psyllium can lower total and LDL cholesterol compared with placebo and arrived at a positive conclusion (Box 2.58).[18]

Box 2.58
Meta-analysis
Psyllium for hyper-cholesterolaemia
Anderson[18]

- Eight RCTs were included

- In total, 656 patients with mild to moderate hypercholesterol-aemia received either psyllium (10.2 g daily) or placebo

- The quality of these trials was, on average, good

- All subjects were taking a low-fat diet concomitantly

- Mean reduction were −0.2 mmol/l, CI −0.2 to −0.3 for total cholesterol and −0.3 mmol/l, CI −0.2 to −0.3 for LDL. There were no effects on HDL and triglycerides

- Psyllium was well tolerated

- Conclusion: psyllium causes a modest reduction of total and LDL cholesterol

Saiko-ka-ryukotsu-borei-to is a herbal mixture used in Kampo medicine and has been suggested to lower total cholesterol and LDL cholesterol levels. An RCT which compared the effects of two Kampo medicines but did not employ a placebo control group and showed no relevant changes in total cholesterol.[19]

Supplements

An RCT (n = 193) tested the effects of 1 and 2 g daily of elemental **calcium** on total serum cholesterol levels.[20] There were no substantial effects on total or HDL cholesterol compared with placebo.

A review of the cholesterol-lowering properties of **chitosan** identified four double-blind placebo-controlled RCTs.[21] It reported a reduction of total serum cholesterol levels ranging between 5.8 to 42.6% and a reduction of LDL cholesterol by 15.1 to 35.1%.

In a double-blind, placebo-controlled RCT 60 mg **Co-enzyme Q10** was given orally to 47 patients with slightly elevated levels of lipoprotein (a) and coronary heart disease.[22] This regimen did not alter total cholesterol but increased HDL cholesterol and lowered LDL cholesterol and lipoprotein (a).

A Cochrane review assessed the effects of **fish oil** on cholesterol levels in patients with type 2 diabetes mellitus.[23] Fish oil reduced triglyceride levels but there was no effect on total or HDL cholesterol and a slight increase was noted in LDL cholesterol levels. In hypercholesterolaemic patients supplementation with omega-3 fatty acids administered either as fish oil capsules or fish powder showed mixed results in RCTs.[24,25] Another RCT reported a reduction in triglyceride levels and an improvement in large artery endothelium dependent dilation.[26]

A small (n = 22) double-blind RCT investigated **konjac glucomannan** in hyperlipidaemic type 2 diabetic patients.[27] Compared with placebo, konjac glucomannan reduced total and LDL-cholesterol, but not triglyceride levels.

The effects of milk products fermented by the **probiotic** *Bifidobacterium longum* strain BL1 was studied in an RCT.[28] Patients (n = 32) with serum total cholesterol ranging from 220 to 280 mg/dl received either low-fat drinking yogurt prepared with *Streptococcus thermophilus* and *Lactobacillus delbrueckii* subsp. *bulgaricus* or low-fat drinking yogurt prepared with *B. longum*. Reduction of serum total cholesterol was observed particularly among subjects with moderate hypercholesterolaemia (> 240 mg/dl). For the commercially available yogurt Benecol reduction compared with baseline are reported for total and LDL cholesterol levels.[29]

Four RCTs of **red yeast rice** conducted in patients with hyperlipidaemia (n = 695) were identified by a systematic review.[3] In all studies reductions in total serum cholesterol levels compared with either control or baseline were reported.

CONDITIONS

An RCT (n = 120) found that neither **seal oil** nor cod-liver oil (15 ml each) administered for 14 months had any effects on the levels of serum total cholesterol, HDL cholesterol or postprandial triacylglycerol.[30]

A systematic review of the effects of **soy** protein on the lipid profile identified 23 RCTs.[31] Soy protein was associated with decreases in serum total cholesterol (by 0.22 mmol/l, or 3.77%), LDL cholesterol (by 0.21 mmol/l, or 5.25%), and triacylglycerols (by 0.10 mmol/l, or 7.27%) and increases in serum HDL cholesterol (by 0.04 mmol/l, or 3.03%). Additional evidence supports these findings,[32] although other RCTs suggest otherwise.[33,34] Endothelial function as assessed by flow-mediated dilation of the brachial artery was improved when soy was administered compared with caseinate,[35] while endothelium-dependent dilator responses to hyperaemia in the brachial artery was not affected compared with placebo.[36]

Hypercholesterolaemia increased circulating vascular cell adhesion molecule-1 and reduced nitric concentrations, which are early characteristics of atherosclerosis. **Vitamin E** supplementation was found to counteract these alterations, representing a potential tool for endothelial protection in hypercholesterolaemic patients.[37]

Other therapies

Ozone therapy was tested in 21 patients with a history of myocardial infarction who were treated with ozone autohaemotherapy in an uncontrolled study.[38] A decrease in total and LDL cholesterol was observed.

A systematic review assessed **yoga therapy** for treating risk factors of cardiovascular disease.[39] It identified four RCTs, which assessed lipid levels in hypercholesterolaemic patients. Overall these data suggest that yoga is beneficial for lowering cholesterol levels.

Overall recommendation

CAM offers several options for reducing total cholesterol levels. Fibre supplements are effective but may be seen as conventional dietary treatment. Compelling evidence exists also for guar gum and soy. The evidence for guggul and garlic is less convincing. Yoga may also be beneficial. The effect size of these therapies is modest and considerably less than that of synthetic lipid-lowering drugs. The exception may be red yeast rice, but more data are required for this food supplement. The bottom line therefore is that some CAM treatments are associated with modest cholesterol-lowering effects, which, not least because of their relative safety, warrants their consideration in cases where diet alone is not sufficiently effective.

Table 2.46
**Summary of
clinical evidence for
hypercholesterol-
aemia**

Treatment	Weight of evidence	Direction of evidence	Serious safety concerns
Herbal medicine			
Aloe vera	O	⇩	Yes (see p 364)
Artichoke	OO	⬈	Yes (see p 368)
Dai-saiko-to	O	⬈	Yes (see p 5)
Fenugreek	OO	⇧	Yes (see p 478)
Garlic	OOO	⬈	Yes (see p 398)
Ginseng	O	⬊	Yes (see p 407)
Green tea	O	⬈	Yes (see p 417)
Guar gum	OOO	⇧	Yes (see p 419)
Guggul	OO	⬈	Yes (see p 478)
Oat	OOO	⇧	Yes (see p 5)
Psyllium	OOO	⬈	Yes (see p 480)
Saiko-ka-ryukotsu-borei-to	O	⬊	Yes (see p 5)
Supplements			
Calcium	O	⬊	Yes (see p 5)
Chitosan	OO	⇧	Yes (see p 380)
Co-enzyme Q10	O	⬈	No (see p 385)
Fish oil	OO	⬈	Yes (see p 483)
Konjac glucomannan	O	⇧	Yes (see p 478)
Probiotics	O	⬈	Yes (see p 5)
Red yeast rice	OO	⬈	Yes (see p 484)
Seal oil	O	⇩	Yes (see p 5)
Soy	OOO	⇧	Yes (see p 450)
Vitamin E	O	⇧	Yes (see p 5)

CONDITIONS

REFERENCES

1 Nasiff H A, Fajardo F, Velez F. Effecto del aloe sobre la hiperlipidemia en pacientes refractarios a la dieta. Rev Cuba Med Gen Integr 1993;9:43–51

2 Pittler M H, Thompson Coon J, Ernst E. Artichoke leaf extract for treating hypercholesterolaemia. Cochrane Database Syst Rev 2002, Issue 3. Art. No.: CD003335

3 Thompson Coon J S, Ernst E. Herbs for serum cholesterol reduction: a systematic review. J Fam Pract 2003;52:468–478

4 Saku K, Hirata K, Zhang B, Liu R, Ying H, Okura Y, Yoshinaga K, Arakawa K. Effects of Chinese herbal drugs on serum lipids, lipoproteins and apolipoproteins in mild to moderate essential hypertensive patients. J Hum Hypertens 1992;6:393–395

5 Singh R B, Niaz M A, Rastogi V, Singh N, Postiglione A, Rastogi S S. Hypolipidemic and antioxidant effects of fenugreek seeds and triphala as adjuncts to dietary therapy in patients with mild to moderate hypercholesterolemia. Perfusion 1998;11:124–130

6 Prasanna M. Hypolipidemic effects of fenugreek: a clinical study. Indian J Pharmacol 2000;32:34–36

7 Silagy C, Neil A. Garlic as a lipid lowering agent – a meta-analysis. J Roy Coll Physicians Lond 1994;28:39–45

8 Ernst E, Stevinson C, Pittler M H. Meta-analyses of garlic for hypercholesterolemia. In: Schulz V, Rietbrock N, Roots I, Loew D. Phytopharmaka VII. Darmstadt: Steinkopff; 2002

9 Satitvipawee P, Rawdaree P, Indrabhakti S, Ratanasuwan T, Getn-gern P, Viwatwongkasem C. No effect of garlic extract supplement on serum lipid levels in hypercholesterolemic subjects. J Med Assoc Thai 2003;86:750–757

10 Peleg A, Hershcovici T, Lipa R, Anbar R, Redler M, Beigel Y. Effect of garlic on lipid profile and psychopathologic parameters in people with mild to moderate hypercholesterolemia. Isr Med Assoc J 2003;5:637–640

11 Sotaneimi E A, Haapakoski E, Rautio A. Ginseng therapy in non-insulin-dependent diabetic patients. Diabetes Care 1995;18:1373–1375

12 Maron D J, Lu G P, Cai N S, Wu Z G, Li Y H, Chen H, Zhu J Q, Jin X J, Wouters B C, Zhao J. Cholesterol-lowering effect of a theaflavin-enriched green tea extract: a randomized controlled trial. Arch Intern Med 2003;163:1448–1453

13 Brown L, Rosner B, Willet W W, Sacks F M. Cholesterol-lowering effects of dietary fiber: a meta-analysis. Am J Clin Nutr 1999;69:30–42

14 Knopp R H, Superko H R, Davidson M, Insull W, Dujovne C A, Kwiterovich P O, Zavoral J H, Graham K, O'Connor R R, Edelman D A. Long-term blood cholesterol-lowering effects of a dietary fiber supplement. Am J Prev Med 1999;17:18–23

15 Zunft H J, Luder W, Harde A, Haber B, Graubaum H J, Koebnick C, Grunwald J. Carob pulp preparation rich in insoluble fibre lowers total and LDL cholesterol in hypercholesterolemic patients. Eur J Nutr 2003;42:235–242

16 Ripsin C M, Keenan J M, Jacobs D R Jr, Elmer P J, Welch R R, Van Horn L, Liu K, Turnbull W H, Thye F W, Kestin M. Oat products and lipid lowering. A meta-analysis. JAMA 1992;267: 3317–3325

17 Brown L, Rosner B, Willett W W, Sacks F M. Cholesterol-lowering effects of dietary fiber: a meta-analysis. Am J Clin Nutr 1999;69:30–42

18 Anderson J W, Allgood L D, Lawrence A, Altringer L A, Jerdack G R, Hengehold D A, Morel J G. Cholesterol-lowering effects of psyllium intake adjunctive to diet therapy in men and women with hypercholesterolemia: meta-analysis of 8 controlled trials. Am J Clin Nutr 2000;71:472–479

19 Nomura K, Hayashi K, Kuga Y, Okura Y, Tanaka K, Yasunobu Y, Shingu T, Ohtani H, Kajiyama G. Hypolipidemic effect of Saiko-ka-ryukotsu-borei-to (TJ-12) in patients with type II or type IV hyperlipidemia. Curr Ther Res Clin Exp 1997;58:446–453

20 Bostick R M, Fosdick L, Grandits G A, Grambsch P, Gross M, Louis T A. Effect of calcium supplementation on serum cholesterol and blood pressure. A randomized, double-blind, placebo-controlled, clinical trial. Arch Fam Med 2000;9:31–38

21 Ylitalo R, Lehtinen S, Wuolijoki E, Ylitalo P, Lehtimaki T. Cholesterol-lowering properties and safety of chitosan. Arzneimittelforschung 2002;52:1–7

22 Singh R B. Serum concentration of lipoprotein (a) decreases on treatment with hydrosoluble coenzyme Q10 in patients with coronary artery disease: discovery of a new role. Int J Cardiol 1999;68:23–29

23 Farmer A, Montori V, Dinneen S, Clar C. Fish oil in people with type 2 diabetes mellitus. Cochrane Database Syst Rev 2001, Issue 3. Art. No.: CD003205

24 Pirich C, Gaszo A, Granegger S, Sinzinger H. Effects of fish oil supplementation on platelet survival and ex vivo platelet function in hypercholesterolemic patients. Thromb Res 1999;96:219–227

25 Nenseter M S, Osterud B, Larsen T, Strom E, Bergei C, Hewitt S, Holven K B, Hagve T A, Mjos S A, Solvang M, Pettersen J, Opstvedt J, Ose L. Effect of Norwegian fish powder on risk factors for coronary heart disease among hypercholesterolemic individuals. Nutr Metab Cardiovasc Dis 2000;10:323–330

26 Goodfellow J, Bellamy M F, Ramsey M W, Jones C J, Lewis M J. Dietary supplementation with marine omega-3 fatty acids improve systemc large artery endothelial function in subjects with hypercholesterolemia. J Am Coll Cardiol 2000;35:265–270

27 Chen H L, Sheu W H, Tai T S, Liaw Y P, Chen Y C. Konjac supplement alleviated hypercholesterolemia and hyperglycemia in type 2 diabetic subjects – a randomized double-blind trial. J Am Coll Nutr 2003;22:36–42

28 Xiao J Z, Kondo S, Takahashi N, Miyaji K, Oshida K, Hiramatsu A, Iwatsuki K, Kokubo S, Hosono A. Effects of milk products fermented by Bifidobacterium longum on blood lipids in rats and healthy adult male volunteers. J Dairy Sci 2003;86:2452–2461

29 Algorta Pineda J, Chinchetru Ranedo M J, Aguirre Anda J, Francisco Terreros S. Hypocholesteremic effectiveness of a yogurt containing plant stanol esters. Rev Clin Esp 2005;205:63–66

30 Brox J, Olaussen K, Osterud B, Elvevoll E O, Bjornstad E, Brattebog G, Iversen H. A long-term seal- and cod-liver-oil supplementation in hypercholesterolemic subjects. Lipids 2001;36:7–13

31 Zhan S, Ho S C. Meta-analysis of the effects of soy protein containing isoflavones on the lipid profile. Am J Clin Nutr 2005;81:397–408

32 Bricarello L P, Kasinski N, Bertolami M C, Faludi A, Pinto L A, Relvas W G, Izar M C, Ihara S S, Tufik S, Fonseca F A. Comparison between the effects of soy milk and non-fat cow milk on lipid profile and lipid peroxidation in patients with primary hypercholesterolemia. Nutrition 2004;20:200–204

33 Lissin L W, Oka R, Lakshmi S, Cooke J P. Isoflavones improve vascular reactivity in post-menopausal women with hypercholesterolemia. Vasc Med 2004;9:26–30

34 West S G, Hilpert K F, Juturu V, Bordi P L, Lampe J W, Mousa S A, Kris-Etherton P M. Effects of including soy protein in a blood cholesterol-lowering diet on markers of cardiac risk in men and in postmenopausal women with and without hormone replacement therapy. J Womens Health 2005;14:253–262

35 Cuevas A M, Irribarra V L, Castillo O A, Yanez M D, Germain A M. Isolated soy protein improves endothelial function in postmenopausal hypercholesterolemic women. Eur J Clin Nutr 2003;57:889–894

36 Blum A, Lang N, Vigder F, Israeli P, Gumanovsky M, Lupovitz S, Elgazi A, Peleg A, Ben-Ami M. Effects of soy protein on endothelium-dependent vasodilatation and lipid profile in postmenopausal women with mild hypercholesterolemia. Clin Invest Med 2003;26:20–26

37 Desideri G, Marinucci M C, Tomassoni G, Masci P G, Santucci A, Ferri C. Vitamin E supplementation reduces plasma vascular cell adhesion molecule-1 and von Willebrand factor levels and increases nitric oxide concentrations in hypercholesterolemic patients. J Clin Endocrinol Metab 2002;87:2940–2945

38 Hernandez F, Menendez F, Wong R. Decrease of blood cholesterol and stimulation of antioxidative response in cardiopathy patients treated with endovenous ozone therapy. Free Radical Biol Med 1995;19:115–119

39 Hutchinson S, Ernst E. Yoga therapy for coronary heart disease: a systematic review. Perfusion 2004;17:44–51

HYPERTENSION

Synonyms Arterial hypertension, essential hypertension, primary hypertension.

Definition Elevation of systolic or diastolic blood pressure that is not due to other causes, e.g. specific disease or medication. Mild hypertension (grade 1) = 140–159 mmHg systolic and 90–99 mmHg diastolic, moderate (grade 2) = 160–179 systolic and 100–109 diastolic, severe (grade 3) = 180 systolic and = 110 diastolic. Malignant hypertension = 200 systolic and = 130 diastolic plus encephalopathy or nephropathy. Elevated blood pressure is an important, independent cardiovascular risk factor.

Related conditions Secondary hypertension, pregnancy-induced hypertension.

CAM usage A recent survey suggested that 64% of hypertensives use some form of CAM, mostly herbal medicines.[1]

Clinical evidence Numerous interventions affect blood pressure. Some of them, such as lifestyle changes, exercise, cognitive–behavioural techniques, dietary measures or minerals are considered mainstream and are by and large excluded here.

Acupuncture

The results of RCTs have been mixed. One RCT with ten hypertensive menopausal women found no effect of acupuncture on 24-hour ambulatory blood pressure compared with sham acupuncture.[2] Another, similar RCT included ten patients with diastolic hypertension and demonstrated short-term hypotensive effects after electroacupuncture.[3]

Autogenic training

A systematic review of five CCTs found encouraging evidence for hypotensive effects of autogenic training. Due to methodological limitations, however, firm conclusions were not possible.[4] A subsequent meta-analysis confirmed these findings.[5]

Biofeedback

A large volume of RCTs have shown that biofeedback lowers both systolic and diastolic blood pressure to a clinically relevant extent. A meta-analysis of these data arrived at a positive conclusion (Box 2.59).[6]

Box 2.59
Meta-analysis
Biofeedback for hypertension
Nakao[6]

- 22 RCTs with a total of 905 patients were included

- Methodological quality varied; some RCTs were rigorous

- Compared with sham biofeedback or other control interventions, both systolic and diastolic blood pressure were reduced

- Conclusion: biofeedback is effective in lowering blood pressure

Chiropractic

Chiropractic adjustments plus massage therapy were followed by a reduction in blood pressure in a small RCT (n = 30) with hypertensive patients.[7] However, a more definitive RCT with 140 individuals with stage 1 hypertension showed that 12 sessions of spinal manipulation during 4 weeks had no effect on blood pressure.[8]

Herbal medicine

Achillea wilhelmsii, a popular folk remedy in Iran, was tested against placebo in a CCT with 120 hypotensive patients.[9] After 2 and 6 months of treatment, reductions in both systolic and diastolic blood pressure were described.

A small CCT (n = 14) tested *Adenia cissampeloides* against no treatment.[10] The results imply that this herbal remedy lowers systolic blood pressure, however, without bringing it into the normal range and without positive effects on elevated diastolic blood pressure.

Various **Chinese herbal medicines** have been tested for hypertension. Except for the only study published in a non-Chinese journal,[11] the results were all positive (Table 2.47).[12-15]

Table 2.47 **RCTs of Chinese herbal medicines for hypertension**

Author	Sample size	Intervention	Main result	Comment
Black[11]	45	A) Chinese herbal mixture of 12 herbs B) Diuretics + propranolol	B had superior hypotensive effects	
Lu[12]	389	A) Cucumber vine compound B) Western antihypertensive medication	A had superior hypotensive effects	Independent replication required
Liu[13]	80	A) Xianbai ruyang huanwu decoction B) Combination of Western medication	A had superior hypotensive effects	Independent replication required
Kim[14]	90	A) Luohuo capsule B) Beijing hypertension No 0	A reduced systolic blood pressure more than B	Quality of preparation?
Yu[15]	90	A) Luohuo capsule B) Beijing hypertension No 0	A reduced systolic blood pressure more than B	Quality of preparation?

Garlic (*Allium sativum*) is often recommended for hypertension. A meta-analysis of eight RCTs (all conducted with the same commercial preparation) found a small pooled effect size and the authors concluded that the evidence was insufficient for treatment recommendations.[16]

No hypotensive effects of **ginkgo** (*Ginkgo biloba*) were noted in a small RCT with healthy volunteers.[17]

Ginseng (*Panax ginseng*) was tested in two small RCTs[18,19] with patients who were either hypertensive or had blood pressures in the high-normal range. Both studies found blood pressure normalising effects of *Panax ginseng*.

Hawthorn (*Crataegus*) is usually used for chronic heart failure (see p 92, 421). Trials with patients only suffering from hypertension are rare and have generated both encouraging[20] and negative results.[21] One reason for this apparent contradiction could be that different species were used. Extrapolating from results obtained in other patient populations, one would expect hawthorn to lower blood pressure.

Hibiscus sabdariffa was tested in two placebo-controlled RCTs including 54 and 75 patients with mild to moderate hypertension. Both studies concur that hibiscus has clinically relevant hypotensive effects.[22,23]

Pycnogenol, a **maritime pine bark extract** (*Pinus pinaster*) was investigated in a placebo-controlled trial with 58 hypertensives.[24] Both groups simultaneously received calcium antagonists for blood pressure control. The experimental group was able to reduce their antihypertensive medication more than the placebo group and also exhibited improvements in endothelial function.

Olive leaf (*Olea europea*) (400 mg extract/day for 3 months) had no effect on blood pressure in a small RCT.[25]

Pomegranate (*Punica granatum*) was tested in a study with ten hypertensive patients.[26] The patients consumed 50 ml concentrated pomegranate juice/day for 2 weeks. This resulted in reductions of angiotensin converting enzyme and systolic blood pressure.

Red clover (*Trifolium subterraneum*) or placebo was administered for 8 weeks to 59 volunteers with high normal blood pressure. The results failed to show meaningful effects on blood pressure.[27]

Homeopathy

A small RCT (n = 32) tested Baryta carbonica 15 CH against placebo on elderly, immobilised hypertensive patients.[28] No effects beyond a placebo response were noted.

Hypnotherapy

Two small CCTs suggested that hypnotherapy may have hypotensive effects in patients suffering from hypertension.[29,30]

Meditation

A systematic review of six RCTs of transcendental meditation[31] failed to find convincing evidence that this approach is a useful option to treat hypotension (Box 2.60).

Box 2.60
Systematic review
Transcendental meditation for hypertension
Canter[31]

- Six RCTs including hypertensive patients or healthy volunteers

- Methodological quality mostly poor; two RCTs reasonable

- Three RCTs reported antihypertensive effects

- Conclusion: insufficient good quality evidence

Relaxation

A meta-analysis of nine RCTs found only very small and therefore clinically probably not relevant pooled effects of stress reduction programmes on systolic (−1.0 mmHg) and diastolic (−1.1 mmHg) blood pressure.[32]

Qigong

Encouraging results of RCTs have emerged from China[33] and from one group in Korea.[34,35] They suggest that the regular practice of qigong for 8–10 weeks normalises elevated systolic and diastolic blood pressure.

Supplements

A systematic review of four RCTs found that 100–200 mg **Coenzyme Q10**/day for 8–12 weeks decreases systolic blood pressure by 6–12 mmHg and systolic blood pressure by 2–16 mmHg.[36]

Fish oil (omega-3 fatty acids) is often used for hypertension. A meta-analysis found clinically relevant reductions in systolic and diastolic blood pressure (Box 2.61).[37] Subsequent trial data have generated both positive[38,39] as well as negative results.[40,41]

Box 2.61
Meta-analysis
**Fish oil
supplementation
for hypertension**
Appel[37]

- Seventeen controlled clinical trials were included

- Doses were generally high (> 3 g/day)

- Methodological quality was usually good

- No relevant BP reduction in normotensives

- Average reductions of 5.5 mmHg systolic and 3.5 mmHg diastolic in untreated hypertension

- Conclusion: high doses of omega-3 fatty acids reduce blood pressure in untreated hypertensives

Green algae (*Chlorella*) have been tested in a small placebo-controlled trial with 33 hypertensives.[42] Patients took the extract for two months. No convincing effects on blood pressure were demonstrated.

L–arginine has, according to one small crossover study, hypertensive effects on systolic (–6 mmHg) and diastolic (–5 mmHg) blood pressure.[43]

Melatonin (2.5 mg at bedtime) was tested in a placebo-controlled RCT including 16 men with untreated hypertension.[44] Intake for 3 weeks reduced systolic and diastolic blood pressures during sleep by an average of 6 and 4 mmHg.

Reishi mushroom (*Ganoderma lucidum*) has been shown to reduce diastolic blood pressure by an amazing 19 mmHg in a Japanese placebo-controlled RCT.[45]

A placebo-controlled RCT showed that 500 mg/day of **vitamin C** taken for 30 days lowered systolic blood pressure by an average of 13 mmHg.[46]

Encouraging findings have also been reported for **vitamin E** (300 mg/day).[47] and for a mixture of antioxidants including vitamin E.[48]

Yoga

A systematic review[49] suggested that adherence to a yoga regimen has positive effects on a range of cardiovascular risk factors, including hypertension. These findings are collectively encouraging but not compelling.

Other therapies

An RCT of regular **Tai Chi** exercises for 12 weeks has suggested that this approach normalises blood pressure in individuals with high–normal values.[50] **Spiritual healing** was investigated for blood pressure lowering activity in patients with hypertension; no such effect was demonstrated.[51]

Overall recommendation

Hypotensive effects have been described for autogenic training, biofeedback, garlic, hibiscus, relaxation, qigong and fish oil. All of these treatments are relatively safe. However, for none is the effect size comparable to conventional treatments of hypertension. The above-named CAM therapies might be recommended as adjuncts to conventional care or for patients unwilling or unable to comply with drug treatment, for instance, because of adverse effects.

Table 2.48
Summary of clinical evidence for hypertension

Treatment	Weight of evidence	Direction of evidence	Serious safety concerns
Acupuncture	O	⇨	Yes (see p 294)
Autogenic training	OO	⤴	No (see p 305)
Biofeedback	OOO	⇧	No (see p 310)
Chiropractic	OO	⤵	Yes (see p 316)
Herbal medicine			
Achillea wilhelmsii	O	⇧	Yes (see p 481)
Adenia cissampeloides	O	⤴	Yes (see p 5)
Chinese herbal medicines	OO	⇨	Yes (see p 5)
Garlic	OOO	⤴	Yes (see p 398)
Ginkgo	O	⇩	Yes (see p 404)
Ginseng	OO	⤴	Yes (see p 407)
Hawthorn	O	⇨	Yes (see p 422)
Hibiscus	OO	⇧	Yes (see p 478)
Maritime pine	O	⇧	Yes (see p 478)
Olive leaf	O	⇩	Yes (see p 480)
Pomegranate	O	⇧	Yes (see p 480)
Red clover	O	⇩	Yes (see p 456)
Homeopathy	O	⇩	No (see p 327)
Hypnotherapy	O	⤴	Yes (see p 331)
Meditation	OO	⇨	No (see p 338)
Relaxation	OOO	⤴	No (see p 348)
Qigong	OO	⇧	No (see p 360)
Supplements			
Co-enzyme Q10	OOO	⇧	Yes (see p 385)
Fish oil	OOO	⤴	Yes (see p 483)

Treatment	Weight of evidence	Direction of evidence	Serious safety concerns
Green algae	O	⇩	Yes (see p 5)
L-Arginine	O	⇧	Yes (see p 482)
Melatonin	O	⇧	Yes (see p 435)
Reishi	O	⇧	Yes (see p 480)
Vitamin C	O	⇧	No (see p 5)
Vitamin E	O	⇧	No (see p 5)
Yoga	OO	⬀	No (see p 356)

CONDITIONS

REFERENCES

1   Shafiq N, Gupta M, Kumari S, Pandhi P. Prevalence and pattern of use of complementary and alternative medicine (CAM) in hypertensive patients of a tertiary care center in India. Int J Clin Pharmacol Ther 2003;41:294–298

2   Kraft K, Coulon S. [Effect of a standardized acupuncture treatment on complaints, blood pressure and serum lipids of hypertensive, postmenopausal women. A randomized, controlled clinical study] Forsch Komplementarmed 1999;6:74–79

3   Williams T, Mueller K, Cornwall M W. Effect of acupuncture-point stimulation on diastolic blood pressure in hypertensive subjects: a preliminary study. Phys Ther 1991;71:523–529

4   Kanji N, White A R, Ernst E. Anti-hypertensive effects of autogenic training: A systematic review. Perfusion 1999;12:279–282

5   Stetter F, Kupper S. Autogenic training: a meta-analysis of clinical outcome studies. Appl Psychophysiol Biofeedback 2002;27:45–98

6   Nakao M, Yano E, Nomura S, Kuboki T. Blood pressure-lowering effects of biofeedback treatment in hypertension: a meta-analysis of randomized controlled trials. Hypertens Res 2003;26:37–46

7   Plaugher G, Long C R, Alcantara J, Silveus A D, Wood H, Lotun K, Menke J M, Meeker W C, Rowe S H. Practice-based randomized controlled-comparison clinical trial of chiropractic adjustments and brief massage treatment at sites of subluxation in subjects with essential hypertension: pilot study. J Manipulative Physiol Ther 2002;25:221–239

8   Goertz C H, Grimm R H, Svendsen K, Grandits G. Treatment of hypertension with alternative therapies: a randomized clinical trial. J Hypertens 2002;20:2063–2068

9   Asgary S, Naderi G H, Sarrafzadegan N, Mohammadifard N, Mostafavi S, Vakili R. Antihypertensive and antihyperlipidemic effects of Achillea wilhelmsii. Drugs Exp Clin Res 2000;26:89–93

10 Nyarko A A, Addy M E. Effect of aqueous extract of Adenia cissampeloides on blood pressure and serum analytes of hypertensive patients. Phytother Res 1990;4:25–28

11 Black H R, Ming S, Poll D S, Wen Y F, Zhou H Y, Zhang Z Q, Chung Y K, Wu Y S. A comparison of the treatment of hypertension with Chinese herbal and Western medication. J Clin Hypertens 1986;2:371–378

12 Lu G L, Yuan W X, Fan Y J. [Clinical and experimental study of tablet cucumber vine compound in treating essential hypertension] Zhong Xi Yi Jie He Za Zhi 1991;11:274–276, 260–261

13 Liu H, Zhou J F. [Xianhai buyang Huanwu decoction used for treating hypertension with kidney qi deficiency and blood stasis]. Zhongguo Zhong Xi Yi Jie He Za Zhi 1993;13:714–717

14 Kim R, Zhou W Q. [Clinical study on effect of luohuo capsule in treating essential hypertension of phlegm-stasis blocking collateral type]. Zhongguo Zhong Xi Yi Jie He Za Zhi 2004;24:610–612

15 Yu X D, Zhou W Q, Cui L. [Hypotensive action of luohuo capsule and its effect on plasma adrenal medullin and tissue factor pathway inhibitor]. Zhongguo Zhong Xi Yi Jie He Za Zhi 2004;23:668–672

16 Silagy C A, Neil H A. A meta-analysis of the effect of garlic on blood pressure. J Hypertens 1994;12:463–468

17 Kalus J S, Piotrowski A A, Fortier C R, Liu X, Kluger J, White C M. Hemodynamic and electrocardiographic effects of short-term Ginkgo biloba. Ann Pharmacother 2003;37:345–349

18 Han K H, Choe S C, Kim H S, Sohn D W, Nam K Y, Oh B H, Lee M M, Park Y B, Choi Y S, Seo J D, Lee Y W. Effect of red ginseng on blood pressure in patients with essential hypertension and white coat hypertension. Am J Chin Med 1998;26:199–209

19 Stavro P M, Vuksan V. Effect of Korean red ginseng extract with escalating doses of ginsenoside Rg3 on blood pressure in individuals with high normal blood pressure or hypertension. Diabetes 2003;52:A554–A555

20 Asgary S, Naderi G H, Sadeghi M, Kelishadi R, Amiri M. Antihypertensive effect of Iranian Crataegus curvisepala Lind.: a randomized, double-blind study. Drugs Exp Clin Res 2004;30:221–225

21 Walker A F, Marakis G, Morris A P, Robinson P A. Promising hypotensive effect of hawthorn extract: a randomized double-blind pilot study of mild, essential hypertension. Phytother Res 2002;16:48–54

22 Haji Faraji M, Haji Tarkhani A. The effect of sour tea (Hibiscus sabdariffa) on essential hypertension. J Ethnopharmacol 1999;65:231–236

23 Herrera-Arellano A, Flores-Romero S, Chavez-Soto M A, Tortoriello J. Effectiveness and tolerability of a standardized extract from Hibiscus sabdariffa in patients with mild to moderate hypertension: a controlled and randomized clinical trial. Phytomedicine 2004;11:375–382

24 Liu X, Wei J, Tan F, Zhou S, Wurthwein G, Rohdewald P. Pycnogenol, French maritime pine bark extract, improves endothelial function of hypertensive patients. Life Sci 2004;74:855–862

25 Cherif S, Rakal N, Haouala M. A clinical trial of a titrated olea extract in the treatment of essential hypertension. Pharm Belg 1996;51:69–71

26 Aviram M, Dornfeld L. Pomegranate juice reduces blood pressure in hypertensive patients in small study. Atherosclerosis 2001;158:195–198

27 Hodgson J M, Puddey I B, Beilin L J, Mori T A S, Burke V, Croft K D, Rogers P B. Effects of isoflavonoids on blood pressure in subjects with high-normal ambulatory blood pressure levels. Am J Hypertens 1999;12:47–53

28 Bignamini M, Bertoli A, Consolandi A M, Dovera N, Saruggia M, Taino S, Tubertini A. Controlled double-blind trial with Baryta carbonica 15 CH versus placebo in a group of hypertensive subjects confined to bed in two old people's homes. Br Homeopath J 1987;76:114–119

29 Friedman H, Taub H A. A six-month follow-up of the use of hypnosis and biofeedback procedures in essential hypertension. Am J Clin Hypn 1978;20:184–188

30 Raskin R, Raps C, Luskin F, Carlson R, Cristal R. Pilot study of the effect of self-hypnosis on the medical management of essential hypertension. Stress Med 1999;15:243–247

31 Canter P H, Ernst E. Insufficient evidence to conclude whether or not Transcendental Meditation decreases blood pressure: results of a systematic review of randomized clinical trials. J Hypertens 2004;22:2049–2054

32 Ebrahim S, Smith G D. Lowering blood pressure: a systematic review of sustained effects of non-pharmacological interventions. J Pub Health Med 1998;20:441–448

33 Li W, Xin Z, Pi D. [Effect of qigong on sympathetico-adrenomedullary function in patients with liver yang exuberance hypertension] Zhong Xi Yi Jie He Za Zhi 1990;10:283–285, 261

34 Lee M S, Lee M S, Kim H J, Moon S R. Qigong reduced blood pressure and catecholamine levels of patients with essential hypertension. Int J Neurosci 2003;113:1691–1701

35 Lee M S, Lee M S, Kim H J, Choi E S. Effects of qigong on blood pressure, high-density lipoprotein cholesterol and other lipid levels in essential hypertension patients. Int J Neurosci 2004;114:777–786

36 Rosenfeldt F, Hilton D, Pepe S, Krum H. Systematic review of effect of coenzyme Q10 in physical exercise, hypertension and heart failure. Biofactors 2003;18:91–100

37 Appel L J, Miller E R 3rd, Seidler A J, Whelton P K. Does supplementation of diet with 'fish oil' reduce blood pressure? A meta-analysis of controlled clinical trials. Arch Intern Med 1993;153:1429–1438

38 Bao D Q, Mori T A, Burke V, Puddey I B, Beilin L J. Effects of dietary fish and weight reduction on ambulatory blood pressure in overweight hypertensives. Hypertension 1998;32:710–717

39 Lungershausen Y K, Abbey M, Nestel P J, Howe P R. Reduction of blood pressure and plasma triglycerides by omega-3 fatty acids in treated hypertensives. J Hypertens 1994;12:1041–1045

40 Sacks F M, Hebert P, Appel L J, Borhani N O, Applegate W B, Cohen J D, Cutler J A, Kirchner K A, Kuller L H, Roth K J. Short report: the effect of fish oil on blood pressure and high-density lipoprotein-cholesterol levels in phase I of the Trials of Hypertension Prevention. J Hypertens 1994;12:209–213

41 Gray D R, Gozzip C G, Eastham J H, Kashyap M L. Fish oil as an adjuvant in the treatment

of hypertension. Pharmacotherapy 1996;16:295–300

42 Merchant R E, Andre C A, Sica D A. Nutritional supplementation with Chlorella pyrenoidosa for mild to moderate hypertension. J Med Food 2002;5:141–152

43 Sinai A, Pagano E, Iacone R. Blood pressure and metabolic changes during dietary L-arginine supplementation in humans. Am J Hypertens 2000;13:547–551

44 Scheer F A J L, Van Montfrans G A, van Someren E J W, Mairuhu G, Buijs R M. Daily nighttime melatonin reduces blood pressure in male patients with essential hypertension. Hypertension 2004;43:192–197

45 Kanmatsuse K, Kajiwara N, Hayashi K, Shimogaichi S, Fukinbara I, Ishikawa H, Tamura T. [Studies on Ganoderma lucidum. I. Efficacy against hypertension and side effects] Yakugaku Zasshi 1985;105:942–947

46 Khosh F, Khosh M. Natural approach to hypertension. Altern Med Rev 2001;6:590–600

47 Palumbo G, Avanzini F, Alli C, Roncaglioni M C, Ronchi E, Cristofari M, Capra A, Rossi S,

Nosotti L, Costantini C, Cavalera C. Effects of vitamin E on clinic and ambulatory blood pressure in treated hypertensive patients. Collaborative Group of the Primary Prevention Project (PPP)–Hypertension study. Am J Hypertens 2000;13:564–567

48 Galley H F, Thornton J, Howdle P D, Walker B E, Webster N R. Combination oral antioxidant supplementation reduces blood pressure. Clin Sci (Lond) 1997;92:361–365

49 Hutchinson S, Ernst E. Yoga therapy for coronary heart disease: a systematic review. Perfusion 2004;17:44–51

50 Tsai J C, Wang W H, Chan P, Lin L J, Wang C H, Tomlinson B, Hsieh M H, Yang H Y, Liu J C. The beneficial effects of Tai Chi Chuan on blood pressure and lipid profile and anxiety status in a randomized controlled trial. J Altern Complement Med 2003;9:747–754

51 Beutler J J, Attevelt J T, Schouten S A, Faber J A, Dorhout Mees E J, Geijskes G G. Paranormal healing and hypertension. BMJ (Clin Res Ed) 1988;296:1491–1494

INSOMNIA

Synonyms Sleeplessness, sleep disturbance.

Definition Poor sleep quality with difficulties in initiating or maintaining sleep, waking too early or failing to feel refreshed. Insomnia is considered chronic if it occurs at least three nights a week or for at least one month.

CAM usage According to a US survey insomnia is a common reason for using CAM with relaxation and herbal medicine being the most popular therapies.[1]

Clinical evidence

Acupuncture
A systematic review included 11 studies regardless of methodological rigour and concluded that the evidence is currently not convincing (Box 2.62).[2]

Box 2.62
Systematic review
Acupuncture for insomnia
Sok[2]

- Eleven clinical trials of any type
- Poor methodological quality
- Only English literature was considered
- All studies reported positive results
- Conclusion: evidence is inconclusive

CONDITIONS

Autogenic training

An RCT compared autogenic training (n = 71) with progressive muscle relaxation (n = 80) and standard rehabilitation (n = 78) for cancer patients suffering from insomnia.[3] Both experimental groups showed better results than patients in the control group in a wide range of sleep-related parameters. The effectiveness is further supported by other studies with less scientific rigour.[4]

Biofeedback

Several controlled trials have found no or only minimal improvement in sleep with biofeedback compared with other interventions, no treatment or sham feedback.[5-8] However, in two RCTs[7,8] positive results were reported in patients for whom the particular form of feedback was appropriate. For example, EEG feedback benefited those with anxiety-related insomnia and sensorimotor rhythm feedback helped non-anxious insomniacs. Collectively the evidence remains inconclusive.[9]

Exercise

A large body of evidence from healthy volunteers suggests that exercise can have small to moderate positive effects on sleep duration and quality.[10] A systematic review of RCTs of exercise for the elderly arrived at a cautiously positive conclusion.[11]

Herbal medicine

Kava (*Piper methysticum*) was shown to improve subjective and objective measures of sleep after acute administration (300 mg) in healthy volunteers (n = 12) in a placebo-controlled trial.[12] A comparative study of kava and valerian suggested that both improve sleep in individuals with stress-induced insomnia.[13]

A systematic review of nine placebo-controlled RCTs of the effects of **valerian** (*Valeriana officinalis*) on sleep reported some positive findings of acute and cumulative effects in patients with insomnia and healthy volunteers (Box 2.63).[14] There was little consistency between studies, though, and the body of evidence is far from compelling. A further RCT (n = 75) reported similar results for valerian and oxazepam in improving the sleep quality of insomniacs.[15] Subsequent RCTs of valerian have generated positive results[15-20] with only one exception.[21] Moreover, a small RCT (n = 9) suggested that, by comparison to triazolam, valerian causes fewer changes in cognitive function.[22]

Hypnotherapy

Positive results with hypnosis have been reported versus no treatment in a non-randomised trial of 37 female patients[23] and several comparison and placebo interventions in RCTs.[24-26] Taking into account various methodological limitations of these studies, hypnotherapy appears to have some promise in improving sleep.

Box 2.63
Systematic review
Valerian for insomnia
Stevinson[14]

- Nine double-blind, placebo-controlled RCTs including 390 volunteers

- Volunteers were insomniacs (four trials) or healthy sleepers (five trials)

- Valerian given as single dose (six trials) or for several weeks (three trials)

- Trial quality generally low

- Some positive results but totality of evidence not conclusive

Light therapy

Exposure to bright light may regulate the circadian rhythm, an approach used for light therapy. Systematic reviews of RCTs found no such studies in the elderly,[27] and five trials in dementia patients.[28] No convincing support for light therapy as a treatment of insomnia emerged.

Relaxation

A large number of clinical trials have suggested that relaxation training can improve sleep, but few are controlled studies and even fewer are randomised. One RCT (n = 22) reported that progressive relaxation training (ten sessions over 2 weeks) was superior to no treatment for alcoholic insomniacs,[29] while another (n = 53) found it as effective as stimulus control.[30] A further RCT (n = 75) suggested that cognitive–behavioural therapy is superior to progressive relaxation training in treating chronic primary insomnia.[31] An additional RCT (n = 26) reported that compared with no treatment, relaxation and sleep hygiene alone produced better long-term results than when hypnotic drugs were also allowed.[32] Specific programmes that generated encouraging results include mindfulness-based stress reduction[33] and relaxation tapes.[34,35] Two meta-analyses of non-pharmacological treatments for insomnia have concluded that relaxation techniques are effective therapies.[36,37]

Supplements

Melatonin has been submitted to a systematic review which suggested that it improves sleep quality (Box 2.64).[38]

The sleep-promoting effects of **vitamin B$_{12}$** have been investigated in an RCT (n = 50) of people with delayed sleep-phase syndrome[39] and in a small non-randomised trial (n = 10) of shift workers.[40] Neither found any superiority over placebo.

Other therapies

An **aromatherapy** study with healthy volunteers under stressful conditions indicated that sleep latency was reduced by the odor of bitter orange essential oil, but not by five other oils including lavender and valerian.[41] The first RCT of **craniosacral therapy** (n = 20) ever published suggested that this approach can alter

Box 2.64
Systematic review
Melatonin for insomnia
Olde Rikkert[38]

- Six RCTs were included

- Review focused on elderly patients

- Methodological quality was variable

- Dose ranged from 0.51 mg to 6 mg before bedtime

- Sleep latency decreased in four studies

- Conclusion: sufficient evidence that low doses of melatonin improve initial sleep quality

sleep latency. These results are clearly preliminary and require confirmation.[42] A placebo-controlled RCT with 100 army recruits suffering from sleep problems, showed encouraging results for **magnetic field therapy**.[43] When **massage therapy** was compared with relaxation therapy in an RCT of stress-induced insomnia, no differences in sleep parameters emerged, but patients strongly preferred massage therapy.[44] Encouraging results emerged from two Chinese studies of **music** therapy for cancer patients and elderly people with sleep problems.[45,46] **Yoga** was compared in a CCT (n = 39) to no treatment for cancer patients with sleep problems. Improvements in sleep-related outcomes were noted.[47]

Overall recommendation

Evidence exists to suggest that regular physical exercise, hypnotherapy, relaxation, and melatonin can improve sleep. Considering that these approaches are not associated with adverse effects as regularly as conventional drug therapy, they deserve a positive recommendation.

Table 2.49
Summary of clinical evidence for insomnia

Treatment	Weight of evidence	Direction of evidence	Serious safety concerns
Acupuncture	OOO	⇨	Yes (see p 294)
Autogenic training	OO	⬈	Yes (see p 305)
Biofeedback	OOO	⇨	No (see p 310)
Exercise	OO	⇧	Yes (see p 5)
Herbal medicine			
Kava	OO	⇧	Yes (see p 429)
Valerian	OOO	⬈	Yes (see p 469)
Hypnotherapy	OO	⬈	Yes (see p 331)
Light therapy	OO	⇨	No (see p 5)
Relaxation	OOO	⇧	No (see p 348)
Supplements			
Melatonin	OOO	⇧	Yes (see p 435)
Vitamin B$_{12}$	O	⇩	No (see p 5)

REFERENCES

1 Eisenberg D M, Davis R B, Ettner S L, Appel S, Wilkey S, Rompay M V, Kessler R C. Trends in alternative medicine use in the United States, 1990–1997. JAMA 1998;280:1569–1575

2 Sok S R, Erlen J A, Kim K B. Effects of acupuncture therapy on insomnia. J Adv Nurs 2003;44:375–384

3 Simeit R, Deck R, Conta-Marx B. Sleep management training for cancer patients with insomnia. Support Care Cancer 2004;12:176–183

4 Stetter F, Kupper S. Autogenes Training – Qualitative Meta-Analyse kontrollierter klinischer Studien und Beziehungen zur Naturheilkunde. Forsch Komplementarmed 1998;5:211–223

5 Freedman R, Papsdorf J D. Biofeedback and progressive relaxation treatment of sleep-onset insomnia: a controlled all-night investigation. Biofeedback Self Regulation 1976;1:253–271

6 Nicassio P M, Boylan M B, McCabe T G. Progressive relaxation, EMG biofeedback and biofeedback placebo in the treatment of sleep-onset insomnia. Br J Med Psychol 1982;55:159–166

7 Hauri P. Treating psychophysiologic insomnia with biofeedback. Arch Gen Psychiatr 1981;38:752–758

8 Hauri P J, Percy L, Hellekson C, Hartmann E, Russ D. The treatment of psychophysiologic insomnia with biofeedback: a replication study. Biofeedback Self Regulation 1982;7:223–235

9 Ernst E. Systematic reviews of biofeedback. Phys Med Rehab Kuror 2003;13:321–324

10 Kubitz K A, Landers D M, Petruzzello S J, Han M. The effects of acute and chronic exercise on sleep. Sports Med 1996;21:277–291

11 Montgomery P, Dennis J. Physical exercise for sleep problems in adults aged 60+. The Cochrane Database of Systematic Reviews 2002, Issue 4. Art No: CD003404

12 Emser W, Bartylla K. Verbesserung der Schlafqualität: Zur Wirkung von Kava-Extrakt WS 1490 auf das Schlafmuster bei Gesunden. Neurologie/Psychiatrie 1991;5:636–642

13 Wheatley D. Kava and valerian in the treatment of stress-induced insomnia. Phytother Res 2001;15:549–551

14 Stevinson C, Ernst E. Valerian for insomnia: a systematic review of randomized clinical trials. Sleep Med 2000;1:91–99

15 Dorn M. Baldrian versus oxazepam: efficacy and tolerability in non-organic and non-psychiatric insomniacs: a randomized, double-blind, clinical comparative study. [Article in German] Forsch Komplementärmed Klass Naturheilkd 2000;7:79–84

16 Fussel A, Wolf A, Brattstrom A. Effect of a fixed valerian-Hop extract combination (Ze 91019) on sleep polygraphy in patients with non-organic insomnia: a pilot study. Eur J Med Res 2000;5:385–390

17 Herrera-Arellano A, Luna-Villegas G, Cuevas-Uriostegui M L, Alvarez L,Vargas-Pineda G, Zamilpa-Alvarez A, Tortoriello J. Polysomnographic evaluation of the hypnotic effect of Valeriana edulis standardized extract in patients suffering from insomnia. Planta Med 2001;67:695–699

18 Ziegler G, Ploch M, Miettinen-Baumann A, Collet W. Efficacy and tolerability of valerian extract LI 156 compared with oxazepam in the treatment of non-organic insomnia – a randomized, double-blind, comparative clinical study. Eur J Med Res 2002;7:480–486

19 Farag N H, Mills P J. A randomised-controlled trial of the effects of a traditional herbal supplement on sleep onset insomnia. Complement Ther Med 2003;11:223–225

20 Poyares D R, Guilleminault C, Ohayon M M, Tufik S. Can valerian improve the sleep of insomniacs after benzodiazepine withdrawal? Prog Neuropsychopharmacol Biol Psychiatry 2002;26:539–545

21 Coxeter P D, Schluter P J, Eastwood H L, Nikles C J, Glasziou P P. Valerian does not appear to reduce symptoms for patients with chronic insomnia in general practice using a series of randomised n-of-1 trials. Complement Ther Med 2003;11:215–222

22 Hallam K T, Olver J S, McGrath C, Norman T R. Comparative cognitive and psychomotor effects of single doses of Valeriana officinalis and triazolam in healthy volunteers. Hum Psychopharmacol 2003;18:619–625

23 Borkovec T D, Fowles D C. Controlled investigation of the effects of progressive and hypnotic relaxation on insomnia. J Abnormal Psychol 1973;82:153–158

24 Anderson J A, Dalton E R, Basker M A. Insomnia and hypnotherapy. J Roy Soc Med 1979;72:734–739

25 Barabasz A F. Treatment of insomnia in depressed patients by hypnosis and cerebral electrotherapy. Am J Clin Hypnos 1976;19:120–122

26 Stanton H E. Hypnotic relaxation and the reduction of sleep onset insomnia. Int J Psychosom 1989;36:64–68

27 Montgomery P, Dennis J. Bright light therapy for sleep problems in adults aged 60+. The Cochrane Database of Systematic Reviews 2002, Issue 2. Art No: CD003403

CONDITIONS

28 Forbes D, Morgan D G, Bangma J, Peacock S, Pelletier N, Adamson J. Light therapy for managing sleep, behaviour, and mood disturbances in dementia. The Cochrane Database of Systematic Reviews 2004, Issue 2. Art No: CD003946

29 Greeff A P, Conradie W S. Use of progressive relaxation training for chronic alcoholics with insomnia. Psychol Reps 1998;82:407–412

30 Engle Friedman M, Bootzin R R, Hazlewood L, Tsao C. An evaluation of behavioural treatments for insomnia in the older adult. J Clin Psychol 1992;48:77–90

31 Edinger J D, Wohlgemuth W K, Radtke R A, Marsh G R, Quillian R E. Cognitive behavioral therapy for treatment of chronic primary insomnia: a randomized controlled trial. JAMA 2001;285:1856–1864

32 Hauri P J. Can we mix behavioural therapy with hypnotics when treating insomniacs? Sleep 1997;20:1111–1118

33 Shapiro S L, Bootzin R R, Figueredo A J, Lopez A M, Schwartz G E. The efficacy of mindfulness-based stress reduction in the treatment of sleep disturbance in women with breast cancer: an exploratory study. J Psychosom Res 2003;54:85–91

34 Pallesen S, Nordhus I H, Kvale G, Nielsen G H, Havik O E, Johnsen B H, Skjotskift S. Behavioral treatment of insomnia in older adults: an open clinical trial comparing two interventions. Behav Res Ther 2003;41:31–48

35 Rybarczyk B, Lopez M, Benson R, Alsten C, Stepanski E. Efficacy of two behavioral treatment programs for comorbid geriatric insomnia. Psychol Aging 2002;17:288–298

36 Morin C M, Culbert J P, Schwartz S M. Non-pharmacological interventions for insomnia: a meta-analysis of treatment efficacy. Am J Psychiatr 1994;151:1172–1180

37 Murtagh D R, Greenwood K M. Identifying effective psychological treatments for insomnia: a meta-analysis. J Consult Clin Psychol 1995;63:79–89

38 Olde Rikkert M G, Rigaud A S. Melatonin in elderly patients with insomnia. A systematic review. Z Gerontol Geriatr 2001;34:491–497

39 Okawa M, Takahashi K, Egashira K, Furuta H, Higashitani Y, Higuchi T, Ichikawa H, Ichimaru Y, Inoue Y, Ishizuka Y, Ito N, Kamei K, Kaneko M, Kim Y, Kohsaka M, Komori T, Kotorii T, Matsumoto M, Mishima K, Mizuki Y, Morimoto K, Nagayama H, Ohta T, Okamoto N, Takahashi S. Vitamin B12 treatment for delayed sleep phase syndrome: a multi-centre double-blind study. Psychiatr Clin Neurosci 1997;51:275–279

40 Bohr K C. Effect of vitamin B12 on sleep quality and performance of shift workers. Wien Medizin Wochenschr 1996;146:289–291

41 Miyake Y, Nakagawa M, Asakura Y. Effects of odors on humans (I). Effects on sleep latency. Chemical Senses 1991;16:183

42 Cutler M J, Holland B S, Stupski B A, Gamber R G, Smith M L. Cranial manipulation can alter sleep latency and sympathetic nerve activity in humans: a pilot study. J Altern Complement Med 2005;11:103–108

43 Pelka R B, Jaenicke C, Gruenwald J. Impulse magnetic-field therapy for insomnia: a double-blind, placebo-controlled study. Adv Ther 2001;18:174–180

44 Hanley J, Stirling P, Brown C. Randomised controlled trial of therapeutic massage in the management of stress. Br J Gen Pract 2003;53:20–25

45 Cai G R, Li P W, Jiao L P. Clinical observation of music therapy combined with anti-tumor drugs in treating 116 cases of tumor patients. [Article in Chinese] Zhongguo Zhong Xi Yi Jie He Za Zhi 2001;21:891–894

46 Lai H L, Good M. Music improves sleep quality in older adults. J Adv Nurs 2005;49:234–244

47 Cohen L, Warneke C, Fouladi R T, Rodriguez M A, Chaoul-Reich A. Psychological adjustment and sleep quality in a randomized trial of the effects of a Tibetan yoga intervention in patients with lymphoma. Cancer 2004;100:2253–2260

IRRITABLE BOWEL SYNDROME

Synonyms Irritable colon, mucous colitis, spastic colitis, spastic colon.

Definition Irritable bowel syndrome (IBS) is a chronic non-inflammatory condition characterised by abdominal pain, altered bowel habit such as diarrhoea or constipation, and abdominal bloating, but with no identifiable structural or biochemical disorder.

CAM usage According to surveys from North America herbal medicine, relaxation and homeopathy are most frequently used for irritable bowel syndrome.[1]

Clinical evidence

Acupuncture
There are few data from rigorous trials of acupuncture for this condition. One RCT reported beneficial effects compared with sham acupuncture[2] but important details are missing, preventing full appraisal of the report. Another RCT concluded that, although the results of acupuncture at LI4 seemed beneficial, there was no difference compared with sham acupuncture at BL60.[3] In an uncontrolled study, the results suggested an improvement in general well-being and in symptoms of bloating.[4] Further studies assessing visceral perception reported mixed results.[5,6]

Biofeedback
Two controlled studies (n = 122) assessed a multi-component treatment consisting of thermal biofeedback, relaxation and cognitive therapy and found no advantage over attention control for overall symptom scores.[7] An RCT sought to determine whether biofeedback could be implemented with patients who were diagnosed with functional disorders (IBS, fibromyalgia/chronic fatigue syndrome, myofascial pain, anxiety, or non-cardiac chest pain) and whether there were cost savings through reduced use of medical services.[8] Medical costs were reduced in the treatment group compared with a no biofeedback group.

Herbal medicine
Appital, a combination preparation containing various herbal extracts, e.g. caraway oil, was tested in a double-blind RCT, which included 59 patients who were diagnosed according to the Manning criteria.[9] At the end of an 8-week treatment period, there were no differences in symptom scores in the treatment group compared with placebo.

A double-blind placebo-controlled RCT assessed the effects of **Asa foetida** (0.1% alcoholic dilution) and asa foetida in a combination preparation also containing **Nux vomica** (0.01% alcoholic dilution).[10] The results indicate some beneficial effect in the global improvement of symptoms in the active groups, but there was no difference compared with placebo.

CONDITIONS

In a placebo-controlled, double-blind RCT, 169 patients were treated for 6 weeks with either standard therapy consisting of clidinium bromide, chlordiazepoxide and psyllium or an **Ayurvedic herbal preparation** containing *Aegle marmelos correa* and *Bacopa monniere*.[11] Long-term results show that neither form of therapy was better than placebo.

A double-blind RCT compared individualised **Chinese herbal formulations** with standard Chinese herbal formulations and placebo in 116 patients.[12] After 16 weeks global improvements in symptoms were reported in both treatment groups compared with placebo. Individualised treatment was no better than standard Chinese herbal formulation. An RCT testing the Chinese compound changjitai reported that it was superior compared with pinaverium bromide for a number of outcomes including reduction of defecation in patients with diarrhoea.[13]

A systematic review found some encouraging data for the combination prepapration **Iberogast**, containing extracts of bitter candytuft, matricaria flower, peppermint leaves, caraway fruit, licorice root and melissa balm.[14] A further rigorous double-blind RCT which assessed 203 patients reported that the preparation is more effective than placebo for abdominal pain.[15]

Padma lax, a complex Tibetan herbal formula was evaluated in treating constipation-predominant IBS in a 3-month double-blind RCT.[16] Patients (Padma lax n = 34, placebo n = 27) experienced an improvement after 3 months in the Padma lax group compared with placebo for constipation, severity of abdominal pain, and its effect on daily activities, incomplete evacuation, abdominal distension and flatus/flatulence. Adverse events consisted mostly of loose stools and responded well to the lowering of dosage.

A meta-analysis assessed the available evidence for **peppermint** oil.[17] Of eight RCTs of peppermint oil monopreparations, seven trials included patients who were not diagnosed according to accepted criteria. Although the meta-analysis suggested beneficial effects, it was concluded that the effectiveness of peppermint oil for IBS is not established beyond reasonable doubt (Box 2.65). A further double-blind RCT, reported beneficial effects for abdominal pain, distension and stool frequency, but also failed to diagnose patients according to the accepted Rome or Manning criteria.[18]

A double-blind RCT compared two different preparations of a fixed combination of **peppermint and caraway oil**.[19] Two hundred and twenty-three patients with non-ulcer dyspepsia in combination with IBS received either enteric-coated capsules or an enteric-soluble formulation. The results indicate a reduction in pain intensity compared with baseline and equivalent effectiveness of the preparations.

Three RCTs have assessed preparations containing **psyllium** (*Plantago ovata*) (Table 2.50).[20-22] Two trials reported beneficial

Box 2.65
Meta-analysis
**Peppermint oil for
irritable bowel
syndrome**
Pittler[17]

- Eight RCTs (seven double-blind) including 295 patients

- The only study that diagnosed patients according to accepted criteria (Manning) was negative

- Dosage was 3×0.2–0.4 ml/d for 2–4 w

- Global improvement of symptoms (odds ratio 0.20; CI 0.04 to 0.89, n = 5)

- Two of three studies not subjected to meta-analysis were positive

- Adverse effects included heartburn, perianal burning, blurred vision, nausea and vomiting

- Conclusion: The role of peppermint in irritable bowel syndrome is not established beyond reasonable doubt

effects, while one study found no global improvement of symptoms compared with placebo. Overall, the evidence is encouraging, but the heterogeneity of the available data in terms of medication used, dosage and treatment period prevents any firm judgement.

Table 2.50 **Double-blind RCTs of psyllium (ispaghula husk) for irritable bowel syndrome**

Reference	Sample size	Interventions [dosage]	Result	Comment
Ritchie[20]	96	A) Psyllium [2 × 1 sachet/d for 3 mo] B) Hyoscine butylbromide (Buscopan) [4 × 10 mg/d] C) Lorazepam [2 × 1 mg/d] D) Placebo	A superior to D for global improvement	The only difference was between psyllium and placebo
Golechha[21]	26	A) Psyllium [2.5 g/d for 3 w] B) Placebo	A superior to B for global improvement	Patients with additional psychiatric symptoms had the least improvement
Arthurs[22]	80	A) Psyllium poloxamer [two sachets/d for 4 w] B) Placebo	No intergroup differences including global improvement	All patients received 30 g dietary fibre

Hypnotherapy

A review assessed a total of 14 published studies (n = 644) on the efficacy of hypnosis in treating IBS (eight with no control group and six with a control group). The authors concluded that hypnosis consistently produces significant results and improves the cardinal symptoms of IBS in the majority of patients, as well as positively affecting non-colonic symptoms.[23]

Supplements

A systematic review aimed to quantify the effect of different types of **fibre** on global and symptom relief from IBS (Box 2.66).[24] It concluded that there is only marginal benefit for global symptom improvement.

Box 2.66
Systematic review
Fibre for irritable bowel syndrome
Bijkerk[24]

- 17 RCTs were included (seven double-blind) including 295 patients

- Fibre, in general, for global symptom relief (relative risk 1.33, CI 1.19–1.50)

- Soluble fibre (psyllium, calcium polycarbophil) for global symptom relief (relative risk 1.55, CI 1.35–1.78)

- Insoluble fibre (corn, wheat bran) compared with placebo (relative risk 0.89, CI 0.72–1.11)

- Conclusion: The benefits of fibre in the treatment of irritable bowel syndrome are marginal for global irritable bowel syndrome symptom improvement and irritable bowel syndrome-related constipation.

A multicentre RCT[25] investigated the effectiveness of the supplement **Florelax**, which contains yeast, vitamin B, nicotinamide, folic acid and herbal extracts of camomile, angelica, valerian and peppermint. Three hundred and eighty patients received either two tablets of the supplement plus a high-fibre diet daily or diet alone for 6 weeks. The results indicate a reduction of the intensity, frequency and duration of the symptoms in the treatment group compared with diet alone.

Several RCTs tested **probiotics** for IBS. The results suggested beneficial effects using *Lactobacillus plantarum* for pain and overall symptom improvement compared with placebo.[26,27] Another RCT suggested beneficial differences for flatulence compared with placebo.[28] Two smaller RCTs (n = 25) did not suggest beneficial effects for pain, urgency, bloating or global symptom relief.[29,30]

Other therapies

Single RCTs have tested **charcoal tablets**,[31] **cognitive–behaviour therapy**,[32] **meditation**[33] and **yoga**.[34] All of these studies require independent replication before any firm judgements can be made.

Overall recommendation

The evidence suggests that fibre supplements are effective for patients with IBS. The size of the effect however seems small. The evidence of hypnotherapy looks promising making it a possible treatment option. For other complementary treatments, the evidence of effectiveness is not compelling, which also applies to most conventional therapies although smooth muscle relaxants have shown to be beneficial for abdominal pain. The data for peppermint oil and the combination preparation Iberogast are encouraging and given the few treatment options available and their favourable safety profiles, these options may be worth considering. Other treatments with encouraging data include Chinese herbal formulations, probiotics and acupuncture.

Table 2.51
Summary of clinical evidence for irritable bowel syndrome

Treatment	Weight of evidence	Direction of evidence	Serious safety concerns
Acupuncture	OO	↗	Yes (see p 294)
Biofeedback	OO	⇒	No (see p 310)
Herbal medicine			
Appital	O	⇓	Yes (see p 5)
Asa foetida	O	↘	Yes (see p 478)
Ayurveda	O	⇓	Yes (see p 5)
Chinese herbs	OO	⇑	Yes (see p 5)
Iberogast	OOO	↗	Yes (see p 5)
Psyllium	OO	↗	Yes (see p 480)
Padma lax	O	⇑	Yes (see p 5)
Peppermint	OOO	↗	Yes (see p 448)
Hypnotherapy	OOO	↗	Yes (see p 331)
Supplements			
Fibre	OOO	⇑	Yes (see p 5)
Florelax	O	⇑	Yes (see p 5)
Probiotics	OO	↗	Yes (see p 5)

CONDITIONS

REFERENCES

1 Eisenberg D M, Davis R B, Ettner S L, Appel S, Wilkey S, Rompay M V, Kessler R C. Trends in alternative medicine use in the United States, 1990–1997. JAMA 1998;280:1569–1575

2 Kunze M, Seidel H-J, Stübe G. Vergleichende Untersuchung zur Effektivität der kleinen Psychotherapie, der Akupunktur und der Papaverintherapie bei Patienten mit Colon irritabile. Z Gesamte Inn Med 1990;45:625–627

3 Fireman Z, Segal A, Kopelman Y, Sternberg A, Carasso R. Acupuncture treatment for irritable bowel syndrome. A double-blind controlled study. Digestion 2001;64:100–103

4 Chan J, Carr I, Mayberry J F. The role of acupuncture in the treatment of irritable bowel syndrome: a pilot study. Hepato-Gastroenterol 1997;44:1328–1330

5 Rohrbock R B, Hammer J, Vogelsang H, Talley N J, Hammer H F. Acupuncture has a placebo effect on rectal perception but not on distensibility and spatial summation: a study in health and IBS. Am J Gastroenterol 2004;99:1990–1997

6 Xing J, Larive B, Mekhail N, Soffer E. Transcutaneous electrical acustimulation can reduce visceral perception in patients with

the irritable bowel syndrome: a pilot study. Altern Ther Health Med 2004;10:38–42

7   Blanchard E B, Schwartz S P, Suls J M et al. Two controlled evaluations of multicomponent psychological treatment of irritable bowel syndrome. Behav Res Ther 1992;30:175–189

8   Ryan M, Gevirtz R. Biofeedback-based psychophysiological treatment in a primary care setting: an initial feasibility study. Appl Psychophysiol Biofeedback 2004;29:79–93

9   Pedersen B S, Helø O H, Jørgensen F B, Kromann-Andersen H. Behandling af colon irritabile med kosttilskuddet Appital. Ugeskr Lœger 1998;160:7259–7262

10 Rahlfs V W, Mössinger P. Zur Behandlung des Colon irritabile. Arzneim-Forsch Drug Res 1976;26:2230–2234

11 Yadav S K, Jain A K, Tripathi S N, Gupta J P. Irritable bowel syndrome: therapeutic evaluation of indigenous drugs. Ind J Med Res 1989;90:496–503

12 Bensoussan A, Talley N J, Hing M, Menzies R, Guo A, Ngu M. Treatment of irritable bowel syndrome with Chinese herbal medicine. A randomized controlled trial. JAMA 1998;280:1585–1589

13 Shen Y, Cai G, Sun X. Randomized controlled clinical study on effect of Chinese compound changjitai in treating diarrheic irritable bowel syndrome. Zhongguo Zhong Xi Yi Jie He Za Zhi 2003;23:823–825

14 Saller R, Pfister-Hotz G, Iten F, Melzer J, Reichling J. Iberogast: a modern phytotherapeutic combined herbal drug for the treatment of functional disorders of the gastrointestinal tract (dyspepsia, irritable bowel syndrome) – from phytomedicine to 'evidence based phytotherapy.' A systematic review. Forsch Komplementarmed Klass Naturheilkd 2002;9(Suppl 1):1–20

15 Madisch A, Holtmann G, Plein K, Hotz J. Treatment of irritable bowel syndrome with herbal preparations: results of a double-blind, randomized, placebo-controlled, multi-centre trial. Aliment Pharmacol Ther 2004;19:271–279

16 Sallon S, Ben-Arye E, Davidson R, Shapiro H, Ginsberg G, Ligumsky M. A novel treatment for constipation-predominant irritable bowel syndrome using Padma Lax, a Tibetan herbal formula. Digestion 2002;65:161–171

17 Pittler M H, Ernst E. Peppermint oil for irritable bowel syndrome: a critical review and meta-analysis. Am J Gastroenterol 1998;93:1131–1135

18 Liu J-H, Chen G-H, Yeh H-Z, Huang C-K, Poon S-K. Enteric-coated peppermint-oil capsules in the treatment of irritable bowel syndrome: a prospective, randomized trial. J Gastroenterol 1997;32:765–768

19 Freise J, Köhler S. Pfefferminzöl/Kümmelöl-Fixkombination bei nicht-säurebedingter Dyspepsie – Vergleich der Wirksamkeit und Verträglichkeit zweier galenischer Zubereitungen. Pharmazie 1999;54:210–215

20 Ritchie J A, Truelove S C. Treatment of irritable bowel syndrome with lorazepam, hyoscine butylbromide, and ispaghula husk. BMJ 1979;1:376–378

21 Golechha A C, Chadda V S, Chadda S, Sharma S K, Mishra S N. Role of ispaghula husk in the management of irritable bowel syndrome (a randomized double-blind crossover study). J Assoc Physicians India 1982;30:353–355

22 Arthurs Y, Fielding J F. Double blind trial of ispaghula/poloxamer in the Irritable Bowel Syndrome. Ir Med J 1983;76:253

23 Tan G, Hammond D C, Joseph G. Hypnosis and irritable bowel syndrome: a review of efficacy and mechanism of action. Am J Clin Hypn 2005;47:161–178

24 Bijkerk C J, Muris J W, Knottnerus J A, Hoes A W, de Wit N J. Systematic review: the role of different types of fibre in the treatment of irritable bowel syndrome. Aliment Pharmacol Ther 2004;19:245–251

25 Grattagliano A, Anti M, Luchetti R, Marino P, Gasbarrini G. Studie clinico randomizzato sull'efficacia di un integratore biologico nei pazienti affetti da sindrome dell'intestino irritabile. Minerva Gastroenterol Dietol 1998;44:51–55

26 Niedzielin K, Kordecki H, Birkenfeld B. A controlled, double-blind, randomized study on the efficacy of Lactobacillus plantarum 299V in patients with irritable bowel syndrome. Eur J Gastroenterol Hepatol 2001;13:1143–1147

27 Saggioro A. Probiotics in the treatment of irritable bowel syndrome. J Clin Gastroenterol 2004;38:S104–106

28 Nobaek S, Johansson M L, Molin G, Ahrne S, Jeppsson B. Alteration of intestinal microflora is associated with reduction in abdominal bloating and pain in patients with irritable bowel syndrome. Am J Gastroenterol 2000;95:1231–1238.

29 Kim H J, Camilleri M, McKinzie S, Lempke M B, Burton D D, Thomforde G M, Zinsmeister A R. A randomized controlled trial of a probiotic, VSL#3, on gut transit and symptoms in diarrhoea-predominant irritable bowel syndrome. Aliment Pharmacol Ther 2003;17:895–904

30 O'Sullivan M A, O'Morain C A. Bacterial supplementation in the irritable bowel

syndrome. A randomised double-blind placebo-controlled crossover study. Dig Liver Dis 2000;32:294–301

31 Hubner W D, Moser E H. Charcoal tablets in the treatment of patients with irritable bowel syndrome. Adv Ther 2002;19:245–252

32 Boyce P M, Talley N J, Balaam B, Koloski N A, Truman G. A randomized controlled trial of cognitive behavior therapy, relaxation training, and routine clinical care for the irritable bowel syndrome. Am J Gastroenterol 2003;98:2209–2218

33 Keefer L, Blanchard E B. The effects of relaxation response meditation on the symptoms of irritable bowel syndrome: results of a controlled treatment study. Behav Res Ther 2001;39:801–811

34 Taneja I, Deepak K K, Poojary G, Acharya I N, Pandey R M, Sharma M P. Yogic versus conventional treatment in diarrhea-predominant irritable bowel syndrome: a randomized control study. Appl Psychophysiol Biofeedback 2004;29:19–33

LABOUR

Synonyms   Childbirth; parodynia.

Definition   Labour is the act of giving birth to a baby. Labour pains are rhythmical uterine contractions which under normal conditions increase in intensity, frequency, and duration, culminating in vaginal delivery of the infant.

CAM usage   Hypnosis, acupuncture and some herbal medicines (particularly raspberry leaves) are commonly used non-pharmacological therapies.

Clinical evidence   Several systematic reviews of complementary therapies for pain management or induction of labour have been published.[1-3]

Acupuncture
A systematic review of acupuncture for labour pain management (Box 2.67) concluded that the evidence for acupuncture as an adjunct to conventional pain control during labour is encouraging but, because of the paucity of trial data, not convincing.[4]

Box 2.67
Systematic review
Acupuncture for pain management in labour
Lee[4]

- Three trials including 496 parturients

- All trials were of good quality

- Two RCTs compared adjunctive acupuncture with usual care and reported a reduction of meperidine and/or epidural analgesia

- One placebo-controlled RCT showed differences in both subjective and objective outcome measures of pain

- No adverse events were reported in any of the trials

- Conclusion: the evidence for acupuncture is promising but, because of the paucity of trial data, not convincing

CONDITIONS

A systematic review of acupuncture for the induction of labour including one RCT stated that there is insufficient evidence as data from the trial were unsuitable for analysis.[5]

Two RCTs assessed the effect of acupressure during labour: one (n = 127) comparing acupressure at LI4 and BL67 with light skin stroking or no treatment or conversation only indicated decreased labour pain in the acupressure group but found no effects on uterine contractions;[6] the other RCT (n = 75) found SP6 acupressure compared with SP6 touch control to be more effective in reducing pain and shortening labour.[7]

Aromatherapy

A systematic review included one double-blind RCT in which 22 multiparous women with a singleton pregnancy received essential oil of ginger or essential oil of lemongrass baths.[3] There were no differences between groups regarding analgesic consumption or outcome of delivery.

Biofeedback

Two small RCTs tested biofeedback for pain relief during labour; one found it to lower pain and shorten labour compared with controls[8] while the other one found no difference between effectively trained electromyographic, ineffectively trained skin-conductance and standard antenatal classes.[9]

Herbal medicine

The Chinese herbal medicine mixture, **Chanlibao**, was compared with oxytocin and no intervention in an RCT (n = 161) and was suggested to accelerate the second stage of labour.[10]

In a double-blind, placebo-controlled RCT (n = 192), **raspberry leaf** (*Rubus idaeus*) tablets were found to shorten the second but not the first stage of labour and no differences were found in birth outcome.[11]

Homeopathy

A systematic review (Box 2.68) of two trials with 133 women found no differences between the treatment and control groups in cervical ripening or labour induction and concluded that there was not enough evidence to show an effect of homeopathy for inducing labour.[12]

Hypnosis

A systematic review of hypnosis (Box 2.69) in pain relief in labour included four randomised and two non-randomised clinical trials and found that fewer parturients receiving hypnosis required analgesia.[13] A subsequent large RCT (n = 520) reported fewer complications at birth in women receiving prenatal hypnosis compared with attention-only or no-contact.[14]

Box 2.68
Systematic review
Homeopathy for induction of labour
Smith[12]

- Two trials with 133 women were included

- Both were placebo-controlled and double-blind but quality was not high

- One trial used *Caulophyllum*, the other five different homeo-pathic preparations of *Caulophyllum, Arnica, Actaea racemosa, Pulsatilla* and geranium

- No differences were found in any primary or secondary outcome between the treatment and control groups

- Conclusion: there is not enough evidence to show the effect of homeopathy for inducing labour

Box 2.69
Meta-analysis
Hypnosis for pain management in labour
Cyna[13]

- Four RCTs of 224 women and two non randomised CTs were included

- Meta-analysis of three RCTs showed that fewer parturients receiving hypnosis required analgesia (relative risk = 0.51, CI 0.28 to 0.95); one RCT rated poor on quality assessment

- Of the two non-randomised CTs included, one showed lower pain ratings and the other reduced opioid and pharmacological analgesia requirements with hypnosis

- Conclusion: hypnosis alone or in combination with other anaesthetic techniques, may offer advantages over conven-tional analgesia alone

Intracutaneous sterile water injections

Four RCTs compared low back pain in labouring women receiv-ing intracutaneous sterile water injections with controls receiv-ing a saline placebo[15-17] or TENS, movement, massage, and baths.[18] All four found it to be effective in decreasing severe low back pain within minutes although no decrease in the request for other pain medication was reported in three studies assessing pain relief consumption.

Massage

Two RCTs were included in a systematic review.[2] One included 28 women receiving massage in addition to coaching in breathing or coaching in breathing alone, the other (n = 60) massage or attention control. Both trials found massage to provide pain relief and psy-chological support during labour. A further RCT (n = 40) reported nurse- and self-administered massage in combination with breathing techniques to be effective in reducing the perception of pain.[19]

Music

An RCT (n = 110) of the effects of music on sensation and distress of pain during labour reported less sensation and distress of pain in the music group and a delayed increase of affective pain for 1 hour.[20] One small RCT (n = 30) examining the effect of standard psychoprophylactic child birth instruction antenatally combined with music compared with standard psychoprophylactic alone found no difference in the frequency of analgesia use between groups.[21] Music did not have an effect on analogued labour pain using nulliparous volunteers in two small trials when compared with no-treatment control or various forms of imagery.[22]

Water immersion

A systematic review[23] of eight RCTs (Box 2.70) comparing any kind of bath tub or pool use with no immersion during pregnancy, labour or birth found that water immersion during the first stage of labour reduced the use of analgesia and reported maternal pain without adverse outcome of operative delivery rates or neonatal well-being. A subsequent RCT reported similar findings.[24]

Box 2.70
Meta-analysis
Immersion in water in labour and birth
Cluett[23]

- Eight RCTs (n = 2939) comparing any kind of bath tub or pool use with no immersion during pregnancy, labour or birth

- Reduction in the use of epidural/spinal/paracervical analgesia/anaesthesia amongst women allocated to water immersion during the first stage of labour (odds ratio 0.84, 95% CI 0.71 to 0.99, n = 4)

- Less pain reported by women who used water immersion during the first stage of labour (OR 0.23, 95% 0.08 to 0.63, n = 1)

- Labour duration, operative delivery rates or neonatal well-being were not adversely affected and did not differ between groups

- Conclusion: There is evidence that water immersion during the first stage of labour reduces the use of analgesia and reported maternal pain without adverse outcomes; further research is needed to assess the effect of immersion in water on neonatal and maternal morbidity

Overall recommendation

Labour pain is arguably one of the most severe pains a woman experiences in her life yet pain management during childbirth has always been controversial. The possible effects of anaesthesia on progress of labour and on the neonate continue to concern healthcare professionals and patients. Epidural anaesthesia, the current gold standard for pain relief during childbirth, is not acceptable for all women and many are drawn to non-pharmacological interventions. Patients should, however, always be advised of safety issues associated with complementary therapies. Particularly during pregnancy the precautionary principle that a treatment is not considered risk-free unless evidence suggests otherwise should be applied.

Hypnosis and immersion in water, as well as intracutaneous sterile water injections and massage seem to be effective in reducing pain during labour and are not associated with serious safety concerns. The evidence for acupuncture is encouraging but further research is required. There is not enough evidence for any other complementary therapy to make any firm recommendations.

Table 2.52
Summary of clinical evidence for labour

Treatment	Weight of evidence	Direction of evidence	Serious safety concerns
Acupuncture			Yes (see p 294)
(pain)	OO	⤴	
(induction)	O	⇨	
Acupressure			Yes (see p 294)
(pain)	OO	⤴	
(induction)	OO	⇨	
Aromatherapy	O	⇨	Yes (see p 301)
Biofeedback (pain)	O	⇨	No (see p 310)
Herbal medicine			
Chanlibao (induction)	O	⤵	Yes (see p 5)
Raspberry leaf (induction)	O	⤴	Yes (see p 480)
Homeopathy (induction)	OO	⇩	No (see p 327)
Hypnosis (pain)	OOO	⇧	Yes (see p 331)
Intracutaneous sterile water injections (pain)	OO	⤴	Yes (see p 361)
Massage (pain)	OO	⇧	No (see p 334)
Music (pain)	OO	⤵	No (see p 360)
Water immersion (pain)	OOO	⇧	No (see p 5)

REFERENCES

1 Simkin P, Bolding A. Update on non-pharmacologic approaches to relieve labor pain and prevent suffering. J Midwifery Womens Health 2004;49:489–504

2 Huntley A L, Coon J T, Ernst E. Complementary and alternative medicine for labor pain: a systematic review. Am J Obstet Gynecol 2004;191:36–44

CONDITIONS

3   Smith C A, Collins C T, Cyna A M, Crowther C A. Complementary and alternative therapies for pain management in labour. The Cochrane Database of Systematic Reviews 2003, Issue 2. Art. No.: CD003521

4   Lee H, Ernst E. Acupuncture for labor pain management: A systematic review. Am J Obstet Gynecol 2004;191:1573–1579

5   Smith C A, Crowther C A. Acupuncture for induction of labour. The Cochrane Database of Systematic Reviews 2004, Issue 1. Art. No.: CD002962

6   Chung U L, Hung L C, Kuo S C, Huang C L. Effects of LI4 and BL 67 acupressure on labor pain and uterine contractions in the first stage of labor. J Nurs Res 2003;11:251–260.

7   Lee M K, Chang S B, Kang D H. Effects of SP6 acupressure on labor pain and length of delivery time in women during labor. J Altern Complement Med 2004;10:959–965

8   Duchene P. Effects of biofeedback on childbirth pain. J Pain Symptom Manage 1989;4:117–123

9   St James-Roberts I, Chamberlain G, Haran F J, Hutchinson C M. Use of electromyographic and skin-conductance biofeedback relaxation training of facilitate childbirth in primiparae. J Psychosom Res 1982;26:455–462

10 Qiu H, Zhu H, Ouyang W, Wang Z, Sun H. Clinical effects and mechanism of chanlibao in accelerating second stage of labor. J Tongji Med Univ 1999;19:141–144

11 Simpson M, Parsons M, Greenwood J, Wade K. Raspberry leaf in pregnancy: its safety and efficacy in labor. J Midwifery Womens Health 2001;46:51–59

12 Smith C A. Homoeopathy for induction of labour. The Cochrane Database of Systematic Reviews 2003, Issue 4. Art. No.: CD003399

13 Cyna A M, McAuliffe G L, Andrew M I. Hypnosis for pain relief in labour and childbirth: a systematic review. Br J Anaesth 2004;93:505–511

14 Mehl-Madrona L E. Hypnosis to facilitate uncomplicated birth. Am J Clin Hypn 2004;46:299–312

15 Martensson L, Wallin G. Labour pain treated with cutaneous injections of sterile water: a randomised controlled trial. Br J Obstet Gynaecol 1999;106:633–637

16 Ader L, Hansson B, Wallin G. Parturition pain treated by intracutaneous injections of sterile water. Pain 1990;41:133–138

17 Trolle B, Moller M, Kronborg H, Thomsen S. The effect of sterile water blocks on low back labor pain. Am J Obstet Gynecol 1991;164:1277–1281

18 Labrecque M, Nouwen A, Bergeron M, Rancourt J F. A randomized controlled trial of non-pharmacologic approaches for relief of low back pain during labor. J Fam Pract 1999;48:259–263

19 Yildirim G, Sahin N H. The effect of breathing and skin stimulation techniques on labour pain perception of Turkish women. Pain Res Manag 2004;9:183–187

20 Phumdoung S, Good M. Music reduces sensation and distress of labor pain. Pain Manag Nurs 2003;4:54–61

21 Durham L, Collins M. The effect of music as a conditioning aid in prepared childbirth education. J Obstet Gynecol Neonatal Nurs 1986;15:268–270

22 Geden E A, Lower M, Beattie S, Beck N. Effects of music and imagery on physiologic and self-report of analogued labor pain. Nurs Res 1989;38:37–41

23 Cluett E R, Nikodem V C, McCandlish R E, Burns E E. Immersion in water in pregnancy, labour and birth. The Cochrane Database of Systematic Reviews 2004, Issue 1. Art. No.: CD000111

24 Cluett E R, Pickering R M, Getliffe K, St George Saunders N J. Randomised controlled trial of labouring in water compared with standard of augmentation for management of dystocia in first stage of labour. BMJ 2004;328:314

MENOPAUSE

Synonyms   Climacteric.

Definition   The physiologic cessation of menstruation often characterised by symptoms such as hot flushes, insomnia, night sweats, dizziness, palpitations, low energy, decreased sexual interest, vaginal dryness, urinary symptoms, depression and other mood changes.

CAM usage   The CAM modalities most popular with menopausal women have been identified as dietary or nutritional supplements, spiritual approaches, exercise, herbal medicine and homeopathy.[1]

Clinical evidence

Acupuncture
RCTs of different forms of acupuncture for alleviating menopausal symptoms have reached both positive[2–4] and negative conclusions.[5] A systematic review[6] found no evidence for the effectiveness of acupuncture for menopausal symptoms.

Herbal medicine
A systematic review of any herbal medicine for the treatment of menopausal symptoms found no convincing evidence for any product.[7]

A systematic review of its pharmacological effects concluded that **black cohosh** (*Actaea racemosa* L) possesses central rather than hormonal activity.[8] A systematic review of RCTs found that its clinical efficacy has not been convincingly established (Box 2.71).[9] Two more RCTs, however, did yield encouraging results. An RCT (n = 62) lasting 3 months suggested black cohosh to be equipotent with conjugated oestrogen for symptom control and bone metabolism.[10] Another RCT compared two doses of black cohosh extract and found that the normal dose of 39 mg/day is adequate for symptom control.[11] A large RCT (n = 304) with a treatment period of 12 weeks found that black cohosh (40 mg/day) improved menopausal symptoms better than placebo.[12] On balance, therefore, the evidence seems encouraging.

Box 2.71
Systematic review
Black cohosh for menopausal symptoms
Borelli[9]

- Four RCTs including 226 women
- Methodological quality mixed
- Best RCT was negative
- Conclusion: overall no conclusive evidence for efficacy

A double-blind RCT (n = 71) of **dong quai** (*Angelica sinensis*) found no superiority over placebo in reducing menopausal symptoms and no oestrogenic effects after 6 months of treatment.[13]

The efficacy of oil of **evening primrose** (*Oenothera biennis*) for alleviating hot flushes was examined in a double-blind RCT (n = 56).[14] No benefit over placebo was demonstrated for the frequency of night or daytime flushes.

Ginkgo *(Ginkgo biloba)* was tested against placebo in a small RCT (n = 31).[15] Modest effects were noted on cognitive function of post-menopausal women. A larger RCT (n = 87) found positive effects on mental flexibility which were, however, limited to patients with initially poorer performance.[16]

Ginseng *(Panax ginseng)* was investigated in a double-blind RCT (n = 384) for its effects on quality of life.[17] Results were not different from placebo for quality of life or hot flushes and no effects on vaginal cytology were observed.

Two double-blind, placebo-controlled RCTs (n = 40) of kava *(Piper methysticum)* (300 mg daily for 2–3 months) suggested that it is effective in alleviating menopausal symptoms.[18,19] A further RCT suggested that adding kava to conventional therapy improves mood in menopausal women.[20]

The Chinese herbal medicine **Kudzu** *(Pueraria lobata)* was tested in an RCT (n = 129) against hormone replacement therapy.[21] No improvements in the health of postmenopausal women were noted.

Red clover *(Trifolium pratense)* was tested in 17 RCTs of which 11 could be submitted to a systematic review.[22] It concluded that there is evidence for a small effect on hot flushes (Box 2.72).

Box 2.72
Systematic review
Red clover for menopausal symptoms
Thompson Coon[22]

- Eleven RCTs including 1160 women

- Five RCTs were suitable for meta-analysis

- Small reduction of hot flushes was noted (WMD = −1.45 hot flushes/day, 95% CI −2.94 to 0.03, p = 0.05)

- No serious adverse effects

- No long-term data

- Conclusion: evidence of small effect

Other isoflavones or phytoestrogens have shown positive results in terms of cardiovascular benefit,[23,24] fluid retention,[25] endothelial function,[26] and bone metabolism[27–29]while the data on menopausal symptoms are controversial.[30–33] A systematic review[34] concluded that phytoestrogens do not improve hot flushes or other menopausal symptoms (Box 2.73).

Box 2.73
Systematic review
Phytoestrogens for menopausal symptoms
Krebs[34]

- 25 RCTs including 2348 women

- Methodological quality was mixed but some trials were rigorous

- No clear effect on hot flushes

- Conclusion: phytoestrogens do not improve symptoms of menopause

St John's wort (*Hypericum perforatum*) (900 mg daily for 3 months) produced positive results on psychological symptoms in an uncontrolled study[35] and in an RCT when combined with black cohosh.[36]

Wild yam (*Dioscorea villosa*) cream was tested against placebo in 23 postmenopausal women.[37] No convincing symptomatic effects were noted.

Three RCTs of Chinese or Kampo herbal mixtures are available. One study showed encouraging results for **Jai-Wey Shiau-You San;**[38] in another trial no effects were noted for a herbal formula.[39] An RCT of the Kampo medicine **Unkei-to** showed encouraging results for depressive mood.[40]

Relaxation

Three small RCTs have suggested that relaxation training can have positive effects on hot flush symptoms (Table 2.53).[41–43] The results are inconsistent regarding the best type of relaxation method, with progressive muscle relaxation proving effective in two studies but no better than the control intervention in the other one where a breathing technique produced positive results.

Table 2.53 **RCTs of relaxation training for menopause**

Reference	Sample size	Interventions [regimen]	Result	Comment
Germaine[41]	14	A) Muscle relaxation [1 h/w for 6 w] B) EEG biofeedback	A superior to B in hot flush frequency	Hot flushes assessed by self-report 1 & 6 mo after treatment
Freedman[42]	33	A) Paced respiration [1 h/fortnight for 16 w] B) Muscle relaxation C) EEG biofeedback	A superior to B & C in hot flush frequency	Hot flushes assessed by ambulatory monitoring of skin conductance for 24 h
Irvin[43]	45	A) Relaxation training [20 min/d for 7 w] B) Attention control C) Reading	A superior to B & C in hot flush intensity and depression/ anxiety	Hot flush assessed by daily charting; drop-out rate of over 25%

Spinal manipulation

An RCT (n = 30) compared the effects of **osteopathy** (once weekly for 10 weeks) with sham treatment.[44] Superior results were reported for osteopathy on several menopausal symptoms including depression and hot flushes.

Supplements

Dietary **linseed, soy** and **wheat** reduced hot flushes in comparative RCTs.[45,46] A systematic review[47] of soy supplements found some encouraging but no conclusive evidence (Box 2.74). A further placebo-controlled RCT (n = 202) found no evidence that soy protein has beneficial effects on vascular function in menopausal women.[48]

Box 2.74
Systematic review
Soy for menopausal symptoms
Huntley[47]

- 13 RCTs were found, ten were included

- Methodological quality was mixed but some studies were rigorous

- Four RCTs were negative and six RCTs were positive

- Conclusion: heterogeneity of primary data prohibits a definitive judgement

Vitamin E was reported useful for reducing hot flushes according to uncontrolled studies (e.g.[49]). However, a placebo-controlled trial found no specific effect of the treatment.[50]

Other therapies

The results of case–control and uncontrolled studies suggest that aerobic **exercise** training is associated with a reduction in menopausal symptoms.[51–53] Another study found no correlation between energy expenditure and menopausal symptoms.[54] An RCT suggested that regular **tai chi** retards bone loss in menopausal women.[55] **Reflexology** was not superior to sham treatment for menopausal symptoms control in an RCT with 76 women.[56]

Overall recommendation

There is no fully convincing evidence for the efficacy of any complementary treatment for alleviating menopausal symptoms. Red clover looks more encouraging than other treatments in this respect and has a favourable safety profile. Soy, other phyto-estrogens and black cohosh may have potential. Relaxation techniques also appear to have some benefits. Hormone replacement therapy has stronger effects on menopausal symptoms than any CAM option. However, none of the CAM approaches is associated with the recently discovered adverse effects of hormone replacement therapy. On balance, therefore, some CAM options may be worth trying, particularly in patients who are anxious about hormone replacement therapy.

Table 2.54
Summary of clinical evidence for menopause

Treatment	Weight of evidence	Direction of evidence	Serious safety concerns
Acupuncture	OO	⇨	Yes (see p 294)
Herbal medicine			
Black cohosh	OOO	⬈	Yes (see p 373)

Treatment	Weight of evidence	Direction of evidence	Serious safety concerns
Dong quai	O	⇩	Yes (see p 478)
Evening primrose oil	O	⇩	Yes (see p 393)
Ginkgo	OO	⇗	Yes (see p 404)
Ginseng	O	⇘	Yes (see p 407)
Jai-Wey Shiau-You San	O	⇗	Yes (see p 5)
Kava	O	⇧	Yes (see p 429)
Pueraria lobata	O	⇩	Yes (see p 479)
Red clover	OOO	⇧	Yes (see p 456)
St John's wort	O	⇗	Yes (see p 463)
Unkei-to	O	⇗	Yes (see p 5)
Wild yam	O	⇩	Yes (see p 481)
Various herbal mixtures	O	⇘	Yes (see p 5)
Relaxation	OO	⇧	No (see p 348)
Spinal manipulation			
Osteopathy	O	⇧	Yes (see p 343)
Supplements			
Soy	OOO	⇨	No (see p 450)
Vitamin E	O	⇨	No (see p 5)

REFERENCES

1 Kass-Annese B. Alternative therapies for menopause. Clin Obstet Gynecol 2000;43: 163–183

2 Wyon Y, Lindgren R, Hammar M, Lundeberg T. Acupuncture against climacteric disorders? Lower number of symptoms after menopause. Lakartidningen 1994;91:2318–2322

3 Kraft K, Coulon S. Effect of a standardised acupuncture treatment on complaints, blood pressure and serum lipids of hypertensive postmenopausal women. A randomized controlled clinical study. Forsch Komplementärmed 1999;6:74–79

4 Cohen S M, Rousseau M E, Carey B L. Can acupuncture ease the symptoms of menopause? Holist Nurs Pract 2003;17:295–299

5 Sandberg M, Wijma K, Wyon Y, Nedstrand E, Hammar M. Effects of electro-acupuncture on psychological distress in postmenopausal women. Complement Ther Med 2002;10:161–169

6 White A R. A review of controlled trials of acupuncture for women's reproductive healthcare. J Fam Plann Reprod Health Care 2003;29: 233–236

7 Huntley A L, Ernst E. A systematic review of herbal medicinal products for the treatment of menopausal symptoms. Menopause 2003;10:465–476

8 Borrelli F, Izzo A A, Ernst E. Pharmacological effects of Cimicifuga racemosa. Life Sci 2003;73:1215–1229

9 Borrelli F, Ernst E. Cimicifuga racemosa: a systematic review of its clinical efficacy. Eur J Clin Pharmacol 2002;58:235–241

10 Wuttke W, Seidlova-Wuttke D, Gorkow C. The Cimicifuga preparation BNO 1055 vs. conjugated estrogens in a double-blind placebo-controlled study: effects on menopause symptoms and bone markers. Maturitas 2003;44(Suppl1):S67–S77

11 Liske E, Hanggi W, Henneicke-von Zepelin H H, Boblitz N, Wustenberg P, Rahlfs V W.

Physiological investigation of a unique extract of black cohosh (Cimicifugae racemosae rhizoma): a 6-month clinical study demonstrates no systemic estrogenic effect. J Womens Health Gend Based Med 2002;11:163–174

12 Osmers R, Friede M, Liske E, Schnitker J, Freudenstein J, Henneicke-von Zepelin H H. Efficacy and safety of isopropanolic black cohosh extract for climacteric symptoms. Obstet Gynecol 2005;105:1074–1083

13 Hirata J D, Swiersz L M, Zell B, Small R, Ettinger B. Does dong quai have estrogenic effects in postmenopausal women? A double-blind placebo controlled trial. Fertil Steril 1997;68:981–986

14 Chenoy S, Hussain S, Tayob Y, O'Brien P M S, Moss M Y, Morse P F. Effect of oral gamolenic acid from evening primrose oil on menopausal flushing. BMJ 1994;308:501–503

15 Hartley D E, Heinze L, Elsabagh S, File S E. Effects on cognition and mood in postmenopausal women of 1-week treatment with Ginkgo biloba. Pharmacol Biochem Behav 2003;75:711–720

16 Elsabagh S, Hartley D E, File S E. Limited cognitive benefits in Stage +2 postmenopausal women after 6 weeks of treatment with Ginkgo biloba. J Psychopharmacol 2005;19:173–181

17 Wiklund I K, Mattsson L A, Lindgren R, Limoni C. Effects of a standardized ginseng extract on quality of life and physiological parameters in symptomatic postmenopausal women: a double-blind, placebo-controlled trial. Int J Clin Pharmacol Res 1999;19:89–99

18 Warnecke G, Pfaender H, Gerster G, Gracza E. Wirksamkeit von Kawa-Kawa-Extrakt beim klimakterischen Syndrom. Zeitschr für Phytotherapie 1990;11:81–86

19 Warnecke G. Psychosomatische Dysfunktionen im weiblichen Klimakterium: Klinische Wirksamkeit und Verträglichkeit von Kava-Extrakt WS 1490. Fortschr der Medizin 1991;109:119–122

20 De Leo V, La Marca A, Lanzetta D, Palazzi S, Torricelli M, Facchini C, Morgante G. Valutazione dell'associazione di estratto do Kava-Kava e terpia ormoale sostitutiva nel tratta mento d'ansia in postmenpausa. Minerva Ginecol 2000;52:263–267

21 Woo J, Lau E, Ho S C, Cheng F, Chan C, Chan A S, Haines C J, Chan T Y, Li M, Sham A. Comparison of Pueraria lobata with hormone replacement therapy in treating the adverse health consequences of menopause. Menopause 2003;10:352–361

22 Thompson Coon J, Pittler M H, Ernst E. The role of red clover (Trifolium pratense) isoflavones in women's reproductive health: a systematic review and meta-analysis of randomised clinical trials. (Submitted for publication)

23 Lissin L W, Oka R, Lakshmi S, Cooke J P. Isoflavones improve vascular reactivity in post-menopausal women with hypercholesterolemia. Vasc Med 2004;9:26–30

24 Goodman-Gruen D, Kritz-Silverstein D. Usual dietary isoflavone intake is associated with cardiovascular disease risk factors in postmenopausal women. J Nutr 2001;131:1202–1206

25 Christie S, Walker A F, Hicks S M, Abeyasekera S. Flavonoid supplement improves leg health and reduces fluid retention in pre-menopausal women in a double-blind, placebo-controlled study. Phytomedicine 2004;11:11–17

26 Hale G, Paul-Labrador M, Dwyer J H, Merz C N. Isoflavone supplementation and endothelial function in menopausal women. Clin Endocrinol 2002;56:693–701

27 Katase K, Kato T, Hirai Y, Hasumi K, Chen J T. Effects of ipriflavone on bone loss following a bilateral ovariectomy and menopause: a randomized placebo-controlled study. Calcif Tissue Int 2001;69:73–77

28 Atkinson C, Compston J E, Day N E, Dowsett M, Bingham S A. The effects of phytoestrogen isoflavones on bone density in women: a double-blind, randomized, placebo-controlled trial. Am J Clin Nutr 2004;79:326–333

29 Lucas E A, Wild R D, Hammond L J, Khalil D A, Juma S, Daggy B P, Stoecker B J, Arjmandi B H. Flaxseed improves lipid profile without altering biomarkers of bone metabolism in postmenopausal women. J Clin Endocrinol Metab 2002;87:1527–1532

30 Sammartino A, Di Carlo C, Mandato V D, Bifulco G, Di Stefano M, Nappi C. Effects of genistein on the endometrium: ultrasonographic evaluation. Gynecol Endocrinol 2003;17:45–49

31 Baber R J, Templeman C, Morton T, Kelly G E, West L. Randomized placebo-controlled trial of an isoflavone supplement and menopausal symptoms in women. Climacteric 1999;2:85–92

32 Russo R, Corosu R. The clinical use of a preparation based on phyto-oestrogens in the treatment of menopausal disorders. Acta Biomed Ateneo Parmense 2003;74:137–143

33 Lemay A, Dodin S, Kadri N, Jacques H, Forest J C. Flaxseed dietary supplement versus

hormone replacement therapy in hypercholesterolemic menopausal women. Obstet Gynecol 2002;100:495–504

34 Krebs E E, Ensrud K E, MacDonald R, Wilt T J. Phytoestrogens for treatment of menopausal symptoms: a systematic review. Obstet Gynecol 2004;104:824–836

35 Grube B, Walper A, Wheatley D. St. John's wort extract: efficacy for menopausal symptoms of psychological origin. Adv Ther 1999;16:177–186

36 Boblitz N, Schrader E, Henneicke-von Zepelin H H, Wüstenberg P. Benefit of a fixed drug combination containing St John's wort and black cohosh for climacteric patients – results of a randomized clinical trial. Focus Alt Complement Ther 2000;5:85–86

37 Komesaroff P A, Black C V, Cable V, Sudhir K. Effects of wild yam extract on menopausal symptoms, lipids and sex hormones in healthy menopausal women. Climacteric 2001;4:144–150

38 Chen L C, Tsao Y T, Yen Y K, Chen Y F, Chou M H, Lin M F. A pilot study comparing the clinical effects of Jia-Wey Shiau-Yau San, a traditional Chinese herbal prescription, and a continuous combined hormone replacement therapy in postmenopausal women with climacteric symptoms. Maturitas 2003;44:55–62

39 Davis S R, Briganti E M, Chen R Q, Dalais F S, Bailey M, Burger H G. The effects of Chinese medicinal herbs on postmenopausal vasomotor symptoms of Australian women. A randomised controlled trial. Med J Aust 2001;174:68–71

40 Koike K, Ohno S, Takahashi N, Suzuki N, Nozaki N, Murakami K, Sugiura K, Yamada K, Inoue M. Efficacy of the herbal medicine Unkei-to as an adjunctive treatment to hormone replacement therapy for postmenopausal women with depressive symptoms. Clin Neuropharmacol 2004;27:157–162

41 Germaine L M, Freedman R R. Behavioral treatment of menopausal hot flashes: evaluation by objective methods. J Consult Clin Psychol 1984;52:1072–1079

42 Freedman R R, Woodward S. Behavioral treatment of menopausal hot flushes: evaluation by ambulatory monitoring. Am J Obstet Gynecol 1992;167:436–439

43 Irvin J H, Domar A D, Clark C, Zuttermeister P C, Friedman R. The effects of relaxation response training on menopausal symptoms. J Psychosom Obstet Gynaecol 1996;17:202–207

44 Cleary C, Fox J P. Menopausal symptoms: an osteopathic investigation. Complement Ther Med 1994;2:181–186

45 Murkies A L, Lombard C, Strauss B J, Wilcox G, Burger H G, Morton M S. Dietary flour supplementation decreases post-menopausal hot flushes: effect of soy and wheat. Maturitas 1995;21:189–195

46 Dalais F S, Rice G E, Wahlqvist M L, Grehan M, Murkies A L, Medley G, Ayton R, Strauss B J. Effects of dietary phytoestrogens in postmenopausal women. Climacteric 1998;1:124–129

47 Huntley A H, Ernst E. Soy for the treatment of perimenopausal symptoms – a systematic review. Maturitas 2004;47:1–9

48 Kreijkamp-Kaspers S, Kok L, Bots M L, Grobbee D E, Lampe J W, van der Schouw Y T. Randomized controlled trial of the effects of soy protein containing isoflavones on vascular function in postmenopausal women. Am J Clin Nutr 2005;81:189–195

49 McLaren H C. Vitamin E in the menopause. BMJ 1949;2:1378–1382

50 Blatt M H G, Weisbader H, Kupperman H S. Vitamin E and climacteric syndrome. Arch Intern Med 1953;91:792–799

51 Hammar M, Berg G, Lindgren R. Does physical exercise influence the frequency of postmenopausal hot flushes? Acta Obstet Gynecol Scand 1990;69:409–412

52 Wallace J P, Lovell S, Talano C, Webb M L, Hodgson J L. Changes in menstrual function, climacteric syndrome and serum concentrations of sex hormones in pre and post-menopausal women following a moderate intensity conditioning program. Med Sci Sports Exer 1982;14:154

53 Slaven L, Lee C. Mood and symptom reporting among middle-aged women: the relationship between menopausal status, hormone replacement therapy and exercise participation. Health Psychol 1997;16:203–208

54 Wilbur J, Holm K, Dan A. The relationship of energy expenditure to physical and psychologic symptoms in women at midlife. Nurs Outlook 1992;40:269–275

55 Chan K, Qin L, Lau M, Woo J, Au S, Choy W, Lee K, Lee S. A randomized, prospective study of the effects of Tai Chi Chun exercise on bone mineral density in postmenopausal women. Arch Phys Med Rehabil 2004;85:717–722

56 Williamson J, White A, Hart A, Ernst E. Randomised controlled trial of reflexology for menopausal symptoms. BJOG 2002;109: 1050–1055

CONDITIONS

MIGRAINE

Synonyms

Vascular headache, bilious headache, sick headache, blind headache, hemicrania. May also be named according to associated symptom, e.g. hemiplegic, ophthalmoplegic and ophthalmic nerve migraines.

Definition

Migraine is a primary headache disorder manifesting as recurring attacks usually lasting for 4–72 hours and involving pain of moderate to severe intensity, often with nausea, sometimes vomiting, and/or sensitivity to light, sound, and other sensory stimuli. Patients with this chronic complaint are very likely to seek help from CAM, the commonest forms being herbal medicine, spinal manipulation, acupuncture, homeopathy and reflexology.[1]

Clinical evidence

The available evidence relates mostly to prevention of migraine rather than treatment of an acute attack.

Acupuncture

A systematic review[2] (Box 2.75) concluded cautiously in favour of acupuncture for prevention of migraine. However, the generally modest quality of studies prevented a firm conclusion. Since then, the trial data have generated mixed results. In one RCT, 160 patients received either acupuncture or oral flunarizine.[3] After 2 and 4 months' treatment, the frequency of attacks was lower in the acupuncture group, while at 6 months there was no longer a difference. An RCT involving 179 patients in the early stages of acute migraine, suggested that acupuncture reduces the number of patients who develop a full migraine within 48 hours compared with placebo; the effect was similar to sumatriptan.[4] Comparing TENS, low dose laser therapy and acupuncture for 4 months, acupuncture proved to be best for migraine-prevention.[5] When 401 patients with chronic headache, predominantly migraine, were randomised to either receive advice to consult an acupuncturist or to have the usual treatment, acupuncture led to a persistent reduction in headache scores.[6] A small RCT (n = 28) found no differences in the prevention of menstrually-related migraine between real and sham acupuncture.[7] A large, high quality RCT (n = 302) showed no differences between sham and real acupuncture in preventing migraine attacks but both treatments yielded better results than no treatment at all.[8] On balance therefore the evidence is encouraging but not fully convincing.

Biofeedback and relaxation

Meta-analysis suggests that these therapies generate benefits for adults with migraine[9] (Box 2.76) but the conclusions must be cautious since appropriate controls are difficult to arrange. Moreover, the review included any type of prospective study.

Box 2.75
Systematic review
Acupuncture for migraine
Melchart[2]

- Twenty-six RCTs involving 1151 with idiopathic headache patients (16 RCTs of migraine)

- Quality of studies was variable and often poor

- Sixteen sham-controlled RCTs showed efficacy of acupuncture

- Conclusion: the existing evidence supports the value of acupuncture

More recent RCTs show positive results for a multidisciplinary approach, including stress-management,[10] as well as for thermal biofeedback,[11] and for a complex relaxation programme.[12]

Box 2.76
Meta-analysis
Biofeedback/relaxation for migraine (adults)
Holroyd[9]

- Thirty-five prospective trials of relaxation and/or biofeedback (sample sizes not quoted)

- Simultaneous analysis of 25 trials of propranolol, for comparison

- Overall, effect size similar to propranolol: 43% reduction in headache activity (improvement as a percentage of baseline symptoms)

- Effect size for those who received placebo medication was 14% and for untreated group 0%

- Conclusion: evidence provides substantial support for effectiveness of relaxation/biofeedback and for propranolol

A 1995 NIH Technology Assessment Panel found moderate evidence in support of the hypothesis that biofeedback is more effective than either relaxation or no treatment in relieving migraine headache.[13] The evidence was less clear when biofeedback was compared with placebo.

Prospective studies in pediatric migraine[14] suggest effectiveness of biofeedback, either alone or in combination with relaxation, with a similar effect to propranolol, though the result is not supported by the evidence from controlled studies (Box 2.77).

Diet

Of 88 children with severe, frequent migraine, 93% improved on a low-allergen diet. The role of foods provoking migraine was established by double-blind challenge in 40 of the children.[15] Confirmation of the role of food allergy in causing migraine was

Box 2.77
Meta-analysis
**Biofeedback/relaxa-
tion for migraine
(children)**
Hermann[14]

- Twenty-nine prospective investigations of behavioural inter-ventions, mainly biofeedback and/or relaxation, involving 471 subjects

- Investigations of drug therapy (n = 556) used for comparison

- Effect sizes (measured in standard deviations): biofeedback, 2.6; relaxation, 1.0; biofeedback combined with relaxation, 3.1; placebo, 0.6; waiting list, 0.6; propranolol, 2.8; ergotamine 1.6: clonidine, 1.5

- Further analysis restricted to controlled trials found no dif-ferences compared with various control interventions

- Conclusion: cautiously positive, lack of good-quality studies

provided by a study of 43 adults with migraine who were skin tested for allergies.[16] Those who were positive were more likely to respond to dietary manipulation than those who were nega-tive. Attacks were provoked in several cases (71%) by blinded food challenge but not by placebo. Clearly, if trigger foods such as chocolate, cheese, shellfish or red wine are identified, these should be avoided. No rigorous studies of other nutritional approaches are available.

Herbal medicine

Butterbur (*Petasites hybridus*) was compared with placebo in a 12-week RCT with 60 migraineurs.[17] The frequency of migraine attacks proved to be lower in the verum group. A re-analysis of these data showed that the responder rate with butterbur was 45%, while that of the placebo group was 15%.[18]

A systematic review[19] of **feverfew** (*Tanacetum parthenium*) (Box 2.78), found three positive studies but there are weaknesses in most of these and the evidence was not considered to be con-clusive in favour of feverfew.

Box 2.78
Systematic review
**Feverfew for
migraine**
Pittler[19]

- Five RCTs including 343 subjects

- Results favoured feverfew over placebo for migraine-preven-tion but had limitations, in particular short duration

- No major safety problems emerged

- Conclusion: the evidence is insufficient

Encouraging results were also reported for a Chinese patent medicine (shutianning granule)[20] and for a combination of soy isoflavones, dong quai and black cohosh (for menstrual migraine).[21]

Homeopathy

A systematic review[22] of homeopathy for chronic headache, mainly migraine (Box 2.79), found that the evidence suggests that this therapy is not superior to placebo. More recently, a double-blind, placebo-controlled RCT (n = 73) of individualised homeopathy showed a trend in favour of homeopathy in migraine prevention.[23]

Box 2.79
Systematic review
Homeopathy for migraine
Ernst[22]

- Four RCTs including 294 subjects

- One study also included patients with other forms of chronic headache

- One RCT, the lowest quality, found improvement in frequency, duration and intensity of attacks

- The remaining three RCTs were negative for attack frequency, severity and intensity, although in one, the neurologist's assessment favoured homeopathy

- Conclusion: homeopathy is not superior to placebo

Spinal manipulation

Two systematic reviews of spinal manipulation for various forms of headache are available.[24,25] They include three RCTs on migraine patients. Their results suggest effectiveness of this treatment for migraine (Box 2.80).

Box 2.80
Systematic reviews
Spinal manipulation for migraine
Bronfort[24], Astin[25]

- Eight RCTs including patients with various forms of headache

- Three RCTs on migraine including a total of 430 patients

- Quality was satisfactory to moderate

- Conclusion: overall these studies imply effectiveness

Supplements

A small placebo-controlled RCT (n = 42) suggested that **Coenzyme Q10** (3 × 100 mg/day) is effective in reducing the number of migraine attacks of chronic migraine sufferers.[26]

Two RCTs (n = 27 and n = 196) tested the effects of **fish oil** (omega-3 fatty acid) in migraine prevention. In the smaller study[27] no effect was found, yet a slight reduction (by 1.1 attacks per 4 months) was noted in the larger trial.[28]

Other therapies

No benefits were demonstrated in an RCT of **hyperbaric oxygen therapy**.[29] A double-blind, placebo-controlled RCT of impulse **magnetic-field therapy** generated encouraging results,[30] which, however, require independent replication.

In an RCT involving 20 subjects with mixed migraine and tension headache over 4 months, **yoga** in addition to standard medication produced reduction in headache activity in contrast to standard medication alone.[31]

Overall recommendation

Reasonable choices for prevention of migraine are acupuncture, biofeedback (either alone or with relaxation) or exclusion diets (in suitable patients). For acupuncture, the evidence is encouraging but not fully convincing. Some herbal remedies, such as feverfew or butterbur, may also be beneficial. The results with Co-enzyme Q10 are encouraging but require independent confirmation. Compared with conventional treatments, these CAM therapies seem similarly effective in the prevention of migraine attacks. None of the CAM therapies is associated with major risks and thus may be preferable to long-term use of conventional preventive drugs. The role of CAM therapies in treatment of acute migraine attacks has not been investigated or compared with modern medications such as triptans.

Table 2.55
Summary of clinical evidence for migraine

Treatment	Weight of evidence	Direction of evidence	Serious safety concerns
Acupuncture	OOO	↗	Yes (see p 294)
Biofeedback	OOO	⇧	No (see p 310)
Diet	OO	⇧	No (see p 5)
Herbal medicine			
Butterbur	O	⇧	Yes (see p 477)
Feverfew	OO	↗	Yes (see p 396)
Homeopathy	OO	↘	No (see p 327)
Relaxation	OO	↗	No (see p 348)
Spinal manipulation	OO	↗	Yes (see p 316)
Supplements			
Co-enzyme Q10	O	⇧	Yes (see p 385)
Fish oil	O	↗	Yes (see p 483)

REFERENCES

1 Eisenberg D M, Davis R, Ettner S L, Appel S, Wilkey S, Rompay M V. Trends in alternative medicine use in the United States, 1990–1997. JAMA 1998;280:1569–1575

2 Melchart D, Linde K, Fischer P, Berman B, White A, Vickers A, Allais G. Acupuncture for idiopathic headache. The Cochrane Database of Systematic Reviews 2001, Issue 1. Art No.: CD001218

3 Allais G, De Lorenzo C, Quirico P E, Airola G, Tolardo G, Mana O, Benedetto C. Acupuncture in the prophylactic treatment of migraine without aura: a comparison with flunarizine. Headache 2002;42:855–861

4 Melchart D, Thormaehlen J, Hager S, Liao J, Linde K, Weidenhammer W. Acupuncture versus placebo versus sumatriptan for early treatment of acute migraine attacks – a randomized controlled trial. J Intern Med 2003;253:181–188

5 Allais G, De Lorenzo C, Quirico P E, Lupi G, Airola G, Mana O, Benedetto C. Non-pharmacological approaches to chronic headaches: transcutaneous electrical nerve stimulation, lasertherapy and acupuncture in transformed migraine treatment. Neurol Sci 2003;24: S138–S142

6 Vickers AJ, Rees R W, Zollman C E, McCarney R, Smith C M, Ellis N, Fisher P, Van Haselen R. Acupuncture for chronic headache in primary care: large, pragmatic, randomised trial. BMJ 2004;328:744

7 Linde M, Fjell A, Carlsson J, Dahlof C. Role of the needling per se in acupuncture as prophylaxis for menstrually related migraine: a randomized placebo-controlled study. Cephalal 2005;25:41–47

8 Linde K, Streng A, Jurgens S, Hoppe A, Brinkhaus B, Witt C, Wagenpfeil S, Pfaffenrath V, Hammes M G, Weidenhammer W, Willich S N, Melchart D. Acupuncture for patients with migraine: a randomized controlled trial. JAMA 2005;293:2118–2125

9 Holroyd K A, Penzien D B. Pharmacological versus non-pharmacological prophylaxis of recurrent migraine headache: a meta-analytic review of clinical trials. Pain 1990;42:1–13

10 Lemstra M, Stewart B, Olszynski W P. Effectiveness of multidisciplinary intervention in the treatment of migraine: a randomized controlled trial. Headache 2002;42:845–854

11 Scharff L, Marcus D A, Masek B J. A controlled study of minimal-contact thermal biofeedback treatment in children with migraine. J Pediatr Psychol 2002;27:109–119

12 Fichtel A, Larsson B. Relaxation treatment administered by school nurses to adolescents with recurrent headaches. Headache 2004;44: 545–554

13 NIH Technology Assessment Statement Integration of behavioral and relaxation approaches into the treatment of chronic pain and insomnia. NIH Technol Assess Statement 1995;16–18:1–34

14 Hermann C, Kim M, Blanchard E B. Behavioral and prophylactic pharmacological

intervention studies of pediatric migraine: an exploratory meta-analysis. Pain 1995;60:239–256

15 Egger J, Carter C M, Wilson J, Turner M W, Soothill J F. Is migraine food allergy? A double-blind controlled trial of oligoantigenic diet treatment. Lancet 1983;2:865–869

16 Mansfield L E, Vaughan T R, Waller S F, Haverly R W, Ting S. Food allergy and adult migraine: double-blind and mediator confirmation of an allergic etiology. Ann Allergy 1985;55:126–129

17 Grossman M, Schmidramsl H. An extract of Petasites hybridus is effective in the prophylaxis of migraine. Int J Clin Pharmacol Ther 2000;38:430–435

18 Diener H C, Rahlfs V W, Danesch U. The first placebo-controlled trial of a special butterbur root extract for the prevention of migraine: reanalysis of efficacy criteria. Eur Neurol 2004;51:89–97

19 Pittler M H, Ernst E. Feverfew for preventing migraine. The Cochrane Database of Systematic Reviews 2004, Issue 1. Art No.: CD002286

20 Hu Z Q, Song L G, Mei T. Clinical and experimental study on treatment of migraine with shutianning granule. [Article in Chinese] Zhongguo Zhong Xi Yi Jie He Za Zhi 2002;22:581–583

21 Burke B E, Olson R D, Cusack B J. Randomized, controlled trial of phytoestrogen in the prophylactic treatment of menstrual migraine. Biomed Pharmacother 2002;56:283–288

22 Ernst E. Homeopathic prophylaxis of headaches and migraine? A systematic review. J Pain Symptom Manage 1999;18:353–357

23 Straumsheim P, Borchgrevink C, Mowinckel P, Kierulf H, Hafslund O. Homeopathic treatment of migraine: a double-blind, placebo controlled trial of 68 patients [see comment]. Br Homeopath J 2000;89:4–7

24 Bronfort G, Assendelft W J, Evans R, Haas M, Bouter L. Efficacy of spinal manipulation for chronic headache: a systematic review. J Manipulative Physiol Ther 2001;24:457–466

25 Astin J A, Ernst E. The effectiveness of spinal manipulation for the treatment of headache disorders: a systematic review of randomized clinical trials. Cephalalgia 2002;22:617–623

26 Sándor P S, Di Clemente L, Coppola G, Saenger U, Magis D, Seidel L, Agosti R M, Schoenen J. Efficacy of coenzyme Q10 in migraine prophylaxis: a randomized controlled trial. Neurol 2005;64:713–715

27 Harel Z, Gascon G, Riggs S, Vaz R, Brown W, Exil G. Supplementation with omega-3

polyunsaturated fatty acids in the management of recurrent migraines in adolescents. J Adolesc Health 2002;31:154–161

28 Pradalier A, Bakouche P, Baudesson G, Delage A, Cornaille-Lafage G, Launay J M, Biason P. Failure of omega-3 polyunsaturated fatty acids in prevention of migraine: a double-blind study versus placebo. Cephalalgia 2001;21:818–822

29 Eftedal O S, Lydersen S, Helde G, White L, Brubakk A O, Stovner L J. A randomized,

double blind study of the prophylactic effect of hyperbaric oxygen therapy on migraine. Cephalalgia 2004;24:639–644

30 Pelka R B, Jaenicke C, Gruenwald J. Impulse magnetic-field therapy for migraine and other headaches: a double-blind, placebo-controlled study. Adv Ther 2001;18:101–109

31 Latha, Kaliappan K V. Efficacy of yoga therapy in the management of headaches. J Indian Psychol 1992;10:41–47

MULTIPLE SCLEROSIS

Synonyms/ subcategories
Disseminated, focal or insular sclerosis, demyelinating disease.

Definition
A common demyelinating disorder of the central nervous system, causing patches of sclerosis (plaques) in the brain and spinal cord.

Related conditions
None, but numerous other conditions can mimic the extremely variable symptoms of multiple sclerosis (MS), particularly in the early stages.

CAM usage
Survey data suggest that between 41% and 64% of MS patients use CAM.[1,2] Relaxation techniques, homeopathy, herbal medicines and dietary treatments are amongst the most common modalities. In our survey of CAM organisations (see p 4), the following treatments were recommended: aromatherapy, hypnotherapy, massage, reflexology and yoga.

Clinical evidence

Feldenkrais method
In a small (n = 20) crossover RCT, MS patients were allocated to Feldenkrais or sham sessions for 8 weeks.[3] Patients reported less stress and anxiety with Feldenkrais compared with sham.

Herbal medicine
Two small RCTs suggest that pure compounds from cannabis (*Cannabis sativa*) can reduce pain in MS patients.[4,5] A large RCT showed that cannabinoids do not reduce spasticity in MS patients but some improvement in mobility was noted.[6] A small RCT produced no evidence that cannabis extract reduces MS-associated tremor.[7]

Imagery
An RCT with ambulatory MS patients tested imagery versus no treatment.[8] Its results demonstrated a reduction in state anxiety, but no change in depression or physical symptoms associated with MS.

Magnetic field therapy

Two sham-controlled RCTs of magnetic field therapy for the symptoms of MS are available.[9,10] One trial (n = 38) demonstrated an improvement in spasticity but not in other symptoms.[9] The other study (n = 30) showed improvement in the combined rating for bladder control, cognitive function, fatigue level, mobility, spasticity and vision.[10] There was, however, no change in the overall symptom score and some patients in the treatment group had increased headaches during the initial treatment phases. A follow-up RCT of the latter trial (n = 117) showed improvements in fatigue and quality of life but no effects on bladder control or disability.[11]

Massage

Twenty-four MS patients were randomised to receive either regular massage therapy or no treatment in addition to standard care.[12] At the end of the 5 week treatment period the former group had lower anxiety levels and were less depressed. Moreover, they had improved self-esteem, body image and social functioning.

Music therapy

Two small RCTs of active music therapy showed positive trends for respiratory muscle strength[13] or self-esteem, depression and anxiety in MS patients.[14] However, possibly because of too small sample sizes, the effects failed to reach statistical significance.

Neural therapy

The treatment was tested in a small (n = 21) double-blind RCT against placebo.[15] A larger proportion improved in the actively treated compared with the control group according to validated outcome scales measuring subjective symptoms.

Reflexology

Seventy-one MS patients were randomised to receive either 11 weeks of regular (foot) reflexology or non-specific (sham) massage of the calf.[16] Improvements were noted in terms of paresthesiae, urinary symptoms, muscle strength and spasticity.

Supplements

An RCT investigated the effects of **eicosapentaenic** (EPA) and **docosahexaenic** (DHA) acids on the symptoms of 312 MS patients.[17] There were no differences between patients taking 20 capsules of fish oil per day or those taking placebo in terms of clinical improvements.

Epidemiological studies (e.g.[18]) suggest the effectiveness of **linoleic acid** in MS. In the first RCT 87 patients with MS were randomised to receive twice-daily supplements of vegetable oil mixture containing either a total of 17.2 g linolate or 7.6 g oleate (control) for 2 years.[19] The results suggest a greater severity of clinical relapses in patients taking oleate than those receiving the linolate. The second study[20] involved 116 MS patients in an RCT of polyunsaturated fatty acids taken for 2 years. Patients were randomly allocated to one of four groups. Two groups received linoleic acid either as a spread (23 g of linoleic acid) or in nau-dicelle capsules (2.92 g of linoleic acid and 0.34 g of gamma-linoleic acid). Two control groups received oleic acid (16 g and 4 g daily). Rates of clinical deterioration and frequencies of attacks were not different between treated and control groups. Exacerbations were marginally shorter and less severe in patients receiving the higher dose of linoleic acid than controls. In the third RCT,[21] 96 patients were randomised to receive either a dose of 17 g/day of linoleic acid or 21 g/day of oleic acid. The trial results showed no therapeutic benefit from the use of linoleic acid during the 30-month period.

Epidemiological data suggest that regular intake of **vitamin D** from supplements but not from food may protect against developing MS.[22]

Yoga

An RCT compared regular yoga exercise with conventional aerobic exercise (both for 6 months) with a waiting list control. Both types of exercise improved fatigue but not cognitive function.[23]

Overall recommendation

There is some encouraging evidence that several CAM modalities alleviate the symptoms of MS. In as far as these are not associated with risks, they can be endorsed for the use of patients who are keen to try CAM and are probably best used as adjunctive forms of treatment. Whether magnetic field therapy or food supplements like linoleic acid delay the course of the disease is unclear at present. Compared with conventional treatments, CAM might prove useful for improving quality of life of MS patients. None of the CAM treatments offers the prospect of a cure for MS.

Table 2.56
Summary of clinical evidence for multiple sclerosis

Treatment	Weight of evidence	Direction of evidence	Serious safety concerns
Feldenkrais	O	↗	No (see p 359)
Herbal medicine			
Cannabis	OO	↗	Yes (see p 5)
Imagery	O	↗	No (see p 359)
Magnetic field therapy	OO	↗	No (see p 359)
Massage	O	↗	No (see p 334)
Music therapy	O	⇨	No (see p 360)

Treatment	Weight of evidence	Direction of evidence	Serious safety concerns
Neural therapy	O	⬈	Yes (see p 360)
Reflexology	O	⬆	No (see p 345)
Supplements			
EPA/DHA	O	⬇	No (see p 5)
Linoleic acid	OO	⇨	No (see p 5)
Vitamin D (prevention)	O	⬈	No (see p 5)
Yoga	O	⬈	No (see p 356)

REFERENCES

1 Sastre-Garriga J, Munteis E, Rio J, Pericot I, Tintore M, Montalban X. Unconventional therapy in multiple sclerosis. Mult Scler 2003;9:320–322

2 Winterholler M, Erbguth F, Neudorfer B. Use of alternative medicine by patients with multiple sclerosis – users characterisation and patterns of use. Fortschr Neurol Psychiatr 1997;65:555–561

3 Johnson S K, Frederick J, Kaufman M, Mountjoy B. A controlled investigation of body work in multiple sclerosis. J Alt Complement Med 1999;5:237–243

4 Wade D T, Robson P, House H, Makela P, Aram J. A preliminary controlled study to determine whether whole-plant cannabis extracts can improve intractable neurogenic symptoms. Clin Rehabil 2003;17:21–29

5 Svendsen K B, Jensen T S, Bach F W. Does the cannabinoid dronabinol reduce central pain in multiple sclerosis? Randomised double blind placebo controlled crossover trial. BMJ 2004;329:253

6 Zajicek J, Fox P, Sanders H, Wright D, Vickery J, Nunn A, Thompson A; UK MS Research Group. Cannabinoids for treatment of spasticity and other symptoms related to multiple sclerosis (CAMS study): multicentre randomised placebo-controlled trial. Lancet 2003;362:1517–1526

7 Fox P, Bain P G, Glickman S, Carroll C, Zajicek J. The effect of cannabis on tremor in patients with multiple sclerosis. Neurology 2004;62: 1105–1109

8 Maguire B L. The effects of imagery on attitudes and moods in multiple sclerosis patients. Alt Ther Health Med 1996;2:75–79

9 Nielson J F, Sinkjaer T, Jakobsen J. Treatment of spasticity with repetitive magnetic stimulation; a double-blind placebo-controlled study. Multiple Sclerosis 1996;2:227–232

10 Richards T L, Lappin M S, Acosta Urquidi J, Kraft G H, Heide A C, Lawrie F W, Merrill T E, Melton G B, Cunningham C A. Double-blind study of pulsing magnetic field effects on multiple sclerosis. J Alt Complement Med 1997;3:21–29

11 Lappin M S, Lawrie F W, Richards T L, Kramer E D. Effects of a pulsed electromagnetic therapy on multiple sclerosis fatigue and quality of life: a double-blind, placebo controlled trial. Altern Ther Health Med 2003;9:38–48

12 Hernandez-Reif M, Field T, Field T, Theakston H. Multiple sclerosis patients benefit from massage therapy. J Bodywork Movement Ther 1998;2:168–174

13 Wiens M E, Reimer M A, Guyn H L. Music therapy as a treatment method for improving respiratory muscle strength in patients with advanced multiple sclerosis: a pilot study. Rehabil Nurs 1999;24:74–80

14 Schmid W, Aldridge D. Active music therapy in the treatment of multiple sclerosis patients: a matched control study. J Music Ther 2004;41:225–240

15 Gibson R G, Gibson S L M. Neural therapy in the treatment of multiple sclerosis. J Alt Complement Med 1999;5:543–552

16 Siev-Ner I, Gamus D, Lerner-Geva L, Achiron A. Reflexology treatment relieves symptoms of multiple sclerosis: a randomized controlled study. Mult Scler 2003;9:356–361

17 Bates D, Cartlidge N E, French J M, Jackson M J, Nightingale S, Shaw D A, Smith S, Woo E, Hawkins S A, Millar J. A double-blind controlled trial of long chain n-3 polyunsaturated

fatty acids in the treatment of multiple sclerosis. J Neurol Neurosurg Psychiatr 1989;52:18–22

18 Agranoff B W, Goldberg D. Diet and the geographical distribution of multiple sclerosis. Lancet 1974;2:1061–1066

19 Millar J H, Zilkha K J, Langman M J, Wright H P, Smith A D, Belin J, Thompson R H. Double-blind trial of linoleate supplementation of diet in multiple sclerosis. BMJ 1973;1:765–768

20 Bates D, Fawcett P R, Shaw D A, Weightman. Polyunsaturated fatty acids in treatment of acute remitting multiple sclerosis. BMJ 1978;2:1390–1391

21 Paty D W. Double-blind trial of linoleic acid in multiple sclerosis. Arch Neurol 1983;40:693–694

22 Munger K L, Zhang S M, O'Reilly E, Hernan M A, Olek M J, Willett W C, Ascherio A. Vitamin D intake and incidence of multiple sclerosis. Neurology 2004;62:60–65

23 Oken B S, Kishiyama S, Zajdel D, Bourdette D, Carlsen J, Haas M, Hugos C, Kraemer D F, Lawrence J, Mass M. Randomized controlled trial of yoga and exercise in multiple sclerosis. Neurology 2004;62:2058–2064

NAUSEA AND VOMITING

Definition

Vomiting is the ejection of matter through the mouth from the stomach and nausea is the inclination to vomit or the sensation associated with vomiting. Nausea and vomiting associated with pregnancy, surgery, chemotherapy and motion will be considered.

CAM usage

Acupuncture and acupressure are commonly used for nausea in early pregnancy, commercial acupressure wrist-bands for sea-sickness and various CAM methods may be used as adjuncts in cancer therapy. Ginger (*Zingiber officinale*) is also used for nausea and vomiting of pregnancy, postoperative nausea and vomiting (PONV) and motion sickness.

Clinical evidence

Acupuncture

Stimulation at the relevant point (known as PC6) by acupuncture, acupressure wrist-bands and electrical apparatus are often regarded as so similar that they can be combined in reviews. A systematic review included 33 RCTs and CCTs of acupuncture and related forms of stimulation, mostly given as an adjunct to standard treatment, for postoperative, early pregnancy or chemotherapy-induced nausea and vomiting.[1] Twenty-seven trials were positive: in four negative trials the acupuncture was given after the emetic stimulus and under general anaesthetic.

For **nausea of pregnancy**, subsequent studies allow a positive conclusion. Although a Cochrane review reported mixed results for four RCTs comparing acupressure with placebo or sham treatment[2] (see Box 2.81), the results of eight subsequent trials have generally been positive. Three trials on acupressure (n = 454)[3–5] reported beneficial effects, one RCT (n = 36) concluded that both acupuncture and acupressure were effective in the treatment of hyperemesis gravidarum (n = 36),[6] two RCTs of acupuncture (n = 593, n = 55) reported positive yet non-specific effects[7,8] and an RCT of low level nerve stimulation at acupoint PC6 also came to a positive conclusion.[9]

Box 2.81
Systematic review
**Acupoint
stimulation for
nausea and
vomiting
(pregnancy)**
Jewell[2]

- Four RCTs including 661 women

- Acupressure reduced the proportion of women reporting morning sickness

- Two trials were positive; the two trials which were not included in the summary calculation found no evidence of effect

- Conclusion: women appear to benefit, though this has not been fully demonstrated to be more than a placebo effect

For preventing **postoperative nausea and vomiting** (PONV), a Cochrane review of PC6 acupoint stimulation came to a strongly positive conclusion (Box 2.82).[10] Compared with antiemetic prophylaxis, PC6 acupoint stimulation seems to reduce the risk of nausea but not vomiting. Three RCTs published since this review corroborate this conclusion,[11-13] yet four trials of acupressure reported no positive findings.[14-17] An RCT of acustimulation administered in addition to ondansetron in patients undergoing plastic surgery found it to be most effective when administered after compared with before or during surgery.[18] One double-blind RCT found that a capsicum plaster at the Korean hand acupuncture point KD2 or at PC6 reduced PONV in patients undergoing abdominal hysterectomy.[19]

Box 2.82
Meta-analysis
**Acupoint
stimulation for
nausea and
vomiting
(postoperative)**
Lee[10]

- Twenty-six RCTs involving 3347 participants

- Overall quality score was average, trials were heterogeneous, none reported adequate allocation concealment

- Acupuncture reported as better than sham treatment in the incidence risk of nausea and vomiting

- Acupuncture seems comparable to standard antiemetic medication

- When different antiemetics were pooled: acupuncture superior at reducing risk of nausea but not vomiting

- Conclusion: the use of P6 acupoint stimulation can reduce the risk of postoperative nausea and vomiting with minimal adverse events

For **chemotherapy-induced nausea**, the five CCTs in the original review[1] were all positive. A more recent systematic review of acupressure including two trials came to a cautiously positive conclusion for preventing nausea and vomiting (Box 2.83).[20] In subsequent single RCTs, electrical stimulation of PC6 reduced the

Box 2.83
Systematic review
Acupoint stimulation for nausea and vomiting (chemotherapy)
Klein[20]

- Two RCTs including 483 participants
- The results of the larger study are considerably less positive than for the smaller one
- Conclusion: Acupressure may have positive effects but no firm conclusions can be drawn due to the quality of reporting of these trials

severity of nausea induced by chemotherapy in a double-blind trial among 42 gynaecological cancer patients,[21] adjunctive electroacupuncture in patients with breast cancer had a positive yet short-term effect,[22] and TENS was beneficial as an adjunct to ondansetron therapy.[23] A further RCT suggests that in combination with ondansetron i.v., invasive needle acupuncture at PC6 has no additional effect.[24] In nausea in terminally ill hospice care patients, a small crossover study with six patients found no effect of acupressure wrist-bands.[25]

In **motion sickness** (Table 2.57), three out of four RCTs investigating acupuncture stimulation in the laboratory for experimentally induced symptoms were positive.[26-29] Korean hand acupressure at K-K9 was effective in reducing nausea and subjective symptoms of motion sickness in emergency trauma transport of ten geriatric patients.[30]

A small RCT including 40 patients testing the anti-gagging effects of acupuncture and acupressure during dental procedures was inconclusive.[31] Also inconclusive was a partially blinded and partially randomised trial of PC6 wristband acupressure for relief of nausea and vomiting associated with acute myocardial infarction.[32]

Biofeedback

After early promising case studies, an RCT compared electromyographic and galvanic response biofeedback with relaxation and no treatment for nausea in 81 patients undergoing cancer chemotherapy.[33] Biofeedback was not effective compared with relaxation. Another RCT found no effect of biofeedback compared with placebo feedback or no treatment in laboratory-induced motion sickness.[34]

Herbal medicine

A systematic review of **Chinese medical herbs** for chemotherapy induced nausea and vomiting was inconclusive (Box 2.84).[35]

A systematic review (Box 2.85) of **ginger** (*Zingiber officinale*) as an antiemetic found encouraging results for its use in nausea and vomiting of pregnancy yet no clear evidence for its efficacy in the treatment of PONV or kinestosis.[36] This confirms the results of a systematic review of ginger in

Table 2.57 **RCTs of acupoint stimulation for nausea and vomiting (motion sickness)**

Reference	Sample size	Interventions [regimen]	Result	Comment
Warwick-Evans[26]	36	A) Acupressure [bilateral wrist band for 15 min] B) Placebo stimulation	No difference	Double-blind, experimentally induced nausea
Hu[27]	64	A) Acupressure [unilateral finger pressure 1 Hz for 12 min] B) Dummy-point acupressure C) Placebo acupressure D) No treatment	A superior to all other groups	Experimentally induced nausea
Hu[28]	45	A) Electrical stimulation [unilateral 10 Hz for 15 min] B) Sham stimulation C) Control	A superior to both other groups	Experimentally induced nausea
Stern[29]	25	A) Acupressure [unilateral acuband on wrist 24 min] B) Acupressure [unilateral acuband on forearm 24 min] C) Control [no acuband]	A and B superior to C	Experimentally induced nausea
Bertalanffy[30]	100	A) Non-invasive Korean hand acupressure at K-K9 B) Sham acupressure	A superior to B	Motion sickness in emergency trauma transport

Box 2.84
Systematic review
Chinese medical herbs for nausea and vomiting (chemotherapy)
Taixiang[35]

- Four RCTs involving 342 patients

- All trials were of low quality, none used primary outcome using Common Toxicity Criteria

- All trials used a decoction containing Huangqi compounds

- Huangqi treated patients did experience less nausea and vomiting, no adverse events were reported

- Conclusion: due to the methodological limitations there is no robust demonstration of benefit

pregnancy-induced nausea and vomiting (Box 2.86)[37] and of a systematic review of ginger in PONV which found ginger not a clinically relevant antiemetic for PONV (Box 2.87).[38] One double-blind RCT found ginger to be beneficial for motion sickness.[39]

Peppermint oil was superior to placebo and no treatment when given preoperatively in an RCT.[40]

Hypnotherapy

Self-hypnosis has been described as helpful for both anticipatory and post-chemotherapy nausea and vomiting in children and adolescents and several controlled trials support this view.[41-43]

CONDITIONS

Box 2.85
Systematic review
**Ginger for nausea
and vomiting**
Betz[36]

- Twenty-four RCTs including 1073 patients; 16 contained details of antiemetic activity against pregnancy-induced nausea and vomiting, PONV and motion sickness

- Overall study quality was good

- Encouraging results for treatment of pregnancy induced nausea and vomiting (n = 4)

- No clear evidence for the efficacy in the treatment of PONV (n = 6) and seasickness (n = 6)

- Mild adverse effects (gastrointestinal complaints) were reported in 3.3% of patients and one severe adverse event (abortion) occurred

- Conclusion: ginger is a promising antiemetic herbal remedy, but data are insufficient for firm conclusions

Box 2.86
Systematic review
**Ginger for nausea
and vomiting in
pregnancy**
Borrelli[37]

- Six RCTs (n = 675) and one prospective observational cohort study (n = 175) were included

- Methodological quality of four out of five RCTs was high

- Four of the six trials (n = 246) showed superiority of ginger over placebo, the other two RCTs (n = 429) indicated that ginger was as effective as the reference drug (vitamin B_6) in relieving the severity of nausea and vomiting episodes

- All clinical data were included in a safety review which showed the absence of adverse effects on pregnancy outcome in the above effectiveness trials and found no spontaneous or case reports of adverse events during ginger treatment in pregnancy

- Conclusion: ginger may be an effective treatment for nausea and vomiting in pregnancy; more observational studies with a larger sample size are need to confirm the data on safety

Box 2.87
Systematic review
**Ginger for
postoperative
nausea and
vomiting**
Morin[38]

- Six RCTs involving 538 patients

- Trials of good quality

- Relative risk to suffer from PONV after pre-treatment with ginger was 0.84 (95% CI 0.60 to 1.03), NNT 11 (95% CI 6 to 250)

- Conclusion: ginger is not a clinically relevant antiemetic for postoperative nausea and vomiting

Hypnotherapy may be less effective in adults according to one RCT, but the intervention used may have been little more than relaxation.[44] Hypnotherapy was found to be effective against postoperative nausea and vomiting in women undergoing breast surgery.[45] An RCT of tape-recorded hypnosis instructions, however, reported an increased incidence of vomiting in the hypnosis group compared with the no-tape-group.[46]

Massage
A systematic review included two trials of **massage** for symptom relief in cancer patients.[47] Both trials found massage to be effective for chemotherapy induced nausea. An RCT (n = 230) found no beneficial effects of therapeutic massage and healing touch on chemotherapy-induced nausea.[48]

Relaxation
On balance, the evidence from a dozen RCTs shows that relaxation is effective in preventing nausea and vomiting before, during and after chemotherapy.[33,43,49–58] Research from one centre was summarised by the principal investigator,[59] who found that relaxation appears to be more effective if it is learnt before treatment with chemotherapy starts.

Supplements
A systematic review of **vitamin B$_6$** (Box 2.88)[2] in pregnancy drew a cautiously positive conclusion.

Box 2.88
Systematic review
Vitamin B6 for nausea and vomiting in pregnancy
Jewell[2]

- Two RCTs involving 416 women
- Pyridoxine (vitamin B$_6$) 75 mg or 30 mg/day respectively
- Quality not specifically reported
- No effect on vomiting
- Results suggest an effect on nausea, but there is insufficient evidence for firm conclusions

Other therapies
Peppermint **aromatherapy** reduced the perceived severity of PONV in a small RCT but had no specific effects compared with alcohol and saline control.[60]

A systematic review of **guided imagery** as an adjuvant cancer therapy found no compelling evidence to suggest positive effects on nausea and vomiting.[61]

CONDITIONS

A single RCT of 33 patients suggests that **music** may have some benefit in the management of chemotherapy induced nausea in addition to standard therapy,[62] while four RCTs report no beneficial effects of music on PONV.[63-66]

Overall recommendation

For nausea and vomiting of **pregnancy**, where no conventional drug therapy is acceptable, vitamin B_6 has a role. Acupressure is known to be useful and safe, but the effect may be non-specific. Ginger, although most likely effective is contraindicated.

For nausea and vomiting in other circumstances, some forms of CAM appear to offer a role as adjuncts to conventional therapies. In **postoperative nausea and vomiting**, conventional therapies are effective but expensive and have known adverse effects; acupressure bands are cheap, safe and easy to administer; the results for peppermint and hypnotherapy are encouraging but further evidence of effectiveness is required before any recommendations can be made. For nausea induced by **chemotherapy**, effective conventional drugs will usually be available because of the high incidence and severity of symptoms. However, both acupoint stimulation and relaxation are useful adjuncts. Hypnotherapy appears to have a useful preventive role, particularly in children, for nausea and vomiting before, during and after chemotherapy. The place of hypnotherapy for adults is less certain.

For **motion sickness**, ginger and acupuncture are worth using since conventional drugs, although effective, may have adverse effects.

Table 2.58
Summary of clinical evidence for nausea and vomiting

Treatment	Weight of evidence	Direction of evidence	Serious safety concerns
Nausea of pregnancy			
Acupoint stimulation	OOO	⇧	Yes (see p 294)
Herbal medicine			
Ginger	OO	⇧	Yes (see p 401)
Supplements			
Vitamin B_6	O	⬈	Yes (see p 5)
Postoperative nausea and vomiting			
Acupoint stimulation	OOO	⬈	Yes (see p 294)
Herbal medicine			
Ginger	OO	⬊	Yes (see p 401)
Peppermint	O	⇧	Yes (see p 448)
Hypnotherapy	O	⬈	Yes (see p 331)
Music therapy	OO	⇩	Yes (see p 360)

Treatment	Weight of evidence	Direction of evidence	Serious safety concerns
Nausea and vomiting induced by chemotherapy			
Acupoint stimulation	OO	↗	Yes (see p 294)
Biofeedback	O	⇩	No (see p 310)
Chinese herbal medicine	O	⇨	Yes (see p 5)
Hypnotherapy	OO	↗	Yes (see p 331)
Relaxation	OOO	⇧	No (see p 348)
Motion sickness			
Acupoint stimulation	OO	↗	Yes (see p 294)
Biofeedback	O	⇩	No (see p 310)
Herbal medicine			
Ginger	O	⇧	Yes (see p 401)

CONDITIONS

REFERENCES

1 Vickers A. Can acupuncture have specific effects on health? A systematic review of acupuncture antiemesis trials. J Roy Soc Med 1996;89:303–311

2 Jewell D, Young G. Interventions for nausea and vomiting in early pregnancy. The Cochrane Database of Systematic Reviews 2003, Issue 4. Art. No.: CD000145

3 Norheim A J, Pedersen E J, Fonnebo V, Berge L. Acupressure treatment of morning sickness in pregnancy. A randomised, double-blind, placebo-controlled study. Scand J Prim Health Care 2001;19:43–47

4 Steele N M, French J, Gatherer-Boyles J, Newman S, Leclaire S. Effect of acupressure by Sea-Bands on nausea and vomiting of pregnancy. J Obstet Gynecol Neonatal Nurs 2001;30:61–70

5 Werntoft E, Dykes A K. Effect of acupressure on nausea and vomiting during pregnancy. A randomized, placebo-controlled, pilot study. J Reprod Med 2001;46:835–839

6 Habek D, Barbir A, Habek J C, Janculiak D, Bobic-Vukovic M. Success of acupuncture and acupressure of the Pc 6 acupoint in the treatment of hyperemesis gravidarum. Forsch Komplementärmed Klass Naturheilkd 2004;11: 20–23

7 Smith C, Crowther C, Beilby J. Acupuncture to treat nausea and vomiting in early pregnancy: a randomized controlled trial. Birth 2002;29:1–9

8 Knight B, Mudge C, Openshaw S, White A, Hart A. Effect of acupuncture on nausea of pregnancy: a randomized, controlled trial. Obstet Gynecol 2001;97:184–188

9 Rosen T, de Veciana M, Miller H S, Stewart L, Rebarber A, Slotnick R N. A randomized controlled trial of nerve stimulation for relief of nausea and vomiting in pregnancy. Obstet Gynecol 2003;102:129–135

10 Lee A, Done ML. Stimulation of the wrist acupuncture point P6 for preventing postoperative nausea and vomiting. The Cochrane Database of Systematic Reviews 2004, Issue 3. Art.No.: CD003281

11 Gan TJ, Jiao KR, Zenn M, Georgiade G. A randomized controlled comparison of electro-acupoint stimulation or ondansetron versus placebo for the prevention of postoperative nausea and vomiting. Anesth Analg 2004;99:1070–1075

12 Streitberger K, Diefenbacher M, Bauer A, Conradi R, Bardenheuer H, Martin E, Schneider A, Unnebrink K. Acupuncture compared with placebo-acupuncture for postoperative nausea and vomiting prophylaxis: a randomised

placebo-controlled patient and observer blind trial. Anaesthesia 2004;59:142–149

13 Kim Y, Kim C W, Kim K S. Clinical observations on postoperative vomiting treated by auricular acupuncture. Am J Chin Med 2003;31:475–480

14 Klein A A, Djaiani G, Karski J, Carroll J, Karkouti K, McCluskey S, Poonawala H, Shayan C, Fedorko L, Cheng D. Acupressure wristbands for the prevention of postoperative nausea and vomiting in adults undergoing cardiac surgery. J Cardiothorac Vasc Anesth 2004;18:68–71

15 Sakurai M, Suleman M I, Morioka N, Akca O, Sessler D I. Minute sphere acupressure does not reduce postoperative pain or morphine consumption. Anesth Analg 2003;96:493–497

16 Samad K, Afshan G, Kamal R. Effect of acupressure on postoperative nausea and vomiting in laparoscopic cholecystectomy. J Pak Med Assoc 2003;53:68–72

17 Schultz A A, Andrews A L, Goran S F, Mathew T, Sturdevant N. Comparison of acupressure bands and droperidol for reducing post-operative nausea and vomiting in gynecologic surgery patients. Appl Nurs Res 2003;16:256–265

18 White P F, Hamza M A, Recart A, Coleman J E, Macaluso A R, Cox L, Jaffer O, Song D, Rohrich R. Optimal timing of acustimulation for antiemetic prophylaxis as an adjunct to ondansetron in patients undergoing plastic surgery. Anesth Analg 2005;100:367–372

19 Kim K S, Koo M S, Jeon J W, Park H S, Seung I S. Capsicum plaster at the Korean hand acupuncture point reduces postoperative nausea and vomiting after abdominal hysterectomy. Anesth Analg 2002;95:1103–1107

20 Klein J, Griffiths P. Acupressure for nausea and vomiting in cancer patients receiving chemotherapy. Br J Community Nurs 2004;9:383–388

21 Pearl M L, Fischer M, McCauley D L, Valea F A, Chalas E. Transcutaneous electrical nerve stimulation as an adjunct for controlling chemotherapy-induced nausea and vomiting in gynecologic oncology patients. Cancer Nurs 1999;22:307–311

22 Shen J, Wenger N, Glaspy J, Hays R D, Albert P S, Choi C, Shekelle P G. Electroacupuncture for control of myeloablative chemotherapy-induced emesis: A randomized controlled trial. JAMA 2000;284:2755–2761

23 Ozgur Tan M, Sandikci Z, Uygur M C, Arik A I, Erol D. Combination of transcutaneous electrical nerve stimulation and ondansetron in preventing cisplatin-induced emesis. Urol Int 2001;67:54–58

24 Streitberger K, Friedrich-Rust M, Bardenheuer H, Unnebrink K, Windeler J, Goldschmidt H, Egerer G. Effect of acupuncture compared with placebo-acupuncture at P6 as additional antiemetic prophylaxis in high-dose chemotherapy and autologous peripheral blood stem cell transplantation: a randomized controlled single-blind trial. Clin Cancer Res 2003l;9:2538–2544

25 Brown S, North D, Marvel M K, Fons R. Acupressure wrist bands to relieve nausea and vomiting in hospice patients: do they work? Am J Hospice Palliat Care 1992;9:26–29

26 Warwick-Evans L A, Masters I J, Redstone S B. A double-blind placebo controlled evaluation of acupressure in the treatment of motion sickness. Aviat Space Environ Med 1991;62:776–778

27 Hu S, Stritzel R, Chandler A, Stern R M. P6 acupressure reduces symptoms of vection-induced motion sickness. Aviat Space Environ Med 1995;66:631–634

28 Hu S, Stern R M, Koch K L. Electrical acustimulation relieves vection-induced motion sickness. Gastroenterology 1992;102:1854–1858

29 Stern R M, Jokerst M D, Muth E R, Hollis C. Acupressure relieves the symptoms of motion sickness and reduces abnormal gastric activity. Altern Ther Health Med 2001;7:91–94

30 Bertalanffy P, Hoerauf K, Fleischhackl R, Strasser H, Wicke F, Greher M, Gustorff B, Kober A. Korean hand acupressure for motion sickness in prehospital trauma care: a prospective, randomized, double-blinded trial in a geriatric population. Anesth Analg 2004;98:220–223

31 Lu D P, Lu G P, Reed J F 3rd. Acupuncture/acupressure to treat gagging dental patients: a clinical study of anti-gagging effects. Gen Dent 2000;48:446–452

32 Dent H E, Dewhurst N G, Mills S Y, Willoughby M. Continuous PC6 wristband acupressure for relief of nausea and vomiting associated with acute myocardial infarction: a partially randomised, placebo-controlled trial. Complement Ther Med 2003;11:72–77

33 Burish T G, Jenkins R A. Effectiveness of biofeedback and relaxation training in reducing the side effects of cancer chemotherapy. Health Psychol 1992;11:17–23

34 Jozsvai E E, Pigeau R A. The effect of autogenic training and biofeedback on motion sickness tolerance. Aviat Space Environ Med 1996;67:963–968

35 Taixiang W, Munro A, Guanjian L. Chinese medical herbs for chemotherapy side effects in colorectal cancer patients. Cochrane Database Syst Rev 2005; Issue 1. Art. No.: CD004540

36 Betz O, Kranke P, Geldner G, Wulf H, Eberhart L H. [Is ginger a clinically relevant antiemetic? A systematic review of randomized controlled trials] Forsch Komplementärmed Klass Naturheilkd 2005;12:14–23

37 Borrelli F, Capasso R, Aviello G, Pittler M H, Izzo A A. Effectiveness and safety of ginger in the treatment of pregnancy-induced nausea and vomiting. Obstet Gynecol 2005;105:849–856

38 Morin A M, Betz O, Kranke P, Geldner G, Wulf H, Eberhart L H. [Is ginger a relevant antiemetic for postoperative nausea and vomiting?] Anasthesiol Intensivmed Notfallmed Schmerzther 2004;39:281–285

39 Lien H C, Sun W M, Chen Y H, Kim H, Hasler W, Owyang C. Effects of ginger on motion sickness and gastric slow-wave dysrhythmias induced by circular vection. Am J Physiol Gastrointest Liver Physiol 2003;284:G481–489

40 Tate S. Peppermint oil: a treatment for postoperative nausea. J Adv Nurs 1997;26:543–549

41 Jacknow D S, Tschann J M, Link M P, Boyce W T. Hypnosis in the prevention of chemotherapy-related nausea and vomiting in children: a prospective study. J Develop Behav Ped 1994,15.258–264

42 Hawkins P J, Liossi C, Ewart B W, Hatira P, Kosmidis V H, Varvutsi M. Hypnotherapy for control of anticipatory nausea and vomiting in children with cancer: preliminary findings. Psycho-Oncology 1995;4:101–106

43 Zeltzer L K, Dolgin M J, LeBaron S, LeBaron C. A randomized, controlled study of behavioral intervention for chemotherapy distress in children with cancer. Pediatrics 1991;88:34–42

44 Syrjala K L, Cummings C, Donaldson G W. Hypnosis or cognitive behavioral training for the reduction of pain and nausea during cancer treatment: a controlled clinical trial. Pain 1992;48:137–146

45 Enqvist B, Bjorklund C, Engman M, Jakobsson J. Preoperative hypnosis reduces postoperative vomiting after surgery of the breasts. A prospective, randomized and blinded study. Acta Anaesthes Scand 1997;41:1028–1032

46 Ghoneim M M, Block R I, Sarasin D S, Davis C S, Marchman J N. Tape-recorded hypnosis instructions as adjuvant in the care of patients scheduled for third molar surgery. Anesth Analg 2000;90:64–68

47 Fellowes D, Barnes K, Wilkinson S. Aromatherapy and massage for symptom relief in patients with cancer. Cochrane Database Syst Rev 2004; Issue 2. Art. No.: CD002287

48 Post-White J, Kinney M E, Savik K, Gau J B, Wilcox C, Lerner I. Therapeutic massage and healing touch improve symptoms in cancer. Integr Cancer Ther 2003;2:332–344

49 Molassiotis A, Yung H P, Yam B M, Chan F Y, Mok T S. The effectiveness of progressive muscle relaxation training in managing chemotherapy-induced nausea and vomiting in Chinese breast cancer patients: a randomised controlled trial. Support Care Cancer 2002;10:237–246

50 Molassiotis A. A pilot study of the use of progressive muscle relaxation training in the management of post-chemotherapy nausea and vomiting. Eur J Cancer Care (Engl) 2000;9:230–234

51 Arakawa S. Relaxation to reduce nausea, vomiting, and anxiety induced by chemotherapy in Japanese patients. Cancer Nurs 1997;20:342–349

52 Arakawa S. Use of relaxation to reduce side effects of chemotherapy in Japanese patients. Cancer Nurs 1995;18:60–66

53 Syrjala K L, Donaldson G W, Davis M W, Kippes M E, Carr J E. Relaxation and imagery and cognitive-behavioral training reduce pain during cancer treatment: a controlled clinical trial. Pain 1995;63:189–198

54 Razavi D, Delvaux N, Farvacques C, De Brier F, Van Heer C, Kaufman L, Derde M P, Beauduin M, Piccart M. Prevention of adjustment disorders and anticipatory nausea secondary to adjuvant chemotherapy: a double-blind, placebo-controlled study assessing the usefulness of alprazolam. J Clin Oncol 1993;11:1384–1390

55 Vasterling J, Jenkins R A, Tope D M, Burish T G. Cognitive distraction and relaxation training for the control of side effects due to cancer chemotherapy. J Behav Med 1993;16:65–80

56 Lerman C, Rimer B, Blumberg B, Cristinzio S, Engstrom PF, MacElwee N, O'Connor K, Seay J. Effects of coping style and relaxation on cancer chemotherapy side effects and emotional responses. Cancer Nurs 1990;13:308–315

57 Carey M P, Burish T G. Providing relaxation training to cancer chemotherapy patients: A comparison of three delivery techniques. J Consult Clin Psychol 1987;55:732–737

58 Burish TG, Lyles JN. Effectiveness of relaxation training in reducing adverse

reactions to cancer chemotherapy. J Behav Med 1981;4:65–78

59 Burish T G, Tope D M. Psychological techniques for controlling the adverse side effects of cancer chemotherapy: findings from a decade of research. J Pain Symptom Manage 1992;7:287–301

60 Anderson L A, Gross J B. Aromatherapy with peppermint, isopropyl alcohol, or placebo is equally effective in relieving postoperative nausea. J Perianesth Nurs 2004;19:29–35

61 Roffe L, Schmidt K, Ernst E. A systematic review of guided imagery as an adjuvant cancer therapy. Psychooncology 2005;14:607–617

62 Ezzone S, Baker C, Rosselet R, Terepka E. Music as an adjunct to antiemetic therapy. Oncol Nurs Forum 1998;25:1551–1556

63 Nilsson U, Rawal N, Enqvist B, Unosson M. Analgesia following music and therapeutic suggestions in the PACU in ambulatory surgery; a randomized controlled trial. Acta Anaesthesiol Scand 2003;47:278–283

64 Nilsson U, Rawal N, Unestahl LE, Zetterberg C, Unosson M. Improved recovery after music and therapeutic suggestions during general anaesthesia: a double-blind randomised controlled trial. Acta Anaesthesiol Scand 2001;45:812–817

65 Ikonomidou E, Rehnstrom A, Naesh O. Effect of music on vital signs and postoperative pain. AORN J 2004;80:269–278

66 Laurion S, Fetzer SJ. The effect of two nursing interventions on the postoperative outcomes of gynecologic laparoscopic patients. J Perianesth Nurs 2003;18:254–261

NECK PAIN

Synonyms/ subcategories

Mechanical neck disorder.

Definition

Pain in the cervical region, with or without referral to the shoulder and arm. The symptom may arise from a broad range of conditions involving muscle, joint, disc, ligament or degenerative disorders. It may also occur with diffuse connective tissue diseases including rheumatoid arthritis, arthritis associated with spondylitis and a number of other systemic conditions. If symptoms persist for more than three months, the term chronic pain neck pain is used.

CAM usage

According to survey data from the USA,[1] 57% of people with neck pain used CAM in the previous 12 months, two-thirds visiting a practitioner. Manual therapies and acupuncture are commonly used.

Clinical evidence

Acupuncture
The results of a systematic review of RCTs (Box 2.89) do not provide evidence that it is superior to placebo.[2] Subsequent RCTs generated both positive[3-10] and negative results.[11] Other RCTs yielded ambiguous findings: acupuncture turned out to be less effective than spinal manipulation but superior to medication,[12] or acupuncture 'produced a statistically, but not clinically, significant effect compared with placebo'.[13]

Box 2.89
Systematic review
**Acupuncture for
neck pain**
White[2]

- Fourteen RCTs involving 724 subjects with neck pain from various causes

- Seven studies were of good quality

- Acupuncture was superior to waiting list (one study), either no different from or superior to physiotherapy (three studies) and no different from placebo acupuncture (four out of five studies)

- Conclusion: no evidence that acupuncture is superior to placebo

Exercise

Both endurance and strength training exercises[14] but not dynamic muscle training[15] have been shown to alleviate chronic neck pain in large RCTs.

Positive findings were confirmed in an RCT (n = 145) that compared exercise with infrared radiation plus advice. The exercise group was superior in terms of pain and disability both in the short term as well as at 6 months follow-up.[16]

Massage

Regarding the effectiveness of massage for neck pain the trial data are somewhat contradictory. The above-mentioned RCT (n = 177) did not seem to indicate that massage (used as a control intervention) was effective.[4] On the other hand, an RCT with 29 patients suffering from neck or back or shoulder pain showed that massage generated more pain relief at the 3-month follow-up than standard medical care.[17]

Spinal manipulation

A Cochrane Review (Box 2.90) found no strong evidence for spinal manipulation.[18] Systematic reviews authored by chiropractors (e.g.[19]) do, however, arrive at more optimistic conclusions.

Box 2.90
Systematic review
**Spinal
manipulation and
mobilisation for
neck pain**
Gross[18]

- Thirty-three RCTs were included

- 42% were of high methodological quality

- No benefit against placebo, or other treatments for acute, subacute or chronic pain

- Combined with exercise there was evidence of benefit

- Conclusion: the evidence did not favour mobilisation or manipulation done alone

A subsequent large RCT (n = 350) showed that adding manipulative therapy to an exercise regime was not followed by clinical improvements after the end of the 6 weeks intervention nor at 6 months' follow-up.[20]

Other therapies

Bitongxiao is a Chinese herbal decoction that was tested in a CCT (n = 102). The results suggest positive effects on pain.[21]

An RCT (n = 68) of **spiritual healing** for improvement of restricted neck movement found no pain relief through this intervention.[22]

Overall recommendation

The evidence for CAM is either ambiguous or not convincing. Therefore it cannot be recommended as a superior option for treating neck pain. Active physiotherapy is a recognised, effective conventional therapy for neck pain.

Table 2.59
Summary of clinical evidence for neck pain

Treatment	Weight of evidence	Direction of evidence	Serious safety concerns
Acupuncture	OOO	⇨	Yes (see p 294)
Exercise	OO	⬀	Yes (see p 5)
Massage	OO	⇨	No (see p 334)
Spinal manipulation	OOO	⬂	Yes (see p 316)

REFERENCES

1 Eisenberg D M, Davis R, Ettner S L, Appel S, Wilkey S, Rompay M V. Trends in alternative medicine use in the United States, 1990–1997. JAMA 1998;280:1569–1575

2 White A R, Ernst E. A systematic review of randomized controlled trials of acupuncture for neck pain. Rheumatol 1999;38:143–147

3 Heikkila H, Johansson M, Wenngren B I. Effects of acupuncture, cervical manipulation and NSAID therapy on dizziness and impaired head repositioning of suspected cervical origin: a pilot study. Man Ther 2000;5:151–157

4 Irnich D, Behrens N, Molzen H, Konig A, Gleditsch J, Krauss M, Natalis M, Senn E, Beyer A, Schops P. Randomised trial of acupuncture compared with conventional massage and 'sham' laser acupuncture for treatment of chronic neck pain. BMJ 2001;322:1574–1578

5 Seidel U, Uhlemann C. Behandlung der zervikalen Tendomyose. Dt Ztschr Akupunktur 2002;45:258–269

6 Irnich D, Behrens N, Gleditsch J M, Stor W, Schreiber M A, Schops P, Vickers A J, Beyer A. Immediate effects of dry needling and acupuncture at distant points in chronic neck pain: results of a randomized, double-blind, sham-controlled crossover trial. Pain 2002;99:83–89

7 Nabeta T, Kawakita K. Relief of chronic neck and shoulder pain by manual acupuncture to tender points – a sham-controlled randomized trial. Complement Ther Med 2002;10:217–222

8 Konig A, Radke S, Molzen H, Haase M, Muller C, Drezler D, Natalis M, Krauss M, Behrens N, Irnich D. [Randomised trial of acupuncture compared with conventional massage and 'sham' laser acupuncture for treatment of chronic neck pain – range of motion analysis. Z Orthop Ihre Grenzgeb 2003;141:395–400

9 Sator-Katzenschlager S M, Szeles J C, Scharbert G, Michalek-Sauberer A, Kober A, Heinze G, Kozek-Langenecker S A. Electrical stimulation of auricular acupuncture points is more effective than conventional manual auricular acupuncture in chronic cervical pain: a pilot study. Anesth Analg 2003;97:1469–1473

10 He D, Veierstad K B, Hostmark A T, Medbo J I. Effect of acupuncture treatment on chronic neck and shoulder pain in sedentary

female workers: a 6-month and 3-year follow-up study. Pain 2004;109:299–307

11 Zhu X M, Polus B. A controlled trial on acupuncture for chronic neck pain. Am J Chin Med 2002;30:13–28

12 Giles L G, Muller R. Chronic spinal pain: a randomized clinical trial comparing medication, acupuncture, and spinal manipulation. Spine 2003;28:1490–1502

13 White P, Lewith G, Prescott P, Conway J. Acupuncture versus placebo for the treatment of chronic mechanical neck pain: a randomized, controlled trial. Ann Intern Med 2004;141:911–919

14 Ylinen J, Takala EP, Nykanen M, Hakkinen A, Malkia E, Pohjolainen T, Karppi SL, Kautiainen H, Airaksinen O. Active neck muscle training in the treatment of chronic neck pain in women: a randomized controlled trial. JAMA 2003;289:2509–2516

15 Viljanen M, Malmivaara A, Utti J, Kinne M, Palmroos P, Laippala P. Effectiveness of dynamic muscle training, relaxation training, or ordinary activity for chronic neck pain: randomised controlled trial. BMJ 2003;327:475

16 Chiu T T, Lam T H, Hedley A J. A randomized controlled trial on the efficacy of exercise for patients with chronic neck pain. Spine 2005;30:E1–E7

17 Walach H, Guthlin C, Konig M. Efficacy of massage therapy in chronic pain: a pragmatic randomized trial. J Altern Complement Med 2003;9:837–846

18 Gross A R, Hoving J L, Haines T A, Goldsmith C H, Kay T, Aker P, Bronfort G; Cervical Overview Group. A Cochrane review of manipulation and mobilization for mechanical neck disorders. Spine 2004;29:1541–1548

19 Bronfort G, Haas M, Evans RL, Bouter LM. Efficacy of spinal manipulation and mobilization for low back pain and neck pain: a systematic review and best evidence synthesis. Spine J 2004;4:335–356

20 Dziedzic K, Hill J, Lewis M, Sim J, Daniels J, Hay E M. Effectiveness of manual therapy or pulsed shortwave diathermy in addition to advice and exercise for neck disorders: a pragmatic and randomized controlled trial in physical therapy clinics. Arthritis Rheum 2005;53:214–222

21 Li J X, Xiang C J, Liu X Q. [Clinical study on analgesic mechanism of bitongxiao in treating neck pain due to cervical spondylitis][Article in Chinese] Zhongguo Zhong Xi Yi Jie He Za Zhi 2001;2197:516–518

22 Gerard S, Smith B H, Simpson J A. A randomized controlled trial of spiritual healing in restricted neck movement. J Altern Complement Med 2003;9:467–477

NON-ULCER DYSPEPSIA

Synonyms   Indigestion.

Related conditions   Heartburn.

Definition   Dyspepsia is the term used to describe pain and discomfort in the upper abdomen or chest that can develop after a meal. Sometimes there is a burning feeling in the chest, which is known as heartburn. Most people have suffered from indigestion after a large meal at some time, and up to 20% of people suffer from heartburn at least once a week.

CAM usage   Herbal and non-herbal dietary supplements are popular for the relief of dyspepsia symptoms.

Clinical evidence   *Herbal medicine*
          A systematic review of all **herbal medicines** for treating non-ulcer dyspepsia suggested that, in particular peppermint and caraway have effects of similar or greater magnitude to conventional therapies and encouraging safety profiles (Box 2.91).[1]

Box 2.91
Systematic review
**Herbal medicines
for non-ulcer
dyspepsia**
Thompson Coon[1]

- Seventeen RCTs were identified

- Four trials were of monopreparations and involved turmeric (*Curcuma longa*), greater celandine (*Chelidonium majus*), banana (*Musa sapientum*) and *Emblica officinalis*

- Thirteen trials were of combination products, including nine in which peppermint (*Mentha piperitae*) and caraway (*Carum carvi*) were constituent ingredients

- Other herbal medicines assessed were Liu-Jun-Zi-Tang, Shenxiahewining, boldo (*Peumus boldus*), cascara (*Rhamnus purshianus*), gentian (*Gentiana lutea*) and rhubarb (*Rheum sp.*)

- There appear to be few adverse effects associated with these remedies, although, in many cases, comprehensive safety data were not available

- Conclusion: some herbal medicinal products identified, in particular peppermint and caraway, with effects of similar or greater magnitude to conventional therapies and encouraging safety profiles, undoubtedly warrant further investigation, especially in the light of the lack of efficacy of conventional therapies for non-ulcer dyspepsia

Since the publication of this review, an open RCT (n = 516) tested 320 or 640 mg **artichoke** (*Cynara scolymus*) leaf extract over a 2-month period. In both dosage groups there was a reduction of all dyspeptic symptoms compared with baseline. However, there were no differences between the two groups.[2] In a double-blind RCT, the overall change in dyspeptic symptoms was found to be greater with artichoke leaf extract than with the placebo.[3]

For **peppermint and caraway** as constituents in combination preparations the results of the above systematic review[1] were supported by an independent meta-analysis,[4] which relates to a specific proprietary product (Iberogast) and by a further double-blind RCT.[5]

Thirty patients were randomly allocated in a double-blind manner to **red pepper** powder or placebo for 5 weeks.[6] The overall symptom score and the epigastric pain, fullness and nausea scores of the red pepper group were lower than those of the placebo group.

Supplements
Non-ulcer dyspepsia patients (n = 199), with a normal upper endoscopy and a positive (13)C-urea breath test were randomly assigned to either pantoprazole, clarithromycin and metronidazole (PCM) or pantoprazole, clarithromycin and **fish oil** (PCF) for 7 days.[7] In an intention-to-treat analysis, PCM eradicated infection in 78% but PCF in only 34%. It was concluded that fish oil is unlikely to be useful in *Helicobacter pylori* eradication regimens.

Other therapies

In a pilot RCT 60 patients who were receiving conventional treatment chose between **acupuncture** and **homeopathy** and were then allocated to this preference or conventional GP care.[8] At the end of the 6-month intervention period there was no difference or trend between the groups for clinical outcome or costs.

Overall recommendation

There is evidence to suggest that the combination of peppermint and caraway is more effective than placebo and possibly similarly effective as conventional medicines for treating non-ulcer dyspepsia. Another intervention with encouraging data is artichoke but further data from rigorous trials are required. All other interventions are not supported by reasonably conclusive evidence.

CONDITIONS

Table 2.60
Summary of clinical evidence for non-ulcer dyspepsia

Treatment	Weight of evidence	Direction of evidence	Serious safety concerns
Herbal medicine			
Artichoke	OO	⇧	Yes (see p 368)
Chinese herbal medicine	O	⇗	Yes (see p 5)
Peppermint and caraway	OOO	⇧	Yes (see p 448)
Red pepper	O	⇧	Yes (see p 480)
Turmeric	O	⇧	Yes (see p 481)
Supplements			
Fish oil	O	⇩	Yes (see p 483)

REFERENCES

1 Thompson Coon J, Ernst E. Systematic review: herbal medicinal products for non-ulcer dyspepsia. Aliment Pharmacol Ther 2002;16:1689–1699

2 Marakis G, Walker AF, Middleton RW, Booth JC, Wright J, Pike DJ. Artichoke leaf extract reduces mild dyspepsia in an open study. Phytomedicine 2002;9:694–699

3 Holtmann G, Adam B, Haag S, Collet W, Grunewald E, Windeck T. Efficacy of artichoke leaf extract in the treatment of patients with functional dyspepsia: a six-week placebo-controlled, double-blind, multicentre trial. Aliment Pharmacol Ther 2003;18:1099–1105

4 Gundermann KJ, Godehardt E, Ulbrich M. Efficacy of a herbal preparation in patients with functional dyspepsia: a meta-analysis of double-blind, randomized, clinical trials. Adv Ther 2003;20:43–49

5 Madisch A, Holtmann G, Mayr G, Vinson B, Hotz J. Treatment of functional dyspepsia with a herbal preparation. A double-blind, randomized, placebo-controlled, multicenter trial. Digestion 2004;69:45–52

6 Bortolotti M, Coccia G, Grossi G, Miglioli M. The treatment of functional dyspepsia with red pepper. Aliment Pharmacol Ther 2002;16:1075–1082

7 Meier R, Wettstein A, Drewe J, Geiser H R; Swiss Helicobacter-Study Group. Fish oil (Eicosapen) is less effective than metronidazole, in combination with pantoprazole and clarithromycin, for Helicobacter pylori eradication. Aliment Pharmacol Ther 2001;15:851–855

8 Paterson C, Ewings P, Brazier JE, Britten N. Treating dyspepsia with acupuncture and homeopathy: reflections on a pilot study by researchers, practitioners and participants. Complement Ther Med 2003;11:78–84

CONDITIONS

OSTEOARTHRITIS

Synonyms/subcategories

Degenerative arthritis, degenerative arthrosis, degenerative joint disease, hypertrophic arthritis, osteoarthrosis, gonarthrosis, coxarthrosis.

Definition

Osteoarthritis is a heterogeneous condition for which the prevalence, risk factors, clinical manifestations, and prognosis vary according to the joints affected. It most commonly affects hands, knees, hips, and spinal apophyseal joints. It is usually defined by pathological or radiological criteria rather than clinical features, and is characterised by focal areas of damage to the cartilage surfaces of synovial joints, associated with remodeling of the underlying bone and mild synovitis. When severe, there is characteristic joint space narrowing and osteophyte formation, with visible subchondral bone changes on radiography.

CAM usage

In a US survey, 27% of people who described themselves as suffering from 'arthritis' had used CAM in the previous 12 months,[1] a third of them seeing a therapist. Acupuncture, massage, manipulation and homeopathy are the therapies most commonly used.

Clinical evidence

Acupuncture

Acupuncture is widely used for treating the pain of osteoarthritis (OA). A systematic review identified evidence of acupuncture for OA of the knee (Box 2.92).[2] In seven RCTs acupuncture was compared with sham treatments or active therapies or no treatment. The evidence suggested that acupuncture is more effective than sham treatment in alleviating pain. Further evidence from RCTs supports these findings[3–5] and suggests an improvement in function. There is limited evidence that acupuncture is better than conventional treatment. These findings are supported by

Box 2.92
Systematic review
Acupuncture for osteoarthritis
Ezzo[2]

- Seven RCTs or quasi RCTs assessing 393 patients with OA of the knee

- For pain there was strong evidence that real acupuncture is more effective than sham

- For pain and function there was limited evidence of effectiveness

- For function there was inconclusive evidence that real acupuncture is more effective than sham.

- Conclusion: the existing evidence suggests that acupuncture may play a role in OA

systematic reviews assessing CAM therapies for arthritis-related pain[6] and musculoskeletal pain.[7,8]

Balneotherapy

Balneotherapy or spa therapy is used to treat osteoarthritis particularly in European countries. A Cochrane review[9] assessed the evidence and concluded that, although one cannot ignore the positive findings in most trials, due to methodological flaws, firm statements about the efficacy of balneotherapy cannot be provided at present. This corroborated the findings of an earlier systematic review.[10] Additional RCTs suggest beneficial effects of a balneotherapeutic regimen for the Lequesne index,[11] mud compresses for knee pain and the Lequesne index[12] and a hydrotherapy-based strengthening programme for leg strength and distance walked.[13]

Herbal medicine

A Cochrane review assessed all placebo-controlled RCTs of herbal treatments for osteoarthritis.[14] Five trials of four different herbal interventions were identified. The data of the two studies testing **avocado/soybean** unsaponifiables were pooled and provided some positive evidence (Box 2.93). Another systematic review identified four double-blind, placebo-controlled RCTs of avocado/soybean unsaponifiables.[15] It concluded that the clinical evidence is, at present, not fully convincing.

A systematic review assessed the effects of **devil's claw** (*Harpagophytum procumbens*).[16] It included all RCTs, quasi RCTs and CCTs. It concluded that there is limited evidence for an ethanolic extract containing < 30 mg harpagoside per day in the treatment of knee and hip osteoarthritis. There is moderate evidence of effectiveness for the use of a devil's claw powder at 60 mg harpagoside in the treatment of osteoarthritis of the knee, hip and spine.

Box 2.93
Systematic review
Herbal therapy for osteoarthritis
Little[14]

- Five RCTs of four different herbal treatments were identified

- Two studies compared the effects of avocado/soybean unsaponifiables to placebo including 327 patients

- Both studies used 100 mm VAS scales for measuring pain. The weighted mean difference was −7.6, 95% CI −11.8 to −3.4)

- For the Lequesne's functional index the weighted mean difference was −1.7, 95% CI −2.4 to −1.0

- Conclusion: The current evidence for herbal treatment of osteoarthritis is generally sparse and therefore insufficient for a reliable assessment of efficacy

CONDITIONS

A systematic review assessed all RCTs of **ginger** (*Zingiber officinalis*).[17] It identified one double-blind RCT (n = 56), which reported no difference compared with placebo for pain and Lequesne index. A large (n = 247) double-blind RCT found a reduction in pain for the percentage of responders,[18] and another double-blind RCT reported that a ginger extract was as effective as placebo during the first 3 months of the study, but at the end of 6 months the ginger extract group showed a superiority over the placebo group.[19]

The efficacy of **Phytodolor** (a proprietary preparation which contains *Populus tremula*, *Fraxinus excelsior* and *Solidago virgaurea*) in painful arthritic conditions has been assessed in a number of studies. A systematic review identified at least six double-blind RCTs including 322 patients with osteoarthritis.[19] These trials suggest pain reduction, increase in mobility and a reduction of NSAID consumption.

SKI 306X is a purified extract from a mixture of three herbs (*Clematis mandshurica*, *Trichosanthes kirilowii* and *Prunella vulgaris*). It was tested in patients with osteoarthritis of the knee and was found to be superior to placebo for pain VAS and Lequesne index.[20] In a comparative trial against 300 mg diclofenac daily, the preparation showed similar effects for pain VAS.[21]

RCTs, which require further independent replication exist for **willow bark**,[22] **Reumalex** (combination of willow bark, guaiacum resin, black cohosh, sarsaparilla and poplar bark),[23] **Tipi**,[24] a mixture of *Withania somnifera*, *Boswellia serrata* and turmeric, a **herbomineral formulation**[25] and **Gitadyl** (containing feverfew, American aspen and milfoil).[26] Additional single RCTs are available for **Eazmov** (an Ayurvedic herbal preparation),[27] **stinging nettle**,[28] *Boswellia serrata*,[29] **Hyben Vital** (preparation of a subspecies of *Rosa* canina fruits)[30] and **Duhuo Jisheng Wan**.[31]

Homeopathy

A systematic review (Box 2.94) identified four trials of either oral or topically applied homeopathy, which were encouraging but insufficient to draw any conclusions for clinical practice.[32]

Box 2.94
Systematic review
Homeopathy for osteoarthritis
Long[32]

- Four RCTs involving 406 patients with OA

- All trials of high quality

- Two positive and one negative comparison with conventional oral drugs

- Topical homeopathic gel no different effect from conventional non-steroidal gel

Magnets

Static magnets and electromagnetic fields are used to treat the symptoms of osteoarthritis. A Cochrane review assessed the evidence and found limited evidence (Box 2.95).[33] Further trials published since this review are available, which suggest some effects,[34-36] but also those which did not find a specific effect.[37,38]

Box 2.95
Systematic review
Magnetic fields for osteoarthritis
Hulme[33]

- Three RCTs including a total of 259 patients

- For pain relief the meta-analysis of two trials showed a standardised mean difference of −0.74, 95% CI −1.15 to −0.34.

- Joint pain on motion improved (standardised mean difference −0.59, 95% CI −0.98 to −2.0)

- Conclusion: There is a need to confirm in larger trials whether the positive results confer clinically important benefits. The current limited evidence does not show a clinically important benefit for treating knee or cervical osteoarthritis

Supplements

A systematic review assessed all RCTs of **capsaicin cream** (0.025% to 0.075%).[19] It identified three double-blind RCTs (n = 135), which show beneficial effects on pain and articular tenderness. The meta-analysis of these data showed that it was better than placebo for treating OA (OR 4.4, 95% CI 2.8 to 6.9).

Chondroitin sulfate (Box 2.96)[39] and **glucosamine** (Box 2.97)[40] appear to be effective in OA and to have fewer adverse effects than NSAIDs. A meta-analysis[41] has looked at similar data for both supplements and concluded that, although the effect sizes seen in the published studies are likely to be exaggerated by publication bias and quality issues, some degree of effectiveness appears probable for both preparations. A comprehensive meta-analysis suggested structural effectiveness for glucosamine and symptomatic effectiveness for glucosamine and chondroitin in knee osteoarthritis,[42] which is also supported for long-term treatment.[43] Further RCTs support this conclusion[44,45] although negative trials are also available.[46,47] Whether these supplements prevent further cartilage loss in patients is as yet not entirely clear.[48,49]

Green-lipped mussel (*Perna canaliculus*) was investigated in a double-blind controlled trial which included 28 rheumatoid and 38 OA patients, on a waiting list for joint surgery.[50] Full results are not given but 38% of those who received mussel improved compared with 14% of the placebo group. A further study by the same group[51] compared different preparations of the mussel, again including patients with either rheumatoid or osteoarthritis. There were improvements in various outcomes in

Box 2.96
Meta-analysis
Chondroitin sulfate for osteoarthritis
Leeb[39]

- Seven studies (372 patients) with duration of > 3 months included

- Pain scores decreased progressively to 42% over the first 6 months of therapy (compared with 80% in placebo). Increased dosage did not result in better effectiveness

- Required daily dose of analgesic and NSAID medications was reduced

- Conclusion: evidence of clinically relevant efficacy of chondroitin sulfate on pain and function of knee and hip OA, at least when given as an adjunct to standard analgesic and NSAID medications

Box 2.97
Meta-analysis
Glucosamine for osteoarthritis
Towheed[40]

- Twenty RCTs (n = 2570) included

- Analysis restricted to eight studies with adequate allocation concealment failed to show benefit of glucosamine for pain and WOMAC function.

- Analysis of 10 RCTs testing the Rotta brand of glucosamine showed superiority for pain (SMD −1.31, 95% CI −1.99 to −0.64) and function using the Lequesne index (SMD −0.51, 95% CI −0.96 to −0.05) compared with placebo

- Comparing the Rotta brand of glucosamine with an NSAID: results were superior in two, and equivalent in two RCTs

- Glucosamine was as safe as placebo in terms of the number of subjects reporting adverse reactions

- Conclusion: Results from studies using a non-Rotta preparation or adequate allocation concealment failed to show benefit in pain and WOMAC function while those studies evaluating the Rotta preparation show that glucosamine was superior to placebo in the treatment of pain and functional impairment resulting from symptomatic OA

both groups. The evidence that green-lipped mussel has any effect in OA is suggestive but not convincing.

The effectiveness of **s-adenosylmethionine** was assessed in a meta-analysis (Box 2.98).[52] There were beneficial effects when compared with placebo and it appears to be effective in reducing pain and in improving functional limitations.

Box 2.98
Meta-analysis
**S-adenosyl-
methionine for
osteoarthritis**
Soeken[52]

- Eleven RCTs met the inclusion criteria

- When compared with placebo, S-adenosylmethionine is more effective in reducing functional limitation in patients with osteoarthritis (effect size 0.31, 95% CI 0.1 to 0.5)

- No effect for reducing pain (effect size 0.22; 95% CI −0.25 to 0.7) compared with placebo

- Compared with NSAIDs (pain: effect size 0.12, 95% CI −0.03 to 0.3; functional limitation: effect size 0.03; 95% CI, −0.13 to 0.18)

- Conclusion: S-adenosylmethionine appears to be as effective as NSAIDs in reducing pain and improving functional limitation in patients with OA without the adverse effects often associated with NSAID therapies

CONDITIONS

Further RCTs, which require independent replication exist for vitamin E,[53] soy,[54] a milk-based micronutrient beverage[55] and Arthritis Relief Plus (also containing capsaicin 0.015%).[56]

Tai chi

Similar to physical exercise tai chi may be beneficial through maintaining balance and strength and through reducing the risk of falls. Two RCTs report less pain and stiffness in joints and fewer difficulties in physical functioning[57] as well as improved self-efficacy for arthritis symptoms.[58] Further trials are required for any recommendation.

Other therapies

Other RCTs, which require replication in independent trials exist for leech therapy,[59] music,[60] yoga,[61] imagery[62] and therapeutic touch.[63] Despite its use in OA no RCTs are available for dietary changes, massage, manipulation and relaxation and other mind-body approaches.

**Overall
recommendation** There is evidence to suggest that acupuncture is effective for pain control. Whether it is superior to conventional treatment is unclear. Other interventions with good evidence of effectiveness are the supplements chondroitin, glucosamine, s-adenosylmethionine and the herbal mixture phytodolor. Considering the favourable safety profile, tai chi seems to be an option worthy of consideration. For all other interventions more evidence is needed before firm recommendations can be made.

CONDITIONS

Table 2.61
Summary of clinical evidence for osteoarthritis

Treatment	Weight of evidence	Direction of evidence	Serious safety concerns
Acupuncture	OOO	⇧	Yes (see p 294)
Balneotherapy	OO	⬀	Yes (see p 5)
Herbal medicine			
Avocado/soybean unsaponifiables	OO	⬀	Yes (see p 370)
Boswellia serrata	O	⇧	Yes (see p 479)
Devil's claw	OO	⬀	Yes (see p 389)
Duhuo Jisheng Wan	O	⇧	Yes (see p 5)
Eazmov	O	↘	Yes (see p 5)
Ginger	OO	⬀	Yes (see p 401)
Gitadyl	O	⇧	Yes (see p 5)
Herbomineral formulation	O	⬀	Yes (see p 5)
Hyben Vital	O	⬀	Yes (see p 5)
Phytodolor	OOO	⇧	Yes (see p 5)
Reumalex	O	⬀	Yes (see p 5)
SKI 306X	OO	⇧	Yes (see p 5)
Stinging nettle	O	⇧	Yes (see p 444)
Tipi	O	⇩	Yes (see p 5)
Willow bark	O	⇧	Yes (see p 472)
Homeopathy	O	⬀	No (see p 327)
Magnets	OO	⬀	No (see p 359)
Supplements			
Arthritis relief plus	O	⇧	Yes (see p 5)
Capsaicin	OO	⇧	Yes (see p 5)
Chondroitin	OOO	⇧	Yes (see p 382)
Glucosamine	OOO	⇧	Yes (see p 412)
Green-lipped mussel	O	⬀	Yes (see p 483)
Micronutrient beverage	O	⇧	Yes (see p 5)
S-adenosylmethionine	OOO	⇧	Yes (see p 484)
Soy	O	⬀	Yes (see p 450)
Vitamin E	O	⇩	Yes (see p 5)
Tai chi	OO	⇧	No (see p 354)

REFERENCES

1   Eisenberg D M, Davis R, Ettner S L, Appel S, Wilkey S, Rompay M V. Trends in alternative medicine use in the United States, 1990–1997. JAMA 1998;280:1569–1575

2   Ezzo J, Hadhazy V, Birch S, Lao L, Kaplan G, Hochberg M, Berman B. Acupuncture for osteoarthritis of the knee: a systematic review. Arthritis Rheum 2001;44:819–825

3   Berman B M, Lao L, Langenberg P, Lee W L, Gilpin A M, Hochberg M C. Effectiveness of acupuncture as adjunctive therapy in osteoarthritis of the knee: a randomised, controlled trial. Ann Intern Med 2004;141:901–910

4   Vas J, Mendez C, Perea-Milla F, Vega E, Panadero M D, Leon J M, Borge M A, Gaspar O, Sanchez-Rodriguez F, Aguilar I, Jurado R. Acupuncture as a complementary therapy to the pharmacological treatment of osteoarthritis of the knee: randomised controlled trial. BMJ 2004;329:1216

5   Tukmachi E, Jubb R, Dempsey E, Jones P. The effect of acupuncture on the symptoms of knee osteoarthritis – an open randomised controlled study. Acupunct Med 2004;22:14–22

6   Soeken K L. Selected CAM therapies for arthritis-related pain: the evidence from systematic reviews. Clin J Pain 2004;20:13–18

7   Ernst E. Musculoskeletal conditions and complementary/alternative medicine. Best Pract Res Clin Rheumatol 2004;18:539–556

8   Welner D K, Ernst E. Complementary and alternative approaches to the treatment of persistent musculoskeletal pain. Clin J Pain 2004;20:244–255

9   Verhagen A P, de Vet H C, de Bie R A, Kessels A G, Boers M, Knipschild P G. Balneotherapy for rheumatoid arthritis and osteoarthritis. The Cochrane Database of Systematic Reviews 2000, Issue 2. Art. No.:CD000518

10 Ernst E, Pittler M H. How effective is spa treatment? A systematic review of randomized studies. Dtsch Med Wochenschr 1998;123:273–277

11 Sukenik S, Flusser D, Codish S, Abu-Shakra M. Balneotherapy at the Dead Sea area for knee osteoarthritis. Isr Med Assoc J 1999;1:83–85

12 Flusser D, Abu Shakra M, Friger M et al. Therapy with mud compresses for knee osteoarthritis. Comparison of natural mud preparations with mineral-depleted mud. J Clin Rheumatol 2002;8:197–203

13 Foley A, Halbert J, Hewitt T, Crotty M. Does hydrotherapy improve strength and physical function in patients with osteoarthritis – a randomised controlled trial comparing a gym based and a hydrotherapy based strengthening programme. Ann Rheum Dis 2003;62: 1162–1167

14 Little C V, Parsons T, Logan S. Herbal therapy for treating osteoarthritis. The Cochrane Database of Systematic Reviews 2000, Issue 4. Art. No.: CD002947

15 Ernst E. Avocado-soybean unsaponifiables (ASU) for osteoarthritis – a systematic review. Clin Rheumatol 2003;22:285–288

16 Gagnier J J, Chrubasik S, Manheimer E. Harpgophytum procumbens for osteoarthritis and low back pain: a systematic review. BMC Complement Altern Med 2004;4:13

17 Long L, Soeken K, Ernst E. Herbal medicines for the treatment of osteoarthritis: a systematic review. Rheumatology 2001;40:779–793

18 Altman R D, Marcussen K C. Effects of a ginger extract on knee pain in patients with osteoarthritis. Arthritis Rheum 2001;44:2531–2538

19 Wigler I, Grotto I, Caspi D, Yaron M. The effects of Zintona EC (a ginger extract) on symptomatic gonarthritis. Osteoarthritis Cartilage 2003;11:783–789

20 Jung Y B, Roh K J, Jung J A, Jung K, Yoo H, Cho Y B, Kwak W J, Kim D K, Kim K H, Han C K. Effect of SKI 306X, a new herbal anti-arthritic agent, in patients with osteoarthritis of the knee: a double-blind placebo controlled study. Am J Chin Med 2001;29:485–491

21 Jung Y B, Seong S C, Lee M C, Shin Y U, Kim D H, Kim J M, Jung Y K, Ahn J H, Seo J G, Park Y S, Lee C S, Roh K J, Han C K, Cho Y B, Chang D Y, Kwak W J, Jung K O, Park B J. A four-week, randomized, double-blind trial of the efficacy and safety of SKI306X: a herbal anti-arthritic agent versus diclofenac in osteoarthritis of the knee. Am J Chin Med 2004;32:291–301

22 Biegert C, Wagner I, Ludtke R, Kotter I, Lohmuller C, Gunaydin I, Taxis K, Heide L. Efficacy and safety of willow bark extract in the treatment of osteoarthritis and rheumatoid arthritis: results of 2 randomized double-blind controlled trials. J Rheumatol 2004;31:2121–2130

23 Mills S Y, Jacoby R K, Chacksfield M, Willoughby M. Effect of a proprietary herbal medicine on the relief of chronic arthritic pain: a double-blind study. Br J Rheumatol 1996;35: 874–878

24 Bosi Ferraz M, Borges Pereira R, Iwata N M, Atra E. Tipi. A popular analgesic tea:

a double-blind cross-over trial in arthritis. Clin Exper Rheumatol 1991;9:205–212

25 Kulkarni R R, Patki P S, Jog V P, Gandage S G, Patwardhan B. Treatment of osteoarthritis with a herbomineral formulation: a double-blind, placebo-controlled, cross-over study. J Ethnopharmacol 1991;33:91–95

26 Ryttig K, Schlamowitz P V, Warnoe O, Wilstrup F. Gitadyl versus ibuprofen in patients with osteoarthrosis. The result of a double-blind, randomized cross-over study. Ugeskrift for Laeger 1991;153:2298–2299

27 Biswas N R, Biswas K, Pandey M, Pandy R M. Treatment of osteoarthritis, rheumatoid arthritis and non-specific arthritis with a herbal drug: A double-blind, active drug controlled parallel study. JK Pract 1998;5:129–132

28 Randall C, Randall H, Dobbs F, Hutton C, Sanders H. Randomized controlled trial of nettle sting for treatment of base-of-thumb pain. J R Soc Med 2000;93:305–309

29 Kimmatkar N, Thawani V, Hingorani L, Khiyani R. Efficacy and tolerability of Boswellia serrata extract in treatment of osteoarthritis of knee – a randomized double blind placebo controlled trial. Phytomedicine 2003;10:3–7

30 Rein E, Kharazmi A, Winther K. A herbal remedy, Hyben Vital (stand. powder of a subspecies of Rosa canina fruits), reduces pain and improves general wellbeing in patients with osteoarthritis–a double-blind, placebo-controlled, randomised trial. Phytomedicine 2004;11:383–391

31 Teekachunhatean S, Kunanusorn P, Rojanasthien N, Sananpanich K, Pojchamarnwiputh S, Lhieochaiphunt S, Pruksakorn S. Chinese herbal recipe versus diclofenac in symptomatic treatment of osteoarthritis of the knee: a randomized controlled trial. BMC Complement Altern Med 2004;4:19

32 Long L, Ernst E. Homeopathic remedies for the treatment of osteoarthritis: a systematic review. Br Homeopath J 2001;90:37–43

33 Hulme J M, Judd M G, Robinson V A, Tugwell P, Wells G, de Bie R A. Electromagnetic fields for the treatment of osteoarthritis. The Cochrane Database of Systematic Reviews 2002, Issue 1. Art. No.: CD003523

34 Battisti E, Piazza E, Rigato M, Nuti R, Bianciardi L, Scribano A, Giordano N. Efficacy and safety of a musically modulated electromagnetic field (TAMMEF) in patients affected by knee osteoarthritis. Clin Exp Rheumatol 2004;22:568–572

35 Nicolakis P, Kollmitzer J, Crevenna R, Bittner C, Erdogmus CB, Nicolakis J. Pulsed magnetic field therapy for osteoarthritis of the knee – a double-blind sham-controlled trial. Wien Klin Wochenschr 2002;114:678–684

36 Hinman M R, Ford J, Heyl H. Effects of static magnets on chronic knee pain and physical function: a double-blind study. Altern Ther Health Med 2002;8:50–55

37 Harlow T, Greaves C, White A, Brown L, Hart A, Ernst E. Randomised controlled trial of magnetic bracelets for relieving pain in osteoarthritis of the hip and knee. BMJ 2004;329:1450–1454

38 Wolsko P M, Eisenberg D M, Simon L S, Davis R B, Walleczek J, Mayo-Smith M, Kaptchuk T J, Phillips R S. Double-blind placebo-controlled trial of static magnets for the treatment of osteoarthritis of the knee: results of a pilot study. Altern Ther Health Med 2004;10:36–43

39 Leeb B F, Schweitzer H, Montag K, Smolen J S. A metaanalysis of chondroitin sulfate in the treatment of osteoarthritis. J Rheumatol 2000;27:205–211

40 Towheed T E, Anastassiades T P, Shea B, Houpt J, Welch V, Hochberg M C. Glucosamine therapy for treating osteoarthritis. The Cochrane Database of Systematic Reviews 2000, Issue 2. Art. No.: CD002946

41 McAlindon T E, LaValley M P, Gulin J P, Felson D T. Glucosamine and chondroitin for treatment of osteoarthritis. JAMA 2005;283:1469–1475

42 Richy F, Bruyere O, Ethgen O, Cucherat M, Henrotin Y, Reginster JY. Structural and symptomatic efficacy of glucosamine and chondroitin in knee osteoarthritis: a comprehensive meta-analysis. Arch Intern Med 2003;163:1514–1522

43 Poolsup N, Suthisisang C, Channark P, Kittikulsuth W. Glucosamine long-term treatment and the progression of knee osteoarthritis: systematic review of randomized controlled trials. Ann Pharmacother 2005;39:1080–1087

44 Uebelhart D, Malaise M, Marcolongo R, DeVathaire F, Piperno M, Mailleux E, Fioravanti A, Matoso L, Vignon-E. Intermittent treatment of knee osteoarthritis with oral chondroitin sulfate: a one-year, randomized, double-blind, multicenter study versus placebo. Osteoarthritis Cartilage 2004;12:269–276

45 Cohen M, Wolfe R, Mai T, Lewis D. A randomized, double blind, placebo controlled

trial of a topical cream containing glucosamine sulfate, chondroitin sulfate, and camphor for osteoarthritis of the knee. J Rheumatol 2003;30:523–528. Erratum in: J Rheumatol 2003;30:2512

46 Cibere J, Kopec J A, Thorne A, Singer J, Canvin J, Robinson D B, Pope J, Hong P, Grant E, Esdaile J M. Randomized, double-blind, placebo-controlled glucosamine discontinuation trial in knee osteoarthritis. Arthritis Rheum 2004;51:738–745

47 McAlindon T, Formica M, LaValley M, Lehmer M, Kabbara K. Effectiveness of glucosamine for symptoms of knee osteoarthritis: results from an internet-based randomized double-blind controlled trial. Am J Med 2004;117:643–649

48 Cibere J, Thorne A, Kopec J A, Singer J, Canvin J, Robinson D B, Pope J, Hong P, Grant E, Lobanok T, Ionescu M, Poole A R, Esdaile J M. Glucosamine sulfate and cartilage type II collagen degradation in patients with knee osteoarthritis: randomized discontinuation trial results employing biomarkers. J Rheumatol 2005;32:896–902

49 Michel B A, Stucki G, Frey D, De Vathaire F, Vignon-E, Bruehlmann P, Uebelhart D. Chondroitins 4 and 6 sulfate in osteoarthritis of the knee: a randomized, controlled trial. Arthritis Rheum 2005;52:779–786

50 Gibson R G, Gibson S L M, Conway V, Chappell D. Perna canaliculus in the treatment of arthritis. Practitioner 1980;224:955–960

51 Gibson S L M, Gibson R G. The treatment of arthritis with a lipid extract of Perna canaliculus: a randomised trial. Complement Ther Med 1998;6:122–126

52 Soeken K L, Lee W L, Bausell R B, Agelli M, Berman B M. Safety and efficacy of S-adenosylmethionine (SAMe) for osteoarthritis. J Fam Pract 2002;51:425–430

53 Wluka A E, Stuckey S, Brand C, Cicuttini F M. Supplementary vitamin E does not affect the loss of cartilage volume in knee osteoarthritis: a 2 year double blind randomized placebo controlled study. J Rheumatol 2002;29:2585–2591

54 Arjmandi B H, Khalil D A, Lucas E A, Smith B J, Sinichi N, Hodges S B, Juma S, Munson M E, Payton M E, Tivis R D, Svanborg A. Soy protein may alleviate osteoarthritis symptoms. Phytomedicine 2004;11:567–575

55 Colker C M, Swain M, Lynch L, Gingerich D A. Effects of a milk-based bioactive micronutrient beverage on pain symptoms and activity of adults with osteoarthritis: a double-blind, placebo-controlled clinical evaluation. Nutrition 2002;18:388–392

56 Gemmell H A, Jacobson B H, Hayes B M. Effect of a topical herbal cream on osteoarthritis of the hand and knee: a pilot study. J Manipulative Physiol Ther 2003;26:e15

57 Song R, Lee E O, Lam P, Bae SC. Effects of tai chi exercise on pain, balance, muscle strength, and perceived difficulties in physical functioning in older women with osteoarthritis: a randomized clinical trial. J Rheumatol 2003;30:2039–2044

58 Hartman C A, Manos T M, Winter C, Hartman D M, Li B, Smith J C. Effects of T'ai Chi training on function and quality of life indicators in older adults with osteoarthritis. J Am Geriatr Soc 2000;48:1553–1559

59 Michalsen A, Klotz S, Lüdtke R, Moebus S, Spahn G, Dobos G J. Effectiveness of leech therapy in osteoarthritis of the knee: a randomized, controlled trial. Ann Intern Med 2003;139:724–730

60 McCaffrey R, Freeman E. Effect of music on chronic osteoarthritis pain in older people. J Adv Nurs 2003;44:517–524

61 Garfinkel M S, Schumacher H R, Husain A, Levy M, Reshetar R A. Evaluation of a yoga based regimen for treatment of osteoarthritis of the hands. J Rheumatol 1994;21:2341–2343

62 Baird C L, Sands L. A pilot study of the effectiveness of guided imagery with progressive muscle relaxation to reduce chronic pain and mobility difficulties of osteoarthritis. Pain Manag Nurs 2004;5:97–104

63 Eckes Peck S D. The effectiveness of therapeutic touch for decreasing pain in elders with degenerative arthritis. J Holistic Nurs 1997;15:176–198

CONDITIONS

OVERWEIGHT/OBESITY

Synonyms Corpulence, corpulency.

Definition Obesity is a chronic condition characterised by an excess of body fat. It is most often defined by the body mass index (BMI), a mathematical formula that is highly correlated with body fat. BMI is weight in kilograms divided by height in metres squared (kg/m^2). Worldwide, adults with BMIs between 25–30 kg/m^2 are categorised as overweight, and those with BMIs above 30 kg/m^2 are categorised as obese.

CAM usage Complementary therapies commonly used by those attempting to lose weight include acupuncture, dietary supplements and herbal medicine.

Clinical evidence

Acupuncture/acupressure

A systematic review assessed all RCTs and systematic reviews and meta-analyses which were based on the findings of RCTs (Box 2.99).[1] Four sham controlled RCTs, including one trial which assessed an acupressure device, were identified from a previous systematic review. Two of the trials report a reduction in hunger, while two others suggest that there were no differences for body weight compared with sham acupuncture. Three additional RCTs were identified. Overall, the evidence is not convincing that acupuncture or acupressure are effective for reducing body weight.[1] This conclusion is corroborated by another review.[2]

Box 2.99
Systematic review
Acupuncture for reducing body weight
Pittler[1]

- One systematic review of four sham-controlled RCTs including 270 subjects

- Heterogeneous in terms of treatment modality and design

- Two trials assessed hunger (positive) and body weight (negative) as the primary endpoint

- Three additional RCTs reported mixed results

- Conclusion: There is no convincing evidence that acupuncture is effective for reducing body weight

Herbal medicine

A systematic review assessed the evidence for *Citrus aurantium*.[3] One eligible randomised placebo-controlled trial, which followed 20 patients for 6 weeks, demonstrated no benefit for weight loss.

The most rigorous review of *Ephedra sinica* to date assessed studies with at least 8 weeks of follow-up and concluded that *E. sinica* and ephedrine promote a small short-term weight loss of about 0.9 kg per month more than placebo (Box 2.100).[4] This is supported by additional evidence from RCTs.[5,6] However, the intake is associated with an increased risk of psychiatric, autonomic or gastrointestinal symptoms and heart palpitations.

Box 2.100
Meta-analysis
Ephedra and ephedrine for weight loss
Shekelle[4]

- Double-blind RCTs of ephedrine including 524 patients
- Double-blind RCTs of ephedra including 189 patients
- Treatment period was 12 to 24 weeks
- Small effect for ephedrine (mean 0.6, 95% CI 0.2 to 1.0) per month and ephedra (0.8, 0.4 to 1.2)
- Conclusion: Ephedrine and ephedra promote modest short-term weight loss. There are no data regarding long-term weight loss

Garcinia cambogia has been shown to inhibit citrate cleavage enzyme, suppress de novo fatty acid synthesis and food intake, and decrease body weight gain. Four double-blind RCTs of monopreparations were identified (Box 2.101).[1] Overall, the evidence for *G. cambogia* is encouraging and further independent studies are needed.

Box 2.101
Systematic review.
***Garcinia cambogia* for reducing body weight**
Pittler[1]

- Four double-blind RCTs of *Garcinia cambogia* monopreparations including 402 subjects
- Reasonable quality
- Three trials report intergroup differences compared with placebo; the trial with the best methodological quality does not
- Conclusion: Overall, the evidence is encouraging and further independent studies are needed

Glucomannan is a component of konjac root, derived from *Amorphophallus konjac*. Its chemical structure is similar to that of galactomannan from guar gum. Systematic reviews identified one double-blind RCT, which included patients with a body weight of 20% or more over their ideal.[1,7] The report suggests larger weight loss in the treatment group compared with placebo.

Guar gum is a dietary fibre derived from *Cyamopsis tetragonolobus*. Its effectiveness for lowering body weight was assessed in a meta-analysis (Box 2.102).[8] Twenty double-blind, placebo-controlled RCTs were included and the data of 11 trials were analysed. The results of the meta-analysis suggest that guar gum is not effective for reducing body weight. The agreement between the included RCTs confirms the overall result of the meta-analysis.

CONDITIONS

Box 2.102
Meta-analysis
Guar gum for body weight reduction
Pittler[8]

- Eleven trials provided data that were suitable for statistical pooling

- The meta-analysis indicated a non-significant difference compared with placebo (weighted mean difference −0.04 kg; 95% CI −2.2 to 2.1)

- Analysis of six trials with similar methodologic features corroborated these findings (weighted mean difference −0.3 kg; 95% CI −4.0 to 3.5)

- Adverse events most frequently reported were abdominal pain, flatulence, diarrhoea, and cramps

- Conclusion: This meta-analysis suggests that guar gum is not efficacious for reducing body weight

Maté extract was assessed in a small (n = 12) double-blind RCT, which reported a rise in respiratory quotient indicating an increase in the proportion of fat oxidised.[7] Other extracts, such as *Corylus avellana, Crithmum maritinum, Ephedra sinica* and guarana, were reported in the same study to have no such effects.

A systematic review of **psyllium** identified one double-blind RCT.[7] There were no changes in body weight in either the treatment group or the placebo group.

Homeopathy
Two RCTs, which assessed homeopathic preparations were identified in a systematic review.[1] *Helianthus tuberosus* D1 was investigated in patients with a mean BMI of 28. After 3 months, patients in the treatment group had lost on average 7.1 kg, which was different compared with patients in the placebo group. In another trial a single dose of Thyroidinum 30cH was given to fasting patients. Thyroidinum 30cH was not more effective than placebo for increasing the rate of body weight reduction.

Hypnotherapy
A meta-analysis which included six RCTs was identified.[1] The results suggested that the addition of hypnotherapy to cognitive–behavioural therapy leads to a relatively small reduction in body weight (Box 2.103).[9] In a further RCT, hypnotherapy directed at either stress reduction or energy intake was compared with dietary advice.[10] Patients in the hypnotherapy group directed at stress reduction showed a greater weight loss compared with control groups.

Box 2.103
Meta-analysis
Hypnosis for obesity
Allison[9]

- Six RCTs provided data for statistical pooling

- Cognitive–behavioural therapy (self-monitoring, goal setting, stimulus control) and hypnosis was compared with cognitive–behavioural therapy alone

- Analysis of the data suggested an effect size of 0.28 (95% CI 0.23 to 0.33)

- Conclusion: The addition of hypnosis to cognitive–behavioural psychotherapy for weight loss results in, at most, a small enhancement of treatment outcome

Supplements

Beta-hydroxy-beta-methylbutyrate is a metabolite of leucine that has shown anticatabolic actions and is primarily used by bodybuilders as a supportive measure to induce body composition changes. Systematic searches[1,7] yielded two double-blind RCTs, which report differences for fat mass reduction and a trend towards an increase in lean body mass. Thus, there are encouraging data, which require further independent replication.

A double blind RCT investigated whether oral **capsaicin** assists weight maintenance by limiting weight regain after weight loss.[11] After a 4-week very-low-energy diet, a 3-month weight-maintenance period followed. During weight maintenance, weight regain during treatment was not different compared with placebo.

A meta-analysis of RCTs of **chitosan** included 14 RCTs with a minimum duration of 4 weeks (Box 2.104).[12] It concluded that although there seems to be a small effect, high-quality and long-term trials indicate that the effect of chitosan on body weight is substantially less and unlikely to be of clinical significance.

Box 2.104
Meta-analysis
Effect of chitosan on weight loss
Ni Mhurchu[12]

- Fourteen RCT trials involving a total of 1071 participants were included

- Adults who were overweight or obese and/or had hypercholesterolaemia at baseline were included

- The analysis indicated a small but statistically significant greater reduction in body weight (weighted mean difference −1.7 kg; 95% CI −2.1 to −1.3 kg) compared with placebo

- Analyses restricted to high-quality studies showed that reductions in weight [−0.6 (−1.2 to 0.1) kg] were less than in lower quality studies [−2.3 (−2.7 to −1.8) kg]

- Conclusion: Results obtained from high-quality trials indicate that the effect of chitosan on body weight is minimal and unlikely to be of clinical significance

Chromium is a cofactor to insulin and has been reported to increase lean body mass, decrease percentage body fat and increase basal metabolic rate. Chromium picolinate is an organic compound of trivalent chromium and picolinic acid. A meta-analysis included ten double-blind RCTs (Box 2.105).[13] It was concluded that the data suggest a small effect compared with placebo, which has to be interpreted with caution due to the lack of robustness of the effect, which is largely dependent on a single trial. A systematic review[7] identified an additional trial using niacin-bound chromium which reported no effect.

Box 2.105
Meta-analysis
Chromium picolinate for body weight reduction
Pittler[13]

- Ten double-blind, placebo-controlled RCTs were included

- A differential effect was found in favour of chromium picolinate (weighted mean difference: -1.1 kg; 95% CI -1.8 to -0.4 kg, n = 489)

- Sensitivity analysis suggests that this effect is largely dependent on the results of a single trial (weighted mean difference: -0.9 kg; 95% CI -2.0 to 0.2 kg, n = 335)

- Conclusion: A small effect compared with placebo was found. The clinical relevance of the effect is debatable and the lack of robustness means that the result has to be interpreted with caution

A double-blind RCT studied the effects of 13 weeks conjugated **linoleic acid** supplementation in overweight subjects on body-weight maintenance, parameters of appetite and energy intake at breakfast after weight loss.[14] It concluded that appetite (hunger, satiety and fullness) was favourably, dose-independently affected by a 13-week consumption of 1.8 or 3.6 g conjugated linoleic acid daily.

Pyruvate is generated in the body via glycolysis and supplementation with pyruvate seems to enhance exercise performance and improve measures of body composition. Two double-blind RCTs, which included patients with a BMI of 25 and above were identified.[1,7] None of the studies reported greater effects for body weight reduction compared with placebo.

Yohimbine, an alpha-2 receptor antagonist is the main active constituent of the ground bark of *Pausinystalia yohimbe* (yohimbe). Most clinical studies relate to the effects of this isolated constituent of yohimbe bark. Three double-blind RCTs were identified[1,7] which report conflicting results for body weight. At present it is unclear whether yohimbine is effective for reducing body weight.

Other therapies

One double-blind RCT assessed 70 obese subjects who received one of three **Ayurvedic herbal formulations** or indistinguishable placebo for 3 months.[15] All patients entered into the trial were at least 20% in excess of their ideal body weight and non-diabetic. The authors report that patients in the treatment group experienced a significant weight loss compared with those in the placebo group. Further single RCTs, which require independent replication were conducted on a **bean extract,**[16] **grape seed extract,**[17] **green tea,**[18] *Phaseolus vulgaris*[19] and **soy-based meal replacement.**[20]

Overall recommendation

Diet modification, increased physical activity and lifestyle changes are the most effective measures to achieve weight loss. There is little convincing evidence for the effectiveness of complementary therapies for reducing body weight. The exceptions are hypnotherapy, *E. sinica* and other ephedrine-containing dietary supplements, which may lead to small reductions in body weight. The intake of *E. sinica* and ephedrine, however, is associated with an increased risk of adverse events.

Table 2.62
Summary of clinical evidence for overweight/ obesity

Treatment	Weight of evidence	Direction of evidence	Serious safety concerns
Acupuncture / acupressure	OOO	⇨	Yes (see p 294)
Herbal medicine			
Citrus aurantium	O	⇘	Yes (see p 481)
Ephedra sinica	OOO	⇧	Yes (see p 479)
Garcinica cambogia	OO	⬈	Yes (see p 5)
Glucomannan	O	⬈	Yes (see p 478)
Guar gum	OOO	⇩	Yes (see p 419)
Maté	O	⇘	Yes (see p 479)
Psyllium	O	⇩	Yes (see p 480)
Homeopathy	O	⇨	No (see p 327)
Hypnotherapy	OOO	⬈	Yes (see p 331)
Supplements			
Capsaicin	O	⇘	Yes (see p 5)
Chitosan	OOO	⇘	Yes (see p 380)
Chromium	OOO	⇩	Yes (see p 482)
Beta-hydroxy-beta-methylbutyrate	OO	⬈	Yes (see p 5)
Linoleic acid	O	⬈	Yes (see p 5)
Pyruvate	OO	⇘	Yes (see p 484)
Yohimbine	OO	⇨	Yes (see p 474)

CONDITIONS

REFERENCES

1 Pittler M H, Ernst E. Complementary therapies for reducing body weight: a systematic review Int J Obes Relat Metab Disord 2005;29: 1030–1038

2 Lacey J M, Terhakovec A M, Foster G D. Acupuncture for the treatment of obesity: a review of the evidence. Int J Obese 2003;27: 419–427

3 Bent S, Padula A, Neuhaus J. Safety and efficacy of citrus aurantium for weight loss. Am J Cardiol 2004;94:1359–1361

4 Shekelle P G, Hardy M L, Morton S C, Maglione M, Mojica W A, Suttorp M J, Rhodes S L, Jungvig L, Gagne J. Efficacy and safety of ephedra and ephedrine for weight loss and athletic performance: a meta-analysis. JAMA 2003;289:1537–1545

5 Greenway F L, De Jonge L, Blanchard D, Frisard M, Smith S R. Effect of a dietary herbal supplement containing caffeine and ephedra on weight, metabolic rate, and body composition. Obes Res 2004;12:1152–1157

6 Coffey C S, Steiner D, Baker BA, Allison D B. A randomized double-blind placebo-controlled clinical trial of a product containing ephedrine, caffeine, and other ingredients from herbal sources for treatment of overweight and obesity in the absence of lifestyle treatment. Int J Obes Relat Metab Disord 2004;28:1411–1419

7 Pittler M H, Ernst E. Dietary supplements for body-weight reduction: a systematic review. Am J Clin Nutr 2004;79:529–536

8 Pittler M H, Ernst E. Guar gum for body weight reduction: meta-analysis of randomized trials. Am J Med 2001;110:724–730

9 Allison D B, Faith M S. Hypnosis as an adjunct to cognitive–behavioral psychotherapy for obesity: a meta-analytic reappraisal. J Consult Clin Psychol 1996;64:513–516

10 Stradling J, Roberts D, Wilson A, Lovelock F. Controlled trial of hypnotherapy for weight loss in patients with obstructive sleep apnoea. Int J Obesity 1998;28:278–281.

11 Lejeune M P, Kovacs E M, Westerterp-Plantenga M S. Effect of capsaicin on substrate oxidation and weight maintenance after modest body-weight loss in human subjects. Br J Nutr 2003;90:651–659

12 Ni Mhurchu C N, Dunshea-Mooij C, Bennett D, Rodgers A. Effect of chitosan on weight loss in overweight and obese individuals: a systematic review of randomized controlled trials. Obes Rev 2005;6:35–42

13 Pittler M H, Stevinson C, Ernst E. Chromium picolinate for body weight reduction. Meta-analysis of randomized trials. Int J Obese 2003;27:522–529

14 Kamphuis M M, Lejeune M P, Saris W H, Westerterp-Plantenga M S. Effect of conjugated linoleic acid supplementation after weight loss on appetite and food intake in overweight subjects. Eur J Clin Nutr 2003;57:1268–1274

15 Paranjpe P, Patki P, Patwardhan B. Ayurvedic treatment of obesity: a randomised double-blind, placebo-controlled clinical trial. J Ethnopharmacol 1990;29:1–11

16 Birketvedt G S, Travis A, Langbakk B, Florholmen J R. Dietary supplementation with bean extract improves lipid profile in overweight and obese subjects. Nutrition 2002;18:729–733

17 Vogels N, Nijs I M, Westerterp-Plantenga M S. The effect of grape-seed extract on 24 h energy intake in humans. Eur J Clin Nutr 2004;58:667–673

18 Kovacs E M, Lejeune M P, Nijs I, Westerterp-Plantenga M S. Effects of green tea on weight maintenance after body-weight loss. Br J Nutr 2004;91:431–437

19 Udani J, Hardy M, Madsen D C. Blocking carbohydrate absorption and weight loss: a clinical trial using Phase 2 brand proprietary fractionated white bean extract. Altern Med Rev 2004;9:63–69

20 Allison D B, Gadbury G, Schwartz L G, Murugesan R, Kraker J L, Heshka S, Fontaine K R, Heymsfield S B. A novel soy-based meal replacement formula for weight loss among obese individuals: a randomised controlled clinical trial. Eur J Clin Nutr 2003;57:514–522

CONDITIONS

PERIPHERAL ARTERIAL OCCLUSIVE DISEASE

Synonyms
Charcot's syndrome, myasthenia angiosclerotica, intermittent claudication, peripheral vascular disease stage II.

Definition
Peripheral arterial occlusive disease (PAOD) arises when there is significant narrowing of arteries distal to the arch of the aorta. Narrowing can arise from atheroma, arteritis, local thrombus formation, or embolisation from the heart or more central arteries.

CAM usage
Hydrotherapy, chelation therapy, herbal medicine and lifestyle changes are interventions frequently used for the treatment of this condition.

Clinical evidence

Acupuncture
One RCT of acupuncture for treating PAOD was identified in a systematic review;[1] patients with unilateral lower and upper leg amputations due to PAOD were included. The authors suggest intergroup differences in favour of acupuncture. At present therefore few data from rigorous clinical trials exist to suggest that acupuncture is effective for patients with PAOD.

Biofeedback
The same review[1] identified one RCT (n = 12), which tested biofeedback as an adjunctive treatment for patients with intermittent claudication. The treatment consisted of electromyographic feedback and skin temperature feedback from fingers and toes. Compared with baseline, maximal walking time increased, but there was no mention of intergroup differences.

Chelation therapy
A Cochrane review identified five RCTs (Box 2.106).[2] All studies compared chelation using ethylenediaminetetraacetic acid

Box 2.106
Systematic review
Chelation therapy for atherosclerotic cardiovascular disease
Villarruz[2]

- Five double-blind, placebo-controlled RCTs

- Four of the studies (n = 250 patients) showed no difference in the following outcomes: direct or indirect measurement of disease severity and subjective measures of improvement

- For painfree walking distance after 20 infusions, there was an effect in favour of placebo (weighted mean difference −16.4 m, CI −32.0 to −0.8, n = 167)

- Adverse events included faintness, hypocalcaemia, proteinuria and gastrointestinal symptoms

- Conclusion: There is not enough evidence to determine the effectiveness or otherwise of chelation therapy

CONDITIONS

(EDTA) with isotonic NaCl solution or distilled water. There were no differences in favour of chelation therapy. For painfree walking distance after 20 infusions the results of two trials (n = 167) were pooled and suggest an effect in favour of placebo.

CO_2-applications

Subcutaneous CO_2 insufflations are being used as a treatment modality almost exclusively in Europe. A systematic review[3] identified three RCTs, which assessed patients with PAOD. The data from one trial suggested differences for pain-free walking distance compared with patients on a waiting list, while two others reported mixed results compared with waiting list controls and patients receiving CO_2-baths. Another RCT (n = 24) assessed the effects of immersion in CO_2-containing water.[4] It reported an increase in painfree walking distance after immersion of the lower extremities for 30 minutes five times weekly for 4 weeks compared with baseline.

Diet

One double-blind RCT investigated the effects of an **L-arginine-enriched food bar**.[5] After 2 weeks of administering the food bar, the pain-free walking distance had increased by 66% while the maximal walking distance had increased by 23%. These effects were not observed in the placebo group. Cohort studies also suggest beneficial effects of a **Mediterranean diet**[6] and **cereal fibre intake**[7] on PAOD risk.

Herbal medicine

A Cochrane review identified one double-blind RCT for **garlic** (*Allium sativum*) extract (Box 2.107),[8] which suggests that garlic powder given in a daily dose of 800 mg for 12 weeks increases pain-free walking distance more than placebo.[9] The Cochrane review, however, concluded that there is no effect on walking distance.

Box 2.107
Systematic review
Garlic for PAOD
Jepson[8]

- One double-blind, placebo-controlled RCT including 78 patients

- Men and women were included (age range 40–75)

- Treatment period was 12 weeks

- Painfree walking distance increased from 161 to 207 m (garlic) and from 172 to 203 m (placebo)

- Conclusion: One small trial of short duration found no effect on walking distance

The evidence for **ginkgo** (*Ginkgo biloba*) has been assessed in a meta-analysis.[10] According to these data and other evidence from comparative trials (e.g.[11]) ginkgo extract is effective for patients with intermittent claudication. Ginkgo increased pain-free and maximal walking distances to a similar degree compared with other conventional oral treatments. The overall effect, however, is modest. Another systematic review confirms the effectiveness for the special ginkgo extract EGb 761 (Box 2.108).[12]

Box 2.108
Meta-analysis
**Ginkgo extract
EGb 761 for PAOD**
Horsch[12]

- Nine double-blind, placebo-controlled RCTs

- All tested ginkgo extract EGb 761 in patients with PAOD in Fontaine stage II

- Methodological quality and design of the trials were heterogeneous

- The data for pain-free walking distance show a beneficial effect over placebo (theta 1.23, CI 1.16 to 1.31)

- Conclusion: This review confirms the efficacy of Ginkgo biloba special extract EGb 761

Padma 28 is an herbal mixture including 22 different ingredients. Data from five double-blind RCTs measuring maximal walking distance are available.[1] Based on these data, meta-analytical pooling suggests a difference of the change of about 81 m over placebo (Box 2.109). Overall, the evidence suggests that this herbal mixture is an option for patients with PAOD.

Box 2.109
Systematic review
**Padma 28 for
PAOD**
Pittler[1]

- Five double-blind RCTs assessing 333 patients in Fontaine stage IIb

- Patients were treated with 1.5 to 2.3 g for 4 months

- The mean difference was 81.3 m (CI 65.5 to 97.1) in favour of padma 28 compared with placebo

- Adverse events were: exanthema, dermatosis, worsening of symptoms; four serious adverse events, of which none were drug related

- Conclusion: The available evidence suggests that this herbal mixture is an option for patients with PAOD

Supplements

A Cochrane review of **fish oil** (omega-3 fatty acid) included four placebo-controlled RCTs.[13] Two trials, which assessed walking distances suggested no changes for painfree and maximal walking distance. It was concluded that, although omega-3 fatty acids may have some beneficial effects, there is no evidence of improved clinical outcomes in patients with PAOD. Another Cochrane review assessed the evidence for **vitamin E** and identified three double-blind RCTs.[14] The authors concluded that there is insufficient evidence to determine whether vitamin E is effective for treating patients with PAOD. The meta-analysis of two trials, which included one non-randomised trial suggested a relative risk of 0.6 (CI 0.3 to 1.2) for patients' subjective evaluation of the treatment.

Overall recommendation

No therapy is as effective as conventional regular physical exercise. It can be recommended as a beneficial lifestyle change in addition to smoking cessation. Convincing evidence exists for the effectiveness of ginkgo extract, which seems to be as effective as other conventional oral interventions. Although the overall effect seems modest, given the nature and frequency of adverse events, it can be recommended as an oral treatment. Padma 28 also seems to be of benefit. For other interventions such as CO_2-applications, and vitamin E the evidence is encouraging but insufficient for firm recommendations.

Table 2.63
Summary of clinical evidence for peripheral arterial occlusive disease

Treatment	Weight of evidence	Direction of evidence	Serious safety concerns
Acupuncture	O	⬈	Yes (see p 294)
Biofeedback	O	⬈	Yes (see p 310)
Chelation therapy	OOO	⬇	Yes (see p 312)
CO_2-applications	OO	⬈	Yes (see p 5)
Diet			
L-arginine-enriched bar	O	⬈	Yes (see p 5)
Mediterranean diet	O	⬈	Yes (see p 5)
Fibre	O	⬈	Yes (see p 5)
Herbal medicine			
Garlic	O	⇨	Yes (see p 398)
Ginkgo	OOO	⬆	Yes (see p 404)
Padma 28	OOO	⬆	Yes (see p 5)
Supplements			
Fish oil	OO	⬊	Yes (see p 483)
Vitamin E	OO	⬈	Yes (see p 5)

REFERENCES

1 Pittler M H, Ernst E. Complementary therapies for peripheral arterial disease: Systematic review. Atherosclerosis 2005;181:1–7

2 Villarruz M V, Dans A, Tan F. Chelation therapy for atherosclerotic cardiovascular disease. Cochrane Database Syst Rev 2002, Issue 4. Art. No.: CD002785

3 Brockow T, Hausner T, Dillner A, Resch K L. Clinical evidence of subcutaneous CO_2 insufflations: a systematic review. J Altern Comp Med 2000;6:391–403

4 Hartmann B R, Bassenge E, Hartmann M. Effects of serial percutaneous application of carbon dioxide in intermittent claudication: results of a controlled trial. Angiology 1997;48: 957–963

5　Maxwell A J, Anderson B E, Cooke J P. Nutritional therapy for peripheral arterial disease: a double-blind, placebo-controlled, randomized trial of HeartBar. Vasc Med 2000;5:11–19

6　Ciccarone E, Di Castelnuovo A, Salcuni M, Siani A, Giacco A, Donati MB, De Gaetano G, Capani F, Iacoviello L; Gendiabe Investigators. A high-score Mediterranean dietary pattern is associated with a reduced risk of peripheral arterial disease in Italian patients with Type 2 diabetes. J Thromb Haemost 2003;1:1744–1752

7　Merchant A T, Hu F B, Spiegelman D, Willett W C, Rimm E B, Ascherio A. Dietary fiber reduces peripheral arterial disease risk in men. J Nutr 2003;133:3658–3663

8　Jepson R G, Kleijnen J, Leng G C. Garlic for peripheral arterial occlusive disease. Cochrane Database Syst Rev 1997, Issue 2. Art. No.: CD000095

9　Kiesewetter H, Jung F, Jung EM, Blume J, Mrowietz C, Birk A, Koscielny J, Wenzel E.

Effects of garlic coated tablets in peripheral arterial occlusive disease. Clin Invest 1993;71:383–386

10　Pittler M H, Ernst E. Ginkgo biloba extract for the treatment of intermittent claudication: a meta-analysis of randomized trials. Am J Med 2000;108:276–281

11　Böhmer D, Kalinski S, Michaelis P, Szögy A. Behandlung der PAVK mit Ginkgo-biloba-extrakt (GBE) oder Pentoxifyllin. Herz Kreislauf 1988;20:5–8

12　Horsch S, Walther C. Ginkgo biloba special extract EGb 761 in the treatment of peripheral arterial occlusive disease (PAOD) – a review based on randomized, controlled studies. Int J Clin Pharmacol Ther 2004;42:63–72

13　Sommerfield T, Hiatt W R. Omega-3 fatty acids for intermittent claudication. Cochrane Database Syst Rev 2004, Issue 1. Art. No.: CD003833

14　Kleijnen J, Mackerras D. Vitamin E for intermittent claudication. Cochrane Database Syst Rev 1998, Issue 1. Art. No.: CD000987

PREMENSTRUAL SYNDROME

Synonyms/ subcategories　Late luteal phase dysphoric disorder, premenstrual dysphoric disorder, premenstrual tension.

Definition　Recurrence of physical, behavioural and/or psychological symptoms during the luteal phase of the menstrual cycle which disappear after the onset of menstruation.

CAM usage　Surveys from the USA and UK reported the complementary therapies most popular with premenstrual syndrome (PMS) sufferers as exercise, vitamins/supplements, meditation, massage, homeopathy and chiropractic.[1,2]

Clinical evidence　*Acupuncture*
A systematic review included four CCTs of acupuncture or acupressure for dysmenorrhoea.[3] Even though they generated encouraging results, methodological limitations prevented a positive conclusion.

Biofeedback
Vaginal temperature feedback (12 weekly sessions) was compared with no treatment in two identically reported RCTs with 30 women.[4] Biofeedback alleviated both physiological and affective symptoms. However, several shortcomings cast doubt on the validity of the findings.

Herbal medicine

For **chaste tree** (*Vitex agnus-castus*) extract there are several uncontrolled studies with positive results including a large (n = 1634) study in which 81% rated themselves 'much better'.[5] The results of double-blind RCTs (Table 2.64) are, however, not uniform.[6-8]

Table 2.64 **Double-blind RCTs of chaste tree for premenstrual syndrome**

Reference	Sample size	Interventions [dosage]	Result	Comment
Turner[6]	217	A) Chaste tree [1800 mg/d] B) Placebo	A no different from B	Postal study; other treatments not excluded
Lauritzen[7]	127	A) Chaste tree [3.5–4.2 mg/d] B) Vitamin B_6 [200 mg/d]	A no different from B	Sample size lacked statistical power; efficacy of control intervention (B_6) unclear
Schellenberg[8]	170	A) Chaste tree one tab/day B) Placebo	A superior to B	Responder rates were 52% (A) and 24% (B)

A systematic review of **evening primrose** (*Oenothera biennis*) oil included uncontrolled studies as well as randomised and placebo-controlled trials (Box 2.110).[9] None of the trials had large samples. The conclusion drawn from the available evidence was that evening primrose oil is of little, if any, value for PMS.

Box 2.110
Systematic review
Evening primrose oil for premenstrual syndrome
Budeiri[9]

- Eleven trials of any design (four RCTs) including 455 patients
- Trial quality generally low
- Three most rigorous trials had negative results
- Conclusion: evening primrose oil is of little, if any, value in the management of PMS

Ginkgo (*Ginkgo biloba*) (160 mg daily for 2 months) was investigated in a double-blind placebo-controlled RCT with 163 women.[10] The results suggested it may be helpful for breast pain, but not other PMS symptoms.

Homeopathy

Two double-blind, placebo-controlled RCTs of classical homeopathy have been conducted. In the first trial, stringent exclusion criteria led to the sample being too small (n = 10) for meaningful results.[11] The other study included 105 patients treated for

3 months,[12] at which point symptom scores were lower in the homeopathy group. There was also less use of tranquillisers and analgesics and fewer work days lost than in the placebo group.

Massage
An RCT (n = 24) of massage therapy for women with premenstrual dysphoric disorder (PMDD) reported some improvements in symptoms immediately after massage sessions and after one month of treatment. However, the mood symptoms that are central to PMDD were not lowered at one month. Relaxation was used as a control, but intergroup analyses were not conducted.[13]

Reflexology
An RCT (n – 35) of reflexology treatment (once weekly for 2 months) produced superior results on both somatic and psychological PMS symptoms than sham reflexology, which involved treating points unrelated to premenstrual symptoms.[14]

Relaxation
Progressive muscle relaxation training (twice weekly for 3 months) alleviated physical symptoms of PMS in an RCT (n = 46) compared with the control interventions of reading and charting symptoms.[15] For women with severe symptoms, there were also improvements in emotional symptoms.

Spinal manipulation
A crossover RCT (n = 25) of **chiropractic** manipulation reported superior results to a sham device.[16] However, improvements were greatest with whichever intervention was received first and therefore may be due to other than specific effects.

Supplements
Calcium supplementation has been demonstrated to be superior to placebo for most types of PMS symptoms in two double-blind RCTs (Table 2.65).[17,18] The second of these trials is impressive in terms of size (n = 466) and rigour and provides promising evidence in favour of calcium.

Table 2.65 **Double-blind RCTs of calcium for premenstrual syndrome**

Reference	Sample size	Interventions [dosage]	Result	Comment
Thys-Jacobs[17]	33	A) Calcium [1000 mg/d for 3 mo] B) Placebo	A superior in three of four symptom subgroups	Crossover trial; high drop-out rate; non-compliance
Thys-Jacobs[18]	466	A) Calcium [1200 mg/d for 3 mo] B) Placebo	A superior in all symptom subgroups	Trial rigorous but not all other treatments excluded

Two small double-blind RCTs of **magnesium** supplements have indicated some benefits over placebo (Table 2.66).[19,20] However, the type of symptoms that improved was different in each study and the data are not compelling.

Table 2.66 **Placebo-controlled, double-blind RCTs of magnesium for premenstrual syndrome**

Reference	Sample size	Interventions [dosage]	Result	Comment
Facchinetti[19]	28	A) Magnesium [360 mg/d for 2 mo] B) Placebo	A superior overall and for 'negative affect' symptom	Unusual lack of placebo response
Walker[20]	38	A) Magnesium [200 mg/d for 2 mo] B) Placebo	A only superior for fluid retention subgroup	Crossover trial; other treatments allowed

Neptune Krill Oil has been compared with fish oil in an RCT with 70 women.[21] The results suggest that it can reduce dysmenorrhoea and other symptoms of PMS.

Potassium was investigated as a therapy in a non-randomised, placebo-controlled trial.[22] The results showed no effect on PMS symptoms or premenstrual weight gain.

The RCT evidence for **vitamin B$_6$** has been subjected to two systematic reviews. One concluded that there is no evidence of efficacy.[23] The other pooled the data, reporting a greater effect than placebo for overall symptoms and premenstrual depression, but cautioned that conclusions are limited due to the low quality of most trials (Box 2.111). The authors advised that doses in excess of 100 mg per day were not justified due to neurological adverse effects.[24] Combining vitamin B$_6$ and magnesium reduces anxiety-related symptoms of PMS.[25]

Box 2.111
Meta-analysis
Vitamin B$_6$ for premenstrual syndrome
Wyatt[24]

- Nine double-blind, placebo-controlled RCTs including 940 patients
- Three used a multinutrient supplement containing vitamin B$_6$
- Trial quality generally low
- Superior to placebo (odds ratio 2.32; CI 1.95 to 2.54)
- Conclusions limited due to low quality of trials

Vitamin E has been investigated in two double-blind, placebo-controlled RCTs.[26,27] Although both show positive results for some PMS symptoms, the overall evidence is ambiguous.

Other therapies

Evidence from questionnaire studies, non-randomised trials and case control studies suggest **aerobic exercise** training may help prevent or alleviate premenstrual symptoms (e.g.[28-31]). **Qi-therapy** has generated encouraging results in two RCTs from the same research group.[32,33]

Overall recommendation

The evidence is not convincing for any complementary treatment. However, given that some have few risks, that some conventional treatments are associated with adverse events and that there is a substantial placebo response in PMS, such treatments may be worth considering. Supplementation with vitamin B_6, calcium or magnesium has been shown to be beneficial in some women. Other interventions where the preliminary evidence looks encouraging include aerobic exercise, relaxation and acupuncture. These can be encouraged as part of a healthy lifestyle for all women.

Table 2.67
Summary of clinical evidence for premenstrual syndrome

Treatment	Weight of evidence	Direction of evidence	Serious safety concerns
Acupuncture	OO	⬈	Yes (see p 294)
Biofeedback	O	⬈	No (see p 310)
Herbal medicine			
Chaste tree	OO	⇨	Yes (see p 378)
Evening primrose oil	OO	⬊	Yes (see p 393)
Ginkgo	O	⬈	Yes (see p 404)
Homeopathy	∩	⇧	No (see p 327)
Massage	O	⬈	No (see p 334)
Reflexology	O	⇧	No (see p 345)
Relaxation	O	⇧	No (see p 348)
Spinal manipulation			
Chiropractic	O	⬈	Yes (see p 316)
Supplements			
Calcium	OO	⇧	No (see p 5)
Magnesium	O	⬈	Yes (see p 5)
Neptune Krill Oil	O	⬈	Yes (see p 5)
Potassium	O	⇩	Yes (see p 5)
Vitamin B_6	OO	⬈	Yes (see p 5)
Vitamin E	O	⬊	No (see p 5)

CONDITIONS

CONDITIONS

REFERENCES

1 Singh B, Berman B, Simpson R, Annechild A. Incidence of premenstrual syndrome and remedy usage: a national probability sample study. Alt Ther Health Med 1998;4:75–79

2 Corney R H, Stanton R. A survey of 658 women who report symptoms of premenstrual syndrome. J Psychosom Res 1991;35:471–482

3 White A R. A review of controlled trials of acupuncture for women's reproductive health care. J Fam Plann Reprod Health Care 2003;29:233–236

4 Van Zak D B. Biofeedback treatments for the premenstrual and premenstrual affective syndromes. Int J Psychosom 1994;41:53–60

5 Loch E G, Selle H, Boblitz N. Treatment of premenstrual syndrome with a phytopharmaceutical formulation containing Vitex agnus castus. J Wom Health Gender-Based Med 2000;9:315–320

6 Turner S, Mills S. A double-blind clinical trial on a herbal remedy for premenstrual syndrome: a case study. Complement Ther Med 1993;1:73–77

7 Lauritzen C, Reuter H D, Repges R, Bohnert K-J, Schmidt U. Treatment of premenstrual tension syndrome with Vitex agnus castus. Controlled, double-blind study versus pyridoxine. Phytomedicine 1997;4:183–189

8 Schellenberg R. Treatment for the premenstrual syndrome with agnus castus fruit extract: prospective, randomized, placebo controlled study. BMJ 2001;322:134–137

9 Budeiri D, Li Wan Po A, Dornan J C. Is evening primrose oil of value in the treatment of premenstrual syndrome? Control Clin Trials 1996;17:60–68

10 Tamborini A, Taurelle R. Intérêt de l'extrait standardisé de Ginkgo biloba (Egb 761) dans la prise en charge des symptômes congestifs du syndrome prémenstruel. Rev Fr Gynécol Obstét 1993;88:447–457

11 Chapman E H, Angelica J, Spitalny G, Strauss M. Results of a study of the homeopathic treatment of PMS. J Am Inst Homeopath 1994;87:14–21

12 Yakir M, Kreitler S, Bzizinsky A, Bentwich Z, Vithoulkas G. Homeopathic treatment of premenstrual syndrome – repeated study. Proceedings of the Annual Conference of the International Homoeopathic League. Budapest, Hungary, May 2000

13 Hernandez-Reif M, Martinex A, Field T, Quintero O, Hart S, Burman I. Premenstrual symptoms are relieved by massage therapy. J Psychosom Obstet Gynecol 2000;21:9–15

14 Oleson T, Flocco W. Randomized controlled study of premenstrual symptoms treated with ear, hand and foot reflexology. Obstet Gynecol 1993;82:906–907

15 Goodale I L, Domar A D, Benson H. Alleviation of premenstrual syndrome symptoms with the relaxation response. Obstet Gynecol 1990;75:649–655

16 Walsh M J, Polus B I. A randomized, placebo-controlled clinical trial on the efficacy of chiropractic therapy on premenstrual syndrome. J Manip Physiol Ther 1999;22:582–585

17 Thys-Jacobs S, Ceccarelli S, Bierman A, Weisman H, Cohen M A, Alvir J. Calcium supplementation in premenstrual syndrome: a randomized crossover trial. J Gen Intern Med 1989;4:183–189

18 Thys-Jacobs S, Starkey P, Bernstein D, Tian J. Calcium carbonate and the premenstrual syndrome: effects on premenstrual and menstrual symptoms. Premenstrual Syndrome Study Group. Am J Obstet Gynecol 1998;179:444–452

19 Facchinetti F, Borella P, Sances G, Fioroni L, Nappi R E, Genazzani A R. Oral magnesium successfully relieves premenstrual mood changes. Obstet Gynecol 1991;78:177–181

20 Walker A F, De Souza M C, Vickers M F, Abeyasekera S, Collins M L, Trinca L A. Magnesium supplementation alleviates premenstrual symptoms of fluid retention. J Womens Health 1998;7:1157–1165

21 Sampalis F, Bunea R, Pelland M F, Kowalski O, Duguet N, Dupuis S. Evaluation of the effects of Neptune Krill Oil on the management of premenstrual syndrome and dysmenorrhea. Altern Med Rev 2003;8:171–179

22 Reeves B D, Garvin J E, McElin T W. Premenstrual tension: symptoms and weight changes related to potassium therapy. Am J Obstet Gynecol 1971;109:1036–1041

23 Kleijnen J, Ter Riet G, Knipschild P. Vitamin B$_6$ in the treatment of the premenstrual syndrome – a review. Br J Obstet Gynaecol 1990;97:847–852

24 Wyatt K M, Dimmock P W, Jones P W, Shaughn O'Brien P M. Efficacy of vitamin B-6 in the treatment of premenstrual syndrome: systematic review. BMJ 1999;318:1375–1381

25 De Souza M C, Walker A F, Robinson P A, Bolland K. A synergistic effect of a daily

supplement for 1 month of 200 mg magnesium plus 50 mg vitamin B6 for the relief of anxiety-related premenstrual syndrome: a randomized, double-blind, crossover study. J Womens Health Gend Based Med 2000;9:131–139

26 London R S, Sundaram G S, Murphy L, Goldstein P J. The effect of α-tocopherol on premenstrual symptomology: a double-blind study. J Am Col Nutr 1983;2:115–122

27 London R S, Murphy L, Kitlowski K E, Reynolds M A. Efficacy of α-tocopherol in the treatment of premenstrual syndrome. J Reprod Med 1987;32:400–404

28 Choi P Y L, Salmon P. Symptom changes across the menstrual cycle in competitive sportswomen, exercisers and sedentary women. Br J Clin Psychol 1995;34:447–460

29 Aganoff J A, Boyle G J. Aerobic exercise, mood states and menstrual cycle symptoms. J Psychosom Res 1994;38:183–192

30 Steege J F, Blumenthal J A. The effects of aerobic exercise on premenstrual symptoms in middle aged women: a preliminary study. J Psychosom Res 1993;37:127–133

31 Prior J C, Vigna Y, Sciarretta D, Alojada N, Schulzer M. Conditioning exercise decreases premenstrual symptoms: a prospective controlled 6 month trial. Fertil Steril 1987;47:402–408

32 Jang H S, Lee M S. Effects of qi therapy (external qigong) on premenstrual syndrome: a randomized placebo-controlled study. J Altern Complement Med 2004;10:456–462

33 Jang H S, Lee M S, Kim M J, Chong E S. Effects of Qi-therapy on premenstrual syndrome. Int J Neurosci 2004;114:909–921

CONDITIONS

RHEUMATOID ARTHRITIS

Synonyms   Arthritis deformans, arthritis nodosa, nodose rheumatism.

Definition   Rheumatoid arthritis is a chronic inflammatory disorder. It is characterised by a chronic polyarthritis that primarily affects the peripheral joints and related periarticular tissues. It usually starts as an insidious symmetric polyarthritis, often with non-specific systemic symptoms. Diagnostic criteria include arthritis lasting longer than 6 weeks, positive rheumatoid factor, and radiological damage.

Related conditions   Other rheumatic diseases such as ankylosing spondylitis.

CAM usage   Rheumatoid arthritis (RA) is associated with a high level of CAM usage. In particular, patients often try herbal treatments and other nutritional supplements.[1] Modifications of the regular diet are also frequent (e.g. vegetarianism); most of these approaches, however, are considered conventional. In our survey of CAM organisations (see p 4) the following treatments were recommended for arthritis: aromatherapy, homeopathy, hypnotherapy, magnet therapy, massage, nutrition, reflexology and yoga.

Clinical evidence   *Acupuncture*

A Cochrane review[2] evaluated the evidence of acupuncture or electroacupuncture in patients with RA (Box 2.112). Two RCTs, one of each for acupuncture and electroacupuncture were identified. No firm recommendations can be made regarding the effectiveness of acupuncture for treating RA.

Box 2.112
Systematic review
Acupuncture for rheumatoid arthritis
Casimiro[2]

- Two RCTs (n = 84) were included

- One of each assessed acupuncture and electroacupuncture

- For acupuncture, there were no effects on C-reactive protein, pain, and other outcome measures

- For electroacupuncture, a decrease in knee pain was reported compared with placebo

- Conclusion: Although some positive results are reported, the effects were only short-term, not exceeding 24 hours of relief. The poor quality of the trial procludes its recommendation in patients with RA

Diet

Various (mostly conventional) dietary approaches have been tried for RA. Trials from Scandinavia show encouraging effects for fasting followed by a vegetarian diet. A systematic review included four such studies.[3] The meta-analysis of these data suggests long-term improvements in pain and related outcomes. Both fasting and strict vegetarian diets are associated with the risk of malnutrition, thus adequate medical supervision is essential. Further CCTs[4] and RCTs[5,6] support the observed benefits associated with dietary interventions.

Herbal medicine

A systematic review assessed the evidence from all RCTs on the effectiveness of **Ayurvedic medicine** (Box 2.113).[7] It is reported that there is a paucity of RCTs of Ayurvedic medicines for RA.

Box 2.113
Systematic review
Ayurvedic medicine for rheumatoid arthritis
Park[7]

- Electronic databases, the abstract service of the Central Council for Research in Ayurveda and Siddha and one Sri Lankan and three Indian journals were searched

- Seven RCTs met the inclusion criteria

- Three trials tested Ayurvedic medicine against placebo and four tested against other Ayurvedic medicines.

- Conclusion: There is a paucity of RCTs of Ayurvedic medicines for RA. The existing RCTs fail to show convincingly that such treatments are effective therapeutic options for this condition

A Cochrane review of herbal treatments for rheumatoid arthritis concluded that there appears to be some potential benefit for the use of **gamma-linolenic acid** (GLA) in RA although further studies are required to establish optimum dosage and duration of treatment.[8] A more recent assessment of the evidence largely corroborates these findings suggesting moderate support for GLA found in some herbal medicines for reducing pain, tender joint count and stiffness (Box 2.114).[9]

Box 2.114
Systematic review
Herbal medicines for rheumatoid arthritis
Soeken[9]

- Fourteen RCTs were included, all were double-blind

- Meta-analyses of three trials of γ-linoleic acid (n = 117)

- Effect size for pain visual analogue scale was 0.76, 95% CI 0.37 to 1.15

- Effect size for tender joint count was 0.93, 95% CI 0.47 to 1.38

- Effect size for stiffness was 0.23, 95% CI 0.02 to 0.90

- Conclusion: Given the number of herbal medicines promoted for RA, further research is needed to examine their efficacy, safety and potential drug interactions

CONDITIONS

Several European herbal mixtures have been tested in clinical trials with positive results for RA patients. Of these preparations, only **Phytodolor** (a German proprietary medicine containing extracts of *Populus tremula, Fraxinus excelsior and Solidago virgaurea*) has been submitted to independently replicated clinical trials (Box 2.115).[10]

Thunder god vine (*Tripterygium wilfordii* Hook) is recommended in traditional Chinese medicine for a large range of conditions. Four RCTs suggested anti-inflammatory properties and effects in reducing the objective signs and subjective symptoms of RA.[11-14]

Box 2.115
Systematic review
Phytodolor for rheumatoid arthritis
Ernst[10]

- Ten RCTs met the inclusion criteria (n = 1035). Six were conducted against placebo, four against reference medication

- Most studies included patients with various rheumatic diseases

- The quality of these trials was, on average, good

- The results imply that Phytodolor is superior to placebo and equally effective as standard NSAIDs in alleviating arthritic pain and restoring function

- Conclusion: Phytodolor is a safe and effective treatment for musculoskeletal pain

An extract of *Uncaria tomentosa* was tested in 40 patients undergoing sulfasalazine or hydroxychloroquine treatment.[15]

Twenty-four weeks of treatment with the extract resulted in a modest reduction of the number of painful joints compared with placebo. This small preliminary study requires independent replication.

Further single RCTs reporting some positive results, which require replication in independent trials, exist for **garlic** (*Allium sativum*)[16] and **tong luo kai bi** tablets.[17]

Single RCTs reporting negative results exist for **boswellia**[9] (*Boswellia serrata*), **feverfew**[9] (*Tanacetum parthenium*) and **willow** (*Salix* spp) bark extract.[18]

Homeopathy

A review summarised three RCTs (n = 266) of homeopathic treatments of RA.[19] Two studies on RA using only classic individualised homeopathy do not suggest beneficial effects (odds ratio 2.04, 95% CI 0.66 to 6.34), whereas positive effects were reported in the third trial. No single homeopathic remedy emerged as more effective than another. An additional RCT published since this review found no evidence that homeopathy improves the symptoms of RA over 3 months in patients attending a routine clinic who are stabilised on NSAIDs or anti-rheumatic drugs.[20] Another systematic review found little evidence and concluded that high quality research is needed, especially for herbal treatments and homeopathy.[21]

Hypnotherapy

Most clinical trials on hypnotherapy suggest that it can be useful in pain management. In particular, pain perception seems to be influenced positively.[22] However, no rigorous RCTs exist specifically for RA.

Magnets

Two RCTs tested the effects of magnets for patients with RA.[23,24] Both trials reported encouraging results for pain relief. Further independent replication is required before any firm recommendations can be made.

Relaxation

Several relaxation techniques are being advocated for RA. Muscle relaxation training was demonstrated to be superior to no intervention in an RCT with 68 RA patients.[25] Patients received 30 min twice weekly for 10 weeks and subsequently showed improvement in both function and well-being. A systematic review of all RCTs on relaxation for chronic pain arrived at cautiously positive conclusions.[26]

Spa therapy

Balneotherapy for people with arthritis is one of the oldest forms of therapy. A Cochrane review (Box 2.116) concluded that although one cannot ignore the positive findings reported in most studies, there is insufficient evidence to support these.[27] High quality research is needed in this area.

Box 2.116
Systematic review
Balneotherapy for rheumatoid arthritis
Verhagen[27]

- Six RCTs met the inclusion criteria (n = 355)

- Most studies reported positive findings but were methodologically flawed to some extent

- Three studies compared balneotherapy with other forms of baths

- It is concluded that there is insufficient evidence that one type of baths is more effective compared with another type of baths and when compared with other treatments or no treatment

Spiritual healing

Several RCTs of various forms of spiritual healing have been published.[28] The question of whether spiritual healing alleviates arthritic pain more than placebo does not find a uniform answer in these studies. Firm recommendations are therefore not possible at present.

Supplements

Elk velvet antler as an adjunctive treatment to conventional arthritis medications was compared with placebo.[29] There were no difference in terms of effectiveness and adverse events.

Fish oil is rich in the omega-3 fatty acids eicosapentaenoic acid and docosahexaenoic acid which have anti-inflammatory activity through interfering with prostaglandin metabolism. Several RCTs have shown clinical benefit of regular supplementation with fish oil in RA. The results of a meta-analysis suggested a reduction in tender joint counts and in morning stiffness,[30] which is confirmed by additional double-blind RCTs.[31,32] Another RCT reported no clinical benefit over placebo for a supplement containing omega-3 fatty acids.[33] The overall size of the effect seems modest. Interestingly, alpha-linolenic acid (e.g. from **flaxseed oil**), which is the precursor of these omega-3 polyunsaturated fatty acids, does not seem to have the same clinical effects.[34]

Green-lipped mussel (*Perna canaliculus*) was tested in an RCT in which 30 RA patients took either 1150 mg/day green-lipped mussel powder or 210 mg/day lipid extract of the green-lipped mussel;[35] 76% of the patients had a positive clinical response with no difference between the groups. As the trial did not include a placebo control group, it is not possible to determine whether the two treatments were equally ineffective or effective.

A small (n = 21) RCT tested the effects of **probiotics** using Lactobacillus rhamnosus.[36] There were no differences in clinical examination, Health Assessment Questionnaire index, erythrocyte sedimentation rate and C-reactive protein compared with placebo.

In an open pilot study 20 RA patients received 20 mcg or 1000 mcg **selenium** orally for 4 weeks.[37] At the end of this treatment phase both immunological and clinical outcome variables suggested a positive effect. An RCT tested the effects of selenium-enriched yeast and assessed pain, Ritchie index, number of swollen and painful joints and morning stiffness.[38] There were no differences compared with placebo.

Tai chi

A Cochrane review assessed the evidence of tai chi for patients with RA (Box 2.117).[39] It seems that it has no detrimental effects on the disease activity of RA in terms of swollen/tender joints and activities of daily living and there appears to be a clinically important benefit on the range of motion outcomes of ankle plantar flexion. This is largely supported by another systematic review which assessed the effects of Tai chi on various chronic conditions.[40]

Box 2.117
Systematic review
Tai chi for treating rheumatoid arthritis
Han[39]

- Three CCTs and one RCT met the inclusion criteria (n = 206)

- No clinically important effect on most outcomes including activities of daily living, tender and swollen joints and patient global overall rating

- For range of motion participants had clinically important improvements in ankle plantar flexion

- No adverse events were found

- Conclusion: Tai chi does not exacerbate symptoms of rheumatoid arthritis. In addition, it has benefits on lower extremity range of motion, in particular ankle range of motion

Other therapies

An observational study suggested that **aromatherapy** massage increases the well-being of patients with RA.[41] Children with juvenile RA received **massage** therapy from their parents 15 minutes daily for 30 days.[42] Subsequently, a decrease in self-reported and physician-assessed pain was noted. RCTs of **vedic vibration technology**[43] and the TCM treatment of softening and lubricating the joints[44] reported some positive results. Some encouraging but mostly anecdotal evidence exists to suggest that **yoga** might benefit RA patients.[45] Unfortunately this hypothesis has so far not been tested in rigorous clinical trials.

Overall recommendation

No disease-modifying complementary treatment of RA exists. The evidence for CAM as a symptomatic therapy is mixed. Given the high rates of adverse effects of synthetic drugs used for RA, the following CAM modalities would seem to be reasonable therapeutic options: Phytodolor, thunder god vine, fish oil, and tai chi. With all of these therapies the effect size is usually moderate to small. Thus such CAM treatments would normally be reasonable adjuvant treatments rather than true therapeutic alternatives.

Table 2.68
Summary of clinical evidence for rheumatoid arthritis

Treatment	Weight of evidence	Direction of evidence	Serious safety concerns
Acupuncture	OO	⇨	Yes (see p 294)
Diet	OOO	⇧	Yes (see p 5)
Fasting & vegetarianism	OO	⇧	Yes (see p 5)
Herbal medicine			
Ayurvedic mixtures	OOO	⇘	Yes (see p 5)
Boswellia serrata	O	⇘	Yes (see p 479)
Feverfew	O	⇘	Yes (see p 396)
Garlic	O	⇗	Yes (see p 390)
Gamma-linolenic acid (e.g. Borage)	OO	⇗	Yes (see p 476)
Phytodolor	OOO	⇧	Yes (see p 5)
Thunder god vine	OO	⇧	Yes (see p 5)
Tong luo kai bi	O	⇗	Yes (see p 5)
Uncaria tomentosa	O	⇗	Yes (see p 477)
Willow bark	O	⇘	Yes (see p 472)
Homeopathy	OO	⇨	No (see p 327)
Hypnotherapy	O	⇨	Yes (see p 331)
Magnets	OO	⇗	No (see p 359)
Relaxation	OO	⇗	No (see p 348)
Spa therapy	OO	⇗	No (see p 5)
Spiritual healing	OO	⇨	No (see p 351)
Supplements			
Elk velvet antler	O	⇘	Yes (see p 5)
Fish oil	OOO	⇗	Yes (see p 483)
Flaxseed oil (alpha-linoleic acid)	O	⇩	Yes (see p 478)
Green-lipped mussel	O	⇨	Yes (see p 483)
Probiotics	O	⇘	Yes (see p 5)
Selenium	OO	⇨	Yes (see p 484)
Tai chi	OO	⇧	No (see p 354)

CONDITIONS

REFERENCES

1 Resch K L, Hill S, Ernst E. Use of complementary therapies by individuals with 'arthritis'. Clin Rheumatol 1997;16:391–395

2 Casimiro L, Brosseau L, Milne S, Robinson V, Wells G, Tugwell P. Acupuncture and electroacupuncture for the treatment of RA. Cochrane Database Syst Rev 2002;3: CD003788

3 Müller H, de Toledo FW, Resch KL. Fasting followed by vegetarian diet in patients with rheumatoid arthritis: a systematic review. Scand J Rheumatol 2001;30:1–10.

4 Kjeldsen-Kragh J. Rheumatoid arthritis treated with vegetarian diets. Am J Clin Nutr 1999;70:594S–600S

5 Hafstrom I, Ringertz B, Spangberg A, von Zweigbergk L, Brannemark S, Nylander I, Ronnelid J, Laasonen L, Klareskog L. A vegan diet free of gluten improves the signs and symptoms of rheumatoid arthritis: the effects on arthritis correlate with a reduction in antibodies to food antigens. Rheumatology (Oxford) 2001;40:1175–1179

6 Skoldstam L, Hagfors L, Johansson G. An experimental study of a Mediterranean diet intervention for patients with rheumatoid arthritis. Ann Rheum Dis 2003;62:208–214

7 Park J, Ernst E. Ayurvedic medicine for rheumatoid arthritis: a systematic review. Semin Arthritis Rheum 2005;34:705–713

8 Little C V, Parsons T. Herbal therapy for treating rheumatoid arthritis. The Cochrane Database of Systematic Reviews 2000, Issue 4. Art. No.: CD002948

9 Soeken K L, Miller S A, Ernst E. Herbal medicines for the treatment of rheumatoid arthritis: a systematic review. Rheumatology (Oxford) 2003;42:652–659

10 Ernst E. The efficacy of phytodolor for the treatment of musculoskeletal pain – a systematic review of randomized clinical trials. J Natural Med 1999;2:3–8

11 Tao X L, Sun Y, Dong Y, Xiao Y L, Hu D W, Shi Y P, Zhu Q L, Dai H, Zhang N Z. A prospective, controlled, double-blind, cross-over study of tripterygium wilfordii hook F in treatment of rheumatoid arthritis. Chin Med J 1989;102:327–332

12 Li R L, Liu P L, Wu X C. Clinical and experimental study on sustained release tablet of Tripterygium wilfordii in treating rheumatoid arthritis. Chung-Kuo Chung Hsi I Chieh Ho Tsa Chih 1996;16:10–13

13 Cibere J, Deng Z, Lin Y, Ou R, He Y, Wang Z, Thorne A, Lehman A J, Tsang I K, Esdaile J M. A randomized double blind, placebo controlled trial of topical Tripterygium wilfordii in rheumatoid arthritis: reanalysis using logistic regression analysis. J Rheumatol 2003;30:465–467

14 Tao X, Younger J, Fan F Z, Wang B, Lipsky P E. Benefit of an extract of Tripterygium Wilfordii Hook F in patients with rheumatoid arthritis: a double-blind, placebo-controlled study. Arthritis Rheum 2002;46:1735–1743

15 Mur E, Hartig F, Eibl G, Schirmer M. Randomized double blind trial of an extract from the pentacyclic alkaloid-chemotype of uncaria tomentosa for the treatment of rheumatoid arthritis. J Rheumatol 2002;29:678–681

16 Denisov L N, Andrianova I V, Timofeeva S S. Garlic effectiveness in rheumatoid arthritis. Tereapevticheskii Arkhiv 1999;71:55–58

17 Shi Y, Zhang H, Du X, Zhang M, Yin Y, Zhou C, Song S, Fu X, Li S, Liu Y, Li H, Li X, Wu X, Zhu Y. A double blind observation for therapeutic effects of the tong luo kai bi tablets on rheumatoid arthritis. J Tradit Chin Med 1999;19:166–172

18 Biegert C, Wagner I, Lüdtke R, Kotter I, Lohmüller C, Gunaydin I, Taxis K, Heide L. Efficacy and safety of willow bark extract in the treatment of osteoarthritis and rheumatoid arthritis: results of 2 randomized double-blind controlled trials. J Rheumatol 2004;31:2121–2130

19 Jonas W, Linde L, Ramirez G. Homeopathy and rheumatic disease. Rheum Dis Clin North Am 2000;26:117–123

20 Fisher P, Scott D L. A randomized controlled trial of homeopathy in rheumatoid arthritis. Rheumatology (Oxford) 2001;40:1052–1055

21 Soeken K L. Selected CAM therapies for arthritis-related pain: the evidence from systematic reviews. Clin J Pain 2004;20:13–18

22 Weissenberg M. Cognitive aspects of pain and pain control. Int J Clin Exper Hypnosis 1998;46:44–61

23 Usichenko T I, Ivashkivsky O I, Gizhko V V. Treatment of rheumatoid arthritis with electromagnetic millimeter waves applied to acupuncture points – a randomized double blind clinical study. Acupunct Electrother Res 2003;28:11–18

24 Segal N A, Toda Y, Huston J, Saeki Y, Shimizu M, Fuchs H, Shimaoka Y, Holcomb R, McLean M J. Two configurations of static magnetic fields for treating rheumatoid arthritis of the knee: a double-blind clinical trial. Arch Phys Med Rehabil 2001;82:1453–1460

25 Lundgren S, Stenstrom C H. Muscle relaxation training and quality of life in rheumatoid arthritis. A randomized controlled clinical trial. Scand J Rheumatol 1999;28:47–53

26 Carroll D, Seers K. Relaxation for the relief of chronic pain: a systematic review. J Adv Nurs 1998;27:476–487

27 Verhagen A P, Bierma-Zeinstra S M A, Cardoso J R, de Bie R A, Boers M, de Vet H C W. Balneotherapy for rheumatoid arthritis. The Cochrane Database of Systematic Reviews 2004, Issue 1. Art. No.: CD000518

28 Astin J A, Harkness E, Ernst E. The efficacy of 'distant healing': a systematic review of randomized trials. Ann Intern Med 2000;132:903–910

29 Allen M, Oberle K, Grace M, Russell A. Elk velvet antler in rheumatoid arthritis: phase II trial. Biol Res Nurs 2002;3:111–118

30 Fortin P R, Lew RA, Liang M H, Wright E A, Beckett L A, Chalmers T C, Sperling R I. Validation of a meta-analysis: the effects of fish oil in rheumatoid arthritis. J Clin Epidemiol 1995;48:1379 1390

31 Volker D, Fitzgerald P, Major G, Garg M. Efficacy of fish oil concentrate in the treatment of rheumatoid arthritis. J Rheumatol 2000;27:2343–2346

32 Berbert A A, Kondo C R, Almendra C L, Matsuo T, Dichi I. Supplementation of fish oil and olive oil in patients with rheumatoid arthritis. Nutrition 2005;21:131–136

33 Remans P H, Sont J K, Wagenaar L W, Wouters-Wesseling W, Zuijderduin W M, Jongma A, Breedveld F C, Van Laar J M. Nutrient supplementation with polyunsaturated fatty acids and micronutrients in rheumatoid arthritis: clinical and biochemical effects. Eur J Clin Nutr 2004;58:839–845

34 Nordstrom D C E, Honkanen V E A, Nasu Y, Antila E, Friman C, Konttinen Y T. Alpha-linolenic acid in the treatment of rheumatoid arthritis: a double-blind, placebo-controlled and randomized study: flaxseed vs safflower seed. Rheumatol Int 1995;14:231–234

35 Gibson S L M, Gibson R G. The treatment of arthritis with a lipid extract of Perna canaliculus: a randomized trial. Complement Ther Med 1998;6:122–126

36 Hatakka K, Martio J, Korpela M, Herranen M, Poussa T, Laasanen T, Saxelin M, Vapaatalo H, Moilanen E, Korpela R. Effects of probiotic therapy on the activity and activation of mild rheumatoid arthritis–a pilot study. Scand J Rheumatol 2003;32:211–215

37 Maleitzke R, Gottl K H. Treatment of rheumatoid arthritis with selenium. Therapicwoche 1996;46:1529–1532

38 Peretz A, Siderova V, Neve J. Selenium supplementation in rheumatoid arthritis investigated in a double blind, placebo-controlled trial. Scand J Rheumatol 2001;30:208–212

39 Han A, Judd M G, Robinson V A, Taixiang W, Tugwell P, Wells G. Tai chi for treating rheumatoid arthritis. The Cochrane Database of Systematic Reviews 2004, Issue 3. Art. No.: CD004849

40 Wang C, Collet J P, Lau J. The effect of Tai Chi on health outcomes in patients with chronic conditions: a systematic review. Arch Intern Med 2004;164:493–501

41 Brownfield A. Aromatherapy in arthritis: a study. Nurs Standard 1998;13:34–35

42 Field T, Hernandez-Reif M, Seligman S, Krasnegor J, Sunshine W, Rivas-Chacon R, Schanberg S, Kuhn C. Juvenile rheumatoid arthritis: benefits from massage therapy. J Paediatr Psychol 1997;22:607–617

43 Nader T A, Smith D E, Dillbeck M C, Schanbacher V, Dillbeck S L, Gallois P, Beall-Rougerie S, Schneider R H, Nidich S I, Kaplan G P, Belok S. A double blind randomized controlled trial of Maharishi Vedic vibration technology in subjects with arthritis. Front Biosci 2001;6:H7–H17

44 Yang W, Ouyang J, Zhu K, Zhou S, Peng Z. TCM treatment for 40 cases of rheumatoid arthritis with channel blockage due to yin deficiency. J Tradit Chin Med 2003;23:172–174

45 Haslock I, Monro R, Nagarathna R, Nagendra H R, Raghuram N V. Measuring the effects of yoga in rheumatoid arthritis. Br J Rheumatol 1994;33:787–788

CONDITIONS

SMOKING CESSATION

Synonyms/ subcategories	Nicotine withdrawal, nicotine dependence.
Definition	Desire or need to stop smoking.
CAM usage	Acupuncture and hypnotherapy are common CAM therapies used for smoking cessation.

Clinical evidence

Acupuncture

A systematic review strongly suggested that the effects of acupuncture do not go beyond those of a placebo (Box 2.118).[1]

Box 2.118
Meta-analysis
Acupuncture for smoking cessation
White[1]

- Twenty-two RCTs
- Quality varied from poor to good
- Variety of acupuncture techniques used
- Acupuncture was not superior to sham acupuncture at any time point. The odds ratio for immediate outcomes was 1.22 (CI 0.99 to 1.49)
- No single technique was superior to another method of acupuncture
- Conclusion: No evidence that acupuncture is effective

Electrostimulation

A total of 101 smokers were randomised to daily electrostimulation for 5 days or placebo stimulation.[2] There was no difference between the groups in terms of withdrawal symptoms or successful cessation.

Exercise

A systematic review of 11 RCTs of exercise as an adjunct to a smoking cessation programme generated encouraging but not conclusive evidence (Box 2.119).[3]

Box 2.119
Systematic review
Exercise-based interventions for smoking cessation
Ussher[3]

- Eleven RCTs of exercise as an adjunct to a smoking cessation programme
- Control groups received multisession cognitive–behavioural programme only
- Six trials had fewer than 25 people in each treatment arm
- Three studies suggested positive effects in terms of abstinence rates
- Conclusion: limited evidence that exercise might help

Group behaviour therapy

A systematic review suggested that group behaviour therapy programmes can help smokers to quit (Box 2.120).[4]

- Fifty-two RCTs were included

- Quality was mixed but good for some RCTs

- Group programmes were more effective than self-help programmes (n = 4395)

- Group programmes were more effective than no intervention (n = 7750)

- Group programmes were not more effective than individual counselling

- Conclusion: group behaviour therapy is supported by good evidence

Hypnotherapy

There are many anecdotal reports of individuals stopping smoking with the help of hypnotherapy and rates of abstinence achieved in uncontrolled studies vary between 4% and 88%. A systematic review found no reliable evidence that hypnotherapy is more effective for smoking cessation than the various control methods, which are themselves unproven (Box 2.121).[5]

- Nine RCTs comparing hypnotherapy with a variety of control procedures in 677 smokers, follow-up period of 6 months

- Quality poor: no validation of successful cessation

- Different methods and regimens of hypnotherapy

- Conflicting results when compared with no treatment or advice

- Conclusion: no evidence of effectiveness when compared with rapid smoking or other psychological treatment

Massage

An RCT compared self-massage to no such treatment in 20 smokers.[6] Positive effects were noted on withdrawal symptoms, number of cigarettes smoked and mood. However, cessation rates were not reported.

Relaxation

Relaxation has not been rigorously investigated for smoking cessation itself, but an RCT tested the effect of relaxation with imagery on relapse prevention in 76 recently successful participants in a smoking cessation programme. Relaxation imagery over the following 3 months resulted in reduced stress and improved abstinence, compared with no additional treatment.[7]

Other therapies
The use of **restricted environmental stimulation therapy** (REST) involving 12- or 24-hour residence in special chambers with repeated recorded messages has produced quit rates of 20% or more in smokers in uncontrolled studies (e.g.[8]), but no controlled studies are available. A similar therapy involving time spent with restricted sensory input in **flotation** tanks showed no benefit compared with various control methods.[9]

Overall recommendation

Conventional techniques of smoking cessation achieve higher quit rates than anything CAM has to offer. Group behaviour therapy is effective and exercise may prove to be a valuable adjunct. Many would, however, regard both as orthodox therapies. Patients should be advised to consider these options to complement other mainstream medical treatments.

Table 2.69
Summary of clinical evidence for smoking cessation

Treatment	Weight of evidence	Direction of evidence	Serious safety concerns
Acupuncture	OOO	⇩	Yes (see p 294)
Electrostimulation	O	⇩	Yes (see p 5)
Exercise	OO	⬈	Yes (see p 5)
Group behaviour therapy	OOO	⇧	No (see p 5)
Hypnotherapy	OO	⇩	Yes (see p 331)
Massage	O	⇧	No (see p 334)
Relaxation	O	⇧	No (see p 348)

REFERENCES

1 White AR, Rampes H, Ernst E. Acupuncture for smoking cessation. The Cochrane Database of Systematic Reviews 2002, Issue 2. Art. No.: CD000009

2 Pickworth W B, Fant R V, Butschky M F, Goffman A L, Henningfield J E. Evaluation of cranial electrostimulation therapy on short-term smoking cessation. Biol Psychiatr 1997;42:116–121

3 Ussher M, West R, Taylor A, McEwen A. Exercise interventions for smoking cessation. The Cochrane

Database of Systematic Reviews 2005, Issue 1 Art. No:. CD002295

4 Stead L F, Lancaster T. Group behaviour therapy programmes for smoking cessation. The Cochrane Database of Systematic Reviews 2002, Issue 3. Art No: CD001007

5 Abbot N C, Stead L F, White A R, Barnes J. Hypnotherapy for smoking cessation. The Cochrane Database of Systematic Reviews 1998, Issue 2. Art. No.: CD001008

6 Hernandez-Reif M, Field T, Hart S. Smoking cravings are reduced by self-massage. Prev Med 1999;28:28–32

7 Wynd C A. Relaxation imagery used for stress reduction in the prevention of smoking relapse. J Adv Nurs 1992;17:294–302

8 Suedfeld P, Baker-Brown G. Restricted environmental stimulation therapy of smoking: a parametric study. Addict Behav 1987;12:263–267

9 Forgays D G. Flotation rest as a smoking intervention. Addict Behav 1987;12:85–90

STROKE

Synonyms/ subcategories	Apoplexy, cerebral infarct, cerebral infarction, cerebral thrombosis, cerebral haemorrhage, cerebral embolism, cerebrovascular accident, intracranial haemorrhage, subarachnoid haemorrhage.
Definition	A clinical syndrome characterised by rapidly developing symptoms and/or signs of focal and sometimes global loss of cerebral function, with symptoms lasting more than 24 hours or leading to death and with no apparent cause other than that of vascular origin.
Related conditions	Reversible ischaemic neurological deficit, transient ischaemic attack.
CAM usage	In Western medicine, no single form of CAM is in particularly common use for the management of stroke recovery. In Eastern medicine, acupuncture and Chinese herbs are widely used.

Clinical evidence

Acupuncture

A systematic review (Box 2.122) located several studies which found that acupuncture was superior to no additional therapy, but placebo-controlled RCTs suggest that this effect may not be specifically due to needling but to other factors such as the extra attention received.[1] RCTs published since that report generated both positive[2–4] and negative results,[5–7] but the negative studies tended to be of higher methodological rigour. RCTs specifically aimed at testing whether acupuncture reduces post-stroke leg spasticity found both no evidence for such an effect[8] as well as encouraging results.[9] A further RCT suggested that electro-acupuncture can be an effective adjunctive treatment for post-stroke shoulder subluxation.[10]

Box 2.122
Systematic review
Acupuncture for stroke
Park[1]

- Nine RCTs involving 538 patients with acute, subacute or chronic stroke

- Only two studies were of good quality

- Six studies suggested that acupuncture is effective: the two good-quality studies were negative

- Conclusion: evidence is suggestive but far from compelling

CONDITIONS

Diet

Diets that are cardioprotective, e.g. high intake of fruit and vegetables, complex carbohydrates and oily fish or the Mediterranean diet, are also protective against stroke (e.g.[11]). Vegetarians had a lower death rate from all causes, including cerebrovascular disease, than non-vegetarians in a cohort of 11 000 health-conscious British people followed up for 17 years.[12] In the Framingham Study,[13] a cohort of 832 healthy men experienced a decrease in the risk of stroke with increased vegetable and fruit intake.

A systematic review (Box 2.123)[14] found a convincing inverse correlation between vitamin C intake or blood marker of vitamin C intake and death from stroke (in contrast to a negative association with coronary artery disease). One possible mechanism could be a modest anti-hypertensive effect.

Box 2.123
Systematic review
Dietary vitamin C for stroke
Ness[14]

- Studies quantifying dietary intake of vitamin C or measuring biological markers of vitamin C status

- Two epidemiological studies found strong correlation

- One case–control study (47 cases, 44 controls) found no correlation

- Seven prospective cohort studies (110 506 persons); two found protective association

- Conclusion: the evidence suggests a protective effect: caution because of the limitations of nature, duration and accuracy of these data

An RCT of 459 hypertensive adults found that increasing the intake of fruits and vegetables lowered blood pressure, though not as much as a diet both rich in fruit and vegetables and low in fats.[15] A retrospective epidemiological study found a slightly higher incidence of stroke in men with the highest level of reported fish consumption.[16]

Herbal medicine

Dan shen is a form of herbal medicine widely used for treating acute stroke in China. A systematic review (Box 2.124) found no conclusive evidence for its effectiveness.[17] A subsequent systematic review found no evidence that Dan shen may be beneficial in improving disability after an acute ischaemic stroke.[18]

Garlic (*Allium sativum*) is known to have a modest effect on serum cholesterol concentrations and is believed to reduce platelet aggregation. Its role in stroke prevention has never been tested clinically. However, encouraging results were obtained in a placebo-controlled RCT in 60 adolescent volunteers with increased platelet aggregation who were at risk of cerebral ischaemic episodes.[19]

Box 2.124
Systematic review
Dan shen for acute stroke
Wu[17]

- Three RCTs or quasi-randomised trials involving 304 patients with acute stroke

- All studies were of poor quality

- All trials reported improvement in neurological deficit

- No adverse effects were noted

- Conclusion: no reliable conclusion can be drawn from this data

In a placebo controlled RCT in 50 patients with cerebral insufficiency following surgery for subarachnoid haemorrhage, **ginkgo** (*Ginkgo biloba*) at a dose of 150 mg per day for 12 weeks produced improvements in attention, reaction time and short-term memory.[20] An intravenous preparation of ginkgo was given to 20 patients in an observational study in acute stroke;[21] ten patients recovered completely or almost completely.

Homeopathy
Two double-blind RCTs of homeopathic **arnica** (*Arnica montana*) given immediately after stroke found no difference in mortality, survival or functioning over a 3-month period in comparison with placebo.[22,23]

Imagery
Two small RCTs tested imagery during stroke rehabilitation. Both found encouraging effects on functional recovery.[24,25]

Meditation
Transcendental meditation may lower mild hypertension (e.g.[26]), though a review concluded that earlier positive claims were based on studies which found little difference between meditation and sham techniques.[27] In one RCT comparing meditation with relaxation in 73 elderly persons, meditation was associated with lower blood pressure and improved survival at 3 years, from a figure of 65% for the relaxation group to 100% for the meditation group.[28] The study did not record death from stroke itself. An RCT in which 138 hypertensive subjects either learnt transcendental meditation or received standard health education found that, in those who meditated for at least 6–9 months, the thickness of the intimal lining of the carotid arteries was reduced, compared with controls.[29]

Supplements
In a large RCT in Italy involving 11 324 patients who had survived recent myocardial infarction, supplementation with **n-3**

polyunsaturated fatty acids (PUFA) produced a clinically relevant decline in cardiovascular deaths including stroke.[30]

In an RCT among 29 584 Chinese, principally aimed at reducing cancer rates, supplementation with a combination of **selenium**, **vitamin A** and **vitamin E** was found to be associated with a lower incidence of stroke over 5 years.[31] The bioavailability of selenium is often low in Western diets.[32]

Other therapies

Listening to **music** with a strong rhythmic pulse can be set to match gait tempo in order to improve rehabilitation. Measurements of gastrocnemius EMG show improvements in laboratory studies but no CCTs are available.[33] A small RCT found encouraging effects on functional recovery of subacute stroke patients after **Reiki** treatments.[34]

Overall recommendation

Admission to a specialist stroke unit is known to improve the outcome after acute stroke. Since no individual conventional therapy has been demonstrated unequivocally to improve rehabilitation, it may be a matter of personal preference and individual judgement whether to use those CAM therapies that are associated with encouraging results. The additional attention given as part of an individualised, hands-on treatment may in itself act as a stimulant and aid recovery. Diets high in vegetables, fruits and fish intake can be recommended, together with supplementation by selenium where dietary intake of this mineral is insufficient as preventive measures.

Table 2.70
Summary of clinical evidence for stroke

Treatment	Weight of evidence	Direction of evidence	Serious safety concerns
Acupuncture	OOO	⇨	Yes (see p 294)

Diets
  Vegetarian
  (prevention)
	O	⤴	No (see p 5)

Herbal medicine
  Dan shen
  Garlic (prevention)
  Ginkgo
	
	O
	O
	O
		
		⇨
		⤴
		⤴
			
			Yes (see p 5)
			Yes (see p 398)
			Yes (see p 404)

Homeopathy	O	⇩	No (see p 327)
Imagery	O	⤴	No (see p 359)
Meditation	O	⤴	Yes (see p 338)

Supplements
  n3-PUFA
  (prevention)
  Vitamin E
	
	O
	
	OOO
		
		⇧
		
		⤴
			
			No (see p 5)
			
			Yes (see p 5)

REFERENCES

1 Park J, Hopwood V, White A R, Ernst E. Effectiveness of acupuncture for stroke: a systematic review. J Neurol 2001;248:558–563

2 Li J Y, Peng Y Z, Yang F. [Clinical observation on effect of tongnao huoluo acupuncture therapy in treating acute cerebral infarction at ultra-early or acute stage] Zhongguo Zhong Xi Yi Jie He Za Zhi 2003;23:736–739 [Article in Chinese]

3 Fang B, Zhou S, Wang S, Sun G. Clinical study on the needling and drug treatment of acute cerebral hemorrhage. J Tradit Chin Med 2003;23:191–192

4 Pei J, Sun L, Chen R, Zhu T, Qian Y, Yuan D. The effect of electro-acupuncture on motor function recovery in patients with acute cerebral infarction: a randomly controlled trial. J Tradit Chin Med 2001;21:270–272

5 Johansson B B, Haker E, von Arbin M, Britton M, Langstrom G, Terent A, Ursing D, Asplund K; Swedish Collaboration on Sensory Stimulation After Stroke. Acupuncture and transcutaneous nerve stimulation in stroke rehabilitation: a randomized, controlled trial. Stroke 2001;32:707–713

6 Sze F K, Wong E, Yi X, Woo J. Does acupuncture have additional value to standard poststroke motor rehabilitation? Stroke 2002;33:186–194

7 Schuler M S, Durdak C, Hösl N M, Klink A, Hauer K A, Oster P. Acupuncture treatment of geriatric patients with ischemic stroke: a randomized, double-controlled, single-blind study. J Am Geriatr Soc 2005;53:549–550

8 Fink M, Rollnik J D, Bijak M, Borstadt C, Dauper J, Guergueltcheva V, Dengler R, Karst M. Needle acupuncture in chronic poststroke leg spasticity. Arch Phys Med Rehabil 2004; 85:667–672

9 Moon S K, Whang Y K, Park S U, Ko C N, Kim Y S, Bae H S, Cho K H. Antispastic effect of electroacupuncture and moxibustion in stroke patients. Am J Chin Med 2003;31:467–474

10 Chen C H, Chen T W, Weng M C, Wang W T, Wang Y L, Huang M H. The effect of electroacupuncture on shoulder subluxation for stroke patients. Kaohsiung J Med Sci 2000;16:525–532

11 Bradley S, Shinton R. Why is there an association between eating fruit and vegetables and a lower risk of stroke? J Human Nutr Dietet 1998;11:363–372

12 Key T J A, Thorogood M, Appleby P N, Burr M L. Dietary habits and mortality in 1100 vegetarians and health conscious people: results of a 17 year follow up. BMJ 1996;313:775–779

13 Gillman M W, Cupples A, Gagnon-D, Posner B M, Ellison R C, Castelli W P, Wolf P A. Protective effect of fruits and vegetables on development of stroke in men. JAMA 1995;273:1113–1117

14 Ness A R, Powles J W, Khaw K T. Vitamin C and cardiovascular disease: a systematic review. J Cardiovasc Risk 1996;3:513–521

15 Appel L J, Moore T J, Obarzanek E, Vollmer W M, Svetkey L P, Sacks F M, Bray G A, Vogt T M, Cutler J A, Windhauser M M, Lin P H, Karanja N. A clinical trial of the effects of dietary patterns on blood pressure. DASH Collaborative Research Group. N Engl J Med 1997;336:1117–1124

16 Orencia A J, Daviglus M L, Dyer A R, Shekelle R B, Stamler J. Fish consumption and stroke in men: 30-year findings of the Chicago Western Electric Study. Stroke 1996;27:204–209

17 Wu B, Liu M, Zhang S. Dan Shen agents for acute ischaemic stroke. The Cochrane Database of Systematic Reviews 2002, Issue 3. Art. No.: CD004295

18 Sze K K H, Yeung F F, Wong E, Lau J. Does Danshen improve disability after acute ischaemic stroke? Acta Neurol Scand 2005;111:118–125

19 Kiesewetter H, Jung F, Jung E M, Mroweitz C, Koscielny J, Wenzel E. Effect of garlic on platelet aggregation in patients with increased risk of juvenile ischemic attack. Eur J Clin Pharmacol 1993;45:333–336

20 Maier-Hauff K. LI 1370 nach zerebraler Aneurysma-Operation. Münch Med Wochenschr 1991;133(suppl 1):S34–S37

21 Buttner T, Ruhmann S, Przuntek H. The treatment of acute cerebral ischemia. Ginkgo: free radical scavenger and PAF antagonist. Therapiewoche 1994;44:1394–1396

22 Savage R H, Roe P F. A double blind trial to assess the benefit of Arnica montana in acute stroke illness. Br Homeopath J 1977;66:207–220

23 Savage R H, Roe P F. A further double-blind trial to assess the benefit of Arnica montana in acute stroke illness. Br Homeopath J 1978;67:210–222

24 Page S J, Levine P, Sisto S, Johnston M V. A randomized efficacy and feasibility study of imagery in acute stroke. Clin Rehabil 2001;15:233–240

25 Liu K P, Chan C C, Lee T M, Hui-Chan C W. Mental imagery for promoting relearning for people after stroke: a randomized controlled trial. Arch Phys Med Rehabil 2004;85:1403–1408

CONDITIONS

26 Wenneberg S R, Schneider R H, Walton K G, Maclean C R, Levitsky D K, Salerno J W, Wallace R K, Mandarino J V, Rainforth M V, Waziri R. A controlled study of the effects of transcendental meditation programme on cardiovascular reactivity and ambulatory blood pressure. Int J Neurosci 1997;89:15–28

27 Eisenberg D M, Delbanco T L, Berkey C S, Kaptchuk T J, Kupelnick B, Kuhl J, Chalmers T C. Cognitive behavioral techniques for hypertension: are they effective? Ann Intern Med 1993;118:964–972

28 Alexander C N, Langer E J, Newman R I, Chandler H M, Davies J L. Transcendental meditation, mindfulness, and longevity: an experimental study with the elderly. J Pers Soc Psychol 1989;57:950–964

29 Castillo-Richmond A, Schneider R H, Alexander C N, Cook R, Myers H, Nidich S, Haney C, Rainforth M, Salerno J. Effects of stress reduction on carotid atherosclerosis in hypertensive African Americans. Stroke 2000;31:568–573

30 GSSI Investigators (Gruppo Italiano per lo Studio della Sopravvivenza nell'Infarto miocardico). Dietary supplementation with n-3 polyunsaturated fatty acids and vitamin E after myocardial infarction: results of the GISSI-Prevenzione trial. Lancet 1999;354: 447–455.

31 Mark S D, Wang W, Fraumeni J F Jr, Li J Y, Taylor P R, Wang G Q, Dawsey S M, Li B, Blot WJ. Do nutritional supplements lower the risk of stroke or hypertension? Epidemiology 1998;9:9–15

32 Rayman M P. Dietary selenium: time to act. BMJ 1997;314:387–388

33 Purdie H. Music therapy in neurorehabilitation: recent developments and new challenges. Crit Rev Phys Med Rehabil 1997;9:205–217

34 Shiflett S C, Nayak S, Bid C, Miles P, Agostinelli S. Effect of Reiki treatments on functional recovery in patients in poststroke rehabilitation: a pilot study. J Altern Complement Med 2002;8:755–763

TINNITUS

Definition

The perception of sound which does not arise from the external environment, nor from within the body, nor from auditory hallucination.

CAM usage

According to a Swedish survey, tinnitus sufferers frequently try acupuncture and relaxation.[1]

Clinical evidence

Acupuncture

A systematic review[2] of six RCTs of acupuncture or electro-acupuncture found no convincing evidence of effectiveness (Box 2.125). Two open trials comparing acupuncture with other interventions reported some beneficial effects, but four sham-controlled trials had negative results. Methodological limitations restrict the conclusiveness of the results but current evidence suggests that acupuncture has no specific benefit in tinnitus.

Box 2.125
Systematic review
Acupuncture for tinnitus
Park[2]

- Six RCTs including 185 patients
- Trials of acupuncture (n = 4) and electroacupuncture (n = 2)
- Trial quality generally low
- Four sham-controlled trials had negative results
- Conclusion: efficacy is not sufficiently demonstrated

Biofeedback

Positive results for biofeedback have been reported in RCTs when compared with no treatment,[3] sham feedback[4] and other treatments.[4,5] However, another RCT (n = 26) found no difference between groups receiving biofeedback, 'counterdemand' biofeedback (where patients were told to expect no treatment for the first 5 weeks) or no treatment.[6] The lack of rigour of most studies along with inconsistent results prevents conclusions about the efficacy of biofeedback for tinnitus.

Herbal medicine

Several traditional Chinese herbal formulae have generated encouraging results in CCTs or RCTs.[7,8] These results require independent confirmation in rigorous clinical trials.

A systematic review of five RCTs of **ginkgo** (*Ginkgo biloba*) compared with placebo or pharmacologic treatment concluded that the evidence was favourable, but not fully conclusive, due to a small number of trials and methodological limitations (Box 2.126).[9] A Cochrane review applied stricter entry criteria and therefore included only two RCTs. The authors found no evidence that ginkgo was effective for tinnitus,[10] a conclusion confirmed by a further systematic review.[11]

Box 2.126
Systematic review
Ginkgo for tinnitus
Ernst[9]

- Five RCTs including 541 patients
- Methodological quality generally mixed
- Results consistently positive with one exception that used low dose of ginkgo
- Conclusion: Evidence is favourable, but not fully conclusive

Homeopathy

A double-blind RCT (n = 28) of a homeopathic remedy called 'Tinnitus' found no superiority over placebo for intensity or intrusiveness of tinnitus or audiological measures.[12]

Hypnotherapy

Three RCTs have suggested that hypnotherapy or self-hypnosis is comparable or superior to counselling or masking interventions in reducing subjective tinnitus symptoms (Table 2.71).[13-15] Taking into account some methodological limitations, the evidence can be considered encouraging.

Relaxation

RCTs have suggested that relaxation training may be superior to no treatment[16,17] and as effective as cognitive techniques,[18,19] but in most cases placebo effects can not be discounted. In one

Table 2.71   **RCTs of hypnotherapy for tinnitus**

Reference	Sample size	Interventions [regimen]	Result	Comment
Attias[13]	36	A) Self-hypnosis [4 × 50 min] B) Auditory stimulus C) Waiting list	Tinnitus totally disappeared in 73% of A and 24% of B	Audiological tests showed no change
Attias[14]	45	A) Self-hypnosis [50 min per w for 5 w] B) Masking C) Attention control	Improvement in tinnitus severity with A, partial with C and none with B	No analysis of intergroup differences
Mason[15]	86	A) Hypnotherapy [three sessions] B) Counselling [one session]	A no different from B on tinnitus severity or loudness but superior on sense of improvement	More therapist contact with hypnosis

trial (n = 30) the improvements with two forms of relaxation were no different from that of the control group.[20] On balance the evidence seems to suggest that relaxation may reduce the annoyance of tinnitus, but benefits appear to be quite modest and short term.

Supplements

A double-blind crossover RCT (n = 30) of **melatonin** found no overall superiority over placebo, although a subgroup analysis indicated better results in patients with bilateral than unilateral tinnitus.[21]

Negative findings for **zinc** supplementation were reported from a double-blind, placebo-controlled RCT with 48 patients.[22] However, patients all had normal serum zinc levels before treatment.

Yoga

Yoga proved much less helpful than cognitive–behavioural therapy and no better than a self-monitoring control group on psychoacoustic measures and symptom ratings in an RCT lasting 3 months with 43 patients.[23]

Overall recommendation   There is no convincing evidence for the efficacy of any complementary therapy. However, given the lack of effective conventional treatment options and the placebo responsiveness observed with tinnitus, therapies that have few risks may be worthy of consideration. Both relaxation and hypnosis are associated with some improvements. Whether Chinese herbal formulae generate more good than harm requires further study.

Table 2.72
Summary of clinical evidence for tinnitus

Treatment	Weight of evidence	Direction of evidence	Serious safety concerns
Acupuncture	OO	↘	Yes (see p 294)
Biofeedback	OO	⇨	No (see p 310)
Herbal medicine			
Ginkgo	OO	↘	Yes (see p 404)
Chinese formulae	O	↗	Yes (see p 5)
Homeopathy	O	⇩	No (see p 327)
Hypnotherapy	OO	↗	Yes (see p 331)
Relaxation	O	↗	No (see p 348)
Supplements			
Melatonin	O	⇩	Yes (see p 435)
Zinc	O	⇩	Yes (see p 5)
Yoga	O	⇩	Yes (see p 356)

REFERENCES

1 Andersson G. Prior treatments in a group of tinnitus sufferers seeking treatment. Psychother Psychosom 1997;66:107–110

2 Park J, White A R, Ernst E. Efficacy of acupuncture as a treatment for tinnitus: a systematic review. Arch Otolaryngol Head Neck Surg 2000;126:489–492

3 White T P, Hoffman S R, Gale E N. Psychophysiological therapy for tinnitus. Ear Hearing 1986;7:397–399

4 Podoshin L, Ben-David Y, Fradis M, Gerstel R, Felner H. Idiopathic subjective tinnitus treated by biofeedback, acupuncture and drug therapy. Ear Nose Throat J 1991;70:284–289

5 Erlandsson S I, Rubinstein B, Carlsson S G. Tinnitus: evaluation of biofeedback and stomatognathic treatment. Br J Audiol 1991;25:151–161

6 Haralambos G, Wilson P H, Platt-Hepworth S, Tonkin J P, Hensley R, Kavanagh D. EMG biofeedback in the treatment of tinnitus: an experimental evaluation. Behav Res Ther 1987;25:49–55

7 Xuan W. The therapeutic effect of Chinese traditional medicine formulas on the treatment of sensorineural tinnitus. Assoc Res Otolaryngol 2003;Abs:926

8 Wang Y J, Zhou H D, Li J C. Clinical observation on effect of yangxue qingnao granule in treating patients with cerebral arteriosclerosis. [Article in Chinese] Zhongguo Zhong Xi Yi Jie He Za Zhi 2004;24:202–204

9 Ernst E, Stevinson C. Ginkgo biloba for tinnitus: a review. Clin Otolaryngol 1999;24:164–167

10 Hilton M, Stuart E. Ginkgo biloba for tinnitus. The Cochrane Database of Systematic Reviews 2004, Issue 2. Art No.: CD003852

11 Rejali D, Sivakumar A, Balaji N. Ginkgo biloba does not benefit patients with tinnitus: a randomized placebo-controlled double blind trial and meta-analysis of randomized trials. Clin Otolaryngol 2004;29:226–231

12 Simpson J J, Donaldson I, Davies W E. Use of homeopathy in the treatment of tinnitus. Br J Audiol 1998;32:227–233

13 Attias J, Shemesh Z, Shoham C, Shahar A, Sohmer H Efficacy of self hypnosis for tinnitus relief. Scand Audiol 1990;19:245–249

14 Attias J, Shemesh Z, Sohmer H, Gold S, Shoham C, Faraggi D. Comparison between self-hypnosis, masking and attentiveness for alleviation of chronic tinnitus. Audiology 1993;32:205–212

15 Mason J D, Rogerson D R, Butler J D. Client centred hypnotherapy in the management of tinnitus – is it better than counselling? J Laryngol Otol 1996;110:117–120

16 Lindberg P, Scott B, Melin L, Lyttkens L. The psychological treatment of tinnitus: an experimental evaluation. Behav Res Ther 1989;27:593–603

CONDITIONS

17 Scott B, Lindberg P, Melin L, Lyttkens L. Psychological treatment of tinnitus. An experimental group study. Scand Audiol 1985;14:223–230

18 Jakes S C, Hallam R S, Rachman S, Hinchcliffe R. The effects of reassurance, relaxation training and distraction on chronic tinnitus sufferers. Behav Res Ther 1986;24:497–507

19 Davies S, McKenna L, Hallam R S. Relaxation and cognitive therapy: a controlled trial in chronic tinnitus. Psychol Health 1995;10:129–143

20 Ireland C E, Wilson P H, Tonkin J P, Platt-Hepworth S. An evaluation of relaxation training in the treatment of tinnitus. Behav Res Ther 1985;23:423–430

21 Rosenberg S I, Silverstein H, Rowan P T, Olds M J. Effect of melatonin on tinnitus. Laryngoscope 1998;108:305–310

22 Paaske P B, Pedersen C B, Kjems G, Sam I L. Zinc in the management of tinnitus. Placebo-controlled trial. Ann Otol Rhinol Laryngol 1991;100:647–649

23 Kroner-Herwig B, Hebing G, Van Rijn-Kalkmann U, Frenzel A, Schilkowsky G, Esser G. The management of chronic tinnitus – comparison of a cognitive–behavioural group training with yoga. J Psychosom Res 1995;39:153–165

ULCERATIVE COLITIS

Synonyms Colitis ulcerosa, inflammatory bowel disease.

Related conditions Crohn's disease.

Definition Ulcerative colitis is an inflammatory bowel disease, which affects the rectum and sometimes the colon. Inflammation and ulcers develop on the inside lining of the colon resulting in urgent and bloody diarrhoea, pain and continual tiredness.

CAM usage Herbal medicines and non-herbal dietary supplements such as ginseng, *Aloe vera* and vitamins are often used. Popular therapies are chiropractic, reflexology and homeopathy.[1–3]

Clinical evidence

Acupuncture
A systematic review identified no prospective clinical studies of acupuncture for ulcerative colitis.[4]

Biofeedback
A systematic review assessed the evidence of biofeedback for gastrointestinal conditions.[5] It identified no controlled trials for treating ulcerative colitis.

Herbal medicine
A double-blind RCT tested the effectiveness of *Aloe vera* for treating patients with mild to moderately active ulcerative colitis.[6] Primary outcome measures were the Simple Clinical Colitis Activity Index and histological scores, which decreased during treatment with *Aloe vera*, but not with placebo.

A systematic review assessed the evidence of *Chlorella pyrenoidosa,* a freshwater green algae rich in proteins, vitamins and minerals.[7] It reported data from nine patients with ulcerative colitis assessed in a double-blind placebo-controlled RCT. The reviewers concluded that the beneficial effects observed warranted larger clinical trials.

Evening primrose (*Oenothera biennis*) oil was compared with eicosapentaenoic acid and placebo.[8] Evening primrose oil improved stool consistency compared with control groups at 6 months of treatment. There was no effect on stool frequency, rectal bleeding, disease relapse, sigmoidoscopic appearance and rectal histology in the three groups.

The Chinese herbal medicine **Jian Pi Ling** was administered with retention enemas of *Sophora flavescentis* radix and Flos sophora and compared with placebo and the same retention enemas and salicylazosulfapyridine with retention enemas of dexamethasone.[9] Treatment with Jian Pi Ling was reported to be more beneficial compared with the control groups.

Three RCTs, two of which were double-blind,[10,12] tested the effects of **psyllium** (*Plantago ovata).* Improvement of symptoms was judged consistently superior to placebo in patients in remission.[10] Psyllium might be as effective as mesalamine to maintain remission.[11] In a comparison with wheat fibre, psyllium was found to be less effective in decreasing the concentration of bile acid in faeces and faecal water.[12]

Patients (n = 23) with active distal ulcerative colitis were treated with **wheat grass** juice in a double-blind placebo controlled RCT.[13] Adjuvant treatment with wheat grass was associated with reductions in the overall disease activity index and in the severity of rectal bleeding.

Relaxation

A systematic review of published RCTs assessed the effects of relaxation for the relief of chronic pain.[14] Only trials of relaxation as monotherapy were considered. It identified data from patients with ulcerative colitis and reported evidence in favour of progressive muscle relaxation compared with waiting list controls.

Supplements

Treatment with probiotics using **bifidobacteria** was tested in four small (n = 18 to 30) RCTs.[15-18] Two trials that assessed patients in remission concluded that the probiotic prevented exacerbations and was successful in maintaining remission. Patients with active ulcerative colitis were included in two other RCTs. In the first, patients received either bifidobacteria-fermented milk in addition to conventional treatment or conventional treatment alone. The disease activity index in patients who received the probiotic was lower compared with patients who received conventional treatment alone. In the second, bifidobacteria were combined with a prebiotic, an inulin-oligofructose growth substrate for the probiotic strain. It was concluded that this treatment led to an improvement of the full clinical appearance of chronic inflammation. In an additional RCT, probiotic treatment reduced the occurrence of pouchitis after ileal pouch–anal anastomosis.[19]

Three large (n = 116 to 327) RCTs assessed whether *Escherichia coli* Nissle 1917 is effective in maintaining remission compared with the gold standard mesalazine.[20–22] Relapse rates were similar in both groups in all three trials. It was concluded that *E. coli* Nissle 1917 shows effectiveness and safety in maintaining remission equivalent to mesalazine.

A non-systematic review assessed the effectiveness of **fish oil** for inflammatory bowel disease.[23] It identified eight placebo-controlled trials of which at least four were RCTs including patients with ulcerative colitis. Patients received omega-3 fatty acids for up to 24 months. It was concluded that the data indicate potential effectiveness in the treatment of ulcerative colitis. Further RCTs published since the review reported mixed results.[24–26] Treatment with omega-3 fatty acids resulted in greater disease activity in a comparison with sulfasalazine,[24] whereas there was a decrease in oxidative stress in patients who received sulfasalazine plus omega-3 fatty acids but no improvement in most laboratory parameters, sigmoidoscopy and histology.[25] Another trial assessed the effectiveness of a combination preparation containing fish oil, fructooligosaccharides, gum arabic, vitamin E, vitamin C, and selenium.[26] It found no difference to placebo on the disease activity index compared with placebo but differences in the dose of prednisone required to control clinical symptoms.

Further evidence from RCTs exist for **folic acid,**[27] a supplement containing **gamma-linolenic acid,**[28] eicosapentaenoic acid and docosahexaenoic acid, and for retention enemas with **Kuijie powder.**[29] The supplement containing gamma-linolenic acid was found to be no different from placebo in relapse rates and sigmoidoscopic findings. For folic acid and Kuijie powder positive results are reported.

Overall recommendation

The evidence is not sufficiently compelling to recommend any CAM therapy for treating ulcerative colitis. Good evidence relates to treatment with non-pathogenic *Escherichia coli* Nissle 1917. It seems that few adverse events are associated with this strain of *Escherichia coli* and it may be worth considering for preventing disease relapses. Further encouraging evidence is available for psyllium and treatment with bifidobacteria, but more data are required. For fish oil the data are not entirely convincing.

Table 2.73
Summary of clinical evidence for ulcerative colitis

Treatment	Weight of evidence	Direction of evidence	Serious safety concerns
Acupuncture	O	⇨	Yes (see p 294)
Biofeedback	O	⇨	Yes (see p 310)
Herbal medicine			
Aloe vera	O	⬈	Yes (see p 364)
Chlorella pyrenoidosa	O	⬈	Yes (see p 477)
Evening primrose	O	⬊	Yes (see p 393)
Jian Pi Ling	O	⬈	Yes (see p 5)
Psyllium	OO	⬈	Yes (see p 480)
Wheat grass	O	⬈	Yes (see p 481)
Relaxation	O	⇧	Yes (see p 348)
Supplements			
Bifidobacteria	OO	⬈	Yes (see p 5)
Escherichia coli	OO	⇧	Yes (see p 5)
Fish oil	OOO	⬈	Yes (see p 483)
Folic acid	O	⬈	Yes (see p 5)
Gamma-linolenic acid	O	⬊	Yes (see p 5)
Kuijie powder	O	⬈	Yes (see p 5)

CONDITIONS

REFERENCES

1 Hilsden R J, Meddings J B, Verhoef M J. Complementary and alternative medicine use by patients with inflammatory bowel disease: An Internet survey. Can J Gastroenterol 1999;13:327–332

2 Hilsden R J, Scott C M, Verhoef M J. Complementary medicine use by patients with inflammatory bowel disease. Am J Gastroenterol 1998;93:697–701

3 Verhoef M J, Scott C M, Hilsden R J. A multimethod research study on the use of complementary therapies among patients with inflammatory bowel disease. Altern Ther Health Med 1998;4:68–71

4 Diehl D L. Acupuncture for gastrointestinal and hepatobiliary disorders. J Altern Comp Med 1999;5:27–45

5 Coulter I D, Favreau J T, Hardy M L, Morton S C, Roth E A, Shekelle P. Biofeedback interventions for gastrointestinal conditions: a systematic review. Altern Ther Health Med 2002;8:76–83

6 Langmead L, Feakins R M, Goldthorpe S, Holt H, Tsironi E, De Silva A, Jewell D P, Rampton DS. Randomized, double blind placebo controlled trial of oral aloe vera gel for active ulcerative colitis. Aliment Pharmacol Ther 2004;19:739–747

7 Merchant R E, Andre C A. A review of recent clinical trials of the nutritional supplement Chlorella pyrenoidosa in the treatment of fibromyalgia, hypertension and ulcerative colitis. Altern Ther Health Med 2001;7:79–91

8 Greenfield S M, Green A T, Teare J P, Jenkins A P, Punchard N A, Ainley C C, Thompson R P. A randomized controlled study of evening primrose oil and fish oil in ulcerative colitis. Aliment Pharmacol Ther 1993;7:159–166

9 Chen Z S, Nie Z W, Sun Q L. Clinical study in treating intractable ulcerative colitis with traditional Chinese medicine. Zhongguo Zhong Xi Yi Jie He Za Zhi 1994;14:400–402

10 Hallert C, Kaldma M, Petersson B G. Ispaghula husk may relieve gastrointestinal symptoms in ulcerative colitis in remission. Scan J Gstroenterol 1991;26:747–750

CONDITIONS

11   Fernandez-Banares F, Hinojosa J, Sanchez-Lombrana J L, Navarro E, Martinez-Salmeron J F, Garcia-Puges A, Gonzales-Huix, F, Riera J, Gonzales-Lara V, Dominguez-Abascal F, Gine J J, Moles J, Gomollon F, Gassull M A. Randomized clinical trial of Plantago ovata seeds (dietary fiber) as compared with mesalamine in maintaining remission in ulcerative colitis. Spanish group for the study of Crohn's disease and ulcerative colitis (GETECCU). Am J Gastroenterol 1999;94:427–433

12   Ejderhamm J, Hedenborg G, Strandvik B. Long-term double-blind study on the influence of dietary fibres on faecal bile acid excretion in juvenile ulcerative colitis. Scand J Clin Lab Invest 1992;52:697–706

13   Ben-Ayre E, Goldin E, Wengrower D, Stamper A, Kohn R, Berry E. Wheat grass juice in the treatment of active distal ulcerative colitis: a randomized double-blind placebo-controlled trial. Scand J Gastroenterol 2002;37:444–449

14   Carroll D, Seers K. Relaxation for the relief of chronic pain: a systematic review. J Adv Nurs 1998;27:476–487

15   Ishikawa H, Akedo I, Umesaki Y, Tanaka R, Imaoka A, Otani T. Randomized controlled trial of the effect of bifidobacteria-fermented milk on ulcerative colitis. J Am Coll Nutr 2003;22:56–63

16   Cui H H, Chen C L, Wang J D, Yang Y J Cun Y, Wu J B, Liu Y H, Dan H L, Jian Y T, Chen X Q. Effects of probiotic on intestinal mucosa of patients with ulcerative colitis. World J Gastroenterol 2004;10:1521–1525

17   Kato K, Mizuno S, Umesaki Y, Ishii Y, Sugitani M, Imaoka A, Otsuka M, Hasunuma O, Kurihara R, Iwasaki A, Arakawa Y. Randomized placebo-controlled trial assessing the effect of bifidobacteria-fermented milk on active ulcerative colitis. Aliment Pharmacol Ther 2004;20:1133–1141

18   Furrie E, Macfarlane S, Kennedy A, Cummings J H, Walsh S V, O'Neil D A, Macfarlane G T. Synbiotic therapy (Bifidobacterium longum/Synergy 1) initiates resolution of inflammation in patients with active ulcerative colitis: a randomized controlled pilot trial. Gut 2005;54:242–249

19   Gionchetti P, Rizzello F, Helwig U, Venturi A, Lammers K M, Brigidi P, Vitali B, Poggioli G, Miglioli M, Campieri M. Prophylaxis of pouchitis onset with probiotic therapy: a double-blind, placebo-controlled trial. Gastroenterology 2003;124:1202–1209

20   Rembacken B J, Snelling A M, Hawkey P M, Chalmers D M, Axon A T. Non-pathogenic Escherichia coli versus mesalazine for the treatment of ulcerative colitis: a randomized trial. Lancet 1999;354:635–639

21   Kruis W, Fric P, Pokrotnieks J, Lukas M, Fixa B, Kascak M, Kamm M A, Weismueller J, Beglinger C, Stolte M, Wolff C, Schulze J. Maintaining remission of ulcerative colitis with the probiotic Escherichia coli Nissle 1917 is as effective as with standard mesalazine. Gut 2004;53:1617–1623

22   Kruis W, Schutz E, Fric P, Fixa B, Judmaier G, Stolte M. Double-blind comparison of an oral Escherichia coli preparation and mesalazine in maintaining remission of ulcerative colitis. Aliment Pharmacol Ther 1997;11:853–858

23   Belluzzi A, Boschi S, Brignola C, Munarini A, Cariani G, Miglio F. Polyunsaturated fatty acids and inflammatory bowel disease. Am J Clin Nutr 2000;71(Suppl 1):339S–342S

24   Dichi I, Frenhane P, Dichi J B, Correa C R, Angeleli A Y, Bicudo M H, Rodrigues M A, Victoria C R, Burini R C. Comparison of omega-3 fatty acids and sulfasalazine in ulcerative colitis. Nutrition 2000;16:87–90

25   Barbosa DS, Cecchini R, El Kadri MZ, Rodriguez MA, Burini RC, Dichi I. Decreased oxidative stress in patient with ulcerative colitis supplemented with fish oil omega-3 fatty acids. Nutrition 2003;19:837–842

26   Seidner D L, Lashner B A, Brzezinski A, Banks P L, Goldblum J, Fiocchi C, Katz J, Lichtenstein G R, Anton P A, Kam L Y, Garleb K A, Demichele S J. An oral supplement enriched with fish oil, soluble fiber, and antioxidants for corticosteroid sparing in ulcerative colitis: a randomized, controlled trial. Clin Gastroenterol Hepatol 2005;3:358–369

27   Biasco G, Zannoni U, Paganelli G M, Santucci R, Gionchetti P, Rivolta G, Miniero R, Pironi L, Calabrese C, Di Febo G, Miglioli M. Folic acid supplementation and cell kinetics of rectal mucosa in patients with ulcerative colitis. Cancer Epidemiol Biomarkers Prev 1997;6:469–471

28   Middleton S J, Naylor S, Woolner J, Hunter J O. A double-blind randomized placebo-controlled trial of essential fatty acid supplementation in the maintenance of remission of ulcerative colitis. Aliment Pharmacol Ther 2002;16:1131–1135

29   Zhou Q, Yu J, Gu S. Clinical and experimental study on treatment of retention enema for chronic non-specific ulcerative colitis with quick-acting kuijie powder. Zhongguo Zhong Xi Yi Jie He Za Zhi 1999;19:395–398

UPPER RESPIRATORY TRACT INFECTION

Synonyms/ subcategories	Common cold, upper respiratory infection.
Definition	Inflammation of upper respiratory tract including nose (rhinitis), pharynx (pharyngitis) and larynx (laryngitis) due to viral or bacterial infection. Influenza is excluded from this discussion.
CAM usage	Herbal medicine, dietary supplements and spiritual approaches are commonly used complementary therapies.[1]

Clinical evidence

Exercise

Epidemiological studies have suggested that regular exercise at a moderate intensity is associated with low risk of upper respiratory tract infection, compared with moderate risk for sedentary individuals and high risk with the intense training of elite athletes.[2] The findings from three RCTs suggest that adopting an exercise regimen may result in shorter or fewer infections (Table 2.74).[3-5]

Table 2.74 **RCTs of preventive effects of exercise for upper respiratory tract infection**

Reference	Sample size	Interventions [regiment]	Result	Comment
Nieman[3]	36	A) Brisk walking [5 × 45 min/w for 15 w] B) No intervention	Shorter duration of symptoms with A than B; no difference in frequency of infections	Negative correlation between cardiovascular fitness & duration of infections
Nieman[4]	32	A) Brisk walking [5 × 40 min/w for 12 w] B) Callisthenics	Lower incidence of infections with A than B	Participants were all females aged more than 67 years
Nieman[5]	91	A) Brisk walking [5 × 45 min/w for 12 w] B) Callisthenics C) Walking & diet D) Diet & calisthenics	Shorter duration of symptoms with A & C than B & D	Participants were all obese females

Herbal medicine

Andrographis paniculata has been tested in several CCTs with encouraging results (Box 2.127).[6]

A review of **Chinese herbs** included ten controlled trials on upper respiratory tract infections.[7] Most trials reported superiority over antibiotics, but poor methodological quality rendered the evidence unconvincing. The safety of these herbs was not addressed. Subsequent CCTs also generated encouraging findings.[8-10]

Box 2.127
Systematic review
***Andrographis
paniculata* for
upper respiratory
tract infections**
Thompson Coon[6]

- Seven double-blind, placebo-controlled trials with a total of 896 patients

- Methodological quality was good

- All studies were treatment trials

- Overall *Andrographis paniculata* was better than placebo in reducing symptoms

- No major adverse events

- Conclusion: *Andrographis paniculata* may be safe and efficacious

A systematic review of RCTs of **echinacea** (*Echinacea angustifolia, purpurea, pallida*) extracts (Box 2.128) found mainly positive results for both prevention and treatment of colds, but inconsistencies in the evidence and probable publication bias prevented clinical recommendations. This review included all species of echinacea and did not attempt to differentiate between them.[11] Subsequent RCTs of echinacea have reported mixed results: *E. purpurea* generated both negative[12] and positive treatment effects.[13,14] For *E. angustifolia*, one large rigorous RCT (n = 399) concluded that three *E. angustifolia* root extracts had no effect on rates of infection or severity of symptoms[15] and a further RCT (n = 148) showed no superiority over placebo in treating the common cold.[16] A systematic review of echinacea for treating the common cold found that only two placebo-controlled RCTs were of high enough quality to be included. The authors concluded that the 'therapeutic effectiveness of echinacea in the treatment of colds has not been established'.[17]

Box 2.128
Systematic review
**Echinacea for
upper respiratory
tract infections**
Melchart[11]

- Sixteen RCTs including 3396 patients

- Trials of prevention (n = 8) and treatment (n = 8)

- Included combination or monopreparations of any species

- Comparison with placebo, no treatment or other intervention

- Trial quality ranged from good to poor

- Conclusion: evidence was generally positive, but insufficient for firm recommendations

Garlic (*Allium sativum*) was tested in an RCT (n = 146) for common cold prevention. During the 3-month medication period, fewer infections occurred with garlic than with placebo.[18]

Steam inhalation of **German chamomile** (*Matricaria recutita*) was reported to have a dose-dependent effect on symptoms of the common cold in a placebo-controlled trial.[19]

An RCT of patients receiving a flu vaccine (n = 227) reported that compared with placebo, **ginseng** (*Panax ginseng*) (100 mg daily for 12 weeks) reduced the frequency of colds and flu and increased immune activity.[20]

Homeopathy

Several RCTs have investigated the therapeutic effects of various homeopathic remedies and combinations, with conflicting outcomes. Two trials reported similar results to acetylsalicylic acid,[21,22] while from placebo-controlled studies, there have been both negative[23] and positive[24,25] results.

Supplements

A systematic review of 30 controlled trials of high-dose (≥ 1g daily) **vitamin C** (Box 2.129), concluded that there was no consistent evidence of a prophylactic effect. However, as a treatment, vitamin C shortened the duration of colds by about half a day.[26]

Box 2.129
Systematic review
Vitamin C for respiratory tract infection
Douglas[25]

- Thirty placebo-controlled trials including >8000 patients (children & adults)
- Trial quality generally mixed
- No evidence of protective effect
- Modest reduction of duration of symptoms (8–9%) when taken for treatment purposes

Vitamin E was tested in two RCTs (n = 652 and n = 617) with both studies showing no superiority over placebo regarding the incidence and severity of acute respiratory tract infections.[27,28]

A systematic review of double-blind, placebo-controlled RCTs of treatment with **zinc** lozenges (Box 2.130) found no overall evidence that the duration of colds was shortened.[29] Two other systematic reviews had similar conclusions[30,31] and subsequent RCTs reported both negative[32] and positive results.[33]

A large-scale placebo-controlled RCT (n = 725) reported a preventive role of supplementation with **trace elements** (zinc and selenium) in elderly institutionalised patients, but not with **vitamins** (beta-carotene, vitamin C, vitamin E).[34] A similar study (n = 66) reported preventative effects for an antioxidant formula

CONDITIONS

Box 2.130
Systematic review
Zinc for upper respiratory tract infection
Marshall[29]

- Seven double-blind, placebo-controlled RCTs including 754 patients
- Trial quality generally good
- Positive results from two trials
- Overall, results suggested no superiority over placebo
- Adverse effects associated with zinc administration

containing both zinc and selenium.[35] An RCT (n = 571) showed encouraging treatment effects for probiotics when given to children aged 1–6 years.[36]

Other therapies

Self-performed nasal **acupressure** provided relief of nasal congestion compared with no intervention in a small (n = 20) RCT.[37] A similarly designed RCT (n = 326) suggested that needle acupuncture was associated with fewer symptoms of a common cold than no treatment at all.[38]

Hydrotherapy consisting of hot/cold showers did not prevent common colds in an RCT (n = 81) with young children.[39]

The anthroposophic remedy **Iscador** (mistletoe, *Viscum album*) showed no effect on the frequency or duration of the common cold in a placebo-controlled RCT (n = 32).[40]

A non-randomised trial (n = 50) reported that regular **sauna bathing** (once or twice weekly for 6 months) resulted in a lower incidence of colds, although no difference in their duration or severity, than no intervention.[41]

Overall recommendation

Compelling evidence is scarce for the effectiveness of complementary therapies in relieving symptoms of upper respiratory tract infections. However, given that conventional options are limited, *Andrographis paniculata* or *Echinacea* are probably worth considering and it appears that large doses of vitamin C may have a small therapeutic effect. For the prevention of infections, *Echinacea* may be useful and regular exercise of a moderate intensity appears to reduce the risk.

Table 2.75
Summary of clinical evidence for upper respiratory tract infection

Treatment	Weight of evidence	Direction of evidence	Serious safety concerns
Exercise (prevention)	OO	⇧	Yes (see p 5)
Herbal medicine			
Andrographis paniculata	OO	⇧	Yes (see p 366)
Chinese herbs	O	⬈	Yes (see p 5)
Echinacea (prevention)	OOO	⇨	Yes (see p 391)
(treatment)	OOO	⇨	Yes (see p 391)
Garlic	O	⇧	Yes (see p 398)
German chamomile	O	⇧	Yes (see p 376)
Ginseng (prevention)	O	⇧	Yes (see p 407)
Homeopathy	OO	⇨	No (see p 327)
Supplements			
Vitamin C (prevention)	OOO	⇩	No (see p 5)
(treatment)	OOO	⇧	No (see p 5)
Vitamin E	OO	⇩	Yes (see p 5)
Zinc	OOO	⬊	Yes (see p 5)

CONDITIONS

REFERENCES

1 Pachter L M, Sumner T, Fontan A, Sneed M, Bernstein B A. Home-based therapies for the common cold among European American and ethnic minority families. Arch Pediatr Adolesc Med 1998;152:1083–1088

2 Peters E M. Exercise, immunology and upper respiratory tract infections. Int J Sports Med 1997;18:S69–S77

3 Nieman D C, Nehlsen-Cannarella S L, Markoff P A, Balk-Lamberton A J, Yang H, Chritton D B, Lee J W, Arabatzis K. The effects of moderate exercise training on natural killer cells and acute upper respiratory tract infections. Int J Sports Med 1990;11:467–473

4 Nieman D C, Henson D A, Gusewitch G, Warren B J, Dotson R C, Butterworth D E, Nehlsen-Cannarella S L. Physical activity and immune function in elderly women. Med Sci Sports Exerc 1993;25:823–831

5 Nieman D C, Nehlsen-Cannarella S L, Henson D A, Koch A J, Butterworth D E, Fagoaga O R, Utter A. Immune response to exercise training and/or energy restriction in obese women. Med Sci Sports Exerc 1998,30.679–686

6 Thompson Coon J, Ernst E. Andrographis paniculata in the treatment of upper respiratory tract infections: a systematic review of safety and efficacy. Planta Med 2004;70:293–298

7 Liu C, Douglas R M. Chinese herbal medicines in the treatment of acute respiratory infections: a review of randomised and controlled clinical trials. Med J Aust 1998;169:579–582

8 Li C, Wang X, Chen S. [Clinical study on acute upper respiratory tract infection treated with qingkailing injection]. Zhongguo Zhong Xi Yi Jie He Za Zhi 1999;19:212–214

9 Ma B, Duan X, Wang Z. [Clinical and experimental study on Shuanghua aerosol in treating infantile upper respiratory tract infection] Zhongguo Zhong Xi Yi Jie He Za Zhi 2000;20:653–655

10 Du B, Wang S, Weng W. [Clinical observation on gangrening granule in treating common

cold] Zhongguo Zhong Xi Yi Jie He Za Zhi 2000;20:34-36

11   Melchart D, Linde K, Fischer P, Kaesmayr J. Echinacea for preventing and treating the common cold. The Cochrane Database of Systematic Reviews 1999, Issue 1. Art.No.:CD000530

12   Yale S H, Liu K. Echinacea purpurea therapy for the treatment of the common cold: a randomized, double-blind, placebo-controlled clinical trial. Arch Intern Med 2004;164:1237-1241

13   Schulten B, Bulitta M, Ballering-Bruhl B, Koster U, Schafer M. Efficacy of Echinacea purpurea in patients with a common cold. A placebo-controlled, randomised, double-blind clinical trial. Arzneimittelforschung 2001;51:563-568

14   Goel V, Lovlin R, Barton R, Lyon M R, Bauer R, Lee T D, Basu T K. Efficacy of a standardized echinacea preparation (Echinilin) for the treatment of the common cold: a randomized, double-blind, placebo-controlled trial. J Clin Pharm Ther 2004;29:75-83

15   Turner R B, Bauer R, Woelkart K, Hulsey T C, Gangemi J D. An evaluation of Echinacea angustifolia in experimental rhinovirus infections. N Engl J Med 2005;353:341-348

16   Barrett B P, Brown R L, Locken K, Maberry R, Bobula J A, D'Alessio D. Treatment of the common cold with unrefined echinacea. A randomized, double-blind, placebo-controlled trial. Ann Intern Med 2002;137:939-946

17   Caruso T J, Gwaltney J M. Treatment of the common cold with Echinacea: a structured review. Clin Infect Dis 2005;40:807-810

18   Josling P. Preventing the common cold with a garlic supplement: a double-blind, placebo-controlled survey. Adv Ther 2001;18:189-193

19   Saller R, Beschomer M, Hellenbrecht D, Buhring M. Dose dependency of symptomatic relief of complaints by chamomile steam inhalation in patients with common cold. Eur J Pharm 1990;183:728-729

20   Scaglione F, Cattaneo G, Alessandria M, Cogo R. Efficacy and safety of the standardized ginseng extract G115 for potentiating vaccination against common cold and/or influenza syndrome. Drugs Exper Clin Res 1996;22:65-72

21   Maiwald L, Weinfurtner T, Mau J, Connert W D. Treatment of common cold with a combination homoeopathic preparation compared with acetylsalicylic acid. Controlled randomised single-blind study. Drug Res 1988;38:578-582

22   Gassinger C A, Wuenstel G, Netter P. Controlled clinical trial for testing the efficacy of the homoeopathic drug eupatorium perfoliatum D2 in the treatment of common cold. Drug Res 1981;31:732-736

23   De Lange De Klerk E S M, Blommers J, Kuik D J, Bezemer P D, Feenstra L. Effect of homoeopathic medicines on daily burden of symptoms in children with recurrent upper respiratory tract infections. BMJ 1994;309: 1329-1332

24   Diefenbach M, Schilken J, Steiner G, Becker H J. Homeopathic therapy in respiratory tract diseases. Evaluation of a clinical study in 258 patients. Zeitschr für Allgemeinmedizin 1997;73: 308-314

25   Ferley J P, Zmirou D, D'Adhemar D, Balducci F. A controlled evaluation of a homeopathic preparation in the treatment of influenza-like syndromes. Br J Clin Pharmacol 1989;27:329-335

26   Douglas R M, Hemila H, D'Souza R, Chalker E B, Treacy B. Vitamin C for preventing and treating the common cold. The Cochrane Database of Systematic Reviews 2004, Issue 4. Art No.: CD000980

27   Graat J M, Schouten E G, Kok F J. Effect of daily vitamin E and multivitamin-mineral supplementation on acute respiratory tract infections in elderly persons: a randomized controlled trial. JAMA 2002;288:715-721

28   Meydani S N, Leka L S, Fine B C, Dallal, G E, Keusch G T, Singh M F, Hamer D H. Vitamin E and respiratory tract infections in elderly nursing home residents: a randomized controlled trial. JAMA 2004;292:828-836

29   Marshall I. Zinc for the common cold. The Cochrane Database of Systematic Reviews 1999, Issue 2. Art No.: CD001364

30   Galand M L, Hagmeyer K O. The role of zinc lozenges in treatment of the common cold. Ann Pharmacother 1998;32:63-69

31   Jackson J L, Peterson C, Lesho E. A meta-analysis of zinc salts lozenges and the common cold. Arch Intern Med 1997;157:2373-2376

32   Macknin M L, Piedmonte M, Calendine C, Janosky J, Wald E. Zinc gluconate lozenges for treating the common cold in children. JAMA 1998;279:1962-1967

33   Prasad A S, Fitzgerald J T, Beck F W J, Chandrasekar P H. Duration of symptoms and plasma cytokine levels in patients with the common cold treated with zinc acetate. Ann Intern Med 2000;133:245-252

34 Girodon F, Galan P, Monget A L, Boutron-Ruault M C, Brunet-Lecomte P, Preziosi P, Arnaud J, Manuguerra J C, Herchberg S. Impact of trace elements and vitamin supplementation on immunity and infections in institutionalized elderly patients: a randomized controlled trial. MIN. VIT. AOX. geriatric network. Arch Intern Med 1999;159:748–754

35 Langkamp-Henken B, Bender B S, Gardner E M, Herrlinger-Garcia, K A, Kelley M J, Murasko D M, Shcaller J P, Stechmiller J K, Thomas D J, Wood S M. Nutritional formula enhanced immune function and reduced days of symptoms of upper respiratory tract infection in seniors. J Am Geriatr Soc 2004;52:3–12

36 Hatakka K, Savilahti E, Ponka A, Meurman J H, Poussa T, Nase L, Saxelin M, Korpela R. Effect of long term consumption of probiotic milk on infections in children attending day care centres: double blind, randomised trial. BMJ 2001;322:1327

37 Takeuchi H, Jawad M S, Eccles R. Effects of nasal massage of the 'yingxiang' acupuncture point on nasal airway resistance and sensation of nasal airflow in patients with nasal congestion with acute upper respiratory tract infection. Am J Rhinol 1999;13:77–79

38 Kawakita K, Shichidou T, Inoue E, Nabeta T, Kitakouji H, Aizawa S, Nishida A, Yamaguchi N, Takahashi N, Yano T, Tanzawa S. Preventive and curative effects of acupuncture on the common cold: a multicentre randomized controlled trial in Japan. Complement Ther Med 2004;12:181–188

39 Gruber C, Riesberg A, Mansmann U, Knipschild P, Wahn U, Buhring M. The effect of hydrotherapy on the incidence of common cold episodes in children: a randomised clinical trial. Eur J Pediatr 2003;162:168–176

40 Huber R, Klein R, Ludtke R, Wener M. [Frequency of the common cold in healthy subjects during exposure to a lectin-rich and a lectin-poor mistletoe preparation in a randomized, double-blind, placebo-controlled study] Forsch Komplementärmed Klass Naturheilkd 2001;8:354–358

41 Ernst E, Pecho E, Wirz P, Saradeth T. Regular sauna bathing and the incidence of common colds. Ann Med 1990;22:225–227

CONDITIONS

Therapies

ACUPUNCTURE

Synonyms	Reflexotherapy (in former USSR); sensory stimulation.
Definition	Insertion of a needle into the skin and underlying tissues in special sites, known as points, for therapeutic or preventive purposes.
Related techniques	Point stimulation by electricity (electroacupuncture), laser (laser-acupuncture, low-level laser therapy), heat (moxibustion), pressure (acupressure, shiatsu, tui na) or ultrasound; electroacupuncture after Voll, Ryodoraku; neural therapy.
Background	Acupuncture originated in China and is one part of oriental medicine. Its precise origin is still the subject of scholarly debate. Some experts state that 'at some time in the first century BCE', acupuncture was already a signature therapy of Chinese medicine.[1] Others insist that 'the earliest clear-cut references to human acupuncture can be reliably dated only to the fifth to eighth century CE'.[2] Some authors even speculated that tattoos on human remains may indicate the use of acupuncture in Europe from about 3300 BCE.
	Although acupuncture has been used for years within immigrant communities in the West, interest among Westerners has fluctuated. The most recent wave of interest dates from about 1970.
	Acupuncture is commonly used in China, Taiwan, Japan, Korea, Singapore and other Eastern countries. In the West, its popularity has grown rapidly,[1] particularly as a treatment for pain.
Traditional concepts	The fundamental concept is qi[1] (pronounced 'chee') which is usually, though inadequately, translated as 'energy'. It is believed that qi is inherited at birth and maintained during life by the intake of food and air. Qi is thought to circulate through the body via 12 'meridians' which form channels through limbs, trunk and head. More than 350 acupuncture points are located on these meridians. Other points lie outside the meridian pathways.
	Several different approaches to diagnosis have been developed, but some concepts are basic to all. For example, health is a balance of two opposites, Yin and Yang. Diseases are associated with disturbances, disharmony or imbalance (typically 'blockage' or 'deficiency') of energy.
	The body is believed to correct its own energy flow and balance after stimulation of acupuncture points and ill health is thought to reflect a disturbance of energy. Therefore every medical condition may be amenable to treatment with acupuncture. It is also claimed that disturbances may be detected before they develop into conditions; therefore even healthy individuals might benefit from acupuncture.

Scientific rationale

No evidence has been found to confirm the existence of qi or meridians.[3] Some acupuncture points are sites at which nerves can be stimulated. Acupuncture could thus be a method of affecting the nervous and muscular systems. Considerable differences have been noted between the historical location of points or meridians and current practice.[3] Acupuncture has been found to release various neurotransmitters, including opioid peptides and serotonin.[4,5] Acupuncture may also be used as a form of trigger point therapy.[6]

Practitioners

In the USA, the certificates of the National Certification Commission for Acupuncture and Oriental Medicine (NCCAOM) are accepted for licensure in many states. In some states non-medically qualified practitioners are allowed to see patients without medical referral. In the UK, there are currently no legal restrictions on the practice of acupuncture; statutory regulation has, however, been drafted. In other countries, the practice of acupuncture is officially restricted to medical practitioners but the restrictions may not be applied rigorously. In Germany, it is practised both by doctors and by *Heilpraktiker* (non-medically trained CAM practitioners).

Conditions frequently treated

Addictions and allergies, chronic musculoskeletal pain, digestive disorders, ear nose and throat conditions, infertility and menstrual problems, 'low energy', maintaining health and preventing illness, mental health problems, stress, various pain syndromes. Considerable differences exist between the conditions treated according to the 'school' and the origin of the practitioner.

Typical session

Traditional acupuncturists will take a history and ask about predisposing or psychological factors. Examinations may include inspection of the tongue, palpation of the pulse and abdomen and a search for tender points. Medical acupuncturists will typically incorporate acupuncture into their usual diagnostic and treatment process.

When the diagnosis has been made, needles will be inserted into one to 12 acupuncture points. The needles are typically about 30 mm long, thin (0.3 mm) and disposable. Needles may be placed just under the skin or deeper into muscle and may be stimulated either by repeated manual rotation or electrically. This may cause an aching sensation called *deqi* (pronounced 'der chee'). The needles may be left in position for up to 20 minutes. Occasionally, special needles are left in place for up to 2 weeks. Points in the ear may be used (auriculoacupuncture).

Points may also be stimulated by pressure (acupressure), or in the Japanese form, shiatsu, where pressure is applied by fingers, hands, elbows or other parts of the body. In the Chinese method, tui na, a variety of methods of physical stimulation are used such as pulling and rubbing. In moxibustion, points are heated by smouldering moxa, the leaves of *Artemisia vulgaris*. Points may also be stimulated by laser, ultrasound or injection of substance. Self-treatment versions of acupuncture use pressure pads or electrical apparatus.

Course of treatment

Consultations usually start at weekly intervals. When symptom relief occurs, the interval between treatments may be increased until a course of about 6–8 sessions is completed. For chronic conditions acupuncturists recommend maintenance treatments.

Clinical evidence

Numerous systematic reviews of acupuncture trials have been published. Table 3.1 is a summary of the most up to date systematic reviews by indications.[7–42] According to these data, acupuncture is of documented effectiveness for back pain,[7,8] dental pain,[9] fibromyalgia,[10] for aiding gastrointestinal endoscopy,[11] idiopathic headache,[12] nausea and vomiting,[13] pain relief after oocyte retrieval,[14] as well as osteoarthritis of the knee.[15] It is likely to be ineffective for rheumatoid arthritis,[40] smoking[41] and weight reduction.[42] For the vast majority of conditions, the data are either inconclusive, e.g. chronic pain,[22] cocaine dependence,[18] depression,[23] shoulder pain,[35] acute stroke,[36] analgesia during surgery[37] or non-existent. Because of numerous methodological and other problems, the current evidence allows ample room for interpretations. Thus different experts arrive at different conclusions. For example, Linde *et al* stated in 2001 that 'convincing evidence is available only for postoperative nausea, for which acupuncture appears to be of benefit, and smoking cessation where acupuncture is no more effective than sham acupunture.[43] While Ramey and Simpson, in their review of systematic reviews from the same year, were even more sceptical: 'effectiveness could not be established with confidence for any condition studied'.[44]

Risks

Contraindications
Severe bleeding disorder. Pregnancy (first trimester) and epilepsy are often regarded as contraindications. Indwelling needles should not be used in patients at risk from bacteraemia.

Precautions/warnings
Asepsis is a precondition. Electroacupuncture should be used with caution for patients carrying a pacemaker. Patients should be treated lying down. As acupuncture causes drowsiness in 3% of patients,[45] operating machinery or driving after treatment could be hazardous. Children should be treated with care, if at all. To avoid injury to internal organs, special care should be taken when needling points on the thorax. Close supervision is essential if indwelling needles are used.

Adverse effects
Mild, transient adverse events in about 7–11% of patients.[45–47] Drowsiness, bleeding, bruising, pain on needling and aggravation of symptoms are the most frequent adverse effects. Serious adverse

events, such as pneumothorax or infections, appear to be rare although well-documented cases, including fatalities are on record.[48]

Interactions
Electroacupuncture may interfere with cardiac pacemakers (see above).

Risk–benefit assessment

In cases where conventional medical diagnosis and advice on best management have previously been obtained, competent acupuncture is relatively safe. For some, but by no means all, conditions acupuncture appears to be effective (Table 3.1). Therefore it is worth considering for some indications.

Table 3.1 **Results of systematic reviews of acupuncture**

Positive	Inconclusive	Negative
Chronic back pain[7,8]	Addictions[16,17*,18]	Rheumatoid arthritis[40]
Dental pain[9]	Asthma[19]	Smoking cessation[41]
Fibromyalgia[10]	Bell's palsy[20]	Weight reduction[42]
Gastrointestinal endoscopy[11]	Cancer pain[21]	
Idiopathic headache[12]	Chronic pain[22]	
Postoperative nausea and vomiting [13]¤	Depression[23]	
Oocyte retrieval[14]	Facial pain[24]	
Osteoarthritis of knee[15]	Induction of labour[25]	
	Inflammatory rheumatic diseases[26]	
	Insomnia[27]	
	Labour pain[28]	
	Lateral elbow pain[29]	
	Myofascial pain syndrome[30]	
	Neck pain[31]	
	Osteoarthritis[32]	
	Primary dysmenorrhoea[33]	
	Sciatica[34]	
	Shoulder pain[35]	
	Stroke[36]	
	Surgical pain[37]	
	Temporomandibular joint dysfunction[38]	
	Tinnitus[39]	

¤ = acupressure only
* = ear acupuncture only

THERAPIES

REFERENCES

1   Kaptchuk T J. Acupuncture: theory, efficacy, and practice. Ann Intern Med 2002;136:374–383

2   Imrie R H, Ramey D W, Buell P D et al. Veterinary acupuncture and historical scholarship: claims for the antiquity of acupuncture. Sci Rev Altern Med 2001;5:133–139

3   Ramey D W. Acupuncture points and meridians do not exist. Sci Rev Altern Med 2001;5: 140–145

4   Han J, Terenius L. Neurochemical basis of acupuncture analgesia. Annu Rev Pharmacol Toxicol 1982;22:193–220

5   Andersson S, Lundeberg T. Acupuncture – from empiricism to science: functional background to acupuncture effects in pain and disease. Med Hypotheses 1995;45:271–281

6   Filshie J, Cummings T M. Western medical acupuncture. In: Ernst E, White A (eds). Acupuncture: a scientific appraisal. Oxford: Butterworth Heinemann, 1999, pp 31–59

7   Manheimer E, White A, Berman B, Forys K, Ernst E. Meta-analysis: acupuncture for back pain. Ann Intern Med 2005;142:651–663

8   Furlan A D, van Tulder M W, Cherkin D C, Tsukayama H, Lao L, Koes B W, Berman B M. Acupuncture and dry-needling for low back pain. The Cochrane Database of Systematic Reviews 2005, Issue 1. Art No.: CD001351

9   Ernst E, Pittler M H. The effectiveness of acupuncture in treating acute dental pain: a systematic review. Br Dent J 1998;184:443–447

10 Berman B M, Swyers J P. Complementary medicine treatments for fibromyalgia syndrome. Baillières Best Pract Res Clin Rheumatol 1999;13:487–492

11 Lee H, Ernst E. Acupuncture for GI endoscopy: A systematic review. Gastrointest Endosc 2004;60:784–789

12 Melchart D, Linde K, Fischer P, Berman B, White A, Vickers A, Allais G. Acupuncture for idiopathic headache. The Cochrane Database of Systematic Reviews 2001, Issue 1. Art. No.: CD001218

13 Lee A, Done M L. Stimulation of the wrist acupuncture point P6 for preventing postoperative nausea and vomiting. The Cochrane Database of Systematic Reviews 2004, Issue 3. Art. No.: CD003281.

14 Stener-Victorin E. The pain-relieving effect of electro-acupuncture and conventional medical analgesic methods during oocyte retrieval: a systematic review of randomized controlled trials. Hum Reprod 2005;20:339–349

15 Ezzo J, Hadhazy V, Birch S, Lao L, Kaplan G, Hochberg M et al. Acupuncture for osteoarthritis of the knee: a systematic review. Arthritis Rheum 2001;44:819–825

16 ter Riet G, Kleijnen J, Knipschild P. A meta-analysis of studies into the effect of acupuncture on addiction. Br J Gen Pract 1990;40:379–382

17 Kunz S, Schulz M, Syrbe G, Driessen M. Acupuncture of the ear as therapeutic approach in the treatment of alcohol and substance abuse – a systematic review. Sucht 2004;50:196–203

18 Mills E J, Wu P, Gagnier J, Ebbert J O. Efficacy of acupuncture for cocaine dependence: a systematic review and meta-analysis. Harm Reduct J 2005;2:4

19 Martin J, Donaldson A N, Villarroel R, Parmar M K, Ernst E, Higginson I J. Efficacy of acupuncture in asthma: systematic review and meta-analysis of published data from 11 randomised controlled trials. Eur Respir J 2002;20:846–852

20 He L, Zhou D, Wu B, Li N, Zhou M K. Acupuncture for Bell's palsy. The Cochrane Database of Systematic Reviews 2004, Issue 1. Art. No.: CD002914

21 Lee H, Schmidt K, Ernst E. Acupuncture for the relief of cancer-related pain – a systematic review. Eur J Pain 2005;9:437–444

22 Ezzo J, Berman B, Hadhazy V A, Jadad A R, Lao L, Sing B B. Is acupuncture effective for the treatment of chronic pain? A systematic review. Pain 2000;86:217–225

23 Smith C A, Hay P P J. Acupuncture for depression. The Cochrane Database of Systematic Reviews 2004, Issue 3. Art. No.: CD004046

24 Myers C D, White BA, Heft M W. A review of complementary and alternative medicine use for treating chronic facial pain. Am Dent Assoc 2002;133:1189–1196

25 Smith C A, Crowther C A. Acupuncture for induction of labour. The Cochrane Database of Systematic Reviews 2004, Issue 1. Art. No.: CD002962

26 Lautenschläger J. Akupunktur bei der Behandlung entzündlich – rheumatischer Erkrankungen. Z Rheumatol 1997;56:8–20

27 Sok S R, Erlen J A, Kim K B. Effects of acupuncture therapy on insomnia. J Adv Nurs 2003;44:375–384

28 Lee H, Ernst E. Acupuncture for labor pain management: a systematic review. Am J Obstet Gynecol 2004;191:1573–1579

29 Trinh K V, Phillips S-D, Ho E, Damsma K. Acupuncture for the alleviation of lateral epicondyle pain: a systematic review. Rheumatology (Oxford) 2004;43:1085–1090

30 Cummings T M, White A R. Needling therapies in the management of myofascial trigger point pain: a systematic review. Arch Phys Med Rehabil 2001;82:986–992

31 White A R, Ernst E. A systematic review of randomized controlled trials of acupuncture for neck pain. Rheumatology (Oxford) 1999;38:143–147

32 Ernst E. Acupuncture as a symptomatic treatment of osteoarthritis. Scand J Rheumatol 1997;26:444–447

33 Proctor M L, Smith C A, Farquhar C M, Stones R W. Transcutaneous electrical nerve stimulation and acupuncture for primary dysmenorrhoea. The Cochrane Database of Systematic Reviews 2002, Issue 1. Art. No.: CD002123

34 Longworth W, McCarthy P W. A review of research on acupuncture for the treatment of lumbar disc protrusions and associated neurological symptomatology. J Altern Complement Med 1997;3:55–76

35 Green S, Buchbinder R, Hetrick S. Acupuncture for shoulder pain. The Cochrane Database of Systematic Reviews 2005, Issue 2. Art. No.: CD005319

36 Zhang S H, Liu M, Asplund K, Li L. Acupuncture for acute stroke. The Cochrane Database of Systematic Reviews 2005, Issue 2. Art. No.: CD003317

37 Lee H, Ernst E. Acupuncture analgesia during surgery: a systematic review. Pain 2005;114:511–517

38 Ernst E, White A. Acupuncture as a treatment for temporomandibular joint dysfunction: a systematic review of randomized trials. Arch Otolaryngol Head Neck Surg 1999;125:269–272

39 Park J, White A R, Ernst E. Efficacy of acupuncture as a treatment for tinnitus: a systematic review. Arch Otolaryngol Head Neck Surg 2000;126:489–492

40 Casimiro L, Brosseau L, Milne S, Robinson V, Wells G, Tugwell P. Acupuncture and electroacupuncture for the treatment of RA. The Cochrane Database of Systematic Reviews 2002, Issue 3. Art. No.: CD003788

41 White A R, Rampes H, Ernst E. Acupuncture for smoking cessation. The Cochrane Database of Systematic Reviews 2002, Issue 2. Art. No.: CD 000009

42 Ernst E. Acupuncture/acupressure for weight reduction? A systematic review. Wien Klin Wochenschr 1997;109:60–62

43 Linde K, Vickers A, Hondras M, ter Riet G, Thormahlen J, Berman B, Melchart D. Systematic reviews of complementary therapies – an annotated bibliography. Part 1: acupuncture. BMC Complement Altern Med 2001;1:3

44 Ramey D W, Sampson W. Review of the evidence for the clinical efficacy of human acupuncture. Sci Rev Altern Med 2001;5:195–201

45 MacPherson H, Scullion A, Thomas K J, Walters S. Patient reports of adverse events associated with acupuncture treatment: a prospective national survey. Qual Saf Health Care 2004;13:349–355

46 White A, Hayhoe S, Hart A, Ernst E. Adverse events following acupuncture: prospective survey of 32000 consultations with doctors and physiotherapists. BMJ 2001;323:485–486

47 Melchart D, Weidenhammer W, Streng A, Reitmayr S, Hoppe A, Ernst E, Linde K. Prospective investigation of adverse effects of acupuncture in 97,733 patients. Arch Intern Med 2004;164:104–105

48 Ernst E, White A. Life-threatening adverse reactions after acupuncture? A systematic review. Pain 1997;71:123–126

ALEXANDER TECHNIQUE

Definition Process of psychophysical reeducation to improve postural balance and coordination in order to move with minimal strain and maximum ease.

Related techniques Feldenkrais method, Rolfing, Tragerwork, yoga.

Background The Alexander technique was developed around the turn of the last century by Frederick M Alexander, an Australian actor who suffered a recurring loss of voice. By observing himself in a mirror, he concluded that it was due to the tense position in which

THERAPIES

he habitually held his head. By correcting the relationship between head, neck and spine during activity, he solved the problem over a number of years. This marked the beginning of the Alexander technique.

Traditional concepts

The Alexander technique is based on three principles:

- function is affected by use
- an organism functions as a whole
- the relationship of the head, neck and spine is vital to the organism's ability to function optimally.

Human movement is thought to be most fluent when the head leads and the spine follows. This new experience is practised repeatedly to create new motor pathways, improving proprioception and upright posture and leading to enhanced coordination and balance.

Scientific rationale

The notion that learning the Alexander technique allows the conscious changing of habitual and detrimental physiologic reactions receives some support from psychophysiology research, suggesting that the mind can modulate aspects of the autonomic nervous system. Specific investigations of the Alexander technique have demonstrated that it improves the efficiency of moving from the sitting to standing position.

Practitioners

There are about 2000 Alexander teachers worldwide. They typically come from a background of performing arts, dance, theater and music or, more recently, physical or occupational therapy and massage. Certified teachers undergo at least three years of training on an approved course involving 1600 hours of training.

Conditions frequently treated

Asthma, chronic pain, headaches, osteoarthritis, stress. Also used by performing artists and sportspeople.

Typical session

Sessions last between 45 and 60 minutes and take place in an Alexander studio with the aid of a bodywork table and mirror. The client or student is encouraged to wear loose, comfortable clothing to facilitate movement. The teacher guides the Alexander process using a gentle hands-on approach to teach movements with the head leading and the spine following. Within 5–10 lessons the student is able to experience and recreate an expansive quality of movement known as poise. The skill can then be refined to specialist activities.

Course of treatment

Thirty lessons are recommended in order to learn the basic concepts. Serious students of the technique may undertake up to 100 lessons. Learning the Alexander technique requires commitment and a great deal of practice by the student.

Clinical evidence Controlled trials have reported enhanced respiratory function in healthy volunteers,[1] greater functional reach in elderly women[2] and improvements in performance and anxiety in music students[3] following training in the Alexander technique. An RCT showed that the Alexander technique is effective in reducing the disability of patients suffering from Parkinson's disease.[4] An uncontrolled trial of a multidisciplinary programme for 67 chronic back pain sufferers incorporating lessons in Alexander technique reported improvements in pain which persisted for 6 months.[5] Multiple cases of successful application of the Alexander technique to people with learning difficulties[6] and craniomandibular disorders[7] have also been reported. A systematic review of all clinical trials concluded that Alexander technique is under-researched but held considerable promise for a range of conditions.[8]

Risks *Contraindications*
None known.

Precautions/warnings
None known.

Adverse effects
None known.

Interactions
None known.

Risk–benefit assessment Whether learning the Alexander technique has a specific therapeutic effect is not clear, but since it is almost entirely safe and has been associated with positive outcomes in various conditions, it may be worth considering as an adjunctive or palliative therapy for patients who express a strong interest.

THERAPIES

REFERENCES

1 Austin J H M, Ausubel P. Enhanced respiratory muscular function in normal adults after lessons in proprioceptive musculoskeletal education without exercises. Chest 1992;102:486–490

2 Dennis R J. Functional reach improvement in normal older women after Alexander technique instruction. J Gerontol – Biol Sci Med Sci 1999;54:8–11

3 Valentine E R, Fitzgerald D F P, Gorton T L, Hudson J A, Symonds E R C. The effect of lessons in the Alexander technique on music performance in high and low stress situations. Psychol Music 1995;23:129–141

4 Stallibras C, Chambers C. Randomized controlled trial of the Alexander Technique for idopathic Parkinson's disease. Clin Rehab 2002;16:705–18

5 Elkayam O, Ben Itzhak S, Avrahami E, Meidan Y, Doron N, Eldar I, Keidar I, Liram N, Yaron M. Multidisciplinary approach to chronic back pain: prognostic elements of the outcome. Clin Exp Rheum 1996;14:281–288

6 Maitland S, Horne R, Burton M. An exploration of the application of the Alexander technique for people with learning disabilities. Br J Learning Disabil 1996;24:70–76

7 Knebelman S. The Alexander technique in diagnosis and treatment of craniomandibular disorders. Basal Facts 1982;5:19–22

8 Ernst E, Canter P H. The Alexander technique: a systematic review of controlled clinical trials. Forsch Komplementärmed Klass Naturheilkd 2003;10:325–329.

AROMATHERAPY

Definition	The controlled use of plant essences for therapeutic purposes.
Related techniques	Massage.
Background	The medicinal use of plant oils has a long history in ancient Egypt, China and India. The development of modern aromatherapy is attributed to French chemist René Gattefosse, who burned his hand while working in a perfume laboratory and immediately doused it in some nearby lavender oil. The burn healed quickly without scarring, leading him to study the potential curative powers of plant oils. He coined the term aromatherapy in 1937.
Traditional concepts	Essential oils can be applied directly to the skin through massage or a compress, added to baths, inhaled with steaming water or spread throughout a room with a diffuser. The oils have effects at the psychological, physiological and cellular levels. These effects can be relaxing or stimulating depending on the chemistry of the oil and also the previous associations of the individual with a particular scent.
Scientific rationale	The scent from the oil activates the olfactory sense. This triggers the limbic system, which governs emotional responses and is involved with the formation and retrieval of learned memories. Essential oils are also absorbed through the skin via the dermis and layer of subcutaneous fat to the bloodstream. Laboratory studies suggest that molecules of the oil can affect organ function, although the clinical relevance of these findings is not clear.
Practitioners	In most countries aromatherapy is largely unregulated. In the UK it is in the process of being regulated. Various aromatherapy associations offer courses with the number of hours of training required ranging from 180 to 500. Many nurses and other healthcare professionals routinely seek aromatherapy qualifications.
Conditions frequently treated	Anxiety, headaches, insomnia, musculoskeletal pain, and other stress-related conditions. Some therapists recommend regular aromatherapy as a means of maintaining general health and well-being. A US survey suggests that stress, musculoskeletal problems and pain are the most common condition treated by aromatherapists.[1]
Typical session	During an initial session the aromatherapist will ask about a client's medical history, health and lifestyle and which aromas are liked or disliked. The therapist will then select essential oils deemed appropriate for the client according to this information.

THERAPIES

Treatment would usually consist of an aromatherapy massage and advice may be given about home treatments involving the use of oils in baths or a diffuser. The initial session may last up to 2 hours. Subsequent sessions would typically last 1 hour.

Course of treatment

For chronic conditions, one weekly session would be recommended for several weeks, with fortnightly or monthly follow-ups.

Clinical evidence

A systematic review of all RCTs of aromatherapy was conducted.[2] Based on six trials with hospitalised patients, it was concluded that aromatherapy massage has mild, transient anxiolytic effects. Due to lack of independent replication, the results of six other trials were not considered conclusive. These included positive findings for the treatment of alopecia areata[3] and prevention of bronchitis[4] and negative results for postnatal perineal discomfort.[5] Another systematic review included four RCTs of topical applications of tea tree oil.[6] There was some encouraging but not compelling evidence for acne and fungal infections. A Cochrane review of aromatherapy for dementia found only one RCT with useable data and concluded that 'aromatherapy showed benefit for people with dementia'.[7] Another Cochrane review focused on aromatherapy and massage for symptom relief in patients with cancer. It included ten RCTs and found that 'massage and aromatherapy confer short-term benefits on psychological well-being, with the effect on anxiety supported by limited evidence'.[8] However, it was uncertain whether aromatherapy enhances the effects of massage. More recent CCTs or RCTs suggest that aromatherapy can reduce anxiety during dental procedures,[9] alleviate pruritus in hemodialysis patients,[10] reduce pain of arthritis,[11] and alleviate constipation in the elderly.[12] Other RCTs fail to show benefit in terms of symptom control in cancer patients,[13] pain control, anxiety or quality of life in hospice patients,[14] relieving postoperative nausea,[15] reducing anxiety during radiotherapy[16] or abortion.[17] An RCT testing whether the mere olfactory absorption of lavender or rosemary essential oils affected pain sensitivity in healthy volunteers (n = 26) failed to show such an effect.[18] Similarly, smelling lavender or thyme oils had no effect on agitation of dementia patients in a small CCT (n = 7).[19]

Risks

Contraindications
Pregnancy, contagious diseases, epilepsy, local venous thrombosis, varicose veins, broken skin, recent surgery, circulatory disorders.

Precautions/warnings
Essential oils should not be taken orally or used undiluted on the skin. Some oils cause photosensitive reactions and some have carcinogenic potential. Allergic reactions are possible with all oils. Aromatherapy should generally be considered an adjunctive treatment, not an alternative to conventional care.

THERAPIES

Adverse effects

Allergic reactions, phototoxic reactions, nausea, headache.

Interactions

Many essential oils are believed to have the potential to either enhance or reduce the effects of prescribed medications including antibiotics, tranquillisers, antihistamines, anticonvulsants, barbiturates, morphine, quinidine.

Quality issues

Products marketed as 'aromatherapy oils' may be synthetic or adulterated rather than the pure essential oil.

Risk–benefit assessment

The trial evidence on aromatherapy is confusingly contradictory. Aromatherapy appears to have some benefits as a palliative or supportive treatment, particularly in reducing anxiety. In the hands of a responsible therapist there seem to be few risks. Aromatherapy may thus be worth considering as an adjunctive treatment for chronically ill patients or individuals with psychosomatic illness.

REFERENCES

1 Osborn C E, Barlas P, Baxter G D, Barlow J H. Aromatherapy: a survey of current practice in the management of rheumatic disease symptoms. Complement Ther Med 2001;9:62–67
2 Cooke B, Ernst E. Aromatherapy: a systematic review. Br J Gen Pract 2000;50:493–496
3 Hay I C, Jamieson M, Ormerod A D. Randomised trial of aromatherapy. Successful treatment for alopecia areata. Arch Dermatol 1998;134:1349–1352
4 Ferley J P, Poutignat N, Zmirou D et al. Prophylactic aromatherapy for supervening infections in patients with chronic bronchitis. Statistical evaluation conducted in clinics against a placebo. Phytother Res1989;3:97–100
5 Dale A, Cornwell S. The role of lavender oil in relieving perineal discomfort following childbirth: a blind randomised clinical trial. J Adv Nurs 1994;19:89–96
6 Ernst E, Huntley A. Tea tree oil: a systematic review of randomized clinical trials. Forsch Komple-mentärmed Klass Naturheilkd 2000;7:17–20
7 Thorgrimsen L, Spector A, Wiles A, Orrell M. Aromatherapy for dementia. The Cochrane Database of Systematic Reviews 2003, Issue 3. Art. No.: CD003150
8 Fellowes D, Barnes K, Wilkinson S. aromatherapy and massage for symptom relief in patients with cancer. The Cochrane Database of Systematic Reviews 2004, Issue 3. Art. No.: CD002287
9 Lehrner J, Eckersberger C, Walla P, Pötsch G, Deecke L. Ambient odor of orange in a dental office reduces anxiety and improves mood in female patients. Physiol Behav 2000;71:83–86
10 Ro Y J, Ha H C, Kim C G, Yeom H A. The effects of aromatherapy on pruritus in patients undergoing hemodialysis. Dermatol Nurs 2002;14:231–234
11 Kim M J, Nam E S, Paik S I. [The effects of aromatherapy on pain, depression, and life satisfaction of arthritis patients.] Taehan Kanho Hakhoe Chi 2005;35:186–194 Korean
12 Kim M A, Sakong J K, Kim E J, Kim E H, Kim E H. [Effect of aromatherapy massage for the relief of constipation in the elderly.] Taehan Kanho Hakhoe Chi 2005;35:56–64 Korean
13 Wilcock A, Manderson C, Weller R, Walker G, Carr D, Carey A M, Broadhurst D, Mew J, Ernst E. Does aromatherapy massage benefit patients with cancer attending a specialist palliative care day centre? Palliat Med 2004;18:287–290
14 Soden K, Vincent K, Craske S, Lucas C, Ashley S. A randomized controlled trial of aromatherapy massage in a hospice setting. Palliat Med 2004;18:87–92
15 Anderson L A, Gross J B. Aromatherapy with peppermint, isopropyl alcohol, or placebo is equally effective in relieving postoperative nausea. J Perianesth Nurs 2004;19:29–35

16 Graham P H, Browne L, Cox H, Graham
    J. Inhalation aromatherapy during
    radiotherapy: results of a placebo-controlled
    double-blind randomized trial. J Clin Oncol
    2003;21:2372–2376
17 Wiebe E. A randomized trial of aromatherapy
    to reduce anxiety before abortion. Eff Clin
    Pract 2000;3:166–169

18 Gedney J J, Glover T L, Fillingim R B. Sensory
    and affective pain discrimination after
    inhalation of essential oils. Psychosom Med
    2004;66:599–606
19 Snow A L, Hovanec L, Brandt J. A controlled
    trial of aromatherpay for agitation in nursing
    home patients with dementia. J Altern
    Complement Med 2004;10:431–437

AUTOGENIC TRAINING

Synonyms Autogenic therapy, autogenics.

Definition Autogenic training (AT) refers to a particular technique of mental exercises involving relaxation and autosuggestion practised regularly, which aims to teach individuals to switch off the 'fight/flight/fight' stress response at will. The passive state which results is believed to allow the brain and body to tap into its own spontaneous self-regulatory mechanism, which, in turn, can encourage an awareness of the origin of certain mental and physical disorders within. In the USA, the term 'autogenic' often refers to any method that involves patients using their own resources to help themselves, usually involving relaxation, visualisation or autosuggestion.

Related techniques Relaxation, self-hypnosis.

Background AT developed out of observations in the last decade of the 19th century that people who had previously undergone hypnotic sessions were able to put themselves readily in a state which appeared to be similar to hypnosis and that the regular use of this state reduced stress and improved efficiency. In the 1920s, the German physician Johannes Schultz explored these ideas and added autosuggestion, with the aim of developing a practice that avoided the therapist dependency of hypnosis and gave control to patients themselves. Heaviness and warmth were the two most common sensations during hypnosis, so Schultz taught patients to think about heaviness and warmth in the limbs. These constitute the first two exercises of AT. Four other instructions, relating to heart rate, breathing, warmth in the abdomen and coolness of the forehead, were added to form the six standard exercises.

In the 1940s, Schultz and Thomas developed the Personal and Motivational Formulae (at first known as 'intentional formulae'), which are tailored to the individual experience, and involve repetition of therapeutic suggestions, designed, for example, to correct negative patterns of thought. Later, a series of meditative exercises were added for those who have gained considerable experience.

THERAPIES

In the 1970s, a chest physician, Wolfgang Luthe, developed the Intentional Off-loading Exercises, whereby individuals are taught to off-load emotions. These exercises are thought to enhance the autogenic process by encouraging the release of stored and pent-up feelings that often manifest in psychosomatic 'stress' symptoms.

The method has spread via associations of interested practitioners, arriving in the UK in the late 1970s. It is now widespread through several European countries, although it is not one of the most common complementary therapies.

Scientific rationale

There is little neurophysiological research on AT. It appears to combine the effects of profound relaxation, which probably involve the limbic system and the hypothalamo-pituitary axis, with psychotherapeutic aspects of autosuggestion.

Practitioners

Practitioners of AT frequently have other healthcare training and integrate AT into their practice. German psychiatrists provide an example of this. There is no regulation or restriction on who may practise. In some countries, associations exist which continue to emphasise the classic method of Schultz and Luthe.

Conditions frequently treated

Angina pectoris, anxiety, asthma, chronic pain, depression, dyspepsia, functional disorders of bladder and bowel, headache, hypertension, migraine, phobia, premenstrual syndrome, sleep disorders, stress responses.

Typical session

In a quietened room, patients (training is often carried out in groups) are first instructed in the three recommended postures. Then they learn to concentrate passively on the heaviness of the dominant arm and to generalise this sensation to the rest of the body. This is followed by instruction in the other standard exercises. These should be practised three times daily, for about 10 minutes each time. Students are asked to keep diaries of their experiences in order that the process and reactions can be monitored by the tutor. When the standard exercises have been mastered, Personal and Motivational Formulae will be added, being devised by the client with the help of the therapist. After gaining considerable experience, advanced AT can be learnt, which involves prolonging the autogenic state and performing meditative exercises on increasingly abstract concepts. A second advanced autogenic method, also prolonging the autogenic state and developed by Luthe, is 'Autogenic Neutralisation', a psychotherapeutic method of release or discharge (neutralisation) of the 'disturbing potency of neuronal record.'

Course of treatment

Typically between eight and ten sessions are required to learn the standard exercises. There is no need for further attendance, unless advanced autogenic training work is undertaken.

THERAPIES

Clinical evidence   A systematic review of all controlled trials reached positive conclusions for some conditions (hypertension, asthma, intestinal diseases, glaucoma and eczema) but made no assessment of the quality of studies.[1] In a systematic review of studies of AT for hypertension, four out of five had positive results;[2] in a review of AT for anxiety (including experimentally induced anxiety) seven out of eight studies were positive.[3] However, in both cases, the quality of studies was too poor to allow firm conclusions to be drawn. Recent RCTs or systematic reviews support the view that AT can effectively reduce stress,[4,5] improve sleep in cancer patients,[6] alleviate headaches in a variety of clinical situations,[7,8] reduce labour pain,[9] and treat anxiety.[10,11]

Risks

Contraindications
Severe mental disorders. Latent psychosis and personality disorders, as these may become overt with introspection. Children under 5 years.

Precautions/warnings
For medical conditions, AT should only be used as an adjunct to standard therapy. Some people have difficulty mastering the technique.

Adverse effects
Reactions to AT may occur, such as unusual sensations in the body.

Interactions
Standard therapy (e.g. for hypertension) should be monitored more regularly while learning AT in case alterations of medication are required.

Risk–benefit assessment   AT is likely to be effective and safe for a number of conditions such as stress and anxiety. It can be recommended in suitable cases.

THERAPIES

REFERENCES

1   Stetter F, Kupper S. Autogenes Training – qualitative Meta-Analyse kontrollierter klinischer Studien und Beziehungen zur Naturheilkunde. Forsch Komplementärmed 1998;5:211–223

2   Kanji N, White A R, Ernst E. Antihypertensive effects of autogenic training: a systematic review. Perfusion 1999;12:279–282

3   Kanji N, Ernst E. Autogenic training for stress and anxiety: a systematic review. Complement Ther Med 2000;8:106–110

4   Hidderley M, Holt M. A pilot randomized trial assessing the effects of autogenic training in early stage cancer patients in relation to psychological status and immune system responses. Eur J Oncol Nurs 2004;8:61–65

5   Goldbeck L, Schmid K. Effectiveness of autogenic relaxation training on children and adolescents with behavioral and emotional problems. J Am Acad Child Adolec Psychiatry 2003;42:1046–1054.

6   Simeit R, Deck R, Conta-Marx B. Sleep management training for cancer patients with insomnia. Support Cancer Care 2004;12:176–183

7   Zsombok T, Juhasz G, Budavari A, Vitrai J, Bagdy G. Effect of Autogenic Training on drug consumption in patients with primary

headache: an 8-month follow-up study.
Headache 2003;43:251–257

8   Devineni T, Blanchard E B. A randomized
controlled trial of an internet-based treatment
for chronic headache. Behav Res Ther
2005;43:277–292

9   Huntley A L, Coon J T, Ernst E.
Complementary and alternative medicine for
labor pain: a systematic review. Am J Obstet
Gynecol 2004;191:36–44

10 Kanji N, White A, Ernst E. Autogenic training
reduces anxiety after coronary angioplasty:
A randomized clinical trial. Am Heart J
2004;147:e10

11 Jorm A F, Christensen H, Griffiths K M,
Parslow R A, Rodgers B, Blewitt K A.
Effectiveness of complementary and self-help
treatments for anxiety disorders. Med J Aust
2004;181(7 Suppl):S29–46

(BACH) FLOWER REMEDIES

Synonyms   Flower remedies; flower essence therapy.

Definition   A therapeutic system that uses specially prepared plant infusions to balance physical and emotional disturbances.

Background   Edward Bach was a microbiologist at the Royal London Homeopathic Hospital in the early part of the 20th century. Inspired by Hahnemann and Jung, he developed his own system of medicine. According to Bach, all human disease and suffering are rooted in emotional imbalances. He identified 38 flower remedies which, he believed, could treat most illnesses.

Traditional concepts   The 38 remedies are divided into seven therapeutic groups according to the following emotions: depression, fear, lack of interest in the present, loneliness, overconcern for the welfare of others, oversensitivity, and uncertainty. Bach associated each of these emotions with flowers to be used as remedies.

The remedies are produced by placing freshly picked sun-exposed flowers into spring water, into which brandy is added for preservation. The prescription of these remedies by specialised therapists is highly individualised and intuitive. According to Bach, the remedies work not through their pharmacological actions but through their 'energy'. Thus there are similarities with homeopathy, even though many homeopaths deny this. The term 'Bach' flower remedies is used as a brand name but there are other 'flower remedies' on the market which are produced according to Bach's instructions.

Scientific rationale   'Energy' in this context has not been defined in scientific terms. The method is scientifically implausible.

Practitioners   Therapists employing flower remedies are not usually medically qualified and often use these remedies in conjunction with other forms of CAM. Flower remedies are also popular for self-treatment and are available in many pharmacies and health food stores.

Conditions frequently treated	According to proponents, flower remedies are not targeted at specific medical conditions but at the underlying emotional imbalances. 'Rescue remedy' (Five-Flower Remedy) is promoted as a first aid for emergency situations.
Typical session	Flower remedies are sold over the counter for self-medication. The idea, proponents say, is for people to use them as a means of self-help. Thus many users of these remedies will not see a specialised practitioner. If they do, the therapeutic encounter will entail the taking of a detailed history with little or no physical examination. At the end of the encounter the therapist will prescribe the remedy, or remedies, that is, according to his or her opinion, best suited.
Course of treatment	In many instances, one prescription constitutes a full course of treatment. For persistent complaints several encounters are likely to be deemed necessary. Flower remedies are often recommended for long-term use, e.g. as a means of illness prevention.
Clinical evidence	There are numerous anecdotal reports about therapeutic successes. Very few controlled clinical trials exist and these are inconclusive, not least because of methodological weaknesses. A randomised, placebo-controlled, double-blind trial[1] tested Five-Flower Remedy for examination stress in 100 university students. Its results show no differences in outcome compared with placebo. A similar RCT found that 61 students responded positively to both Rescue Remedies and placebo.[2] The authors therefore concluded that Bach flower remedies are an 'effective placebo for test-anxiety, which do not have a specific effect'. A recent systematic review uncovered no further rigorous studies.[3]
Risks	**Contraindications** None known. **Precautions/warnings** Contain alcohol. **Adverse effects** Because flower remedies contain only very low concentrations of pharmacologically active ingredients (apart from alcohol), there is little risk of adverse effects. **Interactions** None known
Risk–benefit assessment	According to current evidence, flower remedies are not associated with specific therapeutic effects. They are also devoid of direct risks. Thus their usefulness seems to be limited to that of a placebo therapy.

THERAPIES

REFERENCES

1 Armstrong N C, Ernst E. A randomized, double-blind, placebo-controlled trial of Bach Flower Remedy. Perfusion 1999;11:440–446

2 Walach H, Rilling C, Engelke U. Efficacy of Bach-flower remedies in test anxiety: a double-blind,

placebo-controlled, randomized trial with partial crossover. Anxiety Disord 2001;15: 359–366

3 Ernst E, 'Flower remedies': a systematic review of the clinical evidence. Wien Klin Wochenschr 2002;114:963–966

BIOFEEDBACK

Definition

The use of instrumentation to monitor, amplify, and feed back information on physiological responses so that a patient can learn to regulate these responses.[1,2] Biofeedback is a form of psycho-physiological self-regulation. When biofeedback is used to control brain activity, it is called neurofeedback or neurotherapy.[3]

Related techniques

Biofeedback and neurofeedback are frequently used as adjuncts to relaxation, hypnosis, behaviour therapy and psychotherapy.

Background

Biofeedback developed from several streams of research in the 1960s and 1970s: laboratory-based research on voluntary physiological controls, behavioural therapy efforts to identify reliable principles of behaviour change, and the search of humanistic psychology for the higher potentials of human beings.[4,5] Early research showed voluntary control of EEG brain wave activity, internal visceral functioning, and muscle activity. Biofeedback was shown to increase the human being's awareness and control of many bodily processes previously thought to be beyond voluntary control.

Traditional concepts

The basic concept is that the process of becoming aware of physiological responses in the body offers the individual the opportunity to establish control over such processes. Any physiological response that can be monitored is suitable for biofeedback. The most common responses are electrical activity of the brain (EEG), skin temperature (thermal), muscle tension or surface electromyography (SEMG), galvanic skin response or electrodermal response, blood pressure, respiration, heart rate and heart rate variability, and blood volume.[4,6] This information is presented to the patient through visual and/or auditory signals, often through a computer monitor display. The aim of treatment is to establish the patient's mastery over the response independently of the biofeedback instrument. Biofeedback is also helpful in teaching the patient to recognise the linkage between mind and body, and more specifically to recognise the role of specific thoughts and emotions in the onset of physical symptoms. Biofeedback is frequently used as an adjunct to other therapies. Biofeedback assisted relaxation training supports progress in cognitive-behavioural therapy and stress management. Biofeedback is also

THERAPIES

frequently used to monitor signs of affective arousal or disturbance in psychotherapy.

Scientific rationale

Biofeedback can modify physiological processes mediated by the central and peripheral nervous systems, impacting both somatic and autonomic nervous pathways. The relaxation effects of biofeedback affect the limbic brain, the hypothalamic-pituitary-adrenal axis, autonomic control of a variety of internal organs, and muscle function.[7]

Practitioners

Biofeedback is an inter-disciplinary field. Clinical psychologists, health psychologists and behavioural therapists are among those who use biofeedback frequently. Biofeedback procedures are also widely used by physicians, nurses, physical and occupational therapists, sports physiologists, social workers, counselors, teachers, and many others.

Conditions frequently treated

Conditions that can be alleviated by mental calming and/or affected more directly through physiological changes achieved, such as anxiety, asthma, attention deficit disorder, bruxism, encopresis, enuresis, epileptic seizures, essential tremor, headache (tension-type and migraine), hypertension, insomnia, irritable bowel syndrome, occupational cramps, pelvic floor disorders including urinary incontinence and faecal incontinence, Raynaud's, substance abuse, and tinnitus.

Typical session

An initial medical and psychosocial history provides evidence regarding relevant patterns and mechanisms active in the onset and maintenance of the patient's disorder. The practitioner often conducts a psychophysiological profile, assessing the patient's baseline physiological patterns, reactivity under varied conditions such as stressors, and recovery ability and rate. The profile further identifies physiological systems though which this patient reacts, that could be addressed and modified with biofeedback. The practitioner attaches sensors (SEMG, EEG, temperature, etc.) for measuring various physiological responses. The patient observes audiovisual displays and learns to reduce maladaptive responses, correct abnormal physiological reactions and habits, and produce desired physiological changes. The patient learns to recognise the maladaptive psychophysiological functioning such as the physiological responses and symptoms that are linked to thoughts, emotions, postures, and breathing habits.

Course of treatment

Treatments with biofeedback vary, depending on a range of factors. Initial evaluations last typically about 60 to 90 minutes, and subsequent sessions vary from about 45 to 60 minutes. Therapists often recommend home practice such as varied relaxation procedures. Audiotapes or CDs are often used for training.

THERAPIES

Clinical evidence   An overview provided a summary of systematic reviews on biofeedback.[8] According to these data various forms of biofeedback are effective as adjunctive treatments of anismus, faecal incontinence, paediatric migraine, rheumatoid arthritis, stroke rehabilitation and temporomandibular disorders. The evidence is inconclusive for asthma, chronic pain, erectile dysfunction, gastrointestinal disorders, hypertension, insomnia, obstructive pulmonary disease, stress management, and tinnitus. The evidence is negative for atopic eczema, back pain, tension-type headache and cervicogenic headache. Recent RCT evidence confirms the effectiveness of biofeedback for urinary stress incontinence in women,[9,10] urinary incontinence in men with erectile dysfunction,[11] faecal incontinence in women,[12,13] as well as faecal incontinence after surgical sphincter repair.[14]

Risks   ***Contraindications***
Patients with psychiatric conditions, examples include severe depression, acute agitation, acute or fragile schizophrenia, mania, paranoid disorders with delusions of influence, severe obsessive-compulsive disorder, delirium and dissociative reaction.

Precautions/warnings
As with other therapies that induce changes in mental state, biofeedback should be used only under medical supervision in cases of psychosis or personality disorder.

Adverse effects
There are occasional reports of biofeedback being associated with acute anxiety, dizziness, disorientation and floating sensations.

Interactions
In patients taking medication involved in homeostasis, such as insulin or antihypertensive therapies, the dose may need to be altered.

Risk–benefit assessment   Biofeedback is effective for a range of conditions, often as an adjunct to other interventions. The risks are small, and adverse effects are rare.

REFERENCES

1 Schwartz M, Andrasik F (eds). Biofeedback: a practitioner's guide. New York: Guilford Press; 2003
2 Green J A, Shellenberger R. Biofeedback therapy. In: Jonas W B, Levin J S (eds). Essentials of complementary and alternative medicine. Baltimore, MD: Lippincott Williams & Wilkins; 1999:410–425
3 Evans J R, Abarbanel A (eds). Introduction to quantitative EEG and neurofeedback. San Diego: Academic Press; 1999

4 Gilbert C, Moss D. Biofeedback. In: Moss D, Wickramesekera D I, McGrady A, Davies T (eds). Handbook of mind-body medicine in primary care: Behavioral and physiological tools. Thousand Oaks, CA: Sage; 2003:109–122
5 Moss D. Biofeedback. In: Shannon S (ed). Handbook of complementary and alternative therapies in mental health. San Diego, CA: Academic Press; 2001:135–158
6 Lawlis G F. Biofeedback. In: Freeman L W, Lawlis G F (eds). Mosby's complementary and

alternative medicine: a research based approach. St Louis, MO: Mosby; 2001:196–224

7   Everly G S, Lating J M. A clinical guide to treatment of the human stress response. New York: Plenum; 2002

8   Ernst E. Systematic reviews of biofeedback. Phys Med Rehab Kuror 2003;13:321–324

9   Seo J T, Yoon H, Kim Y H. A randomized prospective study comparing new vaginal cone and FES-Biofeedback. Yonsei Med J 2004;45:879–884

10 Aukee P, Immonen P, Laaksonen D E, Laippala P, Penttinen J, Airaksinen O. The effect of home biofeedback training on stress incontinence. Acta Obstet Gynecol Scand 2004;83:973–977

11 Dorey G, Speakman M, Feneley R, Swinkels A, Dunn C, Ewings P. Pelvic floor exercises for treating post-micturition dribble in men with erectile dysfunction: a randomized controlled trial. Urol Nurs 2004;24:490–497

12 Mahony R T, Malone P A, Nalty J, Behan M, O'Connell P R, O'Herlihy C. Randomized clinical trial of intra-anal electromyographic biofeedback physiotherapy with intra-anal electromyographic biofeedback augmented with electrical stimulation of the anal sphincter in the early treatment of postpartum fecal incontinence. Am J Obstet Gynecol 2004;191:885–890

13 Ilnyckyj A, Fachnie E, Tougas G. A randomized-controlled trial comparing an educational intervention alone vs education and biofeedback in the management of faecal incontinence in women. Neurogastroenterol Motil 2005;17:58–63

14 Davis K J, Kumar D, Poloniecki J. Adjuvant biofeedback following anal sphincter repair: a randomized study. Aliment Pharmacol Ther 2004;20:539–549

CHELATION THERAPY

Definition

A method for removing toxins, minerals and metabolic wastes from the bloodstream and vessel walls using intravenous ethylene diamine tetraacetic acid (EDTA) infusions.

Background

The method was introduced in the 1950s. In mainstream medicine it is an established conventional therapy for heavy metal poisoning. Apparently some clinicians noticed that other conditions also improved in patients treated with chelation therapy. Thus it developed as an 'alternative' treatment for a number of conditions unrelated to heavy metal poisoning. Today chelation is popular with many patients[1] yet 41% of US physicians recommend against it.[2]

Traditional concepts and scientific rationale

It has been claimed that this therapy, through the chelating mechanism, removes calcium deposits from arteriosclerotic plaques and thus represents a causal treatment for arteriosclerosis. This rationale is based on an outdated understanding of atherogenesis. Newer theories of how chelation therapy might work for arteriosclerosis relate to other mechanisms including antioxidation, free radical scavenging, inhibition of LDL oxidation, reduction of reperfusion injury or haemorheological activity. While these are sound concepts of ischaemic injury, it is unclear to what extent chelation therapy does produce such effects in vivo and whether these effects contribute to any clinical changes. Most practitioners add minerals and other supplements to their treatment.

THERAPIES

Practitioners

Today, chelation therapy is used in the 'alternative' way by more than 1000 US physicians and numerous practitioners in Europe, most but not all of whom are medically qualified.

Conditions frequently treated

In CAM the method is used predominantly with a view to inducing regression of arteriosclerotic lesions, e.g. in ischaemic heart disease, intermittent claudication or for stroke prevention or as an alternative to bypass surgery. Other conditions claimed to respond are arthritis and other connective tissue diseases, cataracts, diabetes, emphysema, gallstones, hypertension, osteoporosis, Parkinson's disease, renal disease and impaired vision, hearing, memory or sense of smell.

Typical session

The practitioner would normally take a conventional medical history and establish a conventional diagnosis. For treatment, the patient would receive a slow infusion of EDTA usually in combination with vitamins, trace elements and iron supplements. One session might last for about one to three hours.

Course of treatment

One single treatment is rarely deemed sufficient. A course of treatments often involves 10–30 sessions over several months. The costs for a course of treatments are usually around US $3000.

Clinical evidence

One systematic review of all four randomised, placebo-controlled, double-blind trials of chelation therapy for intermittent claudication found no convincing evidence for its efficacy.[3] It concluded, 'Chelation therapy for peripheral arterial occlusive disease is not superior to placebo . . . It should now be considered obsolete'.[3] A Cochrane review stated that there is 'insufficient evidence'.[4]

Another systematic review included all controlled and uncontrolled clinical studies of chelation therapy for ischaemic heart disease regardless of trial design.[5] Numerous case reports and case series but only two controlled clinical trials were found. The latter studies yielded no convincing evidence for efficacy. It concluded, 'This treatment should now be considered obsolete'.[5] A recent study suggested that, in patients with ischaemic heart disease, chelation 'does not provide additional benefits on abnormal vasomotor responses'.[6] More evidence can be expected from the current National Institutes of Health trial lasting 5 years at a cost of US$ 30 million.

Risks

Contraindications
Unstable coronary heart disease, aneurysms.

Precautions/warnings
Renal insufficiency, pregnancy, bleeding abnormalities, surgery within 24 hours of infusion.

Adverse effects

Faintness (RR = 11.44)[4], gastrointestinal symptoms (R = 1.63)[4], proteinuria (RR = 2.60), renal failure, arrhythmias, tetany, hypocalcaemia (RR = 3.12)[4], hypoglycaemia, hypotension, bone marrow depression, prolonged bleeding time, convulsions, respiratory arrest and autoimmune diseases have all been described. Several fatalities have been reported. In addition the procedure can cause phlebitis and pain.[4]

Interactions

Calcium supplementation, renal clearance of drugs.

Risk–benefit assessment

The documented risks of chelation therapy as used in CAM clearly outweigh the benefits. Proponents of chelation therapy might argue that, with more refined treatment regimens, the problems of the 'early days' have been overcome. Yet, in the absence of reliable supporting data, this notion is unconvincing. Thus chelation therapy is not recommended for indications other than heavy metal poisoning.

REFERENCES

1 Quan H, Ghali W A, Verhoef M J, Norris C M, Galbraith P D, Knudtson M L. Use of chelation therapy after coronary angiography. Am J Med 2001;111:686–691

2 Boutin P D, Buchwald D, Robinson L, Collier A C. Use of and attitudes about alternative and complementary therapies among outpatients and physicians at a municipal hospital. J Altern Complement Med 2000;6:335–430

3 Ernst E. Chelation therapy for peripheral arterial occlusive disease. Circulation 1997;96:1031–1033

4 Villarruz M V, Dans A, Tan F. Chelation therapy for atherosclerotic cardiovascular disease. The Cochrane Database of Systematic Reviews 2002, Issue 4. Art. No. CD002785

5 Ernst E. Chelation therapy for coronary heart disease. An overview of all clinical investigations. Am Heart J 2000;140:139–141

6 Anderson T J, Hubacek J, Wyse D G, Knudtson M L. Effect of chelation therapy on endothelial function in patients with coronary artery disease: PATCH substudy. J Am Coll Cardiol 2003;41:420–425

CHIROPRACTIC

Definition

According to the UK General Chiropractic Council, chiropractic is a health profession concerned with the diagnosis, treatment and prevention of mechanical disorders of the musculoskeletal system, and the effects of these disorders on the function of the nervous system and general health. There is an emphasis on manual treatments including spinal manipulation or adjustment.

Related techniques

Osteopathy, manual therapy, spinal manipulation, spinal mobilisation.

Background

Some therapeutic elements which chiropractors use, such as spinal manipulation, go back to antiquity and were used by bone-setters throughout the history of (folk) medicine. Chiropractic was founded in 1895 by the Canadian Daniel David Palmer (1845–1913) and has since developed into a profession practised worldwide. The term chiropractic was derived from the Greek *cheir* (hand) and *praxis* (action).

During subsequent decades, chiropractic had a colourful history with bickering between various subsets of the chiropractic profession. The 'straights' adhered to Palmer's teaching as to a dogma, while the 'mixers' had a more liberal attitude. A fierce debate also raged between mainstream medicine and chiropractic. Today chiropractors are accepted healthcare professionals and their treatments are now being tested according to the principles of evidence-based medicine.

Traditional concepts

Palmer reasoned that pressure on nerves, caused by misalignment of the vertebral joints, produced disease. He surmised that correction of these misalignments was the only way of restoring health. The most important therapeutic method of chiropractors is spinal manipulation. It generally entails high-velocity, low-amplitude manual thrusts applied to spinal joints, which extend them slightly beyond their physiological range of motion. Spinal mobilisation, by contrast, is the application of manual force to such joints without thrust and within the normal passive range of motion.

Scientific rationale

The primary premise that subluxation is the cause of all illness has no scientific rationale. Spinal mobilisation has been shown to have a number of physiological effects (such as reduction of muscle spasm, inhibition of nociceptive transmissions). Spinal manipulation and related techniques are thought to improve joint function and alleviate pain related to spinal abnormalities.

Practitioners

By definition, chiropractic is what chiropractors do. However, spinal manipulation and mobilisation are also used by osteopaths, naturopaths, physical therapists and doctors. Both in the USA and the UK, chiropractors need a licence for practice. In the UK, chiropractors are regulated by statute.

Conditions frequently treated

Asthma, cardiovascular problems, headache, infantile colic, irritable bowel syndrome, migraine, musculoskeletal problems, more specifically spinal pain syndromes. Patients with complaints of apparently visceral origin comprise about 5% of chiropractic practice.

Typical session

A chiropractor takes the patient's case history and conducts a physical examination. In many cases, this is supplemented by spinal X-rays and possibly other diagnostic procedures. The initial encounter can be purely diagnostic. Subsequent treatments involve hands-on techniques, usually with the patient sitting or lying. These may last for 15 minutes or more and include reviews of patient progress, amendment of treatment plans, and appropriate referral when clinically indicated.

Course of treatment

The number of sessions required is highly variable; on average it is seven, ranging between four and 20. Repeat courses of treatments or continuing prophylactic or supportive sessions are often recommended.

Clinical evidence

A systematic review of spinal manipulative therapies for back pain included 39 RCTs,[1] 29 of which assessed patients with acute pain, 29 studies evaluated patients with chronic pain, and 14 studies included patients with mixed or indeterminate durations of pain. For patients with acute low back pain, the only reported clinically significant improvement in short-term pain occurred among patients receiving spinal manipulation as compared with sham therapy. In comparisons with all other conventionally advocated therapies, spinal manipulative therapies showed no statistical or clinical difference among patients with acute low back pain. Similarly, among patients with chronic low back pain, the only clinically significant findings exist in comparison with the sham therapy or, as the authors state, ineffective therapies groups. No differences were found for the outcomes of short-term or long-term function.

As this review includes all manipulative therapies, it is pertinent to systematically review chiropractic spinal manipulation for back pain separately.[2] Twelve RCTs were found including all forms of back pain. Many trials had considerable methodological shortcomings. Some degree of superiority of chiropractic spinal manipulation over control interventions was noted in 5 studies. More recent trials and those with adequate follow-up periods tended to be negative. It was concluded that the effectiveness of chiropractic spinal manipulation for back pain is not supported by compelling evidence from the majority of RCTs.

A Cochrane review of spinal manipulation and mobilisation for neck pain included 33 trials and found that, administered alone, these treatments were not beneficial.[3] Specifically on chiropractic spinal manipulation only four RCTs were located for a systematic review.[4] None of them convincingly demonstrated the superiority of manipulation over control interventions.

Eight RCTs were included in a systematic review of spinal manipulation for headache disorders.[5] The results were inconclusive and no definitive conclusion about the effectiveness of this approach was drawn. Other reviewers stated 'before any firm conclusions can be drawn, further testing should be done in rigorously designed (...) trials.[6]

Other systematic reviews, including Cochrane reviews, generated no sound evidence for the effectiveness of spinal manipulation as a treatment for non-spinal pain,[7] infantile colic,[8] carpal tunnel syndrome,[9] secondary dysmenorrhoea,[10] and asthma.[11]

Finally, a systematic review of all sham-controlled RCTs of spinal manipulation (for any condition) concluded that 'the most rigorous of these studies suggest that spinal manipulation is not associated with clinically relevant specific therapeutic effects.[12]

THERAPIES

THERAPIES

Risks

Contraindications

High-velocity manipulations are contraindicated in advanced osteoporosis, bleeding abnormalities, malignant or inflammatory spinal disease, patients on anticoagulants, fractures, postoperative spinal instability, cervical spondylotic myelopathy, cauda equina syndrome.

Precautions/warnings

Elderly patients, people who feel uncomfortable with close contact. Overuse of X-ray diagnostics, advice of some chiropractors against immunisation, unreliability of diagnostic techniques used by chiropractors.

Adverse effects

Serious adverse effects are probably rare and include arterial dissection and stroke (upper spinal manipulation) and cauda equina syndrome (lower spinal manipulation).[13] Mild and transient adverse effects of high-velocity manipulations, such as local discomfort, are reported by about 50% of all patients.[13]

Interactions

Patients on anticoagulants may be at a higher risk of cerebrovascular accidents after high-velocity manipulations of the upper spine.

Risk–benefit assessment

Chiropractic treatment might be helpful for low back pain, but the evidence is not convincing. In view of the lack of truly effective conventional treatments for this indication, chiropractic might therefore be worth considering for such patients. For all other indications the evidence is even less compelling. Severe adverse events may be infrequent but mild transient complaints are common.

REFERENCES

1 Assendelft W J J, Morton S C, Yu E I, Suttorp M J, Shekelle P G. Spinal manipulation therapy for low back pain. The Cochrane Database of Systematic Reviews 2004; Issue 1. Art. No.: CD000447

2 Ernst E, Canter P H. Chiropractic spinal manipulation for back pain? A systematic review of randomised controlled trials. Phys Ther Rev 2003;8:85–91

3 Gross A R, Hoving J L, Haines T A, Goldsmith C H, Kay T, Aker P, Bronfort G. A Cochrane review of manipulation and mobilization for mechanical neck disorders. Spine 2004;29:1541–1548

4 Ernst E. Chiropractic spinal manipulation for neck pain: a systematic review. J Pain 2003;4:417–421

5 Astin J A, Ernst E. The effectiveness of spinal manipulation for the treatment of

headache disorders: a systematic review of randomized clinical trials. Cephalalgia 2002;22:617–623

6 Bronfort G, Assendelft W J J, Evans R, Haas M, Bouter L. Efficacy of spinal manipulation for chronic headache: a systematic review. J Manip Physiol Ther 2001;24:457–466

7 Ernst E. Chiropractic manipulation for non-spinal pain – a systematic review. NZ Med J 2003:116:1–9

8 Husereau D, Clifford T, Aker P, Leduc D, Mensinkai S. Spinal manipulation for infantile colic. Ottawa: Canadian Coordinating Office for Health Technology Assessment; 2003. Technology report no 42

9 O'Connor D, Marshall S, Massy-Westropp N. Non-surgical treatment (other than steroid injection) for carpal tunnel syndrome. The

Cochrane Database of Systematic Reviews 2003, Issue 1. Art. No.: CD003219

10 Proctor M L, Hing W, Johnson T C, Murphy P A. Spinal manipulation for primary and secondary dysmenorrhoea. The Cochrane Database of Systematic Reviews 2001, Issue 4. Art. No.: CD002119

11 Hondras M A, Linde K, Jones A P. Manual therapy for asthma. The Cochrane Database of Systematic Reviews 2002, Issue 3. Art. No.: CD001002

12 Ernst E, Harkness E. Spinal manipulation: a systematic review of sham-controlled, double-blind, randomized clinical trials. J Pain Symptom Manage 2001;22:879–889

13 Stevinson C, Ernst E. Risks associated with spinal manipulation. Am J Med 2002;112:566–571

CRANIOSACRAL THERAPY

Synonyms/ subcategories
Cranial osteopathy, sacro occipital technique.

Definition
A subtle form of hands-on treatment which is tissue-, fluid-, membrane-, and energy-oriented and very gentle in its application.

Related techniques
Osteopathy.

Background
The original concepts were first put forward in the 1930s by the American William G Sutherland. Initially it was only practised by osteopaths but, in the 1970s, John E Upledger made some refinements and was the first to teach it to non-osteopathic practitioners. Further refinements in both theory and practice continue to occur. Craniosacral therapy became popular first in the USA and subsequently in Europe.

Traditional concepts
Craniosacral therapy is based on the premise that there are micro-rhythmic motions present in the body which play an important role for health. Particular emphasis is placed upon alleged rhythmic motion of tissues and fluids at the core of the body: cerebrospinal fluid, the central nervous system, the intracranial and intraspinal dural membranes, the cranial bones and the sacrum. The unrestricted motion of these subtle rhythms is believed to be fundamental to the self-healing capabilities of the body. According to Upledger,[1] the rhythmic motion of cerebrospinal fluid can be sensed in a similar way to a peripheral pulse. Treatment is based upon the palpation of any strains or restrictions that affect these subtle rhythms and the use of light touch to facilitate natural motion. Craniosacral therapy is thought to help alleviate a wide range of symptoms.

Scientific rationale
Subtle rhythmic motion at cranial bones and the sacrum not directly related to lung respiration or arterial pulse and motion of cerebrospinal fluid have been reported (e.g.[2–4]). However, there is no published evidence that these movements affect health.

THERAPIES

THERAPIES

Practitioners

Craniosacral therapy is practised by chiropractors, osteopaths, naturopaths, physiotherapists, dentists, massage therapists, physicians and other regulated or unregulated healthcare professionals.

Conditions frequently treated

According to Upledger the following conditions respond to craniosacral therapy: birth trauma, cerebral dysfunction, cerebral palsy, chronic pain, colic, depression, dyslexia, ear infections, headaches, learning disabilities, Ménière's disease, migraine, musculoskeletal problems, sinusitis, strabismus, stroke, temporomandibular joint dysfunction, trigeminal neuralgia. Young children are believed to respond particularly well.

Typical session

The initial diagnostic session is conducted by a craniosacral therapist in order to evaluate the nature of the problem. The patient may be lying down or seated. The procedure mainly involves lightly touching the skull and/or the sacrum although the location of treatment is largely determined by physiological requirements of the patient. The first session may take about one hour. Subsequent therapeutic sessions are often shorter.

Course of treatment

The number of sessions required is extremely variable and depends on the nature and severity of the condition(s) treated. Upledger states that if no effect is seen after about six sessions, craniosacral therapy may not be effective.

Clinical evidence

Anecdotal evidence for the effectiveness of craniosacral therapy exists. Upledger claims that craniosacral therapy 'is helpful in at least 90% of the patients'.[1] A systematic review of the evidence however, concluded that there is 'insufficient evidence to support craniosacral therapy'.[4] An independent review supported these findings.[5] An RCT compared osteopathic treatment employing parietal, visceral and craniosacral techniques with orthopaedic treatment using chiropractic techniques, antiphlogistics and cortisone in 53 patients with chronic epicondylopathia humeri radialis.[6] There was no difference between the treatments.

Risks

Contraindications
Intracranial aneurysm, cerebral haemorrhage, subdural or subarachnoid bleeding, increased intracranial pressure, recent skull fractures.

Precautions/warnings
None known.

Adverse effects
Some undesired effects were reported in patients with traumatic brain syndrome;[7] temporary worsening of symptoms and mild discomfort may occur.[1]

Interactions
May increase antidiabetic, antiepileptic or psychoactive medications.[1]

Risk–benefit assessment

There is no convincing evidence for the effectiveness of craniosacral therapy as a treatment of any disease or symptom. Several indirect and direct risks have been associated with craniosacral therapy. On balance therefore, and until further more positive data emerge craniosacral therapy cannot be recommended for any condition.

REFERENCES

1 Upledger J E. Craniosacral therapy. In: Novey D W (ed). The complete reference to complementary and alternative medicine. St Louis: Mosby; 2000
2 Frymann V M. A study of the rhythmic motions of the living cranium. J Am Osteopath Assoc 1971;70:928–945
3 Tettambel M, Cicora A, Lay E. Recording of the cranial rhythmic impulse. J Am Osteopath Assoc 1978;78·149
4 Green C, Martin C W, Bassett K, Kazanjian A. A systematic review of craniosacral therapy: biological plausibility, assessment reliability and clinical effectiveness. Complement Ther Med 1999;7:201–207

5 Hartman S E, Norton J M. Interexaminer reliability and cranial osteopathy. Sci Review Altern Med 2002;6:23–34
6 Geldschlager S. Osteopathic versus orthopedic treatments for chronic epicondylopathia humeri radialis: a randomized controlled trial. Forsch Komplementärmed Klass Naturheilkd 2004;11: 93–97
7 Greenman P E, McPartland J M. Cranial findings and iatrogenesis from craniosacral manipulation in patients with traumatic brain syndrome. J Am Osteopath Assoc 1995;95:182–188

HERBALISM

Synonyms/ subcategories

Ayurveda, botanical medicine, herbalism, traditional Chinese herbalism, Western herbalism, kampo, phytomedicine, phytotherapy.

Definition

The medical use of preparations that contain exclusively plant material.

Background

Plants have been used since the dawn of humanity for medicinal purposes and form the origin of much of modern medicine (e.g. digoxin from *Digitalis purpurea* or artemether from *Artemisia annua* for severe malaria). Modern Western herbalism or phytomedicine as practised in many European countries (e.g. Germany) is integrated into conventional medicine with compulsory education and training for physicians and pharmacists. Other more traditional systems include Chinese herbal medicine, which is based on the concepts of Yin and Yang and qi energy. Ill health is viewed as a pattern of disharmony or imbalance and Chinese herbal medicines are believed to harmonise these energies and ultimately restore health. In Japan this system of traditional herbal medicine has evolved into kampo. Ayurveda, the traditional medical system of India, also frequently uses herbal mixtures.

THERAPIES

THERAPIES

Characteristic of these systems is a high degree of individualisation of treatment, e.g. two patients with the same disease according to Western criteria could receive two different herbal preparations. Contrary to modern phytomedicine, all traditional herbal medicine systems predominantly employ complex mixtures of different herbs.

Traditional concepts

Whole plants, parts of plants or extracts are used. The different constituents of a single plant or of herbal mixtures are claimed to work synergistically to produce a greater effect than the sum of the effects of the single constituents. It is also claimed that the combined actions of the various constituents reduce the toxicity of the extract as compared with the single isolated constituent. These concepts of synergy and buffering extend to the use of different plant extracts in combination preparations. In traditional herbal medicine the diagnostic principles used differ considerably from those in mainstream medicine, with less emphasis on conventional disease categories and modern diagnostic techniques. Phytomedicine as practised in most European countries follows the diagnostic and therapeutic principles of conventional medicine.

Scientific rationale

Herbal extracts contain plant material with pharmacologically active constituents. The active principle(s) of the extract, which is in many cases unknown, may exert its effects on the molecular level and may have, for instance, enzyme-inhibiting effects (e.g. escin). A single main constituent may be active or, more often, a complex mixture of compounds produces a combined effect. Known active constituents or marker substances may be used to standardise preparations.

Practitioners

Most traditional herbalists in the UK and the USA are not medically qualified. In contrast to the situation in continental Europe, there is little integration into the conventional healthcare systems. In countries such as Germany and France much of herbalism, particularly Western phytomedicine, is practised by conventionally trained physicians and integrated into routine medical care. The educational route for practitioners of traditional Chinese medicine in the UK is currently to complete a 3 to 4 year BSc training in acupuncture, followed by 2 to 3 years postgraduate training in Chinese herbal medicine. There is also an MSc option available.

Conditions frequently treated

A wide range of conditions are treated; for instance, anxiety, benign prostatic hyperplasia, depression, digestive complaints, intermittent claudication, menstrual problems, pain, respiratory condition, skin conditions.

Typical session

During an initial treatment session the practitioner will usually take the patient's medical history to get an overall impression of the medical status and to screen for contraindications. Herbalists of the Chinese, Japanese and Indian traditions will also seek information on the patient's personality and background, which may influence the selection of herbs. Individualised combinations of herbs are prescribed and may be taken as extracts, tinctures, infusions or decoctions. Follow-up appointments are arranged as necessary and herbal preparations and regimen reviewed and changed if appropriate. Practitioners may advise on lifestyle factors such as diet and exercise. Consultations and treatment as practised in phytomedicine mainly on the European continent generally follow the principles of a conventional medical appointment.

Course of treatment

Depending largely on the nature and severity of the condition but generally 1–2 appointments per week for a treatment period ranging from one to several weeks.

Clinical evidence

The clinical evidence has to be evaluated according to each individual herbal preparation (see Section 4) or traditional approach. There is clinical evidence from Cochrane and other reviews for the effectiveness of a number of herbal preparations for treating various conditions (see Table 3.2).[1-54] Traditional Chinese herbal mixtures have also been assessed in Cochrane reviews (e.g.[55,56]). Little evidence from systematic reviews is available for the effectiveness of other traditional herbal medical systems. Safety has been assessed in systematic reviews in relation to, for instance, individual herbs (e.g.[57]) organ systems (e.g.[58,59]) or mechanism (e.g.[60,61]).

Risks

Contraindications
Contraindications and precautions vary for each individual herbal preparation (see Section 4) but usually include pregnancy and lactation (see p 5).

Precautions/warnings
Precautions vary for each individual herbal preparation (see Section 4).

Adverse effects
Plant extracts may have powerful pharmacological effects and therefore the risk of adverse effects is probably greater than with most other complementary therapies. The reader is referred to the information on the individual herbs in Section 4.

Interactions
Possible interactions between different herbal preparations or with conventional drugs should generally be assumed and relevant patients should be closely monitored. Patients should be asked about self-prescription drug use.

THERAPIES

Table 3.2 **Results of systematic reviews of herbal medicine**

Plant name	Evidence of effectiveness	Inconclusive evidence	Evidence of ineffectiveness
Aloe vera		Glycaemic control[1]	
		Acute radiation dermatitis[2]	
		Surgical wound healing[3]	
Andrographis	Upper respiratory tract infection[4]		
Artichoke		Hypercholesterolaemia[5]	Alcohol hangover[6]
Avocado/soybean	Osteoarthritis (knee, hip)[7]		
Bilberry		Night vision[8]	
Black cohosh		Menopausal symptoms[9]	
Chaste tree		Pre-menstrual syndrome[10]	
Cranberry	Urinary tract infections (prevention)[11]	Urinary tract infections (treatment)[12]	
Devil's claw	Osteoarthritis[13]		
	Low back pain[14]		
Echinacea		Common cold (prevention, treatment)[15]	
		Common cold (treatment)[16]	
Evening primrose		Menopausal symptoms[17]	
		Schizophrenia[18]	
Feverfew		Migraine prevention[19]	
Garlic		Hyperlipidaemia[20]	Hypertension[22]
		Peripheral arterial disease[21]	*Helicobacter pylori* infections[23]
Ginkgo	Intermittent claudication[24]	Tinnitus[26]	
	Dementia[25]	Macular degeneration[27]	
		Cognitive function[28]	
Ginseng		Any condition[29]	
Ginger	Pregnancy-induced nausea/vomiting[30]	Nausea and vomiting of other origin[31]	
Green tea		Stomach, intestinal cancer[32]	
		Breast cancer[33]	
Guar gum		Cholestasis in pregnancy[34]	Weight reduction[35]
Hawthorn	Chronic heart failure[36]		
Horse chestnut	Chronic venous insufficiency[37]		
Kava kava	Anxiety[38]		
	Menopausal symptoms[39]		

Plant name	Evidence of effectiveness	Inconclusive evidence	Evidence of ineffectiveness
Milk thistle			Alcoholic liver disease[40]
			Hepatitis B or C liver disease[40]
Mistletoe		Cancer[41,42]	
Nettle	Benign prostatic hyperplasia[43]		
Peppermint	Abdominal pain[44]		
	Non-ulcer dyspepsia[45]		
	Irritable bowel syndrome[46]		
Red clover	Hot flushes[47]		
Saw palmetto	Benign prostatic hyperplasia[48]		
St John's wort	Mild to moderate depression[49]		
Tea tree		Vaginitis (yeast, bacterial)[50]	
		Fungal infections[51]	
Valerian		Insomnia[52]	
Yohimbe	Erectile dysfunction[53]	Weight reduction[54]	

Quality issues

The amount of active constituent may vary and depends on a variety of different factors such as time of harvest, type of soil or amount of sunlight and rain. Products may be contaminated with other plant material or adulterated or plants may be misidentified. The Register of Chinese Herbal Medicine in the UK operates an 'approved suppliers scheme' whereby suppliers of herbs and herbal products are assessed by independent auditors.

Indirect risks

In cases where the therapist is not medically qualified, appropriate treatment of a medical condition may be delayed, however referrals by herbal practitioners to general practitioners are not uncommon.

Risk–benefit assessment

The most convincing evidence that exists in the area of complementary medicine probably relates to a number of herbal extracts, suggesting effectiveness for various conditions. The possibility of adverse effects has to be considered and the risk–benefit ratio has to be assessed for each herbal preparation individually (see Section 4). A number of conditions exist for which conventional medical treatment is not satisfactory and herbalism may provide a possible option.

REFERENCES

1 Yeh G Y, Eisenberg D M, Kaptchuk T J, Phillips R S. Systematic review of herbs and dietary supplements for glycemic control in diabetes. Diabetes Care 2003;26:1277–1294

2 Wickline M M. Prevention and treatment of acute radiation dermatitis: a literature review. Oncol Nurs Forum 2004;31:237–247

3 Vermeulen H, Ubbink D, Goossens A, de Vos R, Legemate D. Dressings and topical agents for surgical wounds healing by secondary intention. Cochrane Database Syst Rev 2004; Issue 2. Art. No.: CD003554

4 Coon J T, Ernst E. Andrographis paniculata in the treatment of upper respiratory tract infections: a systematic review of safety and efficacy. Planta Med 2004;70:293–298

5 Pittler M H, Thompson Coon J, Ernst E. Artichoke leaf extract for treating hypercholesterolaemia. Cochrane Database Syst Rev 2002; Issue 3. Art No.: CD003335

6 Pittler M H, Verster J C, Ernst E. Interventions for preventing or treating alcohol hangover. Systematic review of randomized controlled trials. BMJ 2005;331:1515–1518

7 Ernst E. Avocado-soybean unsaponifiables (ASU) for osteoarthritis – a systematic review. Clin Rheumatol 2003;22:285–288

8 Canter P H, Ernst E. Anthocyanosides of Vaccinium myrtillus (bilberry) for night vision – a systematic review of placebo-controlled trials. Surv Ophthalmol 2004;49:38–50

9 Borrelli F, Ernst E. Cimicifuga racemosa: a systematic review of its clinical efficacy. Eur J Clin Pharmacol 2002;58:235–241

10 Fugh-Berman A, Kronenberg F. Complementary and alternative medicine (CAM) in reproductive-age women: a review of randomized controlled trials. Reprod Toxicol 2003;17:137–152

11 Jepson R G, Mihaljevic L, Craig J. Cranberries for preventing urinary tract infections. Cochrane Database Syst Rev 2004; Issue 2. Art. No.: CD001321

12 Jepson R G, Mihaljevic L, Craig J. Cranberries for treating urinary tract infections. Cochrane Database Syst Rev 2000; Issue 2. Art. No.: CD001322

13 Soeken K L. Selected CAM therapies for arthritis-related pain: the evidence from systematic reviews. Clin J Pain 2004;20:13–18

14 Gagnier J J, Chrubasik S, Manheimer E. Harpgophytum procumbens for osteoarthritis and low back pain: a systematic review. BMC Complement Altern Med 200415;4:13

15 Melchart D, Linde K, Fischer P, Kaesmayr J. Echinacea for preventing and treating the common cold. Cochrane Database Syst Rev 2000; Issue 2. Art. No.: CD000530

16 Caruso T J, Gwaltney J M Jr. Treatment of the common cold with echinacea: a structured review. Clin Infect Dis 2005;40:807–810

17 Huntley A L, Ernst E. A systematic review of herbal medicinal products for the treatment of menopausal symptoms. Menopause 2003;10:465–476

18 Joy C B, Mumby-Croft R, Joy LA. Polyunsaturated fatty acid (fish or evening primrose oil) for schizophrenia. Cochrane Database Syst Rev 2003; Issue 2. Art. No.: CD001257

19 Pittler M H, Ernst E. Feverfew for preventing migraine. Cochrane Database Syst Rev 2004; Issue 1. Art. No.: CD002286

20 Alder R, Lookinland S, Berry J A, Williams M. A systematic review of the effectiveness of garlic as an anti-hyperlipidemic agent. J Am Acad Nurse Pract 2003;15:120–129

21 Jepson R G, Kleijnen J, Leng G C. Garlic for peripheral arterial occlusive disease. Cochrane Database Syst Rev 2000; Issue 2. Art. No.: CD000095

22 Silagy C A, Neil H A. A meta-analysis of the effect of garlic on blood pressure. J Hypertens 1994;12:463–468

23 Martin K W, Ernst E. Herbal medicines for treatment of bacterial infections: a review of controlled clinical trials. J Antimicrob Chemother 2003;51:241–246

24 Pittler M H, Ernst E. Ginkgo biloba extract for the treatment of intermittent claudication: a meta-analysis of randomized trials. Am J Med 2000;108:276–281

25 Birks J, Grimley E V, Van Dongen M. Ginkgo biloba for cognitive impairment and dementia. Cochrane Database Syst Rev 2002; Issue 4. Art. No.: CD003120

26 Hilton M, Stuart E. Ginkgo biloba for tinnitus. Cochrane Database Syst Rev 2004; Issue 2. Art. No.: CD003852

27 Evans J R. Ginkgo biloba extract for age-related macular degeneration. Cochrane Database Syst Rev 2000; Issue 2. Art. No.: CD001775

28 Canter P H, Ernst E. Ginkgo biloba: a smart drug? A systematic review of controlled trials of the cognitive effects of ginkgo biloba extracts in healthy people. Psychopharmacol Bull 2002;36:108–123

29 Vogler B K, Pittler M H, Ernst E. The efficacy of ginseng. A systematic review of randomised clinical trials. Eur J Clin Pharmacol 1999;55:567–575

30 Borrelli F, Capasso R, Aviello G, Pittler M H, Izzo A A. Effectiveness and safety of ginger in the treatment of pregnancy-induced nausea and vomiting. Obstet Gynecol 2005;105:849–856

31 Ernst E, Pittler M H. Efficacy of ginger for nausea and vomiting: a systematic review of randomized clinical trials. Br J Anaesth 2000;84:367–371

32 Borrelli F, Capasso R, Russo A, Ernst E. Systematic review: green tea and gastrointestinal cancer risk. Aliment Pharmacol Ther 2004;19:497–510

33 Seely D, Mills E J, Wu P, Verma S, Guyatt G H. The effects of green tea consumption on incidence of breast cancer and recurrence of breast cancer: a systematic review and meta-analysis. Integr Cancer Ther 2005;4:144–155

34 Burrows R F, Clavisi O, Burrows E. Interventions for treating cholestasis in pregnancy. Cochrane Database Syst Rev 2001; Issue 4. Art. No.: CD000493

35 Pittler M H, Ernst E. Guar gum for body weight reduction: meta-analysis of randomized trials. Am J Med 2001;110:724–730

36 Pittler M H, Schmidt K, Ernst E. Hawthorn extract for treating chronic heart failure: meta-analysis of randomized trials. Am J Med 2003;114:665–674

37 Pittler M H, Ernst E. Horse chestnut seed extract for chronic venous insufficiency. Cochrane Database Syst Rev 2004; Issue 2. Art. No.: CD003230

38 Pittler M H, Ernst E. Kava extract for treating anxiety. Cochrane Database Syst Rev 2005 (in press)

39 Huntley A L, Ernst E. A systematic review of herbal medicinal products for the treatment of menopausal symptoms. Menopause 2003;10: 465–376

40 Rambaldi A, Jacobs B, Iaquinto G, Gluud C. Milk thistle for alcoholic and/or hepatitis B or C virus liver diseases. Cochrane Database Syst Rev 2005; Issue 2. Art. No.: CD003620

41 Kienle G S, Berrino F, Bussing A, Portalupi E, Rosenzweig S, Kiene H. Mistletoe in cancer – a systematic review on controlled clinical trials. Eur J Med Res 2003;8:109–119

42 Ernst E, Schmidt K, Steuer-Vogt M K. Mistletoe for cancer? A systematic review of randomised clinical trials. Int J Cancer 2003;107:262–267

43 Dvorkin L, Song K Y. Herbs for benign prostatic hyperplasia. Ann Pharmacother 2002;36:1443–1452

44 Weydert J A, Ball T M, Davis M F. Systematic review of treatments for recurrent abdominal pain. Pediatrics 2003;111:e1–11

45 Thompson Coon J, Ernst E. Systematic review: herbal medicinal products for non-ulcer dyspepsia. Aliment Pharmacol Ther 2002;16: 1689–1699

46 Koretz R L, Rotblatt M. Complementary and alternative medicine in gastroenterology: the good, the bad, and the ugly. Clin Gastroenterol Hepatol 2004;2:957–967

47 Thompson Coon J, Pittler M H, Ernst. Meta-analysis of Trifolium pratense (red clover) isoflavones for treating vasomotor symptoms in menopausal women. (in press)

48 Wilt T, Ishani A, Mac Donald R. Serenoa repens for benign prostatic hyperplasia. Cochrane Database Syst Rev 2002; Issue 3. Art. No.: CD001423

49 Linde K, Mulrow C, Berner M, Egger M. St John's Wort for depression. Cochrane Database Syst Rev 2005; Issue 2. Art. No.: CD000448

50 Van Kessel K, Assefi N, Marrazzo J, Eckert L. Common complementary and alternative therapies for yeast vaginitis and bacterial vaginosis: a systematic review. Obstet Gynecol Surv 2003;58:351–358

51 Martin K W, Ernst E. Herbal medicines for treatment of fungal infections: a systematic review of controlled clinical trials. Mycoses 2004;47:87–92

52 Stevinson C, Ernst E. Valerian for insomnia: a systematic review of randomized clinical trials. Sleep Med 2000;1:91–99

53 Ernst E, Pittler M H. Yohimbine for erectile dysfunction: a systematic review and meta-analysis of randomized clinical trials. J Urol 1998;159:433–436

54 Pittler M H, Ernst E. Dietary supplements for body-weight reduction: a systematic review. Am J Clin Nutr 2004;79:529–536

55 Liu J P, Zhang M, Wang W Y, Grimsgaard S. Chinese herbal medicines for type 2 diabetes mellitus. Cochrane Database Syst Rev 2004, Issue 3. Art No.: CD003642

56 Zhang W, Leonard T, Bath-Hextall F, Chambers C, Lee C, Humphreys R, Williams H. Chinese herbal medicine for atopic eczema. Cochrane Database Syst Rev 2005, Issue 2. Art No.: CD002291

57 Coon J T, Ernst E. Panax ginseng: a systematic review of adverse effects and drug interactions. Drug Saf 2002;25:323–344

58 Pittler M H, Ernst E. Systematic review: hepatotoxic events associated with herbal medicinal products. Aliment Pharmacol Ther 2003;18:451–471

59 Ernst E. Serious psychiatric and neurological adverse effects of herbal medicines – a systematic review. Acta Psychiatr Scand 2003;108:83–91

60 Izzo A A. Drug interactions with St. John's Wort (Hypericum perforatum): a review of the clinical evidence. Int J Clin Pharmacol Ther 2004;42:139–148

61 Zhou S, Chan E, Pan S Q, Huang M, Lee E J. Pharmacokinetic interactions of drugs with St John's wort. J Psychopharmacol 2004;18:262–276

THERAPIES

HOMEOPATHY

Definition	A therapeutic method, often using highly diluted preparations of substances whose effects when administered to healthy subjects correspond to the manifestations of the disorder (symptoms, clinical signs and pathological states) in the unwell patient.
Related techniques	Autoisopathy, biochemic medicine, homotoxicology, isopathy, tautopathy.
Background	Homeopathy was founded by the German physician Samuel Hahnemann (1755-1843) and became popular first in Europe and later in the US during the second half of the 19th century. With the advent of effective drug treatments in the early part of the 20th century, its popularity decreased in most countries. Today, it is again becoming more widely available due to a general trend towards CAM. Many schools of homeopathy exist.
Traditional concepts	Homeopathy is built on two key principles. The law of similars or 'like cures like' principle states that a remedy which causes a certain symptom (e.g. a headache) in healthy volunteers can be used to treat a headache in patients who suffer from it. According to the second principle, homeopathic remedies become stronger rather than weaker when submitted to 'potentisation', which describes the stepwise dilution combined with 'succussion', i.e. vigorous shaking of the mixture. Thus remedies are believed to be clinically effective even if they are so dilute that they are likely not to contain a single molecule of the original substance.
Scientific rationale	Examples can be found where the 'like cures like' principle does apply (e.g. digitalis), but it is not a universal principle or natural law. Presently there is no scientific rationale for understanding how remedies devoid of pharmacologically active molecules produce clinical effects. Homeopathic 'provings', which form the basis for therapeutic selection, often yield negative results or lack scientific rigour.
Practitioners	Homeopathy is practiced by both medically qualified and non-medically qualified practitioners.
Conditions frequently treated	Homeopaths do not usually use conventional disease categories. Their aim is to match a patient's individual symptoms with a 'drug picture' (i.e. a set of symptoms caused by a remedy in healthy volunteers). Homeopaths often see patients with benign chronic conditions, e.g. ear, nose and throat disorders, headaches, musculoskeletal and digestive problems, respiratory and skin complaints, stress and anxiety.[1,2,3]

Typical session   A first consultation might take $1\frac{1}{2}$ hours or longer. Homeopaths take a thorough history and explore the patient's problems in much detail, with a view to finding the optimally matching homeopathic drug ('similimum'). They put less emphasis on physical examination than conventional physicians.

Course of treatment   Homeopaths believe that the treatment of long-standing problems is necessarily prolonged. Thus they would typically insist on several consultations during which their prescriptions can be altered according to the changes in symptomatology.

Clinical evidence   A meta-analysis[4] of all homeopathic, placebo-controlled or randomised trials suggested that the risk ratio for clinical improvement with homeopathy was 2.45 times that with placebo. This publication has attracted much criticism and 6 re-analyses of these data failed to demonstrate efficacy.[5] Similarly, 11 independent systematic reviews of homeopathy did not generate convincing evidence of efficacy[5] and one meta-analytical comparison of 110 homoeopathy trials and 110 matched conventional-medicine trials concluded that the clinical effects of homeopathy were unspecific placebo effects.[6] This includes conditions such as postoperative ileus, delayed onset muscle soreness, migraine prophylaxis, chronic asthma, and osteoarthritis.[3] Only in 2 areas were the conclusions positive: influenza[7] and rheumatic conditions.[8] Since the publication of these systematic reviews, the results of RCTs have been mixed. Encouraging findings were reported for fibromyalgia,[9] low back pain,[10] chronic fatigue syndrome,[11] pain of unwanted lactation,[12] mild traumatic brain injury,[13] childhood diarrhoea,[14] and glue ear.[15] Negative results emerged for rheumatoid arthritis,[16] ankylosing spondylitis,[17] otitis media,[18] generalised anxiety disorder[19] and asthma.[20] Many of the primary studies of homeopathy have serious methodological limitations.[21]

Risks   *Contraindications*
Life-threatening conditions, pregnancy and lactation (see p 5).

Precautions/warnings
Do not expose remedies to bright light or other radiation and pungent smells. Some homeopaths advise their clients against immunisation of children.[22,23]

Adverse effects
In about one quarter of cases, homeopaths observe an aggravation of symptoms (which is believed to be a positive sign indicating that the correct remedy has been given).[24] In low dilutions, homeopathic remedies can have adverse effects such as allergic reactions.

Interactions
Some medicines (e.g. corticosteroids, antibiotics) are believed to block the actions of homeopathic drugs.

THERAPIES

Risk–benefit assessment

Based on the available trial evidence to date, the effectiveness of homeopathic remedies can be neither confirmed nor ruled out. There are few risks associated with homeopathy. Thus the evidence is insufficient for firm recommendations.

REFERENCES

1 Steinsbekk A, Fønnebø V. Users of homeopaths in Norway in 1998, compared to previous users and GP patients. Homeopathy 2003;92:3–10

2 Trichard M, Lamure E, Chaufferin G. Study of the practice of homeopathic general practitioners in France. Homeopathy 2003;92:135–139

3 Becker-Witt C, Lüdtke R, Weisshuhn T E, Willich S N. Diagnoses and treatment in homeopathic medical practice. Forsch Komplementärmed Klass Naturheilkd 2004;11:98–103

4 Linde K, Clausius N, Ramirez G, Melchart D, Eitel F, Hedges L V, Jonas W. Are the clinical effects of homeopathy placebo effects? A meta-analysis of placebo-controlled trials. Lancet 1997;350:834–843

5 Ernst E. A systematic review of homeopathy. Br J Clin Pharmacol 2002:54:577–582

6 Shang A, Huwiler-Muntener K, Nartey L, Juni P, Dorig S, Sterne J A, Pewsner D, Egger M. Are the clinical effects of homoeopathy placebo efects? Comparative study of placebo-controlled trials of homoeopathy and allopathy. Lancet 2005;366:726–732

7 Vickers A J, Smith C. Homeopathic oscillococcinum for preventing and treating influenza and influenza-like syndromes. Cochrane Database Syst Rev 2004, Issue 1. Art. No.: CD001957

8 Jonas W B, Linde K, Ramirez G. Homeopathy and rheumatic disease. Rheum Dis Clin North Am 2000;26:117–123

9 Bell I R, Lewis D A, Brook A J, Schwartz G E, Lewis S E, Walsh B T, Baldwin C M. Improved clinical status in fibromyalgia patients treated with individualized homeopathic remedies versus placebo. Rheumatology (Oxford) 2004;43:577–582

10 Gmünder R, Kissling R. The efficacy of homeopathy in the treatment of chronic low back pain compared to standardized physiotherapy [German]. Z Orthop Ihre Grenzgeb 2002;140:503–508

11 Weatherley-Jones E, Nicholl J P, Thomas K J, Parry G J, McKendrick M W, Green S T, Stanley P J, Lynch S P J. A randomised, controlled, triple-blind trial of the efficacy of homeopathic treatment for chronic fatigue syndrome. J Psychosom Res 2004;56:189–197

12 Berrebi A, Parant O, Ferval F, Thene M, Ayoubi J M, Connan L, Belon P. Treatment of pain due to unwanted lactation with a homeopathic preparation given in the immediate post-partum period [French]. J Gynecol Obstet Biol Reprod (Paris) 2001;30:353–357

13 Chapman E H, Weintraub R J, Milburn M A, Pirozzi T O, Woo E. Homeopathic treatment of mild traumatic brain injury: A randomized, double-blind, placebo-controlled clinical trial. J Head Trauma Rehabil 1999;14:521–542

14 Jacobs J, Jonas W B, Jimémez-Pérez M, Crothers D. Homeopathy for childhood diarrhea: combined results and metaanalysis from three randomized, controlled clinical trials. Pediatr Infect Dis J 2003;22:229–234

15 Harrison H, Fixsen A, Vickers A. A randomized comparison of homeopathic and standard care for the treatment of glue ear in children. Complement Ther Med 1999;7:132–135

16 Fisher P, Scott D L. A randomized controlled trial of homeopathy in rheumatoid arthritis. Rheumatology (Oxford) 2001;40:1052–1055

17 Schirmer K P, Fritz M, Jäckel W H. Wirksamkeit von Formica rufa und Eigenblut-Injektionen bei Patienten mit ankylosierender Spondylitis: eine doppelblinde, randomisierte Studie. Z Rheumatol 2000;59:321–329

18 Jacobs J, Springer D A, Crothers D. Homeopathic treatment of acute otitis media in children: a preliminary randomized placebo-controlled trial. Pediatr Infect Dis J 2001;20:177–183

19 Bonne O, Shemer Y, Goali Y, Katz M, Shalev-Arieh Y. A randomized, double-blind, placebo-controlled study of classical homeopathy in generalized anxiety disorder. J Clin Psychiatry 2003;64:282–287

20 White A, Slade P, Hunt C, Hart C A, Ernst E. Individualised homeopathy as an adjunct in the treatment of childhood asthma: a randomized placebo controlled trial. Thorax 2003;58:317–321

21 Jonas W B, Anderson R L, Crawford C C, Lyons J S. A systematic review of the quality of homeopathic clinical trials. BMC Complement Altern Med 2001;1:12

22 Schmidt K, Ernst E. MMR vaccination advice over the internet. Vaccine 2003;21:1044–1047

23 Lehrke P, Nübling M, Hofmann F, Stössel U. Impfverhalten und Impfeinstellung bei Ärzten mit und ohne Zusatzbezeichnung Homöopathie. Monatsschr Kinderheilkd 2004;152:752–757

24 Thompson E, Barron S, Spence D. A preliminary audit investigating remedy reactions including adverse events in routine homeopathic practice. Homeopathy 2004;93:203–209

HYPNOTHERAPY

Definition

The induction of a trance-like state to facilitate relaxation and make use of enhanced suggestibility to treat psychological and medical conditions and effect behavioural changes.

Related techniques

Self-hypnosis, imagery, autogenic training, meditation, relaxation.

Background

Hypnotic practices have been traced at least as far back as ancient Egypt, but the first therapeutic use has been attributed to charismatic Austrian physician Franz Anton Mesmer in 1778 from whom the word mesmerism came. He devised a treatment based on magnetism that was hugely successful until a Royal Commission investigated the method and concluded that the effects were due entirely to imagination. Mesmerism saw a revival in the 1800s when British surgeon James Esdaile used it as the sole anaesthetic when performing major operations in India. Another British physician, James Braid, is credited with making hypnosis respectable to the medical community and in the 1950s the British and American Medical Associations recognised hypnosis as a legitimate medical procedure.

Traditional concepts

The goal of hypnotherapy is to gain self-control over behaviour, emotions or physiological processes. This is achieved by the induction of the hypnotic trance (often called an altered state of consciousness) where the patients' focus of attention is directed inwards, thereby allowing easier access to the non-critical unconscious mind which is more receptive to suggestion. A good rapport between the therapist and patient or client is vital, but a fundamental principle of hypnotic phenomena is that the hypnotised individual is under his own control and not that of the hypnotist or anyone else. It is argued consequently that all hypnosis is really self-hypnosis and the therapist should actually be called a facilitator.

Scientific rationale

Hypnosis is usually associated with a deep state of relaxation. Whether this represents a specific altered state of consciousness has been the subject of fierce scientific debate. It has repeatedly been shown that analgesia and many other hypnotic phenomena can be achieved by means of suggestion alone without hypnotising

THERAPIES

THERAPIES

individuals. However, in defense of the genuineness and importance of the hypnotic trance it has been argued that highly suggestible (or hypnotisable) individuals are easily able to enter a hypnotic state without requiring formal induction. The means by which hypnotic suggestion enables involuntary processes such as skin temperature, heart rate and gut secretions to be deliberately controlled is not fully understood. It may be that hypnosis is essentially just a specific type of relaxation technique.

Practitioners

The credentials and duration of training of hypnotherapists vary widely. The number of hours of training may range from 300 to 1600. Most therapists are not medically qualified. Many doctors, dentists and psychologists are trained as clinical hypnotherapists and make use of hypnosis during their practice.

Conditions frequently treated

Addictions, anxiety, pain, phobia, post-traumatic stress disorder, psychosomatic conditions, stress.

Typical session

Sessions typically last between 30 and 90 minutes. The initial visit involves the gathering of history and discussion about hypnosis, suggestion and the client's expectations of the therapy. Tests for hypnotic suggestibility may also be conducted. Hypnotic induction may or may not be part of the first session. The hypnotic state is achieved by first relaxing the body, then shifting attention away from the external environment towards a narrow range of objects or ideas suggested by the therapist. Sometimes hypnotherapy is carried out in group settings, e.g. antenatal classes as preparation for labour.

Course of treatment

Varies according to the individual, but an average course is 6–12 weekly sessions.

Clinical evidence

For pain management, a meta-analysis[1] reported moderate to large hypnoanalgesic effects, which are supported by another meta-analysis[2] of controlled trials assessing surgical patients. RCTs suggested that hypnosis reduced chronic pain[3] and pain in patients with osteoarthritis compared with waiting list controls.[4] For burn patients, pain and anxiety caused by physiotherapy decreased compared with the no-hypnotherapy control group.[5] However, this was not supported by a RCT for pain and anxiety caused by dressing changes when compared with stress reducing strategies.[6] In cancer patients receiving radiotherapy, the addition of hypnotherapy had no effect on anxiety and quality of life compared with radiotherapy alone, although some effects were observed for mental and overall well-being.[7] For paediatric oncology patients beneficial effects were reported for procedure-related pain and anxiety.[8] A review of 15 controlled trials of hypnosis in children found promising but not compelling evidence for pain, enuresis and chemotherapy-related distress.[9] For pain relief in labour and childbirth, a meta-analysis including three RCTs reported beneficial effects compared with no-intervention control groups,[10] which is supported to some extend by another RCT.[11] Systematic reviews and Cochrane reviews found no convincing evidence of effectiveness for non-ulcer dyspepsia,[12] vaginismus,[13] schizophrenia,[14] post-traumatic conditions[15] and smoking cessation.[16] Some positive results from RCTs are reported for psoriasis,[17] irritable bowel syndrome,[18,19] conversion disorder of the motor type,[20] wound and bone fracture healing,[21,22] and during percutaneous transluminal coronary angioplasty.[23] Hypnotherapy was not an effective alternative to midazolam during gastroscopy.[24]

Risks

Contraindications
Psychosis, personality disorders.

Precautions/warnings
Information elicited under hypnosis is subject to confabulation; epilepsy, very young children.

Adverse effects
Recovering repressed memories can be painful and psychological problems may be exacerbated. False memory syndrome has been reported. Studies investigating negative consequences of hypnosis have concluded that when practised by a clinically trained professional, it is safe.

Risk–benefit assessment

There is evidence to suggest that hypnotherapy has analgesic effects. There is also some evidence that anxiety associated with pain is reduced with hypnotherapy. Encouraging data are also available for patients with irritable bowel syndrome. Some risks exist, but on balance it appears to be a valuable tool for pain management and conditions with a psychosomatic component, when performed by a qualified and responsible practitioner.

THERAPIES

REFERENCES

1 Montgomery G H, DuHamel K N, Redd W H. A meta-analysis of hypnotically induced analgesia: how effective is hypnosis? Int J Clin Exp Hypn 2000;48:138–153

2 Montgomery G H, David D, Winkel G, Silverstein J H, Bovbjerg D H. The effectiveness of adjunctive hypnosis with surgical patients: a meta-analysis. Anesth Analg 2002;94:1639–1645

3 Ray P, Page A C. A single session of hypnosis and eye movements desensitisation and reprocessing (EMDR) in the treatment of chronic pain. Aust J Clin Exp Hypn 2002;30:170–178

4 Gay M C, Philippot P, Luminet O. Differential effectiveness of psychological interventions for

reducing osteoarthritis pain: a comparison of Erikson [correction of Erickson] hypnosis and Jacobson relaxation. Eur J Pain 2002;6:1–16

5 Amini Harandi A, Esfandani A, Shakibaei F. The effect of hypnotherapy on procedural pain and state anxiety related to physiotherapy in women hospitalized in a burn unit. Contemp Hypn 2004;21:28–34

6 Frenay M C, Faymonville M E, Devlieger S, Albert A, Vanderkelen A. Psychological approaches during dressing changes of burned patients: a prospective randomised study comparing hypnosis against stress reducing strategy. Burns 2001;27:793–799

7 Stalpers L J, da Costa H C, Merbis M A, Fortuin A A, Muller M J, van Dam F S.

Hypnotherapy in radiotherapy patients: a randomized trial. Int J Radiat Oncol Biol Phys 2005;61:499–506

8 Liossi C, Hatira P. Clinical hypnosis in the alleviation of procedure-related pain in pediatric oncology patients. Int J Clin Exp Hypn 2003;51:4–28

9 Milling L S, Costantino C A. Clinical hypnosis with children: first steps toward empirical support. Int J Clin Exp Hypn 2000;48:113–137

10 Cyna A M, McAuliffe G L, Andrew M I. Hypnosis for pain relief in labour and childbirth: a systematic review. Br J Anaesth 2004;93:505–511

11 Mehl-Madrona L E. Hypnosis to facilitate uncomplicated birth. Am J Clin Hypn 2004;46:299–312

12 Soo S, Forman D, Delaney B C, Moayyedi P. A systematic review of psychological therapies for nonulcer dyspepsia. Am J Gastroenterol 2004;99:1817–1822

13 McGuire H, Hawton K. Interventions for vaginismus. The Cochrane Database of Systematic Reviews 2001, Issue 2. Art. No.: CD001760

14 Izquierdo de Santiago A, Khan M. Hypnosis for schizophrenia. The Cochrane Database of Systematic Reviews 2004, Issue 3. Art. No.: CD004160

15 Cardeña E. Hypnosis in the treatment of trauma: a promising, but not fully supported, efficacious intervention. Int J Clin Exp Hypn 2000;48:125–138

16 Abbot N C, Stead L F, White A R, Barnes J. Hypnotherapy for smoking cessation. The Cochrane Database of Systematic Reviews 1998, Issue 2. Art. No.: CD001008

17 Tausk F, Whitmore SE. A pilot study of hypnosis in the treatment of patients with psoriasis. Psychother Psychosom 1999;68:221–225

18 Forbes A, MacAuley S, Chiotakakou-Faliakou E. Hypnotherapy and therapeutic audiotape: effective in previously unsuccessfully treated irritable bowel syndrome? Int J Colorectal Dis 2000;15:328–334

19 Simren M, Ringstrom G, Bjornsson ES, Abrahamsson H. Treatment with hypnotherapy reduces the sensory and motor component of the gastrocolonic response in irritable bowel syndrome. Psychosom Med 2004;66:233–238

20 Moene F C, Spinhoven P, Hoogduin K A, van Dyck R. A randomised controlled clinical trial on the additional effect of hypnosis in a comprehensive treatment programme for in-patients with conversion disorder of the motor type. Psychother Psychosom 2002;71:66–76

21 Ginandes C, Brooks P, Sando W, Jones C, Aker J. Can medical hypnosis accelerate post-surgical wound healing? Results of a clinical trial. Am J Clin Hypn 2003;45:333–351

22 Ginandes C S, Rosenthal D I. Using hypnosis to accelerate the healing of bone fractures: a randomized controlled pilot study. Altern Ther Health Med 1999;5:67–75

23 Baglini R, Sesana M, Capuano C, Gnecchi-Ruscone T, Ugo L, Danzi G B. Effect of hypnotic sedation during percutaneous transluminal coronary angioplasty on myocardial ischemia and cardiac sympathetic drive. Am J Cardiol 2004;93:1035–1038

24 Conlong P, Rees W. The use of hypnosis in gastroscopy: a comparison with intravenous sedation. Postgrad Med J 1999;75:223–225

MASSAGE

Definition A method of manipulating the soft tissue of whole body areas using pressure and traction (primary focus on 'Swedish massage').

Related techniques Aromatherapy, reflexology, shiatsu.

Background Massage is one of the oldest forms of treatment. The development of modern massage is attributed to the Swede Per Henrik Ling, who developed an integrated system consisting of massage and exercises, which was later termed 'Swedish massage'. In the middle of the 19th century it was introduced in the USA and was practised predominantly by physicians until the early 20th century. The interest in massage therapy gradually declined but increased again in the 1970s. Today massage is considered a complementary therapy in many countries and more gentle techniques than the vigorous treatment recommended by Ling are frequently used. In some European countries (e.g. Germany), however, massage continues to be part of conventional medicine.

Traditional concepts

Massage is applied using various manual techniques, applying pressure and traction to manipulate the soft tissues of the body. Touch is fundamental to massage therapy and allows the therapist to locate areas of muscle tension. These areas can be treated, conveying a sense of caring using touch with the optimal amount of pressure for each person.

Scientific rationale

The friction of the hands and the mechanical pressure exerted on cutaneous and subcutaneous structures affect the body. The circulation of blood and lymph is generally enhanced, resulting in increased oxygen supply and allegedly in the removal of waste products. Direct mechanical pressure and effects mediated by the nervous system beneficially affect areas of increased muscular tension.

Practitioners

In the USA, massage is often practised by nurses and a variety of training courses are available aimed specifically at nurses and other healthcare professionals. The number of hours of training required varies greatly and examinations by the International Therapy Examinations Council are the most widely accepted. In other countries such as Germany, massage is fully registered and a recognised profession.

Conditions frequently treated

Anxiety, back pain, constipation, depression, musculoskeletal conditions, stress and many other conditions.

Typical session

During an initial treatment session the therapist will usually take the patient's medical history to get an overall impression of the medical status and screen for contraindications. The duration of individual treatment sessions varies depending on the condition, but will typically be about 30 minutes. Patients are normally treated unclothed with a sheet or towel provided.

Usually the massage is performed on a specially designed massage couch. Therapists often use oil to facilitate movement of their hands over the patient's body. The five fundamental techniques used in massage are effleurage, pétrissage, friction, tapotement and vibration. Sometimes sessions are followed by other treatments such as hot packs, which essentially applies external heat. Most patients are advised to rest for about 20 minutes after a treatment session.

THERAPIES

Course of treatment

Usually, 1–2 sessions per week for a treatment period of 4–8 weeks would be initially recommended.

Clinical evidence

For treating low back pain, a systematic review[1] conducted within the framework of the Cochrane Collaboration Back Review Group extended the findings of an earlier review[2] and concluded cautiously that massage might be beneficial for patients with subacute and chronic non-specific low back pain, especially when combined with exercises and education. Cochrane reviews for treating upper extremity work-related disorders,[3] tendinitis employing deep transverse friction massage,[4] and asthma[5] found insufficient evidence for any firm conclusions. A Cochrane review[6] of massage for promoting growth and development of preterm and or low birth-weight infants concluded that the evidence is weak and does not warrant wider use of preterm infant massage. Another systematic review[7] concluded that for treating cervicogenic headache, massage appears to be less effective than spinal manipulative therapy. In stroke patients an RCT reported reduced levels of pain and anxiety.[8] A meta-analysis of RCTs suggested that the largest effects of massage therapy are on trait anxiety and depression.[9,10] It has also been concluded in a systematic review that vibratory massage might be of benefit for musculoskeletal pain.[11] For treating constipation a systematic review assessed the evidence on abdominal massage and cautiously concluded that it could be a promising treatment option.[12] RCTs report some positive effects of massage on anxiety during labour,[13] for postburn symptoms,[14] on well-being for patients who had undergone coronary artery bypass surgery,[15] and on breast cancer patients.[16,17] Massage did not affect the level or duration of pain or the loss of strength or function following exercise[18] and seemed to be less effective than swaddling for infants with cerebral injuries.[19] In patients with fibromyalgia massage alone and as part of a multidisciplinary programme has been suggested to relieve pain and depression and improve quality of life.[20,21] The safety of massage was systematically reviewed[22] and it was found that the serious adverse events on record were associated mostly with massage techniques other than 'Swedish' massage. The study concluded that although massage is not entirely risk free, serious adverse events are probably true rarities.

Risks

Contraindications
Phlebitis, deep vein thrombosis, burns, skin infections, eczema, open wounds, bone fractures, advanced osteoporosis.

Precautions/warnings
Cancer, myocardial infarction, osteoporosis, pregnancy, individuals who feel uncomfortable with close contact. Massage should generally be considered as an adjunctive treatment, not as an alternative to conventional care.

Adverse effects

Adverse effects are extremely rare. Serious adverse events such as bone fractures and liver rupture have been reported.

Interactions

Interactions and adverse effects attributable to oils, which may be used, are not considered in the assessment of risks involved in massage. The medical history should, however, include questions relating to any allergic predisposition.

Risk–benefit assessment

Massage appears to have some beneficial effects in a number of conditions such as constipation, back pain, anxiety, depression and stress. Given the few risks involved when performed by a responsible, well-trained practitioner, it may be worth considering. Its comparative effectiveness against other complementary therapies or against conventional treatment approaches is unclear. Given its relaxing effects, massage may have some, albeit non-specific, beneficial influence on the well-being of most patients.

REFERENCES

1 Furlan A D, Brosseau L, Imamura M, Irvin E. Massage for low-back pain: a systematic review within the framework of the Cochrane Collaboration Back Review Group. Spine 2002;27:1896–1910

2 Ernst E. Massage therapy for low back pain: a systematic review. J Pain Symptom Manage 1999;17:65–69

3 Verhagen A P, Bierma-Zeinstra S M A, Feleus A, Karels C, Dahaghin S, Burdorf L, de Vet H C W, Koes B W. Ergonomic and physiotherapeutic interventions for treating upper extremity work related disorders in adults. The Cochrane Database of Systematic Reviews 2004, Issue 1. Art. No.: CD003471

4 Brosseau L, Casimiro L, Milne S, Robinson V, Shea B, Tugwell P, Wells G. Deep transverse friction massage for treating tendinitis. The Cochrane Database of Systematic Reviews 2002, Issue 4. Art. No.: CD003528

5 Hondras M A, Linde K, Jones A P. Manual therapy for asthma. The Cochrane Database of Systematic Reviews 2002, Issue 3. Art. No.: CD001002

6 Vickers A, Ohlsson A, Lacy J B, Horsley A. Massage for promoting growth and development of preterm and/or low birth-weight infants. The Cochrane Database of Systematic Reviews 2004, Issue 2. Art. No.: CD000390

7 Bronfort G, Assendelft W J, Evans R, Haas M, Bouter L. Efficacy of spinal manipulation for chronic headache: a systematic review. J Manipulative Physiol Ther 2001;24:457–466

8 Mok E, Woo C P. The effects of slow-stroke back massage on anxiety and shoulder pain in elderly stroke patients. Complement Ther Nurs Midwifery 2004;10:209–216

9 Moyer C A, Rounds J, Hannum J W. A meta-analysis of massage therapy research. Psychol Bull 2004;130:3–18

10 Muller-Oerlinghausen B, Berg C, Scherer P, Mackert A, Moestl H P, Wolf J. Effects of slow-stroke massage as complementary treatment of depressed hospitalized patients. Dtsch Med Wochenschr 2004;129:1363–1368

11 Gottschild S, Kröling P. Vibrationsmassage. Eine Literaturübersicht zu physiologischen Wirkungen und therapeutischer Wirksamkeit. Phys Med Rehab Kuror 2003;13:85–95

12 Ernst E. Abdominal massage therapy for chronic constipation: a systematic review of controlled clinical trials. Forsch Komplementärmed 1999;6:149–151

13 Chang M Y, Wang S Y, Chen C H. Effects of massage on pain and anxiety during labour: a randomized controlled trial in Taiwan. J Adv Nurs 2002;38:68–73

14 Field T, Peck M, Hernandez-Reif M, Krugman S, Burman I, Ozment-Schenck L. Postburn itching, pain, and psychological symptoms are reduced with massage therapy. J Burn Care Rehabil 2000;21:189–193

15 Hattan J, King L, Griffiths P. The impact of foot massage and guided relaxation following cardiac surgery: a randomized controlled trial. J Adv Nurs 2002;37:199–207

THERAPIES

16 Hernandez-Reif M, Ironson G, Field T, Hurley J, Katz G, Diego M, Weiss S, Fletcher M A, Schanberg S, Kuhn C, Burman I. Breast cancer patients have improved immune and neuroendocrine functions following massage therapy. J Psychosom Res 2004;57:45–52

17 Forchuk C, Baruth P, Prendergast M, Holliday R, Bareham R, Brimner S, Schulz V, Chan YC, Yammine N. Postoperative arm massage: a support for women with lymph node dissection. Cancer Nurs 2004;27:25–33

18 Jonhagen S, Ackermann P, Eriksson T, Saartok T, Renstrom P A. Sports massage after eccentric exercise. Am J Sports Med 2004;32:1499–1503

19 Ohgi S, Akiyama T, Arisawa K, Shigemori K. Randomised controlled trial of swaddling versus massage in the management of excessive crying in infants with cerebral injuries. Arch Dis Child 2004;89:212–216

20 Brattberg G. Connective tissue massage in the treatment of fibromyalgia. Eur J Pain 1999;3:235–245

21 Lemstra M, Olszynski W P. The effectiveness of multidisciplinary rehabilitation in the treatment of fibromyalgia: a randomized controlled trial. Clin J Pain 2005;21:166–174

22 Ernst E. The safety of massage therapy. Rheumatology (Oxford) 2003;42:1101–1106

METICATION
MEDITATION

Synonyms Transcendental Meditation (TM), Sahaja Yoga/Meditation, Mindfulness Meditation (MM).

Definition Meditation is a very diverse range of techniques based on listening to the breath, repeating a mantra, detaching from the thought process or other self-directed mental practices which focus the attention and bring about a state of self-awareness and inner calm.

Related techniques Bensons' Relaxation Response, Qigong.

Background Most forms of meditation originated within the major religions, particularly those of the East where the aim is to bring about altered consciousness or 'enlightenment'. Meditation became popular in the West during the 1960s and 1970s when it became associated with the hippie and pop culture of the time. In addition to its spiritual goals, meditation has been increasingly promoted as a means to achieve relaxation, deal with stress and promote general health and well-being. Meditation continues to be taught in religious, cultic and non-cultic contexts. The latter includes forms developed for research or therapeutic purposes.

Scientific rationale Numerous studies appear to demonstrate changes in physiological parameters such as oxygen consumption, respiration rate, heart rate and brain activity (e.g.[1]) during meditation which could be considered characteristic of a state of deep relaxation. This is not the same thing as proving that regular practice of meditation has prophylactic or therapeutic effects. It is feasible that physiological changes which occur during the state of relaxation could have positive health effects, but specific mechanisms remain unknown.

THERAPIES

Practitioners   Meditation is taught mainly by religious or quasi-religious groups. TM, one of the more popular forms, is promoted by a worldwide organisation and instruction is paid for. In contrast, MM was developed within a healthcare context and has been researched and used with a variety of patient groups.

Conditions frequently treated   Anxiety, asthma, stress, drug and alcohol addiction, epilepsy, heart disease, hypertension.

Typical session   After initial instruction carried out over several sessions either in a group or individually with a teacher, the meditator is expected to practise regularly on a daily basis. In the case of TM, new meditators attend an introductory lecture, several group training sessions, an individual initiation ceremony with a teacher and then periodic follow-up sessions to check for correct practice. Expected daily practice is two 15–20 minute sessions.

Course of treatment   The prophylactic and therapeutic effects of meditation are expected to accrue from continuing daily practice.

Clinical evidence   Research on meditation has been beset by methodological problems including highly selected study populations, uncontrolled or inappropriately controlled designs, high drop-out rates and designs using mixed interventions which prevent the isolation of specific effects. Additionally, many studies have been carried out by researchers affiliated to the organisations promoting the particular technique in question. This is particularly so in the case of TM, the subject of over 800 research papers and reviews, many of which have not been peer-reviewed.[2,3] An independent systematic review of TM for its putative effects on cognitive function found that the outcome of RCTs depended on research design and concluded that the positive effects reported in some studies were an artifact of sample selection and non-specific factors including expectation and motivation.[2] Another independent systematic review concluded that there is presently insufficient evidence to conclude whether or not TM is effective in hypertension.[3] RCT evidence for the effectiveness of other types of meditation is very limited: Sahaja meditation improved some outcomes in patients with poorly controlled asthma but differences were not maintained at 2 months;[4] epileptics practising Sahaja showed a reduction in objective stress measures[5] and seizure frequency[6] but adequate intergroup comparisons are missing and there are differences in baseline anxiety levels and seizure frequency between groups. MM is usually practised as one of several co-interventions so that specific effects are difficult to evaluate. A systematic review and meta-analysis of 20 studies of MM conducted by the Institute for Mindfulness Research reports positive effects of similar size in both controlled

THERAPIES

and uncontrolled studies of MM in a wide spectrum of clinical populations.[7] However, in what appears to be an independent review published earlier[8] the finding was that existing research into MM is fraught with methodological problems and evidence for effectiveness is lacking. A recent review of the therapeutic effects of meditation techniques in general concluded that there is at present only weak evidence for the therapeutic effectiveness of any type of meditation and even less evidence for any specific effect above that of credible control interventions.[9]

Risks

Contraindications
There is a theoretical risk that meditation could create conditions in the brain conducive to epilepsy.[10]

Precautions/warnings
People with pre-existing mental health problems should only take up meditation under the supervision of a qualified psychiatrist or psychotherapist experienced in the use of such techniques in a therapeutic context. People diagnosed with epilepsy or at risk of developing epilepsy should consider the theoretical risk of precipitating attacks before proceeding.

Adverse effects
The safety of meditation has not been studied systematically. There are a few isolated reports of adverse events including exacerbation of pre-existing depression and anxiety, depersonalisation, an attempted suicide, and precipitation of schizophrenic episodes.[11,12]

Interactions
None known.

Risk–benefit assessment

Meditation appears to be safe for most people and those with sufficient motivation to practise regularly will probably find it a pleasant and relaxing experience. Evidence for effectiveness in any indication is weak.

REFERENCES

1 Wallace R, Benson H. The physiology of meditation. Sci Am 1972;226:84–90
2 Canter P H, Ernst E. The cumulative effects of Transcendental Meditation on cognitive function – a systematic review of randomised controlled trials. Wien Klin Wochenschr 2003;115:758–766
3 Canter P H, Ernst E. Insufficient evidence to conclude whether or not Transcendental Meditation lowers blood pressure: results of a systematic review of randomised clinical trials. J Hypertens 2004;22:2049–2054
4 Manocha R, Marks G B, Kenchington P, Peters D, Salome C M. Sahaja yoga in the management of moderate to severe asthma: a randomised controlled trial. Thorax 2002;57:110–115
5 Panjwani U, Gupta H L, Singh S H, Selvamurthy W, Rai U C. Effect of Sahaja yoga practice on stress management in patients of epilepsy. Indian J Physiol Pharmacol 1995;39:111–116
6 Panjwani U, Selvamurthy W, Singh S H, Gupta H L, Thakur L, Rai U C. Effect of Sahaja yoga practice on seizure control & EEG changes in

patients of epilepsy. Indian J Med Res 1996;103:165–172

7   Grossman P, Niemann L, Schmidt S, Walach H. Mindfulness-based stress reduction and health benefits: a meta-analysis. J Psychosom Res 2004;51:35–43

8   Bishop S R. What do we really know about mindfulness-based stress reduction. Psychosom Med 2002;64:71–84

9   Canter P H The therapeutic effects of meditation. BMJ 2003;326:1049–1050

10   Jaseja H. Meditation may predispose to epilepsy: an insight into the alteration in brain environment induced by meditation. Med Hypotheses 2005;64:464–467

11   Lazarus A A. Psychiatric problems precipitated by transcendental meditation. Psychol Rep 1976;39:601–602

12   Sethi S, Bhargava S C. Relationship of meditation and psychosis: case studies. Aust NZ J Psychiatry 2003;37:382

NATUROPATHY

THERAPIES

Definition

An eclectic system of healthcare, which integrates elements of complementary and conventional medicine to support and enhance self-healing processes.

Related techniques

Hydrotherapy, Kneippkur (German), physical medicine, physiotherapy, Naturheilverfahren (German).

Background

The 'healing power of nature' to cure ill health gained interest during the 18th and 19th centuries when the Germans Vinzenz Prieanietz (1799–1851) and particularly Sebastian Kneipp (1821–1897) established complex hydrotherapeutic interventions as a cure for many ailments. A disciple of Kneipp, Benedict Lust (1870–1945), introduced hydrotherapy to the USA and later used the term naturopathy to describe the concept that he developed. In the UK one of the early nature cure resorts was established at Champneys near Tring in Hertfordshire in the 1930s.

Traditional concepts

Naturopathy is based on the belief that health is influenced by nature's own healing power (*vis medicatrix naturae*), which is understood as an inherent property of the living organism. Ill health is viewed as a direct result of ignoring or violating general principles of a healthy lifestyle. These principles are thought to be determined by an internal and external environment that optimises the health of an individual. Naturopathy aims to correct and stabilise the condition of the internal and external environment.

Scientific rationale

The general principles of a healthy lifestyle, including a diet that is rich in fresh fruit and vegetables and a sufficient amount of physical exercise, are now well recognised in mainstream medicine. The different therapeutic interventions and techniques that are used include herbal medicine, hydrotherapy and iridology as well as physical treatments (e.g. spinal manipulation) and others. The scientific rationale varies according to each individual treatment. For some interventions a plausible scientific rationale is lacking, while for others the rationale is supported by the results of scientific investigation.

Practitioners

In the USA, licensed naturopaths have completed a training including basic medical sciences and conventional diagnostic techniques. Four accredited colleges of naturopathic medicine exist in the USA and one in Canada, which offer 4-year training programmes, which may lead to licensure. Naturopaths are currently licensed in 13 US states.[1] In the UK, the number of registered naturopaths, a profession not regulated by statute, is about 500.

Conditions frequently treated

Naturopaths treat any condition but are trained to refer patients with serious medical conditions for conventional treatment.

Typical session

During an initial consultation the naturopath will usually take a detailed medical history of the patient to get an overall impression of the medical status and screen for any serious conditions. This will also include questions relating to lifestyle and diet and may be followed by a more conventional diagnostic evaluation, including laboratory analyses. According to the diagnosed condition, the treatment plan will vary but often includes a change in lifestyle. The treatment of a particular condition may vary between practitioners. Follow-up appointments are arranged as necessary and medicines and regimen reviewed and changed if appropriate.

Course of treatment

Depending largely on the nature and severity of the condition but generally 1–2 appointments per week for a treatment period of one to several weeks.

Clinical evidence

The clinical evidence has to be evaluated according to each individual therapy (see respective chapters). There is clinical evidence from RCTs and systematic reviews for some elements of naturopathy, such as certain herbal extracts,[2,3] balneotherapy[4] and speleotherapy.[5] For other elements there is little evidence to support their use (e.g.[6]). The effectiveness of the totality of the naturopathic approach has not been evaluated in RCTs.

Risks

Contraindications
Contraindications and precautions vary for each individual therapy (see respective chapters) and often include pregnancy and lactation.

Precautions/warnings
Precautions may vary for each individual therapy (see respective chapters).

Adverse effects
The risk of adverse effects exists. The reader is referred to the respective chapters in this book and the conventional medical literature.

Interactions
Possible interactions, for instance between different herbal preparations or with conventional drugs or other intervention,

should be considered (see respective chapters) and relevant patients should be closely monitored. Patients should be asked about self-prescription drug use.

Risk–benefit assessment

The possibility of adverse effects exists and the risk–benefit ratio has to be assessed for each treatment individually (see respective chapters). Given a beneficial safety profile elements of naturopathy may be worth considering when performed by a responsible, well-trained and licensed therapist.

REFERENCES

1 Atwood K C 4th. Naturopathy: a critical appraisal. MedGenMed 2003;5:39
2 Pittler M H, Ernst E. Horse chestnut seed extract for chronic venous insufficiency. The Cochrane Database of Systematic Reviews 2004, Issue 2. Art. No.: CD003230
3 Thompson Coon J, Pittler M H, Ernst E. Systematic review and meta-analysis of *Trifolium pratense* (red clover) isoflavones for treating vasomotor symptoms in menopausal women. (in press)
4 Verhagen A P, Bierma Zeinstra S M A, Cardoso J R, de Bie R A, Boers M, de Vet H C W. Balneotherapy for rheumatoid arthritis. The Cochrane Database of Systematic Reviews 2004, Issue 1. Art. No.: CD000518
5 Beamon S, Falkenbach A, Fainburg G, Linde K. Speleotherapy for asthma. The Cochrane Database of Systematic Reviews 2001, Issue 2. Art. No.: CD001741
6 Ernst E. Iridology. Arch Ophthalmol 2000;118:120–121

OSTEOPATHY

Definition

Form of manual therapy (and diagnosis) involving the manipulation of soft tissues and the mobilisation or manipulation of peripheral and spinal joints.

Related techniques

Craniosacral therapy, chiropractic, manual therapy, spinal manipulation and mobilisation.

Background

Osteopathy was founded in the USA by Andrew Taylor Still in 1874, since then it has had a turbulent history. It is now an accepted conventional form of healthcare in the USA and a well-established form of CAM in the UK and many other countries.

Traditional concepts

Osteopaths believe that the primary role of the therapist is to facilitate the body's inherent ability to heal itself, that the structure and function of the body are closely related and that problems of one organ affect other parts of the body.[1] For osteopaths, an adequate alignment of the musculoskeletal system eliminates obstructions in blood and lymph flow which, in turn, maximise health and function. To ensure alignment, osteopaths have developed a range of techniques. These can be grouped into five major categories:

- direct techniques: high-velocity, low-amplitude thrusts; articulatory, general osteopathic techniques, muscle energy techniques

THERAPIES

- indirect techniques: functional techniques, counterstrain, balanced ligamentous tension, ligamentous articulatory strain
- combined techniques: myofascial/fascial release, visceral techniques, osteopathy in the cranial field, involuntary mechanism
- reflex based techniques: Chapman's reflexes, triggerpoints, neuromuscular techniques
- fluid based techniques: lymphatic pump techniques.[1]

Scientific rationale

Some of the traditional osteopathic concepts ring intuitively true, yet their scientific rationale is not fully convincing. In particular, the theory of the overriding importance of alignment lacks a scientific rationale.

Practitioners

In the USA, osteopaths today constitute the smaller of the two major schools of medicine. US osteopaths (doctors of osteopathy, DOs) use most allopathic therapeutic options alongside osteopathic manipulative techniques and are regarded as mainstream healthcare professionals. Outside the USA, osteopaths mainly use spinal manipulation and mobilisation and are usually considered as complementary therapists. In the UK, osteopaths are now regulated by statute. In continental Europe, the title 'DO' has a different meaning and stands for diploma of osteopathy.

Conditions frequently treated

Typically, osteopaths treat patients suffering from musculoskeletal problems, particularly back and neck pain. US osteopaths would treat many other conditions as well, combining allopathic treatments with manual osteopathic techniques. The majority of US osteopaths, however, no longer use manipulative techniques routinely.

Typical session

A visit to an osteopath would normally be very similar to a consultation with a conventional physician. Outside the USA, an osteopath would take a medical history and perform a careful physical examination, particularly of the musculoskeletal system. In most cases this would be followed by treatment consisting of spinal manipulation and mobilisation.

Course of treatment

Depending on the condition and on clinical progress, 3–6 treatments would constitute a full course for acute conditions. More sessions are usually required for chronic conditions.

Clinical evidence

There is some evidence to suggest that osteopathy is helpful for low back pain, particularly acute and subacute stages.[1-3] A systematic review of six RCTs of osteopathic manipulative treatment for low back pain found greater pain reductions with osteopathy compared to active control treatment, placebo or no treatment.[4] A UK cost-utility analysis generated encouragingly positive results for osteopathic treatment of subacute spinal pain.[5] A small (n = 76) CCT suggested that osteopathic treatment after

THERAPIES

knee or hip arthroplasty was superior to conventional care in speeding up postoperative rehabilitation.[6] Two small RCTs did not generate convincing evidence that osteopathic approaches to treating shoulder pain[7] or tennis elbow[8] are superior to standard care. A Cochrane review failed to find reliable evidence that osteopathy is effective in the treatment of primary or secondary dysmenorrhoea.[9] For other indications the clinical trial evidence is also sparse and not compelling.[1,2]

Risks

Contraindications
Osteoporosis, neoplasms, infections, bleeding disorders (depending on the approach used).

Precautions/warnings
None known.

Adverse effects
Spinal trauma after high-velocity thrusts, vertebral artery dissection, stroke.

Interactions
None known.

Risk–benefit assessment

Osteopathic spinal manipulation and mobilisation may be helpful in cases of low back pain. Osteopathic techniques are typically gentler than those used by chiropractors; thus the risk of spinal injury should be smaller. On balance, osteopathy may be worth trying for patients with low back pain. For all other conditions data are insufficient for issuing definitive recommendations.

REFERENCES

1 Lesho E P. An overview of osteopathic medicine. Arch Fam Med 1999;8:477–483
2 Schwerla F, Hass-Degg K, Schwerla B. Evaluierung und kritische Bewertung von in der europäischen Literatur veröffentlichten, osteopathischen Studien im klinischen Bereich und im Bereich der Grundlagenforschung. Forsch Komplementärmed 1999;6:302–310
3 Williams N H, Wilkinson C, Russell I, Edwards R T, Hibbs R, Linck P, Muntz R. Randomized osteopathic manipulation study (ROMANS): pragmatic trial for spinal pain in primary care. Fam Pract 2003;20:662–669
4 Licciardone J C, Brimhall A K, King L N. Osteopathic manipulative treatment for low back pain: a systematic review and meta-analysis of randomized controlled trials. BMC Musculoskelet Disord 2005;6:43
5 Williams N H, Edwards R T, Linck P, Muntz R, Hibbs R, Wilkinson C, Russell I, Russell D, Hounsome B. Cost-utility analysis of osteopathy in primary care: results from a pragmatic

randomized controlled trial. Fam Pract 2004;21:643–650
6 Jarski R W, Loniewski E G, Williams J, Bahu A, Shafinia S, Gibbs K, Muller M. The effectiveness of osteopathic manipulative treatment as complementary therapy following surgery: A prospective match-controlled outcome study. Altern Ther Health Med 2000;6:77–81
7 Knebl J A, Shores J H, Gamber R G, Gray W T, Herron K M. An RCT of osteopathy for shoulder problems. J Am Osteopath Assoc 2002;102:387–396
8 Geldschläger S. Osteopathic versus orthopaedic interventions for chronic epicondylopathia humeri radialis: randomized controlled trial. Forsch Komplementärmed Klass Naturheildkd 2004;11:93–97
9 Proctor M L, Hing W, Johnson T C, Murphy P A. Spinal manipulation for primary and secondary dysmenorrhoea. The Cochrane Database of Systematic Reviews 2001, Issue 4. Art. No.: CD002119

THERAPIES

REFLEXOLOGY

Synonyms

Zone therapy, reflex zone therapy. Note that the term 'reflexology' is sometimes used to describe treatment of segmental nerve reflexes with needles. 'Reflexotherapy' was used historically to describe acupuncture in the former USSR.

Definition

A therapeutic method that uses manual pressure applied to specific areas, or zones, of the feet (and sometimes the hands or ears) that are believed to correspond to other areas or organs of the body, in order to relieve stress and prevent and treat illness.

Related techniques

Reflexology may be used together with other techniques by manual therapists of various disciplines. Other therapies that use the concept of correspondence to parts of the body include acupuncture techniques such as auriculotherapy and Korean hand acupuncture.

Background

Egyptian papyri from about 2500 BCE show manual treatment of the feet and there is evidence that similar treatment was part of Chinese culture. Zone therapy is recorded in various ancient European medical systems and those of the North American Indians. In the early 20th century William Fitzgerald investigated the effects of pressure in inducing analgesia elsewhere in the body and concluded that the body was divided into ten vertical zones, each represented by a part of the foot including one toe. From this concept, the charts of bodily correspondences evolved, initially drawn up by Eunice Ingham and published from the 1930s onwards.

Traditional concepts

The organs, glands and other components of each half of the body are believed to be represented at the foot on that side, mainly on the sole. The health of the body can be assessed by examining the feet to detect imbalances or obstructions to the flow of energy, which are expressed as tenderness or feelings of grittiness or crystal formation. Bodily functions are believed to be influenced by stimulating these areas with pressure or massage. Reflexology is claimed to reduce stress, improve circulation, eliminate toxins and promote metabolic homeostasis.

Scientific rationale

There is no known neurophysiological basis for connections between organs or other body parts and specific areas of the feet. Reflexologists' diagnoses were no better than chance in identifying medical conditions in one blinded study,[1] whereas in another their diagnostic success was better than chance but not clinically relevant.[2] A further study suggested that reflexologists' diagnoses correlate with some organ systems and not with others.[3] Pressure on the specific areas produced changes in renal and intestinal blood flow.[4,5] Foot massage may have general benefits regardless of any reflex correspondences.

Practitioners

Practitioners range from those who teach themselves from books to those who follow training courses and join professional associations. In most countries, no regulatory systems exist, as there are currently no state licensure or training requirements. Reflexology is sometimes used by other health professionals including conventionally trained nurses.

Conditions frequently treated

Asthma, arthritis, back and neck pain, chronic fatigue, digestive problems such as irritable bowel syndrome and constipation, insomnia, migraine and headaches, postmenopausal symptoms, sinusitis, and stress-related disorders.

Typical session

The reflexologist usually takes a full history before examining the bare feet systematically, with the patient lying on a couch or semi-reclining in a chair. Tender or gritty areas will be massaged as soon as they are found. The strength of pressure used varies greatly between practitioners. For lubrication, therapists may use talc or oil. Often the reflexologist and patient will converse throughout. The whole session usually lasts 45–60 minutes. Some practitioners will use sticks or other instruments to treat the feet.

Course of treatment

This varies considerably between practitioners and conditions treated. Often treatment is offered weekly for a course of 6–8 sessions. For chronic conditions follow-up treatments may be offered.

Clinical evidence

One RCT found reflexology to be superior to placebo reflexology for the treatment of premenstrual symptoms, but the protocol included foot, hand and ear treatment so no conclusions can be drawn about any one independently.[6] Other RCTs found no advantage of reflexology over non-specific foot massage in the treatment of menopausal symptoms[7], irritable bowel syndrome[8] or asthma.[9] One RCT showed beneficial effects on blood glucose in diabetics.[10] Another RCT in patients with multiple sclerosis showed improvements of motor, sensory and urinary symptoms after 11 weeks of regular reflexology compared to non-specific foot massage.[11] A large observational study found that 81% of patients with headache reported themselves helped or cured at 3 months follow-up[12] and an RCT found a trend in the same condition.[13] Other RCTs have shown no effect on asthma,[14] on serum cortisol during surgery[15] or leg circumference measurements in pregnant women with leg oedema.[16] It should be noted that the results of the above studies tend to be negative when placebo-effects were adequately controlled for and positive when this was not the case.

Risks

Contraindications
Relevant conditions of the feet such as gout, ulceration or vascular disease.

THERAPIES

Precautions/warnings
Individuals with bone or joint conditions of the feet or lower leg should be treated cautiously. Although professional reflexology associations insist that reflexologists should not make diagnostic claims, there have been incidents where reflexologists have made false-positive or -negative diagnoses and thus interfered with medical management to the patient's detriment.

Adverse effects
Fatigue, changes in micturition or bowel function. Allergy to lubricants.

Interactions
Possible interference with the effects of some drugs, e.g. insulin.

Risk–benefit assessment
In the hands of responsible practitioners, reflexology seems to do little harm and possibly some good in the management of many functional disorders. Reflexology should never be used to make, or suggest, a medical diagnosis.

REFERENCES

1 White A R, Williamson J, Hart A, Ernst E. A blinded investigation into the accuracy of reflexology charts. Complement Ther Med 2000;8:166–172

2 Baerheim A, Algroy R, Skogedal K R, Stephansen R, Sandvik H. Fottene – et diagnostisk hjelpemiddel? Tidsskr Nor Laegeforen 1998;5:753–755

3 Raz I, Rosengarten Y, Carasso R. Correlation study between conventional medical diagnosis and the diagnosis by reflexology (non conventional). Harefuah 2003;142:600–605+646

4 Sudmeier I, Bodner G, Egger I, Mur E, Ulmer H, Herold M. Änderung der Nierendurchblutung durch organassoziierte Reflexzonentherapie am Fua gemessen mit farbkodierter Doppler-Sonographie. Forsch Komplementärmed 1999;6:129–134

5 Mur E, Schmidseder J, Egger I, Bodner G, Eibl G, Hartig F, Pfeiffer K P, Herold M. Influence of reflex zone therapy of the feet on intestinal blood flow measured by color Doppler sonography. Forsch Komplementärmed Klass Naturheilkd 2001;8:86–89

6 Oleson T, Flocco W. Randomised controlled study of premenstrual symptoms treated with ear, hand and foot reflexology. Obstet Gynaecol 1993;82:906–911

7 Williamson J, White A, Hart A, Ernst E. Randomised controlled trial of reflexology for menopausal symptoms. Br J Obstet Gynaecol 2002;109:1050–1055

8 Tovey P A. A single-blind trial of reflexology for irritable bowel syndrome. Br J Gen Pract 2002;52:19–23

9 Brygge T, Heinig J H, Collins P, Ronborg S M, Gehrchen P M, Hilden J, Heegaard S, Poulsen L K. Zoneterapi og asthma. Ugeskr Laeg 2002;164:2405–2410

10 Wang X M. Treating type II diabetes mellitus with foot reflexotherapy [Chinese]. Chung-Kuo Chung Hsi i Chieh Ho Tsa Chih 1993;13:536–538

11 Siev Ner I, Gamus D, Lerner-Geva L, Achiron A. Reflexology treatment relieves symtpoms of multiple sclerosis: a randomized controlled study. Mult Scler 2003;9:356–361

12 Launso L, Brendstrup E, Arnberg S. An exploratory study of reflexological treatment for headache. Alt Ther Health Med 1999;5:57–65

13 Lafuente A, Noguera M, Puy C, Molins A, Titus F, Sanz F. Effekt der Reflexzonenbehandlung am Fuss bezüglich der prophylaktischen Behandlung mit Funarizin bei an Cephalea-Kopfschmerzen leidenden Patienten. Erfahrungsheilkunde 1990;39:713–715

14 Peterson L N, Faurschou P, Olsen O T, Svendsen U G. Reflexology and bronchial asthma. Ugeskr Laeger 1992;154:2065–2068

15 Engquist A, Vibe-Hansen H. Zone therapy and plasma cortisol during surgical stress. Ugeskr Laeger 1977;139:460–462

16 Mollart L. Single-blind trial addressing the differential effects of two reflexology techniques versus rest, on ankle and foot oedema in late pregnancy. Complement Ther Nurs Midwifery 2003;9:203–208

RELAXATION THERAPY

Definition
Techniques for eliciting the 'relaxation response' of the autonomic nervous system.

Related techniques
Autogenic training, biofeedback, hypnotherapy, meditation. Many CAM interventions include an element of relaxation.

Background
One of the most common relaxation techniques is progressive muscle relaxation, pioneered by the American physician Edmund Jacobson in 1930. It has been modified over time by others, but is still based on the original principles. Other relaxation techniques involve passive muscle relaxation, refocusing, breathing control or imagery.

Traditional concepts
Progressive muscle relaxation is based on the notion that it is impossible to be tense in any part of the body where the muscles are completely relaxed. Furthermore, tension in involuntary muscles can be reduced if the associated skeletal muscles are relaxed. The method is learnt by first tensing a muscle before relaxing it, to help recognise the difference between tension and relaxation. Subsequently, it is possible to relax a limb without tensing it first. Systematic relaxation involves a more passive release of tension while focusing on muscle groups. Benson's relaxation response contains an attention control element where the focus is on slow rhythmical breathing combined with repetition of a single word. With imagery-based relaxation, the idea is to imagine oneself in a place or situation associated with relaxation and comfort using visualisation and involving all the other senses in creating a vivid image.

Scientific rationale
Progressive muscle relaxation has been shown to be effective in eliciting the relaxation response, resulting in the normalising of blood supply to the muscles, decreases in oxygen consumption, heart rate, respiration and skeletal muscle activity and increases in skin resistance and alpha brain waves. Other relaxation techniques have also been shown to be effective in diffusing muscle tension.

Practitioners
Relaxation techniques are taught by various complementary practitioners, physicians, psychotherapists, hypnotherapists, nurses, clinical psychologists and sports therapists. There is no formal credentialing for relaxation therapies.

Conditions frequently treated
Anxiety, headaches, musculoskeletal pain, stress disorders.

THERAPIES

THERAPIES

Typical session

With progressive muscle relaxation, subjects usually lie on their back with arms to the side in a quiet environment without bright light. Occasionally a sitting posture in a comfortable chair is adopted instead. Muscle groups are systematically contracted then relaxed in a predetermined order. In the early stages, an entire session will be devoted to a single muscle group. With practice it becomes possible to combine muscle groups and then eventually relax the entire body all at once.

Course of treatment

With progressive muscle relaxation, several months of daily practice is needed in order to be able to evoke the relaxation response within seconds.

Clinical evidence

A large body of evidence suggests that relaxation therapies are useful in anxiety. Positive results from RCTs exist for relaxation in association with desensitisation for agoraphobia and panic disorder (e.g.[1,2]), anxiety associated with cancer[3] and for guided imagery in patients undergoing medical interventions such as radiation therapy.[4] A systematic review included 22 studies of progressive muscle relaxation and reported a moderate effect on trait anxiety in non-psychiatric patients.[5] Systematic reviews of RCTs in both acute[6] and chronic[7] pain have found only weak and contradictory evidence that relaxation is an effective form of treatment on its own. For patients with chronic cancer pain, an RCT reported positive effects of relaxation therapy using music for falling asleep.[8] No difference was reported when relaxation therapy was compared with occlusal appliance in temporomandibular disorder pain.[9] Other conditions for which there is promising evidence from RCTs include depression,[10-12] insomnia,[13-15] menopausal symptoms,[16-18] hypertension,[19] coronary syndrome X,[20] night eating syndrome,[21] cardiac events after myocardial infarction[22] and preterm labour outcome.[23] Relaxation therapy was inferior to cognitive behaviour therapy for chronic fatigue syndrome[24] and as an addition to routine clinical care relaxation therapy was not different to clinical care alone in irritable bowel syndrome.[25] Cochrane reviews reported no convincing evidence for relaxation therapy in non-ulcer dyspepsia[26] and epilepsy.[27]

Risks

Contraindications
Schizophrenic or actively psychotic patients.

Precautions/warnings
Techniques requiring inward focusing may intensify depressed mood.

Adverse effects
None known.

Interactions
Adjunctive relaxation therapy may reduce the required dosage of certain medications, i.e. antihypertensive or anxiolytic drugs.

Risk–benefit assessment

Relaxation techniques may be useful for treating anxiety disorders or states, although they do not appear to be as effective as psychotherapy. For conditions with a strong psychosomatic element, relaxation appears to have some potential benefits although these may not be long term. However, since relaxation therapies are almost risk free, they can be recommended as an adjunctive therapy for most conditions.

REFERENCES

1 Ost L G, Westling B E, Hellstrom K. Applied relaxation, exposure in vivo and cognitive methods in the treatment of panic disorder with agoraphobia. Behav Res Ther 1993;31:383–394

2 Beck J G, Stanley M A, Baldwin L E, Deagle E A 3rd, Averill P M. Comparison of cognitive therapy and relaxation training for panic disorder. J Consult Clin Psychol 1994;62:818–826

3 Bindemann S, Soukop M, Kaye S B. Randomized controlled study of relaxation training. Eur J Cancer 1991;27:170–174

4 Kolcaba K, Fox C. The effects of guided imagery on comfort of women with early stage breast cancer undergoing radiation therapy. Oncol Nurs Forum 1999;26:67–72

5 Eppley K R, Abrams A I, Shear J. Differential effects of relaxation techniques on trait anxiety. J Clin Psychol 1989;45:957–974

6 Seers K, Carroll D. Relaxation techniques for acute pain management: a systematic review. J Adv Nurs 1998;27:466–475

7 Carroll D, Seers K. Relaxation for the relief of chronic pain: a systematic review. J Adv Nurs 1998;27:476–487

8 Reinhardt U. Investigations into synchronisation of heart rate and musical rhythm in a relaxation therapy in patients with cancer pain. Forsch Komplementärmed 1999;6:135–141

9 Wahlund K, List T, Larsson B. Treatment of temporomandibular disorders among adolescents: a comparison between occlusal appliance, relaxation training, and brief information. Acta Odontol Scand 2003;61:203–211

10 Reynolds W M, Coats K I. A comparison of cognitive-behavioural therapy and relaxation training for the treatment of depression in adolescents. J Consult Clin Psychol 1986;54:653–660

11 Broota A, Dhir R. Efficacy of two relaxation techniques in depression. J Pers Clin Stud 1990;6:83–90

12 Murphy G E, Carney R M, Knesevich M A, Wetzel R D, Whitworth P. Cognitive behaviour therapy, relaxation training and tricyclic antidepressant medication in the treatment of depression. Psychol Rep 1995;77:403–420

13 Greeff A P, Conradie W S. Use of progressive relaxation training for chronic alcoholics with insomnia. Psychol Rep 1998;82:407–412

14 Engle Friedman M, Bootzin R R, Hazlewood L, Tsao C. An evaluation of behavioural treatments for insomnia in the older adult. J Clin Psychol 1992;48:77–90

15 Hauri P J. Can we mix behavioural therapy with hypnotics when treating insomniacs? Sleep 1997;20:1111–1118

16 Irvin J H, Domar A D, Clark C, Zuttermeister P C, Friedman R. The effects of relaxation response training on menopausal symptoms. J Psychosom Obstet Gynecol 1996;17:202–207

17 Freedman R R, Woodward S. Behavioural treatment of menopausal hot flushes: evaluation by ambulatory monitoring. Am J Obstet Gynecol 1992;167:436–439

18 Germaine L M, Freedman R R. Behavioural treatment of menopausal hot flashes: evaluation by objective methods. J Consult Clin Psychol 1984;52:1072–1079

19 Yung P, French P, Leung B. Relaxation training as complementary therapy for mild hypertension control and the implications of evidence-based medicine. Complement Ther Nurs Midwifery 2001;7:59–65

20 Tyni-Lenne R, Stryjan S, Eriksson B, Berglund M, Sylven C. Beneficial therapeutic effects of physical training and relaxation therapy in women with coronary syndrome X. Physiother Res Int 2002;7:35–43

21 Pawlow L A, O'Neil P M, Malcolm R J. Night eating syndrome: effects of brief relaxation training on stress, mood, hunger, and eating patterns. Int J Obes Relat Metab Disord 2003;27:970–978

THERAPIES

22 van Dixhoorn J J, Duivenvoorden H J. Effect of relaxation therapy on cardiac events after myocardial infarction: a 5-year follow-up study. J Cardiopulm Rehabil 1999;19:178–185

23 Janke J. The effect of relaxation therapy on preterm labor outcomes. J Obstet Gynecol Neonatal Nurs 1999;28:255–263

24 Deale A, Husain K, Chalder T, Wessely S. Long-term outcome of cognitive behavior therapy versus relaxation therapy for chronic fatigue syndrome: a 5-year follow-up study. Am J Psychiatry 2001;158:2038–2042

25 Boyce P M, Talley N J, Balaam B, Koloski N A, Truman G. A randomized controlled trial of cognitive behavior therapy, relaxation training, and routine clinical care for the irritable bowel syndrome. Am J Gastroenterol 2003;98:2209–2218

26 Soo S, Moayyedi P, Deeks J, Delaney B, Lewis M, Forman D. Psychological interventions for non-ulcer dyspepsia. The Cochrane Database of Systematic Reviews 2004, Issue 3. Art. No.: CD002301

27 Ramaratnam S, Baker GA, Goldstein L H. Psychological treatments for epilepsy. The Cochrane Database of Systematic Reviews 2003, Issue 4. Art. No.: CD002029

SPIRITUAL HEALING

Synonyms/ subcategories	Distant healing, faith healing, intercessory prayer, paranormal healing, psychic healing, Reiki, therapeutic touch.
Definition	The direct interaction between one individual (the healer) and a second (sick) individual with the intention of bringing about an improvement or cure of the illness.[1]
Related techniques	All types of energy healing systems.
Traditional concepts	Spiritual healing can be traced as far back as the Bible (New Testament, *1 Corinthians* 12:9) where it was listed amongst the gifts bestowed on the faithful. It has always had its adherents and in recent years has gained widespread popularity. Spiritual healers believe that the therapeutic effect results from the channelling of healing 'energy' from an assumed source via the healer to the patient. The central claim of healers is that they promote or facilitate self-healing in the patient.
Scientific rationale	There is no scientific evidence to support the existence of this 'energy', nor is there a scientific rationale for any other concept underlying spiritual healing.
Practitioners	In the UK around 14 000 members are today registered in nine separate healing organisations. In the USA its related therapies, therapeutic touch (TT) and Reiki, boast many thousands of healers. TT was developed in the early 1970s by Dora Kunz and Dolores Krieger. The technique is taught at 75 US institutions and universities. Krieger claims she has personally taught TT to more than 48 000 healthcare professionals in 75 countries. Most healers are not medically qualified and there is no mandatory training. Members of the UK Confederation of Healing Organisations

have, however, a minimum of 2 years' training. Most US practitioners of TT are trained nurses.

Conditions frequently treated

Healers do not usually relate to the disease entities of conventional medicine. Their aim is to help the patient in more general terms, for instance by increasing well-being. Many healers treat patients with chronic pain or emotional problems.

Typical session

The healer discusses the problem with the patient in order to gain some understanding of it. Subsequently the patient may be asked to lie or sit down and the therapist may scan the patient's body with his or her hands at a distance and channel healing 'energy' through his or her body towards the patient.

Course of treatment

A typical course may consist of eight or more single sessions. Often several courses of treatment are given within a year.

Clinical evidence

A systematic review[2] of all types of healing included 23 placebo-controlled RCTs involving almost 3000 patients. About half of these studies yielded a positive result, suggesting that spiritual healing is effective. However, due to numerous methodological limitations of these trials, no firm conclusions could be drawn. An update of this review included eight non-randomised and nine randomised clinical trials which had emerged since.[3] These data collectively shift the weight of the evidence against the notion that healing is more than a placebo. Cochrane reviews found no convincing evidence that TT promotes wound healing,[4] or that intercessory prayer alleviates ill health of any type.[5] An RCT (n = 57) suggested that therapeutic touch decreases behavioural symptoms of dementia.[6] Another RCT was unable to show any benefit for intercessory prayer for children in psychiatric care.[7]

Risks

Contraindications
Psychiatric illness.

Precautions/warnings
None known.

Adverse effects
Sensations like heat or tingling are often reported in areas under the hands of the healer. Belief in the occult can undermine rationality in general.

Interactions
None known.

Risk–benefit assessment

Spiritual healing does not seem to be associated with specific therapeutic effects. Healing has some risks. It cannot be recommended as a medical treatment, particularly not as substitute for conventional therapies.

THERAPIES

THERAPIES

REFERENCES

1 Hodges R D, Scofield A M. Is spiritual healing a valid and effective therapy? J Roy Soc Med 1995;88:203–207

2 Astin J, Harkness E, Ernst E. The efficacy of spiritual healing: a systematic review of randomised trials. Ann Intern Med 2000;132:903–910

3 Ernst E. Distant healing – an 'update' of a systematic review. Wien Klin Wochenschr 2003;115:241–245

4 O'Mathuna D P, Ashford R L. Therapeutic touch for healing acute wounds. The Cochrane Database of Systematic Reviews 2003, Issue 4. Art. No.: CD002766

5 Roberts L, Ahmed I, Hall S. Intercessory prayer for the alleviation of ill health. The Cochrane Database of Systematic Reviews 2000, Issue 2. Art. No.: CD000368

6 Woods D L, Craven R F, Whitney J. The effect of therapeutic touch on behavioral symptoms of persons with dementia. Altern Ther Health Med 2005;11:66–74

7 Mathai J, Bourne A. Pilot study investigating the effect of intercessory prayer in the treatment of child psychiatric disorders. Australas Psychiatry 2004;12:386–389

TAI CHI

Definition

A system of movements and postures rooted in ancient Chinese philosophy and martial arts used to enhance mental and physical health.

Related techniques

Qi gong.

Background

Tai chi has a long history in China and is today widely practised there. It has also become increasingly popular in many Western countries. A number of different styles and forms were developed from the original 13 postures, believed to have been created in the early 12th century. The various forms of tai chi comprise a series of postures linked by gentle and graceful movements.

Traditional concepts

Influenced by Confucian and Buddhist philosophy, tai chi is based on the principles of the two opposing life forces, Yin and Yang. Ill-health is viewed as an imbalance between Yin, the female, receptive principle, and Yang, the male, creative principle. The alternating movements and postures are thought to stabilise these flowing energies, create inner and outer harmony and emotional balance.

Scientific rationale

The slow movement between different postures that are normally held for a short period of time are physical stimuli with effects on the cardiovascular and muscular system. These stimuli, much like other physical exercise, result in muscular adaptation, which ultimately leads to increased muscle strength, if performed regularly. In addition to adaptation processes at the level of the nervous system, these effects produce better cardiovascular function,[1] and may enhance strength, balance and coordination.[2]

Practitioners	Teachers should have a basic understanding of human anatomy and physiology and should have some knowledge of the philosophy and historical background of tai chi. Ideally, teachers have had at least 5 years of experience and study with a master before independent teaching. There is, however, no generally acknowledged minimum requirement.
Conditions frequently treated	Depression, high or low blood pressure, osteoporosis, stress-related conditions.
Typical session	Tai chi is usually taught in classes of 5–10 or more people. The atmosphere during practice is usually quiet, relaxed but intense. The student should maintain a level of concentration and should not be distracted by external influences. The movements are performed simultaneously by the group responding to advice and corrections by the teacher. Tai chi is a lifelong endeavour and regular practice is essential in achieving beneficial effects.
Course of treatment	The various forms take between 5 and 30 minutes to complete. Daily practice is ideal but at least twice-weekly exercises are recommended. The best time for practice is said to be early in the morning.
Clinical evidence	The effectiveness of tai chi in older adults was assessed in a systematic review.[3] A total of seven studies were included (n = 505), of whom all but 27 were healthy seniors, between 53 and 96 years of age. All studies mention a beneficial effect of tai chi, but in most studies this conclusion was based on a pre-post analysis. It was concluded that there is limited evidence that tai chi is effective in reducing falls and blood pressure in the elderly. A Cochrane review of interventions for preventing falls in the elderly identified one RCT testing tai chi which suggested a beneficial effect.[4] A systematic review of health outcomes in patients with chronic conditions identified nine RCTs.[5] It concluded that, although tai chi appears to have physiological and psychosocial benefits and also appears to be safe and effective in promoting balance control, flexibility, and cardiovascular fitness in older patients with chronic conditions, limitations or biases exist in most studies, and it is difficult to draw firm conclusions about the benefits reported. As an option for treating rheumatoid arthritis, a Cochrane review suggested that tai chi is beneficial for lower extremity range of motion, particularly ankle range of motion and does not exacerbate the symptoms of rheumatoid arthritis.[6] Other single RCTs suggest a retardation of bone loss in postmenopausal women,[7] increases in distance walked and quality of life in chronic heart failure NYHA stage II,[8] improvement in quality of sleep[9] and quality of life and self-esteem in breast cancer survivors.[10]

THERAPIES

THERAPIES

Risks

Contraindications

Contraindications and precautions are largely based on common sense (e.g. severe osteoporosis, severe heart conditions, acute back pain, knee problems, sprains and fractures). Usually it can be safely practised during pregnancy and lactation.

Precautions/warnings

Before starting tai chi older individuals should be carefully examined for any of the above or other contraindications.

Adverse effects

Adverse effects are rare, but may include delayed-onset muscle soreness, pulled ligaments or ankle sprains.

Interactions

None known.

Indirect risk

Tai chi should be viewed as an adjunctive treatment, not as an alternative to conventional medical care.

Risk–benefit assessment

Tai chi can be recommended for patients with rheumatoid arthritis to increase lower extremity range of motion. For all other indications there is only limited evidence from rigorous clinical trials. It appears that tai chi has a range of beneficial effects similar to those established for other physical exercise. Given the nature and frequency of the risks involved when instructed by a responsible teacher, it is worth considering as a general measure for promoting a healthy lifestyle and may thus benefit most individuals.

REFERENCES

1 Taylor-Piliae R E, Froelicher E S. Effectiveness of Tai Chi exercise in improving aerobic capacity: a meta-analysis. J Cardiovasc Nurs 2004;19:48–57

2 Wolfson L, Whipple R, Derby C, Judge J, King M, Amerman P, Schmidt J, Smyers D. Balance and strength in older adults: intervention gains and tai chi maintenance. J Am Geriatr Soc 1996;44:498–506

3 Verhagen A P, Immink M, van der Meulen A, Bierma-Zeinstra S M. The efficacy of Tai Chi Chuan in older adults: a systematic review. Fam Pract 2004;21:107–113

4 Gillespie L D, Gillespie W J, Robertson M C, Lamb S E, Cumming R G, Rowe B H. Interventions for preventing falls in elderly people. The Cochrane Database of Systematic Reviews 2003, Issue 4. Art. No.: CD000340

5 Wang C, Collet J P, Lau J. The effect of Tai Chi on health outcomes in patients with chronic conditions: a systematic review. Arch Intern Med 2004;164:493–501

6 Han A, Robinson V, Judd M, Taixiang W, Wells G, Tugwell P. Tai chi for treating rheumatoid arthritis. The Cochrane Database of Systematic Reviews 2004, Issue 3. Art. No.: CD004849

7 Chan K, Qin L, Lau M, Woo J, Au S, Choy W, Lee K, Lee S. A randomized, prospective study of the effects of Tai Chi Chun exercise on bone mineral density in postmenopausal women. Arch Phys Med Rehabil 2004;85:717–722

8 Yeh G Y, Wood M J, Lorell B H, Stevenson L W, Eisenberg D M, Wayne P M, Goldberger A L, Davis R B, Phillips R S. Effects of tai chi mind-body movement therapy on functional

status and exercise capacity in patients with chronic heart failure: a randomized controlled trial. Am J Med 2004;117:541–548

9 Li F, Fisher K J, Harmer P, Irbe D, Tearse R G, Weimer C. Tai chi and self-rated quality of sleep and daytime sleepiness in older adults: a randomized controlled trial. J Am Geriatr Soc 2004;52:892–900

10 Mustian K M, Katula J A, Gill D L, Roscoe J A, Lang D, Murphy K. Tai Chi Chuan, health-related quality of life and self-esteem: a randomized trial with breast cancer survivors. Support Care Cancer 2004;12:871–876

YOGA

Definition

A practice of gentle stretching, exercises for breath control and meditation as a mind–body intervention.

Related techniques

Meditation.

Background

The word yoga is derived from the Sanskrit word *yuj*, which means 'to yoke', reflecting its purpose in joining mind and body in harmonious relaxation. Indian symbols dating from 3000 BCE are believed to indicate that yoga was in existence at that time. Records of the Yoga Sutras, the eight aspects of spiritual enlightenment, date from about 2300 years ago and include ethical principles of behaviour. Most widely used in the West is hatha yoga, which includes the poses (*asanas*), breath control (*pranayama*) and meditation, which are aimed at bringing the body to a perfect state of health and stillness, thus achieving heightened awareness. Yoga devotees practise regularly and increase their skills and techniques throughout their lifetime. Yoga is widely practised in both Eastern and Western countries, but yoga masters from India are still held in great reverence.

The practice of yoga does not require spiritual beliefs or religious observances.

Traditional concepts

Yoga is believed to increase the body's stores of *prana*, or vital energy, and to facilitate its flow by improved posture. The body becomes a 'fit vehicle for the spirit'. Poor diet, stress and other factors can block the natural flow of prana, leaving the body vulnerable.

Scientific rationale

The regular practise of yoga induces a deep sense of relaxation which is beneficial in itself, at least temporarily. Physical benefits of regular practice that have been described include bodily suppleness and muscular strength. Mental benefits include feelings of well-being and, possibly, reduction of sympathetic drive. Yoga breathing exercises counter the rapid breathing that accompanies the stress response and may in addition reduce muscular spasm and expand the available lung capacity.

THERAPIES

Practitioners

Although yoga can be self-taught through various media, it is preferable to learn with supervision in classes. Practitioners or teachers should have the knowledge and experience to ensure that benefit is obtained without overstretching joints and muscles. No uniform credentialing exists and no licensure is currently required to teach yoga.

Conditions frequently treated

Anxiety, arthritis, back pain, cardiovascular problems, gastro-intestinal complaints, headaches, insomnia, premenstrual syndrome, respiratory problems, stress. Also used in pregnancy as preparation for childbirth. Yoga can also be used by healthy people to gain self-mastery.

Typical session

Classes last about one hour and involve some theoretical introduction, supervised postures and breathing exercises usually leading to a period of deep relaxation or sometimes meditation. Precise content and form vary considerably.

Course of treatment

Yoga is probably best practised daily for maximum benefit. It should be regarded as a long-term commitment.

Clinical evidence

According to a large UK consumer survey, yoga leads to more patient-satisfaction than any other CAM modality.[1] A systematic review of six RCTs suggested that yoga can normalise cardiovascular risk factors and be a supportive therapy for coronary heart disease.[2] A Cochrane review found no conclusive evidence that it is helpful for epilepsy.[3] Several RCTs generated promising results for depression,[4] obsessive compulsive disorder[5] and attention deficit/hyperactivity disorder.[6] Other RCTs suggested that yoga is an effective symptomatic therapy for multiple sclerosis,[7] back pain,[8] carpal tunnel syndrome,[9] asthma,[10] tuberculosis[11] and diabetes.[12] Controlled trials suggest that yoga reduces anxiety and stress,[13,14] may have a useful long-term effect in the treatment of hypertension,[15] reduce joint stiffness in osteoarthritis,[16] and improves sleep quality for lymphoma patients.[17] Unfortunately, the methodological quality of many yoga studies is poor.

Risks

Contraindications
No absolute contraindications exist, but extreme postures are contraindicated in pregnancy. Meditation may precipitate feelings of unreality and depersonalisation and should therefore not be used by people with a history of psychotic or personality disorder.

Precautions/warnings
Physical damage can occur from overstretching either healthy or, more particularly, diseased joints and ligaments. Those learning yoga for treatment of medical conditions are advised to inform their doctors and to seek supervision by an experienced and knowledgeable teacher who will adapt the postures in appropriate ways.

Adverse effects

Drowsiness may occur, one case is documented where Kapalabhati pranayama has been associated with pneumothorax.[18]

Interactions

None known. Possible additive effects on antihypertensive medication.

Risk–benefit assessment

Regular practice of yoga is a largely safe method of improving general health and well-being. Its role as an adjunct to the management of some medical conditions is reasonably well established.

REFERENCES

1 N N. Healing power. Which 2001;Dec:35–37
2 Hutchinson S, Ernst E. Yoga therapy for coronary heart disease: a systematic review. Perfusion 2004;17:44–51
3 Ramaratnam S, Sridharan K. Yoga for epilepsy. The Cochrane Database of Systematic Reviews 2000, Issue 1. Art. No.: CD001524
4 Janakiramaiah N, Gangadhar B N, Naga-Venkatesha-Murthy P J, Harish M G, Subbakrishna D K, Vedamurthachar A. Antidepressant efficacy of Sunarshan Kriya Yoga (SKY) in melancholia: A randomized comparison with electroconvulsive therapy (ECT) and imipramine. J Affective Dis 2000;57:255–259
5 Shannahoff-Khalsa D S, Ray L E, Levine S, Gallen C C, Schwartz B J, Sidorowich J J. Randomized controlled trial of yogic meditation techniques for patients with obsessive-compulsive disorder. CNS-Spectr 1999;4:34–47
6 Jensen P S, Kenny D T. The effects of yoga on the attention and behavior of boys with Attention-Deficit/Hyperactivity Disorder (ADHD). Atten Disord 2004;7:205–216
7 Oken B S, Kishiyama S, Zajdel D, Bourdette D, Carlsen J, Haas M, Hugos C, Kraemer D, Lawrence F, Mass M. Randomized controlled trial of yoga and exercise in multiple sclerosis. Neurology 2004;62:2058–2064
8 Galantino M L, Bzdewka T M, Eissler-Russo J L, Holbrook M L, Mogck E P, Geigle P, Farrar J T. The impact of modified hatha yoga on chronic low back pain: A pilot study. Altern Ther Health Med 2004;10:56–59
9 Garfinkel M S, Singhal A, Katz W A, Allan D A, Reshetar R, Schumacher H R Jr. Yoga-based intervention for carpal tunnel syndrome: A randomized trial. JAMA 1998;280:1601–1603
10 Manocha R, Marks G B, Kenchington P, Peters D, Salome C M. Sahaja yoga in the management of moderate to severe asthma: a randomised controlled trial. Thorax 2002;57:110–115
11 Visweswaraiah N K, Telles S. Randomized trial of yoga as a complementary therapy for pulmonary tuberculosis. Respirology 2004;9:96–101
12 Kerr D, Gillam E, Ryder J, Trowbridge S, Cavan D, Thomas P. An Eastern art form of a Western disease: Randomised controlled trial of yoga in patients with poorly controlled insulin-treated diabetes. Pract Diabet Int 2002;19:164–166
13 Shannahoff-Khalsa-David S. An introduction to Kundalini yoga meditation techniques that are specific for the treatment of psychiatric disorders. J Altern Complement Med 2004;10:91–101
14 West J, Otte C, Geber K, Johnson J, Mohr D C. Effects of Hatha yoga and African dance on perceived stress, affect, and salivary cortisol. Ann Behav Med 2004;28:114–118
15 Patel C. Twelve month follow up of yoga and bio-feedback in the management of hypertension. Lancet 1975;1:62–64
16 Garfinkel M S, Schumacher H R, Husain A, Levy M, Reshetar R A. Evaluation of a yoga based regimen for treatment of osteoarthritis of the hands. J Rheumatol 1994;21:2341–2343
17 Cohen L, Warneke C, Fouladi RT, Rodriguez MA, Chaoul-Reich A. Psychological adjustment and sleep quality in a randomized trial of the effects of a Tibetan Yoga intervention in patients with Lymphoma. Cancer 2004;100:2253–2260
18 Johnson DB, Tierney MJ, Sadighi PJ. Kapallabhati pranayama: breath of fire or cause of pneumothorax? A case report. Chest 2004;125:1951–1952

THERAPIES

THERAPIES

Table 3.3 **Other therapies which have been tested for effectiveness or are used frequently**

Therapy	Description	Conditions frequently treated	Safety concerns
Anthroposophical Medicine	An approach that integrates conventional medicine with an exploration of inner feelings and the meaning of illness. Treatment may involve both conventional and CAM interventions	Any condition	None other than those of the individual therapies
Art therapy	Use of creative art as a means of expression for rehabilitation and personal development	Adjunct to psychotherapy for many psychological and psychiatric conditions	Use of potentially harmful chemicals, e.g. solvents; problems with disturbed behaviour
Autologous blood therapy	Taking of small amounts of blood, usually from an antecubital vein, and intramuscular reinjection	Asthma, eczema, psoriasis, pemphigus, urticaria and many other chronic conditions	Pain around the injection sites, bruising, infection
Bowen technique	Gentle soft tissue mobilisation procedures using pressure from thumb and fingers	Musculoskeletal conditions; stress-related disorders; symptoms of chronic conditions	None known
Buteyko breathing	A technique that reduces hyperventilation through slow breathing and holding of breath	Asthma	None known
Colonic irrigation, colon therapy, hydrotherapy	Use of standard enemas for rectosigmoid area or apparatus for prolonged irrigation of higher colon. Uses water, sometimes with enzymes, herbs or coffee added	Constipation, diarrhoea, gastrointestinal disorders; removal of 'toxins' in wide range of conditions inc. addictions, allergies	Infections, perforations, electrolyte imbalance and deaths have been reported
Colour (light, photo-) therapy	Single or mixed colours (inc. laser) shone on whole body or particular areas, e.g. chakras	Psychological problems including seasonal affective disorder, attention deficit disorder, visually related disorders; conventional use in skin disease and hyper-bilirubinaemia	Direct eye injury; strobic light may produce seizures; photosensitivity
Crystal therapy, crystal healing, gem therapy	Use of crystals, individually selected for their wavelength, to influence the body's 'energy field'	Wide range of mental and physical conditions	None known

TABLE 3.3 OTHER THERAPIES **359**

Therapy	Description	Conditions frequently treated	Safety concerns
Dance (movement) therapy	Use of dance to express emotions for therapeutic purposes	Communication disorders; physical and learning disabilities; stress and other psychological problems	None known
Di Bella Therapy	A cocktail of natural and synthetic drugs claimed to cure cancer	Cancer	Several ingredients can have toxic effects or interact with prescribed drugs
Enzyme therapy	Plant-derived and pancreatic enzymes given orally with the aim of improving the digestive and immune system	A wide variety of conditions including chronic digestive disorders, inflammatory and viral diseases, multiple sclerosis and cancer	Increased risk of bleeding
Feldenkrais method	A method of relearning dysfunctional movement habits; based on classes of 'awareness through movement' and 'functional integration'	Disabilities from injury, disease or degeneration; anxiety, other psychological and stress-related disorders	Possible exacerbation of symptoms
Flotation therapy	Form of sensory deprivation from lying in a tank filled with saline to counteract gravitational stress, with low or absent light and sound	Stressful states, for relaxation, arthritis and low back pain, drug abuse and smoking cessation	Hygiene problems from reuse of water; frightening for those with claustrophobia
Hellerwork, structural integration	Deep tissue bodywork, movement education and dialogue to improve posture (see Rolfing)	Postural and musculoskeletal conditions; headaches; stress	Possible exacerbation of symptoms
Imagery, guided imagery, visualisation	Controlled use of mental images for therapeutic purposes	Psychological symptoms, especially anxiety, stress-related disorders, depression; physical symptoms, especially pain; cancer	None known (but excessive inward focusing may reveal latent psychoses or personality disorders)
Magnetic field therapy	Permanent or pulsed magnetic fields applied to head or other part of body; often used with acupuncture	Non-union of fracture (FDA approved); wide variety of indications (self-use)	Contraindicated in pregnancy, pacemakers, myasthenia gravis, bleeding disorders

THERAPIES

table continues

THERAPIES

Therapy	Description	Conditions frequently treated	Safety concerns
Mindfulness-based stress reduction	A Zen-like approach to meditation with focus on what occurs at the moment	Stress	None known
Music therapy	Listening to or making music for therapeutic purposes	Communication disorders; stress and other psychological problems; pain; neurological disability	Music should not exceed 90dB as this may lead to hearing impairment
Neural therapy	Injection of 'trigger' areas, usually with local anaesthetic	Chronic conditions, especially pain	Allergy to anaesthetic agent
Neurolinguistic programming	Use of mental strategies and changes to thought patterns in problem solving	Anxiety, stress, other psychological problems; personal development	Abreaction has been reported
Oxygen therapy	Use of oxygen injections; use of hyperbaric oxygen for unconventional indications (sometimes used for ozone therapy)	Stroke and other brain injury; many conditions, especially chronic; physical fitness enhancement	Excess free radicals, peroxidation; risk of embolism or infection with IV injection
Ozone therapy	Injection of ozone (or hydrogen peroxide) or reinjection of own blood enriched with ozone	Degenerative diseases; HIV/AIDS; cancer	Serious complications reported including infections and embolism
Polarity therapy	Use of hands in order to influence flow of body energy; may also involve exercise and lifestyle changes	Anxiety, stress, other psychological and functional physical conditions	None known
Qi gong	Branch of Chinese medicine using meditation to strengthen own qi (see pp 292, 352); also exercises, self-massage; many individual styles; Qi gong masters use 'emitted qi' for healing	Health promotion; wide range of functional disorders; symptom control	Psychosis reported, probably in those with latent condition
Reiki	A form of spiritual healing (see p 350)	Chronic pain, emotional problems	None known
Rolfing, structural integration	Improves posture of body by soft tissue techniques, including strong massage, often in an ordered sequence, designed to free fascia	Postural problems, musculoskeletal conditions; headaches; stress	Possible exacerbation of symptoms, risk of fracturing osteoporotic bones
Shiatsu	Japanese form of massage on acupressure points (see p 292)	Numerous, especially chronic conditions and general ill health	Tissue trauma from excessive force

TABLE 3.3 OTHER THERAPIES **361**

Therapy	Description	Conditions frequently treated	Safety concerns
Stress management	An umbrella term for psychological interventions to reduce stress	Stress	None known
Tragerwork	Use of therapist's hands and mind to communicate lightness and encourage 'playfulness'	Many chronic physical and psychological conditions	None known
Water injection	Subcutaneous injection of sterile water over trigger points	Painful conditions, particularly due to myofascial trigger points	Local pain, bruising, infection

THERAPIES

Herbal and non-herbal medicines

ALOE
(Aloe vera)

Source	*Aloe vera* gel is made of mucilaginous tissue from the centre of the leaf. *Aloe vera* latex (also sap or aloes) is produced from the peripheral bundle sheath cells.
Main constituents	*Aloe vera* gel contains several polysaccharides. *Aloe vera* latex contains aloin, anthraquinones, barbaloine and glycosides.
Background	A cactus-like plant which grows in hot, dry climates, *Aloe vera* has been used in most ancient medical cultures. At present it is heavily promoted for numerous purposes ranging from diabetes to wound healing.
Examples of traditional uses	Alopecia, burns, laxative, various skin problems, wound healing.
Pharmacologic action	*Gel*: antimicrobial, anti-inflammatory, moisturising, antipruritic. *Latex*: laxative, hypoglycaemic, hypolipo-proteinaemic. The best-documented mechanism of action is irritation of the large intestines by a metabolite of aloin, responsible for the laxative properties of *Aloe vera* latex.
Conditions frequently treated	Constipation and dermatologic conditions.
Clinical evidence	A systematic review included ten CCTs, seven with topical and three with oral administration.[1] Taken orally, *Aloe vera* latex might lower blood glucose and blood lipids levels, according to these trials. Applied topically, *Aloe vera* gel might be effective for genital herpes and psoriasis. The evidence for its effects on wound healing is contradictory. Two trials did not show a protective effect of *Aloe vera* gel on radiation-induced skin injury. Three subsequently published controlled trials[2–4] confirm these findings whilst one controlled trial in contrast reports a positive effect on radiation-induced skin injury.[5] For none of these indications is the available evidence compelling. Preliminary evidence from a recent RCT suggests that oral *Aloe vera* gel reduces symptoms in patients with mild to moderate ulcerative colitis.[6]
Dosage	*Gel*: apply liberally to the skin as needed. *Latex* (orally): common laxative dose is 100–200 mg *Aloe vera* daily or 50 mg taken in the evening.
Risks	***Contraindications*** Pregnancy as aloe latex can induce abortions and stimulate menstruation, lactation as genotoxic aloe-emodin might pass into

milk, known allergy to plants from the *Liliaceae* family (e.g. garlic, onions, tulips), intestinal obstruction, acute intestinal inflammation, ulcers and haemorrhoids.

Precautions/warnings
Reflex stimulation of uterus could theoretically cause abortion in pregnant women. *Aloe vera* products should not be injected; this has been associated with serious complications and death. *Aloe vera* should be used cautiously in patients with diabetes or glucose intolerance.

Adverse effects
Allergic skin reactions, damage to intestinal mucosa, delayed healing of deep wounds (topical use), red discoloration of urine, intestinal pain, diarrhoea, fluid or electrolyte loss (frequent oral use).

Overdose
Life-threatening haemorrhagic diarrhoea and kidney damage with oral use have been reported.

Interactions
Increased effects of antiarrhythmics, cardiac glycosides, diuretics and steroids.

Quality issues
Stability of preparations is not established.

Risk–benefit assessment

Topical use has few risks but also few well-documented benefits The oral administration of *Aloe vera* latex is associated with considerable risks and has no benefit over conventional treatments. Its use should therefore be discouraged until compelling evidence to the contrary is available.

REFERENCES

1 Vogler B K, Ernst E. Aloe vera: a systematic review of its clinical effectiveness. Br J Gen Pract 1999;49:823–828

2 Su C K, Mehta V, Ravikumar L, Shah R, Pinto H, Halpern J, Koong A, Goffinet D, Le QT. Phase II double-blind randomized study comparing oral aloe vera versus placebo to prevent radiation-related mucositis in patients with head-and-neck neoplasms. Int J Radiat Oncol Biol Phys 2004;60:171–177

3 Bosley C, Smith J, Baratti P, Pritchard D L, Xiong X, Li C, Merchant T E. A phase III trial comparing an anionic phospholipid-based (APP) cream and aloe vera-based gel in the prevention and treatment of radiation dermatitis. Int J Radiat Oncol Biol Phys 2003;57:S438

4 Heggie S, Bryant G P, Tripcony L, Keller J, Rose P, Glendenning M, Heath J. A Phase III study on the efficacy of topical aloe vera gel on irradiated breast tissue. Cancer Nurs 2002;25:442–451

5 Olsen D L, Raub W, Jr, Bradley C. The effect of aloe vera gel/mild soap versus mild soap alone in preventing skin reactions in patients undergoing radiation therapy. Oncol Nurs Forum 2001;28:543–547

6 Langmead L, Feakins R M, Goldthorpe S, Holt H, Tsironi E, de Silva A, Jewell D P, Rampton D S. Randomized, double-blind, placebo-controlled trial of aloe vera gel for active ulcerative colitis. Aliment Pharmacol Ther 2004;19:739–747

ANDROGRAPHIS
(*Andrographis paniculata*)

Source	Leaf and rhizome.
Main constituents	Diterpenes such as andrographolide and deoxyandrographolide.
Background	Plant belonging to the *Acanthaceae* family native in Asia. Today it is cultivated in many parts of the world.
Examples of traditional uses	In Ayurvedic medicine *Andrographis paniculata* was used for a wide range of conditions but most commonly for infections such as the common cold.
Pharmacologic action	Stimulation of immune response, antibacterial, hepatoprotective, reduction of blood pressure, inhibition of platelet aggregation, abortificiant, reduction of male and female fertility.
Conditions frequently treated	Common cold.
Clinical evidence	A systematic review included seven double-blind CCTs of satisfactory rigour.[1] All of them suggest positive effects in the symptomatic treatment of uncomplicated upper respiratory tract infections. A meta-analysis of four RCTs corroborated these results.[2] More recent trials with *A. paniculata*[3,4] or *A. paniculata* plus echinacea[5] also confirm these findings. Whether it is helpful for HIV-infected individuals is unclear at present.[6]
Dosage	200–400 mg extract daily (standardised to contain 4–5.6 mg andrographolide).
Risks	*Contraindications* Pregnancy and lactation (see p 5); *A. paniculata* was traditionally used as abortificient. *Precautions/warnings* Patients on antiplatelet drugs, immunosuppressants and antihypertensives should use *A. paniculata* with caution. *Adverse effects* Allergic reactions, fatigue, change of taste, lymph node tenderness or swelling. *Interactions* Anticoagulants, antihypertensives, immunosuppressants.

Quality issues
Standardised extract is available.

Risk–benefit assessment

The efficacy for alleviating symptoms of upper respiratory tract infections is reasonably well documented. With short-term use, adverse effects are rare; long-term data are not available. Thus *A. paniculata* can be recommended for the short-term symptomatic treatment of upper respiratory infections.

REFERENCES
1 Thompson Coon J, Ernst E. Andrographis paniculata in the treatment of upper respiratory tract infections: a systematic review of safety and efficacy. Planta Med 2004;70:293–298
2 Poolsup N, Suthisisang C, Prathanturarug S, Asawamekin A, Chanchareon U. Andrographis paniculata in the symptomatic treatment of uncomplicated upper respiratory tract infection: systematic review of randomized controlled trials. J Clin Pharm Therapeut 2004;29:37–45
3 Shakhova EG, Spasov A A, Ostrovskii O V, Konovalova I V, Chernikov M V, Melnikova G I. Effectiveness of using the drug Kan-Yang in children with acute respiratory viral infection. Vestn Otorinolaringol 2003;3:48–50
4 Amaryan G, Asvatsatryan V, Gabrielyan E, Panossian A, Panosyan V, Wikman G. Double-blind, placebo-controlled, randomized, pilot clinical trial of ImmunoGuard – a standardized fixed combination of Andrographis paniculata Nees, with Eleutherococcus senticosus Maxim, Schizandra chinensis Bail. and Glycyrrhiza glabra L. extracts in patients with Familial Mediterranean Fever. Phytomed 2003;10:271–285
5 Sapsov AA, Ostrovskii O F, Chernikov M V, Wikman G. Comparative controlled study of Andrographis paniculata fixed combination, Kan Jang and an Echinacea preparation as adjuvant, in the treatment of uncomplicated respiratory disease in children. Phytother Res 2004;18:47–53
6 Calabrese C, Berman S H, Babish J G, Ma X, Shinto L, Dorr M, Wells K, Wenner C A, Standish L J. A phase I trial of andrographolide in HIV positive patients and normal volunteers. Phytother Res 2000;14:333–338

ARTICHOKE
(Cynara scolymus)

Source

Leaf. Avoid confusion with Jerusalem artichoke (*Helianthus tuberosa* L.), which is a species of sunflower.

Main constituents

Flavonoids, phenolic acids, sesquiterpene lactones.

Background

Artichoke is a herbaceous perennial, which can grow to a height of up to 2 m. The plant is native to southern Europe, northern Africa and the Canary Islands. For pharmaceutical use the first-year rosette of leaves is preferred and harvested from plants especially produced for medicinal purposes.

Examples of traditional uses

As a choleretic and diuretic.

Pharmacologic action

Hepatostimulating, diuretic, lipid lowering, carminative, antiemetic, choleretic. Indirect inhibitory effects at the level of HMG-CoA reductase have been suggested as a possible

HERBAL AND NON-HERBAL MEDICINES

mechanism of action.[1] Cynarine (1.5-di-caffeoyl-D-quinic acid) may be one of the principal active components of artichoke extract. Other findings indicate that the flavonoid luteolin may be responsible for its effects.

Conditions frequently treated

Dyspepsia, hyperlipidaemia.

Clinical evidence

Artichoke extract has been the subject of a small number of clinical trials in patients with hypercholesterolaemia. A systematic review identified two RCTs with a total of 167 participants.[1] It concluded that few data from rigorous clinical trials assessing artichoke extract for treating hypercholesterolaemia exist. The evidence for lowering cholesterol is therefore not compelling. A further double-blind RCT[2] assessed 54 patients with mean total cholesterol levels of 274 mg/dl at baseline. A reduction of total cholesterol levels of 6.8% over placebo was observed in patients who received artichoke, which included those patients who additionally received a fiber supplement. A small (n = 18) uncontrolled study suggested that artichoke positively modulates endothelial function in hypercholesterolaemia.[3] For mild dyspepsia patients were found to experience some benefit from a daily dose of 320 or 640 mg artichoke extract after 2 months of treatment in an open study.[4] A significant effect was reported in a double-blind RCT[5] in which 247 patients with dyspepsia were treated with either 640 mg three times daily of a commercial artichoke extract or placebo for 6 weeks.[5] Overall the dyspeptic symptoms improved compared with placebo. A post hoc subgroup analysis of patients with dyspepsia who were also identified as having irritable bowel syndrome suggested that it might have symptom-ameliorating effects.[6] A double-blind RCT suggests an increase in bile secretion compared with placebo after a single dose of 1.92 g artichoke extract.[7] A double-blind RCT suggests that artichoke extract is not effective in preventing symptoms of alcohol-induced hangover, larger studies are required to confirm this finding.[8]

Dosage

0.5–1.92 g of dry extract daily in divided doses.

Risks

Contraindications
Known allergies to artichoke and related species (*Asteraceae* or *Compositae*), obstruction of bile duct. Pregnancy and lactation (see p 5).

Precautions/warnings
Gallstones, bile duct obstruction.

Adverse effects
Flatulence, allergic reactions.

Interactions

None known.

Quality issues

Standardised extracts contain a 3.8–5.5:1 artichoke extract ratio, which is equivalent to about 1500 mg dried artichoke leaves for a 320 mg capsule.

Risk–benefit assessment

The clinical evidence for the medicinal use of artichoke extract is not compelling for any indication.

REFERENCES

1 Pittler M H, Thompson Coon J, Ernst E. Artichoke leaf extract for treating hypercholesterolaemia. The Cochrane Database of Systematic Reviews 2002, Issue 3. Art. No.: CD003335

2 Schmiedel V. Senkung des Cholesterinspiegels durch Artischocke und Ballaststoffe. Erfahrungsheilkunde 2002;51:405–414

3 Lupattelli G, Marchesi S, Lombardini R, Roscini A R, Trinca F, Gemelli F, Vaudo G, Mannarino F. Artichoke juice improves endothelial function in hyperlipemia. Life Sci 2004;76:775–782

4 Marakis G, Walker A F, Middleton R W, Booth J C L, Wright J, Pike D J. Artichoke leaf extract reduces mild dyspepsia in an open study. Phytomedicine 2002;9:694–699

5 Holtmann G, Adam B, Haag S, Collet W, Grünewald E, Windeck T. Efficacy of artichoke leaf extract in the treatment of patients with

functional dyspepsia: a six-week placebo-controlled, double-blind, multicentre trial. Aliment Pharmacol Ther 2003;18:1099–1105

6 Bundy R, Walker A F, Middleton R W, Marakis G, Booth J C. Artichoke leaf extract reduces symptoms of irritable bowel syndrome and improves quality of life in otherwise healthy volunteers suffering from concomitant dyspepsia: a subset analysis. J Altern Complement Med 2004;10:667–669

7 Kirchhoff R, Beckers C H, Kirchhoff G M, Trinczek-Gärtner H, Petrowicz O, Reimann H J. Increase in choleresis by means of artichoke extract. Phytomedicine 1994;1:107–115

8 Pittler M H, White A R, Stevinson C, Ernst E. Effectiveness of artichoke in preventing alcohol-induced hangovers: a randomized controlled trial. CMAJ 2003;169:1269–1273

AVOCADO-SOYBEAN UNSAPONIFIABLES

Source

Oil from avocado fruit and soy.

Main constituents

Fraction of oils (soy:avocado oil = 3:1) which, after hydrolysis, is not producing soap, e.g. sterols, volatile acids.

Background

Avocado-soybean unsaponifiables (ASU) are a mixture of oils left over after hydrolysis. They are chemically not defined and their pharmacologically active principles are not clearly defined. ASU are sold as a food supplement in most countries.

Examples of traditional uses

Avocado has traditionally been used for a range of medicinal purposes, e.g. aphrodisiac, emmenagogue, promotion of hair growth, wound healing. However, ASU have no traditional use.

HERBAL AND NON-HERBAL MEDICINES

Pharmacologic action	Inhibition of interleukin-1 synthesis, stimulation of collagen synthesis, protective effects on chondrocytes, anti-inflammatory effects, anabolic effects.
Conditions frequently treated	Osteoarthritis.
Clinical evidence	A systematic review included four high quality RCTs.[1] Three of these studies showed efficacy of ASU in the symptomatic treatment of osteoarthritis. A further RCT showed no difference between ASU and placebo in terms of joint space in osteoarthritic hip joints. In a subgroup analysis, however, such a structural change was apparent in patients with advanced disease.[2] The structure-modifying effect of ASU is also supported by in vitro studies on isolated chondrocytes.[3]
Dosage	300–600 mg/day.

Risks

Contraindications
Pregnancy and lactation (see p 5).

Precautions/warnings
None known.

Adverse effects
None known, in the RCTs adverse effect rates were typically as with placebo.

Interactions
None known.

Quality issues
Quality could vary from product to product.

Risk–benefit assessment	Most of the available RCTs suggest efficacy for symptom relief in osteoarthritis. Whether ASU have disease modifying properties is presently not clear. As the risks seem to be minor, ASU are a treatment worth considering for osteoarthritis.

REFERENCES

1 Ernst E. Avocado-soybean unsaponifiables (ASU) for osteoarthritis – a systematic review. Clin Rheumatol 2003;22:285–288

2 Lequesne M, Maheu E, Cadet C, Dreiser RL. Structural effect of avocado/soybean unsaponifiables on joint space loss in osteoarthritis of the hip. Arthritis Rheum 2002;47:50–58

3 Henrotin YE, Sanchez C, Deberg MA, Piccardi N, Guillou GB, Msika P, Reginster JY. Avocado/soybean unsaponifiables increase aggrecan synthesis and reduce catabolic and proinflammatory production by human osteoarthritic chondrocytes. J Rheumatol 2003;30:1825–1834

BILBERRY
(Vaccinium myrtillus)

Source	Fruit, leaves and stems.
Main constituents	Anthocyanosides.
Background	*V. myrtillus* is a deciduous perennial shrub of the *Ericaceae* family. It is native to Europe, North America and Northern Asia. The folk name bilberry is derived from the Danish bollebar meaning dark berry. *V. myrtillus* should not be confused with the related but distinct species *V. corymbosum*, the blueberry.
Examples of traditional uses	Orally for age-related macular degeneration, angina, arthritis, atherosclerosis, cataracts, dermatitis, diabetes, diarrhoea, gastrointestinal disease, glaucoma, gout, haemorrhoids, kidney disease, night blindness, retinopathy, urinary tract disease, varicose veins, venous insufficiency, visual acuity. Topically for mouth and throat inflammation.
Pharmacologic action	Anthocyanosides have antioxidant properties, may accelerate resynthesis of rhodopsin, modulate retinal enzyme activity, improve microcirculation, may stabilise connective tissue and have antiplatelet activity.
Conditions frequently treated	Age-related macular degeneration, diabetes, dysmenorrhoea, glaucoma, night blindness, retinopathy, varicose veins, venous insufficiency, mouth and throat inflammation.
Clinical evidence	Although there is a considerable amount of pre-clinical work demonstrating mechanisms which could plausibly produce beneficial effects in eye disorders and circulatory disorders, clinical evidence for effectiveness is meagre. A systematic review of RCTs testing the use of *V. myrtillus* to improve night vision concluded that the best evidence indicated that the extract had no beneficial effect in healthy subjects.[1] There have, however, been no rigorous clinical trials of the effects in subjects with impaired night vision. For degenerative eye disorders such as glaucoma, retinopathy and cataracts the evidence is limited to single, small-scale, clinical trials or case studies and effectiveness in these or any other indications has not been demonstrated conclusively.
Dosage	Concentrated extracts are standardised to contain 25% anthocyanidins, the equivalent of 37% anthocyanosides. Dose is commonly 80 mg twice daily for ophthalmologic and circulatory indications. Higher doses (up to 480 mg/day) have been recommended in some indications including dysmenorrhoea (160 mg twice daily).

Risks

Contraindications

Based on its use as a food, the fruit is generally considered to be safe unless taken in excessive quantities. Theoretical risk of increased bleeding in those with bleeding disorders or in patients taking anticoagulants. Theoretical risk of hypoglycaemia in diabetics and patients taking hypoglycaemic medications.

Precautions/warnings

Limit dosage to that used in most studies (up to 480 mg/day). Avoid ingesting leaves which may be toxic.

Adverse effects

Pregnancy and lactation (see p 5).

Interactions

Theoretical risk of interaction with NSAIDs, drugs and herbs with anticoagulant activity, antiplatelet agents, and hypoglycaemics.

Quality issues

The anythocyanoside content of *V. myrtillus* comprises 15 different anthocyanosides and although extracts are usually standardised for total anthocyanoside content they probably vary in anthocyanoside composition according to country of origin, time of harvest and other factors.

Risk–benefit assessment

Evidence for effectiveness in any indication is weak. Consumption of *V. myrtillus* extract in quantities similar to the use of the raw fruit as a food is probably safe. People may consider it worth trying in degenerative eye conditions, venous problems and dysmenorrhoea.

REFERENCES

1 Canter P H, Ernst E. Anthocyanosides of Vaccinium myrtillus (bilberry) for night vision – a systematic review of placebo-controlled trials. Surv Ophthalmol 2004;49:38–50

BLACK COHOSH
(*Actaea racemosa*)

Source

Rhizome.

Main constituents

27-deoxyactein, actein, cimicifugoside, salicylic acid, steroidal terpenes tannins.

Background

Black cohosh is a perennial plant and a member of the buttercup family native to the eastern parts of North America. It grows up to a height of 2 m and is found particularly in shady forests. Black cohosh was frequently used by the early settlers in North America as a remedy for rheumatism and rheumatic pain. Today, it is one of the best selling herbal remedies for reducing menopausal symptoms in the USA and other countries.

Examples of traditional uses

Diarrhoea, dysmenorrhoea, induction of labour, inflammation, menopausal symptoms, premenstrual syndrome, promotion of lactation, rheumatism.

Pharmacologic action

Vascular and oestrogen-like activity, hypotensive, anti-inflammatory.

Conditions frequently treated

Climacteric symptoms, dysmenorrhoea, premenstrual syndrome.

Clinical evidence

The efficacy of black cohosh was assessed in a systematic review identifying four RCTs.[1] All trials assessed the effects for treating menopausal symptoms. The data suggest that the evidence is promising but not compelling. Two further systematic reviews, which were conducted independently, assessed the evidence of herbal medicines for menopausal symptoms and corroborated these findings.[2,3] For treating hot flushes in breast cancer survivors, a systematic review reported little clinical benefit from black cohosh,[4] while a subsequent RCT reported that the combined administration of tamoxifen and black cohosh extract is superior to tamoxifen alone for reducing severe hot flushes (n = 136).[5] Two different doses (39 mg and 127 mg daily) were tested in a double-blind RCT, which reported no differences between groups for the Kupperman Menopause Index and the Self Rating Depression Scale but a decrease in symptoms.[6] A double-blind RCT (n = 62) reported an equipotent effect of 40 mg black cohosh extract compared with 0.6 mg of conjugated oestrogens and a superior effect compared with placebo in reducing climacteric complaints.[7] Evidence from another double-blind RCT (n = 179) suggested that a fixed combination of St John's wort and black cohosh administered over a treatment period of 6 weeks reduces psychovegetative complaints compared with placebo.[8] A systematic review of the safety of black cohosh reported that the evidence from uncontrolled reports, post-marketing surveillance, and human clinical trials including more than 2,800 patients demonstrate a low incidence of adverse events (5.4%). Of the reported adverse events, 97% were minor and the only severe events were not attributed to black cohosh treatment.[9] These findings are supported by further systematic reviews.[10,11]

Dosage

Extract: 8 mg of standardised extract (1% 27-deoxyactein) daily in divided doses.
Root: 40 mg of dried rhizome and root daily in divided doses.

Risks

Contraindications
Pregnancy and lactation (see p 5), oestrogen-dependent tumours, allergy to black cohosh or members of the buttercup family.

HERBAL AND NON-HERBAL MEDICINES

Precautions/warnings
Patients receiving antihypertensive medication.

Adverse effects
Gastrointestinal complaints, hepatitis, hypotension, arrhythmia, headache, dizziness, nausea, allergic reactions.

Overdose
A review found no evidence for toxic or mutagenic effects in animal experiments after administering the extract for 6 months at about 90 times the human dose.[12]

Interactions
May interact with antihypertensive agents, may increase the effects of potentially hepatotoxic drugs.

Quality issues
Quality and purity may vary between preparations. The majority of clinical trials were conducted using the same brand (Remifemin).

Risk–benefit assessment

Systematic reviews report promising but not compelling evidence of black cohosh for treating symptoms associated with menopause. Its adverse effects profile for short-term application is encouraging and it seems worth considering for symptoms associated with menopause. However, more clinical data are required. Conflicting evidence exists on its alleged oestrogen-like activity and its effects in oestrogen-dependent tumours. Thus it seems wise to view the latter condition as a contraindication for black cohosh extract.

REFERENCES

1 Borrelli F, Ernst E. Cimicifuga racemosa: a systematic review of its clinical efficacy. Eur J Clin Pharmacol 2002;58:235–241

2 Huntley A L, Ernst. A systematic review of herbal medicinal products for the treatment of menopausal symptoms. Menopause 2003;10: 465–476

3 Kronenberg F, Fugh-Berman A. Complementary and alternative medicine for menopausal symptoms: a review of randomized, controlled trials. Ann Intern Med 2002;137:805–813

4 Simpson B. Hot flash pharmacotherapy in breast cancer survivors: A literature review. Can Pharm J 2004;137:36–45

5 Hernández-Muñoz G, Pluchino S. Cimicifuga racemosa for the treatment of hot flushes in women surviving breast cancer. Maturitas 2003;44(Suppl):59–65

6 Liske E, Hänggi W, Henneicke von Zepelin H H, Boblitz N, Wüstenberg P, Rahlfs V W, Stat C. Physiological investigation of a unique extract of black cohosh (Cimicifugae racemosae rhizoma): A 6-month clinical study demonstrates no systemic estrogenic effect. J Women S Health Gender Med 2002;11:163–174

7 Wuttke W, Seidlová-Wuttke D, Gorkow C. The Cimicifuga preparation BNO 1055 vs. conjugated estrogens in a double-blind placebo-controlled study: Effects on menopause symptoms and bone markers. Maturitas 2003;44(Suppl):67–77

8 Boblitz N, Schrader E, Henneicke-von Zeppelin H-H, Wüstenberg P. Benefit of a drug containing St John's wort and black cohosh for climacteric patients – results of a randomised clinical trial. Focus Altern Complement Ther 2000;5:85–86

9 Dog T L, Powell K L, Weisman S M. Critical evaluation of the safety of Cimicifuga racemosa in menopause symptom relief. Menopause 2003;10:299–313

10 Huntley A. The safety of black cohosh
    (Actaea racemosa, Cimicifuga racemosa).
    Expert Opin Drug Saf 2004;3:615–623
11 Huntley A, Ernst E. A systematic review of
    the safety of black cohosh. Menopause
    2003;10:58–64

12 Beuscher N. Cimicifuga racemosa L. – Die
    Traubensilberkerze. Zeitschr für Phytotherapie
    1995;16:301–310

CHAMOMILE
(Matricaria recutita)

Source	Flowerheads.
Main constituents	Capric acid, coumarins, flavonoids (apigenin), polysaccharides, spiroethers, tannins, terpenoid volatile oils (chamazulene, alpha-bisabolol).
Background	Chamomile is an annual herb belonging to the *Asteraceae* family. It is native to most of Europe and western Asia and naturalised throughout North America and Australia. Along with Roman or English chamomile (*Chamaemelum nobile*), it has been used for medicinal purposes since ancient times due to its reputed anti-inflammatory and antispasmodic properties. It is commonly drunk as a tea.
Examples of traditional uses	Anxiety, colic in babies, gastrointestinal complaints, gum irritations, insomnia, respiratory tract infections, restlessness, skin conditions, teething.
Pharmacologic action	Antibacterial, anti-inflammatory, antispasmodic.
Conditions frequently treated	Anxiety, gastrointestinal complaints, insomnia, skin inflammations.
Clinical evidence	For eczema a commercial topical preparation based on chamomile was reported to be as useful as hydrocortisone in a non-randomised trial (n = 161), although no statistical analysis was conducted.[1] In a subsequent RCT (n = 72) the chamomile cream showed, according to the authors, mild superiority over 0.5% hydrocortisone but little difference compared with placebo.[2] Again there was no statistical analysis. Another non-randomised trial found no superiority of the same preparation over almond oil for skin damage after irradiation for breast cancer treatment.[3] Placebo-controlled RCTs found chamomile mouthwash ineffective in reducing 5-fluorouracil-induced stomatitis (n = 164)[4] and in preventing postoperative sore throat and hoarseness (n = 161).[5] An RCT (n = 79) found that a preparation consisting of chamomile extract and apple pectin reduced the duration of childhood diarrhoea more than placebo.[6] Steam

HERBAL AND NON-HERBAL MEDICINES

inhalation of chamomile extract was reported to have a dose-dependent effect on symptoms of the common cold in a placebo-controlled trial.[7] Double-blind RCTs assessed the same commercially available combination preparation containing chamomile flower and found beneficial effects in patients with functional dyspepsia and irritable bowel syndrome[8,9] compared with placebo. For functional dyspepsia the data from three RCTs (n = 273) were pooled in a meta-analysis, which suggests superiority over placebo.[10]

Dosage

Liquid extract: 1–4 ml of (1:1 in 45% alcohol) three times daily. *Dried flowers:* 3 g in 150 ml hot water (chamomile tea) three times daily.

Risks

Contraindications
Pregnancy and lactation (see p 5).

Precautions/warnings
Known sensitivity to other members of the *Asteraceae* family (e.g. asters, chrysanthemums, sunflowers), asthma or other allergic conditions.

Adverse effects
Allergic reactions (at least three cases of anaphylactic reactions have been reported), vomiting.

Overdose
Emesis has been reported following consumption of large doses.

Interactions
Theoretically, the effects of anticoagulants and central nervous system depressants could be potentiated and the level of drugs metabolised by cytochrome P450 3A4 could be increased.

Quality issues
Some commercially available preparations are standardised (e.g. Kamillosan); Chamazulene and alpha-bisabolol are commonly used as the marker substances.

Risk–benefit assessment

There is little convincing evidence to support the therapeutic effectiveness of chamomile extracts. Encouraging evidence is emerging for a specific combination preparation in patients with functional dyspepsia. Given the risk of allergic reactions and the few rigorous clinical trials that have been conducted, it is not entirely clear whether the potential benefits outweigh the possible risks.

REFERENCES

1 Aertgeerts P, Albring M, Klaschka F, Nasemann T, Patzelt-Wenczler R, Rauhut K, Weigl B. Comparative testing of Kamillosan cream and steroidal (0.25% hydrocortisone, 0.75% fluocortin butyl ester) and non-steroidal (5% bufexamac) dermatologic agents in maintenance therapy of eczematous diseases. Zeitschr für Hautkrankheiten 1985;60:270–277

2 Patzelt-Wenczler R, Ponce-Pöschl E. Proof of efficacy of Kamillosan cream in atopic eczema. Eur J Med Res 2000;5:171–175

3 Maiche A G, Grohn P, Maki-Hokkonen H. Effect of chamomile cream and almond ointment on acute radiation skin reaction. Acta Oncol 1991;30:395–396

4 Fidler P, Loprinzi C, O'Fallon J, Leitch J M, Lee J K, Hayes D L, Novotny P, Clemens-Schutjer D, Bartel J, Michalak J C. Prospective evaluation of a chamomile mouthwash for prevention of 5 FU induced oral mucositis. Cancer 1996;77:522–525

5 Kyokong O, Charuluxananan S, Muangmingsuk V, Rodanant O, Subornsug K, Punyasang W. Efficacy of chamomile-extract spray for prevention of post-operative sore throat. J Med Assoc Thai 2002;85:S180–185

6 De La Motte S, O'Reilly S, Heinisch M, Harrison F. Double-blind comparison of an apple pectin-chamomile extract preparation with placebo in children with diarrhoea. Arzeim-Forsch/Drug Res 1997;47:1247–1249

7 Saller R, Beschomer M, Hellenbrecht D, Bühring M. Dose dependency of symptomatic relief of complaints by chamomile steam inhalation in patients with common cold. Eur J Pharmacol 1990;183:728–729

8 Madisch A, Melderis H, Mayr G, Sassin I, Hotz J. Ein Phytotherapeutikum und seine modifizierte Rezeptur bei funktioneller Dyspepsie. Ergebnisse einer doppelblinden plazebokontrollierten Vergleichsstudie. Z Gastroenterol 2001;39:511–517

9 Madisch A, Holtmann G, Plein K, Hotz J. Treatment of irritable bowel syndrome with herbal preparations: results of a double blind, randomized, placebo-controlled, multi-centre trial. Aliment Pharmacol Ther 2004;19:271–279

10 Melzer J, Rosch W, Reichling J, Brignoli R, Saller R. Meta-analysis: phytotherapy of functional dyspepsia with the herbal drug preparation STW 5 (Iberogast). Aliment Pharmacol Ther 2004;20:1279–1287

CHASTE TREE
(Vitex agnus-castus)

Source	Root, bark and fruit.
Main constituents	Diterpens (clerodadienols), flavonoids, iridoids, linoleic acid, volatile oil.
Background	A member of the *Verbenaceae* family, chaste tree is a deciduous shrub originating in Mediterranean Europe and western Asia. In Greek and Roman times the plant was used for promoting chastity in women and celibacy in monks. The main uses that have persisted to modern times are in women's healthcare.
Examples of traditional uses	Amenorrhoea, diarrhoea, dysmenorrhoea, epilepsy, infertility, injuries, inflammation, premenstrual and menopausal symptoms, snake bite, women's health, i.e. insufficient lactation.
Pharmacologic action	Hypoprolactinaemic, dopaminergic, anti-inflammatory, anti-androgenic, antimicrobial.
Conditions frequently treated	Female infertility, menopausal complaints, premenstrual syndrome.

HERBAL AND NON-HERBAL MEDICINES

Clinical evidence

Double-blind placebo-controlled RCTs have suggested that chaste tree extracts are effective for cyclical mastalgia,[1–3] luteal phase deficiency[4] and female infertility due to secondary amenorrhoea or luteal insufficiency.[5–7] For premenstrual syndrome, uncontrolled trials have produced positive results[8] and placebo-controlled RCTs generated both negative[9] as well as positive results with the latter trial being more rigorous than the former.[10] An RCT comparing chaste tree and vitamin B_6 had an ambiguous result,[11] and an RCT comparing it with fluoxetine in the treatment of premenstrual dysphoric disorder yielded a responder rate of 58% for chaste tree and 68% for fluoxetine.[12] No positive results were found for chaste tree as a 'bust-enhancing' herbal medicine.[13]

Dosage

40 mg of standardised extract daily in divided doses.

Risks

Contraindications
Pregnancy and lactation (see p 5).

Precautions/warnings
Increases in menstrual flow and changes in cycle are possible.

Adverse effects
Adverse effects are usually mild and transient[14] and include acne, agitation, allergic reaction, alopecia, dry mouth, fatigue, gastrointestinal problems, headache, intra-menstrual bleeding, nausea, and tachycardia.[15] According to a large observational study (n = 1634), they occur in only 1.2% of patients.[8]

Overdose
Studies with male volunteers have found no adverse effects with doses 12 times higher than the recommended dose. Routine animal toxicology studies have revealed no specific risks of large doses.

Interactions
Theoretically, interactions are possible with oral contraceptives, hormone replacement therapy and dopamine agonists and antagonists.

Quality issues
The whole plant extract is considered necessary for a therapeutic action. Authenticity is usually measured by agnuside content.

Risk–benefit assessment

There are encouraging results for a range of indications. The safety profile of chaste tree is encouraging. As a monotherapy, therefore, the potential benefits of this herb can probably outweigh the risks.

REFERENCES

1 Wuttke W, Splitt G, Gorkow C. Sieder C. Behandlung zyklusabhängiger Brustschmerzen mit einem Agnus castus-haltigen Arzneimittel. Ergebnisse einer randomisierten, plazebokontrollierten Doppelblindstudie. Geb Fra 1997;57:569–574

2 Kubista E, Müller G, Spona J. Behandlung der Mastopathie mit zyklischer Mastodynie. Klinische Ergebnisse und Hormonprofile. Gynak Rdsch 1986;26:65–79

3 Halaska M, Beles P, Gorkow C, Sieder C. Treatment of cyclical mastalgia with a solution containing an extract of Vitex agnus castus: recent results of a placebo-controlled double-blind study. Breast 1999;8:175–181

4 Milewicz A, Gejdel E, Sworen H, Sienkiewicz K, Jedrzejak J, Teucher T, Schmitz H. Vitex agnus castus extract in the treatment of luteal phase defects due to latent hyperprolactinemia: results of a randomised, placebo-controlled, double-blind study. Arzneim-Forsch/Drug Res 1993;43:752–756

5 Gerhard I, Patek A, Monga B, Blank A, Gorkow C. Mastodynon bei weiblicher Sterilität. Randomisierte, plazebokontrollierte klinische Doppelblindstudie. Forsch Komplementärmed 1998;20:272–278

6 Westphal L M, Polan M L, Trant A S, Mooney S B. A nutritional supplement for improving fertility in women: a pilot study. J Reprod Med 2004;49:289–293

7 Bergmann J, Luft B, Boehmann S, Runnebaum S, Gerhard B. The efficacy of the complex medication Phyto-Hypophyson L in female, hormone-related sterility. A randomized, placebo-controlled clinical double-blind study. Forsch Komplementärmed Klass Naturheilkd 2000;7:190–199

8 Loch E G, Selle H, Boblitz N. Treatment of premenstrual syndrome with a phytopharmaceutical formulation containing Vitex agnus castus. J Wom Health Gender-Based Med 2000;9:315–320

9 Turner S, Mills S. A double blind clinical trial on a herbal remedy for premenstrual syndrome: a case study. Complement Ther Med 1993;1:73–77

10 Schellenberg R. Treatment for the premenstrual syndrome with agnus castus fruit extract: prospective, randomised, placebo controlled study. BMJ 2001;322:134–137

11 Lauritzen C H, Reuter H D, Repges R, Bohnert K J, Schmidt U. Treatment of premenstrual tension syndrome with Vitex agnus castus. Controlled, double-blind study versus pyrodoxine. Phytomedicine 1997;4:183–189

12 Atmaca M, Kumru S, Tezcan E. Fluoxetine versus Vitex agnus castus extract in the treatment of premenstrual dysphoric disorder. Hum-Psychopharmacol 2003;18:191–195

13 Fugh-Berman A. 'Bust enhancing' herbal products. Obstet Gynecol 2003;101:1345–1349

14 Daniele C, Thompson Coon J, Pittler M H, Ernst E. Vitex agnus castus: a systematic review of adverse events. Drug Saf 2005;28:319–332

15 Chasteberry monograph. Natural Medicines Comprehensive Database, *www.naturaldata-base.com*, accessed 05/10/04

CHITOSAN

Source	Shells of crustacea and various fungi.
Main constituent	Chitosan is a hydrophilic, positively charged polysaccharide.
Background	Chitosan is the N-deacetylated form of chitin, which is extracted from the shells of crustaceans. It is used, for instance, in the cosmetic and textile industries but also as an ingredient in over-the-counter remedies.
Examples of traditional uses	Chitosan has only relatively recently been used for medicinal purposes.

HERBAL AND NON-HERBAL MEDICINES

Pharmacologic action	Hypocholesterolaemic, hypolipidaemic, fat binding (in vitro and, according to manufacturers' claims, in human intestines), haemostatic, wound healing.
Conditions frequently treated	Hypercholesterolaemia, obesity, overweight, peridontitis, tissue regeneration.
Clinical evidence	A meta-analysis assessed five double-blind RCTs of chitosan for body weight reduction including 386 patients who were described as either obese, overweight or with 10% to 25% excess body weight.[1] A positive effect was identified, but due to methodological limitations it was concluded that the effectiveness of chitosan for lowering body weight is not established beyond reasonable doubt. In subsequent systematic reviews at least five additional double-blind RCTs were identified assessing overweight or obese patients.[2,3] The findings of both independent systematic reviews indicate that there is considerable doubt that chitosan is effective for reducing body weight in humans. An additional independent systematic review of 14 RCTs (n = 1071) supports the earlier findings and concludes that the results obtained from high-quality trials indicate that the effect of chitosan on body weight is minimal and unlikely to be of clinical significance.[4] Several clinical RCTs, which administered calorie-restricted diets (1000–1200 kcal/day)[5,6] corroborated findings from animal experiments and suggested cholesterol-lowering effects in hypercholesterolaemic patients. This is confirmed by the findings of other RCTs.[7,8] However, other double-blind RCTs found no relevant effects on total cholesterol levels.[9–11] Conflicting results exist for the effects on low-density lipoprotein levels.[8,11] No significant effects on fat-soluble vitamins are reported. Some positive findings from an RCT exist for chitosan as a mouth rinse to reduce dental plaque formation.[12]
Dosage	2 g of deacetylated chitin biopolymer daily in divided doses.
Risks	*Contraindications* Pregnancy and lactation (see p 5). *Precautions/warnings* There is a lack of relevant safety data relating to effects in women taking oral contraceptives. *Adverse effects* Constipation, flatulence, diarrhoea, nausea. *Interactions* May slow the absorption of oral contraceptives.

Quality issues
Products may vary in their content of deacetylated chitin.

Risk–benefit assessment

Clinical studies report mixed findings on the effects of chitosan for cholesterol reduction. The effectiveness of chitosan for hyper-cholesterolaemia is therefore not established beyond reasonable doubt. Similarly, there is considerable doubt that chitosan is effective for reducing body weight. It may reduce dental plaque formation. Chitosan seems to be relatively safe but it is costly.

REFERENCES

1 Ernst E, Pittler M H. Chitosan as a treatment for body weight reduction? A meta-analysis. Perfusion 1998;11:461–465
2 Pittler M H, Ernst E. Dietary supplements for body-weight reduction: a systematic review. Am J Clin Nutr 2004;79:529–536
3 Lenz T L, Hamilton W R. Supplemental products used for weight loss. J Am Pharm Assoc 2004;44:59–67
4 Mhurchu C N, Dunshea-Mooij C, Bennett D, Rodgers A. Effect of chitosan on weight loss in overweight and obese individuals: a systematic review of randomized controlled trials. Obes Rev 2005;6:35–42
5 Veneroni G, Veneroni F, Contos S, Tripodi S, de Bernardi M, Guarino C, Marleti A M. Effect of a new chitosan dietary integrator and hypocaloric diet on hyperlipidemia and overweight in obese patients. Acta Toxicol Ther 1996;17:53–70
6 Sciutto A M, Colombo P. Lipid-lowering effect of chitosan dietary integrator and hypocaloric diet in obese patients. Acta Toxicol Ther 1995;16:215–230
7 Bokura H, Kobayashi S. Chitosan decreases total cholesterol in women: a randomized, double-blind, placebo-controlled trial. Eur J Clin Nutr 2003;57:721–725

8 Tai T S, Sheu W H, Lee W J, Yao H T, Chiang M T Effect of chitosan on plasma lipoprotein concentrations in type 2 diabetic subjects with hypercholesterolemia. Diabetes Care 2000;23:1703–1704
9 Pittler M H, Abbot N C, Harkness E F, Ernst E. Randomised, double blind trial of chitosan for body weight reduction. Eur J Clin Nutr 1999;53:379–381
10 Wuolijoki E, Hirvela T, Ylitalo P. Decrease in serum LDL cholesterol with microcrystalline chitosan. Methods Find Exp Clin Pharmacol 1999;21:357–361
11 Metso S, Ylitalo R, Nikkilä M, Wuolijoki E, Ylitalo P, Lehtimäki T. The effect of long-term microcrystalline chitosan therapy on plasma lipids and glucose concentrations in subjects with increased plasma total cholesterol: a randomised placebo-controlled double-blind crossover trial in healthy men and women. Eur J Clin Pharmacol 2003;59:741–746
12 Sano H, Shibasaki-Ken I, Matsukubo T, Takaesu Y. Effect of chitosan rinsing on reduction of dental plaque formation. Bull Tokyo Dent Coll 2003;44:9–16

CHONDROITIN

Source

Bovine tracheal cartilage.

Main constituents

Glycosaminoglycans, principally chondroitin-4-sulfate and chon-droitin-6-sulfate, and disaccharide polymers composed of equi-molar amounts of D-glucuronic acid. N-acetylgalactosamine and sulfates in 30 to 100 disaccharide units.

Background

Chondroitin is thought to rebuild cartilage and is promoted as a treatment for conditions associated with cartilage degeneration.

Examples of traditional uses	Joint pain, osteoarthritis.
Pharmacologic action	Chondroitin has anti-inflammatory activity, controls the formation of new cartilage matrix, inhibits leukocyte elastase and hyaluronidase. It also stimulates production of highly polymerised hyaluronic acid in synovial cells, thus increasing synovial viscosity and therefore possibly contributing to a 'lubrication effect'. Furthermore, it reduces inflammatory activity by inhibiting the recognition process of complement. These actions are believed to work in concert and constitute chondroitin's complex mechanisms of action.
Conditions frequently treated	Osteoarthritis.
Clinical evidence	Several good-quality trials suggest symptomatic improvement in patients suffering from osteoarthritis (e.g.[1]). A meta-analysis of seven RCTs, including 372 patients in total, also came to a cautiously positive conclusion.[2] Yet it also pointed to the lack of long-term data. Three further meta-analysis of chondroitin and glucosamine for treatment of osteoarthritis all arrived at positive conclusions.[3-5] Further trial data suggest positive effects on osteoarthritis even in the long-term[6] and confirm that chondroitin has structure-modulating properties in osteoarthritic joints.[7] This notion was recently confirmed in two RCTs (n = 100 and 300) showing that long-term medication of chondroitin and glucosamine sulfate prevents joint space narrowing in patients with knee osteoarthritis.[8,9] One RCT also suggests that a preparation of topical chondroitin and glucosamine is effective in relieving pain of knee osteoarthritis.[10] Other indications for chondroitin might be erosive osteoarthritis of the hands,[11] low back pain[12] and temperomandibular joint disorder.[13]
Dosage	800–1200 mg of chondroitin sulfate daily in divided doses.
Risks	*Contraindications* Pregnancy and lactation (see p 5). *Precautions/warnings* Bleeding disorders, asthma can be exacerbated. *Adverse effects* Dyspepsia, headache, euphoria, nausea. *Interactions* Potentiation of anticoagulants theoretically possible. *Quality issues* Many commercially available products do not contain the stated dosage.

| **Risk–benefit assessment** | Effectiveness of chondroitin is well documented and risks seem to be minor. The size of the symptomatic effects is usually such that it is best used as an adjuvant to other interventions for osteoarthritis. |

REFERENCES

1 Morreale P, Manopulo R, Galati M. Boccanera L, Saponati G, Bocchi L. Comparison of the anti-inflammatory efficacy of chondroitin sulfate and diclofenac sodium in patients with knee osteoarthritis. J Rheumatol 1996;23:1385–1391

2 Leeb B F, Scweitzer H, Montag K, Smolen J S. A metaanalysis of chondroitin sulfate in the treatment of osteoarthritis. J Rheumatol 2000;27:205–211

3 McAlindon T E, LaValley M P, Gulin J P, Felson D T. Glucosamine and chondroitin for treatment of osteoarthritis. A systematic quality assessment and meta-analysis. JAMA 2000;283:1469–1475

4 Häuselmann H J. Nutripharmaceuticals for osteoarthritis. Best Pract Res Clin Rheumatol 2001;15:595–607

5 Richy F, Bruyere O, Ethgen O, Cucherat M, Henrotin Y, Reginster JY. Structural and symptomatic efficacy of glucosamine and chondroitin in knee osteoarthritis: a comprehensive meta-analysis. Arch Intern Med 2003;163:1514–1522

6 Uebelhart D, Malaise M, Marcolongo R, DeVathaire F, Piperno M, Mailleux E, Fioravanti A, Matoso L, Vignon E. Intermittent treatment of kne osteoarthritis with oral chonidroitin sulfate: a one-year, randomized, double-blind, multicenter study versus placebo. Osteoarthritis Cartilage 2004;12:269–276

7 Mathieu P. Radiological progression of internal femoro-tibial osteoarthritis in gonarthrosis. Chondro-protective effect of chondroitin sulfates ACS4-ACS6. Presse Med 2002;31:1386–1390

8 Rai J, Pal S K, Gul A, Senthil R, Singh H. Efficacy of chondroitin sulfate and glucosamine sulfate in the progression of symptomatic knee osteoarthritis: a randomized, placebo-controlled, double blind study. Bull Postgrad Inst Med Educ Res Chandigarh 2004;38:18–22

9 Michel B A, Stucki G, Frey D, De Vathaire F, Vignon E, Bruehlmann P, Uebelhart D. Chondroitins 4 and 6 sulfate in osteoarthritis of the knee: a randomized, controlled trial. Arthritis Rheum 2005;52:779–786

10 Cohen M, Wolfe R, Mai T, Lewis D. A randomized, double blind, placebo controlled trial of a topical cream containing glucosamine sulfate, chondroitin sulfate, and camphor for osteoarthritis of the knee. J Rheumatol 2003;30:2512

11 Rovetta G, Monteforte P, Molfetta G, Balestra V. Chonidroitin sulfate in erosive osteoarthritis of the hands. Int J Tissue React 2002;24:29–32

12 Leffler CT, Philippi AF, Leffler SG, Mosure JC, Kim PD. Glucosamine, chondroitin, and manganese ascorbate for degenerative joint disease for the knee or low back: a randomized, double-blind, placebo-controlled pilot study. Mil Med 1999;164:85–91

13 Nguyen P, Mohamed SE, Gardiner D, Salinas L. A randomized double blind clinical trial of the effect of chondroitin sulfate and glucosamine hydrochloride on temporomandibular joint disorders: a pilot study. Cranio 2001;19:130–139

COENZYME Q10

| **Source** | Coenzyme Q10 is produced by the human body. It is present in most cells and the highest concentrations are found in the heart, liver, kidneys and pancreas. Today it is synthesised in large quantities for the food supplement market by fermenting sugar beets and sugar cane with special strains of yeast. |

| **Main constituent** | Ubiquinones. |

| **Background** | The compound is thought to enhance cell function. Patients with congestive heart failure have low levels of coenzyme Q10. It is |

commercially produced according to a Japanese patent and marketed for a wide range of conditions.

Examples of traditional uses

Oral supplementation with coenzyme Q10 has been promoted for a wide variety of indications ranging from heart failure to general tonic.

Pharmacologic action

On the cellular level coenzyme Q10 participates in the electron transfer within the oxidative respiration chain in the mitochondria, thus preventing adenosine triphosphate depletion as well as oxidant and ischaemic cellular damage. It also acts as a membrane stabiliser and free radical scavenger and is a co-factor in many metabolic processes.

Conditions frequently treated

Alzheimer's, breast cancer, chronic heart failure, hypertension, immune deficiency, neuromuscular disorders and periodontal disease.

Clinical evidence

The evidence for coenzyme Q10 in heart failure remains controversial. A meta-analysis of eight double-blind, placebo-controlled RCTs[1] and one subsequently published RCT[2] suggest that, in addition to conventional treatments, coenzyme Q10 improves functional status, clinical symptoms and quality of life in patients with chronic heart failure. Yet a more recent meta-analysis including nine double-blind, placebo-controlled RCTs did not confirm these findings and concluded that there were insufficient numbers of patients for meaningful results.[3] Controversial evidence also exists for the role of coenzyme Q10 in myocardial protection[4-6] and aerobic exercise.[3] A systematic review of eight RCTs (n = 397) shows positive effects on blood pressure.[3] A systematic review of six studies on tolerability of cancer treatments suggests some protection against cardiotoxicity and liver toxicity; the results are, however, not conclusive mainly due to methodological weaknesses in the original studies.[7] Evidence from single RCTs shows a decrease of risk of cardiac events in patients with recent myocardial infarction who are at risk of atherothrombosis,[8] an improvement in mitochondrial function in patients receiving coenzyme Q10 before cardic surgery,[9] a reduction of attack-frequency, headache-days and days-with-nausea in migraine patients,[10] slower progressive deterioration of function in Parkinson's disease in patients who received a high dosage of coenzyme Q10 (1200 mg daily – an effect which has not been noted with lower dosages),[11] and improvement in renal functions in patients with chronic renal failure.[12] Two RCTs showed positive effects for muscular dystrophy.[13] No positive effects have been found for Huntington's disease,[14] periodontal disease[15] and cocaine dependence.[16]

Dosage

50–300 mg of coenzyme Q10 daily, higher dosages of up to 3000 mg daily have been used.

Risks

Contraindications

Pregnancy and lactation (see p 5), known allergy (probably rare).

Precautions/warnings

Excessive exercise should be avoided while taking coenzyme Q10 supplements.

Adverse effects

Diarrhoea and other gastrointestinal complaints such as nausea, vomiting, occur in less than 1% of patients.

Interactions

Theoretically it could decrease the effects of warfarin; HMG-CoA reductase inhibitors might decrease coenzyme Q10 levels; might have additional blood pressure lowering effects when used with antihypertensive drugs.

Quality issues

Products should state concentration and purity.

Risk–benefit assessment

The effectiveness of coenzyme Q10 for chronic heart failure is uncertain but risks are few. Several effective conventional treatments exist for this condition, so coenzyme Q10 cannot be recommended as therapy for chronic heart failure. Promising evidence exists for a blood pressure lowering effect of coenzyme Q10 when administered with other antihypertensives. No conclusive evidence from large trials exists for any other indications.

REFERENCES

1 Soja A M, Mortensen S A. Treatment of congestive heart failure with coenzyme Q10 illuminated by meta-analyses of clinical trials. Mol Aspects Med 1997;18:S159–168

2 Berman M, Erman A, Ben-Gal T, Dvir D, Georghiou G P, Stamler A, Vered Y, Vidne B A, Aravot D. Coenzyme Q10 in patients with end-stage heart failure awaiting cardiac transplantation: a randomized, placebo-controlled study. Clin Cardiol 2004;27:295–299

3 Rosenfeldt F, Hilton D, Pepe S, Krum H. Systematic review of effect of coenzyme Q10 in physical exercise, hypertension and heart failure. BioFactors 2003;18:91–100

4 Chello M, Mastroroberto P, Romano R, Castaldo P, Bevacqua E, Marchese A R. Protection by coenzyme Q10 of tissue reperfusion injury during abdominal aortic cross-clamping. J Cardiovasc Surg (Torino) 1996;37:229–235

5 Chello M, Mastroroberto P, Romano R, Bevacqua E, Pantaleo D, Ascione R, Marchese

AR, Spampinato N. Protection by coenzyme Q10 from myocardial reperfusion injury during coronary artery bypass grafting. Ann Thorac Surg 1994;58:1427–1432

6 Taggart DP, Jenkins M, Hooper J, Hadjinikolas L, Kemp M, Hue D, Bennett G. Effects of short-term supplementation with coenzyme Q10 on myocardial protection during cardiac operations. Ann Thorac Surg 1996;61:829–833

7 Roffe E A, Schmidt K, Ernst E. Efficacy of coenzyme Q10 for improved tolerability of cancer treatments: a systematic review. J Clin Oncol 2004;22:4418–4424

8 Singh R B, Neki N S, Kartikey K, Pella D, Kumar A, Niaz M A, Thakur A S. Effect of coenzyme Q10 on risk of atherosclerosis in patients with recent myocardial infarction. Mol Cell Biochem 2003;246:75–82.

9 Rosenfeldt F, Marasco S, Lyon W, Wowk M, Sheeran F, Bailey M, Esmore D, Davis B, Pick A, Rabinov M, Smith J, Nagley P, Pepe S. Coenzyme Q10 therapy before cardiac surgery

improves mitochondrial function and in vitro contractility of myocardial tissue. J Thorac Cardiovasc Surg 2005;129:25–32

10 Sandor P S, Di Clemente L, Coppola G, Saenger U, Fumal A, Magis D, Seidel L, Agosti R M, Schoenen J. Efficacy of coenzyme Q10 in migraine prophylaxis: a randomized controlled trial. Neurology 2005;64:713–715

11 Shults C W, Oakes D, Kieburtz K, Beal M F, Haas R, Plumb S, Juncos J L, Nutt J, Shoulson I, Carter J, Kompoliti K, Perlmutter J S, Reich S, Stern M, Watts R L, Kurlan R, Molho E, Harrison M, Lew M; Parkinson Study Group. Effects of coenzyme Q10 in early Parkinson disease: evidence of slowing of the functional decline. Arch Neurol 2002;59:1541–1550

12 Singh R B, Khanna H K, Niaz M A. Randomized, double-blind placebo-controlled trial of coenzyme Q10 in chronic renal failure: discovery of a new role. J Nutr Environ Med 2000;10:281–288

13 Folkers K, Simonsen R. Two successful double-blind trials with coenzyme Q10 (vitamin Q10) on muscular dystrophies and neurogenic atrophies. Biochem Biophys Acta 1995;1271: 281–286

14 Huntington Study Group. A randomized, placebo-controlled trial of coenzyme Q10 and remacemide in Huntington's disease. Neurology 2001;57:397–404

15 Hanioka T, Tanaka M, Ojima M, Shizukuishi S, Folkers K. Effect of topical application of coenzyme Q10 on adult periodontitis. Molec Aspects Med 1994;15:S241–S248

16 Reid MS, Casadonte P, Baker S, Sanfilipo M, Braunstein D, Hitzemann R, Montgomery A, Majewska D, Robinson J, Rotrosen J. A placebo-controlled screening trial of olanzapine, valproate, and coenzyme Q10/L-carnitine for the treatment of cocaine dependence. Addiction 2005;100 (Suppl 1):43–57

CRANBERRY
(Vaccinium macrocarpon)

Source	Berries.
Main constituents	Catechin, flavone glycosides, fructose, organic acids, proanthocyanidins, vitamin C.
Background	Cranberries are evergreen shrubs which grow in most temperate climates. Since German scientists postulated in 1840 that cranberry juice had antibacterial activity, it has been advocated as a remedy for urinary tract infections. It is, however, now clear that cranberry has no antibacterial activity.
Examples of traditional uses	Urinary tract infection.
Pharmacologic action	The current theory suggests that cranberry's mode of action is the inhibition of the adhesion of bacteria to the uroepithelial surface by proanthycanidin and fructose. It does not, however, seem to have the ability to release bacteria which are already adhered to the urinary tract epithelial cells.
Conditions frequently treated	Prevention of recurrent urinary tract infections.
Clinical evidence	A Cochrane review[1] included seven RCTs. In two good quality RCTs, cranberry products reduced the incidence of urinary tract

infections at 12 months in women. There was no difference in the incidence between cranberry juice versus cranberry capsules. Five of the included trials suffered from methodological flaws or lack of available data. Only one reported a positive result for the outcome of symptomatic urinary tract infections. Side effects were common in all trials, and dropouts/withdrawals in several of the trials were numerous (up to 55%). In two subsequently published placebo-controlled RCTs[2,3] of individuals with neurogenic bladders secondary to spinal cord injury cranberry tablets were not found to be effective for preventing urinary tract infections. A further RCT[4] showed no difference in the urinary symptoms experienced during external beam radiation therapy for prostate cancer related to the consumption of cranberry juice compared with apple juice.[4] A Cochrane review concluded that cranberry juice is not an effective therapy for manifest infections.[5] No convincing evidence exists in support of cranberry for any other indication.

Dosage

There are no clear dosing guidelines; recommended doses range from 90–480 ml of cranberry juice twice daily; 300–400 mg of standardised extract twice daily.

Risks

Contraindications
Pregnancy and lactation (see p 5).

Precautions/warnings
Cranberry should not be taken as a substitute for antibiotic treatment; diabetics must consider the sugar content of the juice.

Adverse effects
None known.

Overdose
Doses of over 3l daily may cause gastrointestinal distress and diarrhoea. Toxicity in infants and young children.

Interactions
Theoretically cranberry juice could enhance the elimination of drugs excreted in urine or increase effects of some antibiotics in the urinary tract. A preliminary report suggests a potential interaction between cranberry and warfarin.

Quality issues
Standardised extracts or juice should be used for medicinal purposes; diabetics should use sugar-free preparations.

Risk–benefit assessment

On balance, the evidence is only marginally in favour of cranberry in preventing urinary tract infections. However, its safety profile is excellent so it might be considered as a preventive in patients prone to such infections who prefer such an approach, particularly as long-term antibiotic prophylaxis has significant adverse effects. No evidence supports its use for the treatment of urinary tract infections.

REFERENCES

1 Jepson R G, Mihaljevic L, Craig J. Cranberries for preventing urinary tract infections. The Cochrane Database of Systematic Reviews 2004, Issue 2. Art. No.: CD001321

2 Linsenmeyer T A, Harrison B, Oakley A, Kirshblum S, Stock J A, Millis S R. Evaluation of cranberry supplement for reduction of urinary tract infections in individuals with neurogenic bladders secondary to spinal cord injury. A prospective, double-blinded, placebo-controlled, crossover study. J Spinal Cord Med 2004;27:29–34

3 Waites K B, Canupp K C, Armstrong S, DeVivo M J. Effect of cranberry extract on bacteriuria and pyuria in persons with neurogenic bladder secondary to spinal cord injury. J Spinal Cord Med 2004;27:35–40

4 Campbell G, Pickles T, D'yachkova Y. A randomised trial of cranberry versus apple juice in the management of urinary symptoms during external beam radiation therapy for prostate cancer. Clin Oncol (R Coll Radiol) 2003;15: 322–328

5 Jepson R G, Mihaljevic L, Craig J C. Cranberries for treating urinary tract infections. The Cochrane Database of Systematic Reviews 1998, Issue 4. Art. No.: CD001322

DEVIL'S CLAW
(Harpagophytum procumbens)

Source	Tuberous roots.
Main constituents	The major active ingredient is harpagoside. Other compounds are beta-sitosterol, flavonoids, procumbides, stigmasterol, triterpenes.
Background	The name devil's claw is derived from the plant's unique fruits which are covered with claw-like hooks. It grows wild in South Africa and the recent popularity of devil's claw has nearly resulted in it becoming an endangered species.
Examples of traditional uses	Digestive problems, dysmenorrhoea, gastrointestinal complaints, headaches, liver and kidney diseases, malaria, menopausal symptoms, nicotine poisoning, rheumatic conditions, skin cancer.
Pharmacologic action	Anti-inflammatory, analgesic, negative chronotropic, positive inotropic, antiarrhythmic.
Conditions frequently treated	Arthritic and musculoskeletal pain.
Clinical evidence	A recent systematic review of RCTs, quasi-randomised clinical trials and controlled clinical trials for devil's claw in the treatment of various forms of musculoskeletal pain assessed five RCTs including 385 patients with osteoarthritis of the hip or the knee, four RCTs including 505 patients with acute exacerbations of chronic non-specific low back pain and three placebo-controlled trials including

215 patients with various forms of musculoskeletal pain.[1] The review reports positive evidence from placebo- or conventional treatment-controlled trials for an aqueous extract of devil's claw in the treatment of acute exacerbations of chronic non-specific low back pain; best results were obtained with a daily dose equivalent of 50 mg harpagosides. It also shows encouraging evidence for devil's claw powder at 60 mg harpagosides in the treatment of osteoarthritis of the spine, hip and knee.

Dosage

400–500 mg of dried extract three times daily.

Risks

Contraindications
Pregnancy, due to uterus stimulating effects of devil's claw, lactation (see p 5), gastric or duodenal ulcer, gallstones.

Precautions/warnings
Insufficient reliable information is available about the safety of topical or long-term oral use. Might lower blood sugar levels.

Adverse effects
Gastrointestinal symptoms, allergic skin reactions.

Overdose
Cardiac effects.

Interactions
May increase anticoagulation effects of warfarin; theoretically it could interact with cardiac drugs.

Quality issues
The harpagoside content and pharmacokinetic profile have been shown to vary considerably between commercial preparations.

Risk–benefit assessment

Effectiveness for musculoskeletal pain related to osteoarthritis and non-specific low back pain is reasonably well documented and only mild adverse effects are on record. The effectiveness of devil's claw has been compared with conventional treatment options (e.g. NSAIDs) in four of the trials which suggests that it is better or not worse than conventional treatment options. Thus devil's claw can be tried in selected cases but the risks of herb/drug interactions must be considered.

HERBAL AND NON-HERBAL MEDICINES

REFERENCES
1 Gagnier JJ, Chrubasik S, Manheimer E. Harpagophytum procumbens for osteoarthritis and low back pain: a systematic review. BMC Complement Altern Med 2004;4:13

ECHINACEA
(*Echinacea* spp)

Source	Roots of *E. angustifolia* and *E. pallida*, roots and other parts of *E. purpurea*.
Main constituents	Alkylamides, caffeic acid derivatives, glycoproteins, ketoalkenes/ketoalkynes (*E. pallida* only), polysaccharides.
Background	Echinacea was used for medicinal purposes by the American Indians. It started to be scientifically investigated in the late 19th century, mainly in Germany, and is now one of the most popular herbal remedies on the US and European markets. Three different species are used for medicinal purposes.
Examples of traditional uses	Externally for burns, eczema, mouth sores, toothache, wound healing. Internally for fever, prevention of infections, snake bites, urinary tract infections, varicose ulcers.
Pharmacologic action	Modulates cellular and hormonal immune defence, local anesthetic, anti-inflammatory, activation of adrenal cortex, antiviral, antifungal, free radical scavenger. Alkylamides found in echinacea are reported to modulate the expression of the tumour necrosis factor alpha in primary human monocytes/macrophages.
Conditions frequently treated	Prevention and treatment of common infections such as respiratory tract infections.
Clinical evidence	The evidence regarding echinacea in the treatment and prevention of upper respiratory tract infections remains mixed. A Cochrane review of the effects of echinacea in preventing or treating the common cold summarised 16 RCTs with a total of 3396 patients.[1] Although most trials reported results in favour of echinacea preparations, variations in the products used, methodological weaknesses and suspected publication bias prevented the authors from making clinical recommendations. Two other reviews have reached similarly favourable but cautious conclusions.[2,3] A large rigorous RCT (n = 399) concluded that three *E. angustifolia* root extracts had no effect on rates of infection or severity of symptoms.[4] One recent review focused only on **treatment** of the common cold and concluded that due to the limited information available, the possible value of echinacea in treating the common cold was not established.[5] Two subsequently published CCTs of echinacea in the treatment of upper respiratory tract infections found it not to be effective.[6,7] Three trials investigating the effectiveness of echinacea in the **prevention** of respiratory tract infections found it not to be effective.[8–10] Two CCTs using combination products reported positive findings: one used *E. purpurea*, white cedar and wild indigo for

the treatment of the common cold,[11] the other echinacea, propolis and vitamin C in the prevention of common colds in children.[12]

One small RCT found echinacea not to be effective in the treatment of genital herpes.[13] In one RCT *E. purpurea* juice failed to stimulate the nonspecific immune response in healthy young men.[14]

Dosage

Capsules of powdered herb: 500–1000 mg three times daily.
Juice: 6–9 ml daily in divided doses.
Tincture (1:5): 0.75–1.5 ml 2–5 times daily.
Tea: 4 g of echinacea in one cup of water.

Risks

Contraindications
Pregnancy and lactation (see p 5).

Precautions/warnings
Patients suffering from progressive systemic diseases such as AIDS/HIV, multiple sclerosis, tuberculosis, collagen or autoimmune diseases and leukoses should not use echinacea. Drug-free intervals are recommended when used for prolonged periods of time (over 8 weeks).

Adverse effects
Allergic reactions, rash in children, gastrointestinal complaints.

Interactions
Could theoretically decrease effects of immunosuppressants.

Quality issues
Cold-pressed juice of *E. purpurea* seems to be the most active preparation for prevention of upper respiratory tract infections. Controversy continues as to which parts of the plants are best suited for medicinal use. *Echinacea* spp products are highly variable.

Risk–benefit assessment

There is some encouraging evidence relating to the treatment of the common cold particularly when started in the very early stages of the condition. The results from clinical trials are, however, mixed and the methodologically best trials tend not to support efficacy. Echinacea seems not effective in the **prevention** of upper respiratory tract infections. No serious risks have been reported and adverse events in adults seem to be rare. Echinacea was of no benefit in treating the common cold in children and associated with an increased risk of rash. Its use can therefore not be recommended in this patient group.

REFERENCES

1 Melchart D, Linde K, Fischer P, Kaesmayr J. Echinacea for preventing and treating the common cold. The Cochrane Database of Systematic Reviews 1999, Issue 1. Art. No.: CD000530

2 Giles J T, Palat C T 3rd, Chien S H, Chang Z G, Kennedy D T. Evaluation of echinacea for treatment of the common cold. Pharmacotherapy 2000;20:690–697

3   Barrett B, Vohmann M, Calabrese C. Echinacea for upper respiratory infection. J Fam Pract 1999;48:628–635

4   Turner R B, Bauer R, Woelkart K, Hulsey T C, Gangemi J D. An evaluation of Echinacea angustifolia in experimental rhinovirus infections. N Engl J Med 2005;353:341–348.

5   Caruso T J, Gwaltney J M Jr. Treatment of the common cold with Echinacea: a structured review. Clin Infect Dis 2005;40:807–810

6   Yale S H, Liu K. Echinacea purpurea therapy for the treatment of the common cold: a randomized, double-blind, placebo-controlled clinical trial. Arch Intern Med 2004;164:1237–1241

7   Spasov A A, Ostrovskij O V, Chernikov M V, Wikman G. Comparative controlled study of Andrographis paniculata fixed combination, Kan Jang and an Echinacea preparation as adjuvant, in the treatment of uncomplicated respiratory disease in children. Phytother Res 2004;18:47–53

8   Grimm W, Müller H H. A randomized controlled trial of the effect of fluid extract of Echinacea purpurea on the incidence and severity of colds and respiratory infections. Am J Med 1999;106:138–143

9   Sperber S J, Shah L P, Gilbert R D, Ritchey T W, Monto A S. Echinacea purpurea for prevention of experimental rhinovirus colds. Clin Infect Dis 2004;38:1367–1371

10 Turner R B, Riker D K, Gangemi J D. Ineffectiveness of echinacea for prevention of experimental rhinovirus colds. Antimicrob Agents Chemother 2000;44:1708–1709.

11 Henneicke-von Zepelin H, Hentschel C, Schnitker J, Kohnen R, Kohler G, Wüstenberg P. Efficacy and safety of a fixed combination phytomedicine in the treatment of the common cold (acute viral respiratory tract infection): results of a randomised, double blind, placebo-controlled, multicentre study. Curr Med Res Opin 1999;15:214–227.

12 Cohen H A, Varsano I, Kahan E, Sarrell E M, Uziel Y. Effectiveness of an herbal preparation containing echinacea, propolis, and vitamin C in preventing respiratory tract infections in children: a randomized, double-blind, placebo-controlled, multicenter study. Arch Pediatr Adolesc Med 2004;158:217–221

13 Vonau B, Chard S, Mandalia S, Wilkinson D, Barton S E. Does the extract of the plant Echinacea purpurea influence the clinical course of recurrent genital herpes? Int J STD AIDS 2001;12:154–158

14 Schwarz E, Metzler J, Diedrich J P, Freudenstein J, Bode C, Bode J C. Oral administration of freshly expressed juice of Echinacea purpurea herbs fail to stimulate the nonspecific immune response in healthy young men: results of a double-blind, placebo-controlled crossover study. J Immunother 2002;25:413–420

EVENING PRIMROSE
(*Oenothera biennis*)

Source	Oil from seeds.
Main constituents	The seeds contain 14% fixed oil comprising approximately 70% cis-linoleic acid (LA), 9% cis-gamma-linolenic acid (GLA), 2–16% oleic acid, 7% palmitic acid, 3% stearic acid.
Background	Evening primrose is not actually a primrose but belongs to the fuchsia (*Onagraceae*) family. It is native to North America and naturalised in western Europe and parts of Asia and blooms in early summer, producing large yellow flowers which open in the evenings – hence its name. Originally the root was used as a vegetable for culinary purposes and the whole plant was used for its medicinal properties to treat a wide range of conditions. Today it is mainly the oil that is used for therapeutic purposes. Survey data suggest that it is popular, particularly with menopausal women.[1]
Examples of traditional uses	Asthma, gastrointestinal disorders, neuralgia, whooping cough.

Pharmacologic action	For individuals in whom the conversion of LA to GLA by the enzyme delta-6 desaturase is impaired, the rich GLA content of evening primrose oil allows this conversion to be bypassed.
Conditions frequently treated	Cardiovascular conditions, dermatological conditions (atopic eczema, psoriasis), female conditions (premenstrual syndrome, menopausal complaints, mastalgia), inflammatory/autoimmune conditions (rheumatoid arthritis, multiple sclerosis), psychiatric conditions (schizophrenia, hyperactivity, dementia).
Clinical evidence	Positive results from a meta-analysis of nine controlled trials of atopic eczema[2] have been contradicted by subsequent RCTs.[3-5] A systematic review of premenstrual syndrome trials suggested that evening primrose oil had little value for treating this condition.[6] A recent RCT failed to show any benefit for bone mineral density in peri- or postmenopausal women.[7] A large range of other conditions have been investigated, including asthma,[8,9] psoriasis,[10,11] cellulite,[12] hyperactivity,[13,14] multiple sclerosis,[15,16] menopausal flushing,[17] schizophrenia,[18] obesity,[19,20] chronic fatigue syndrome,[21,22] fatigue associated with primary Sjörgren's syndrome,[23] rheumatoid arthritis,[24-26] and mastalgia.[27-30] Results have been largely negative or ambiguous. Diabetic neuropathy and uraemic pruritus are conditions where results appear promising.[31-33]
Dosage	*Mastalgia:* 3–4 g (8% GLA) daily in divided doses. *Atopic eczema:* 6–8 g (adults), 2–4 g (children) daily in divided doses.
Risks	**Contraindications** Pregnancy and lactation (see p 5), mania, epilepsy. **Precautions/warnings** There is a risk of undiagnosed temporal lobe epilepsy being manifested in schizophrenics or other patients taking epileptogenic agents. **Adverse effects** Gastrointestinal symptoms, headache. **Overdose** Gastrointestinal symptoms have been observed with large doses. **Interactions** Theoretically, interactions with anti-inflammatory drugs, corticosteroids, beta-blockers, antipsychotics and anticoagulants are possible. Concomitant use with epileptogenic agents such as phenothiazines may increase the risk of seizures. **Quality issues** Standardised preparations usually contain 8% GLA. Some products contain a combination of evening primrose oil and fish oil (omega-3 fatty acids).

HERBAL AND NON-HERBAL MEDICINES

Risk–benefit assessment

Despite having been subjected to a relatively large number of clinical trials, evening primrose oil has not been established as an efficacious treatment for any condition. It appears to be generally safe. For conditions where preliminary evidence offers some promise (e.g. diabetic neuropathy and uraemic pruritus), it may therefore merit consideration.

REFERENCES

1 Mahady G B, Parrot J, Lee C, Yun G S, Dan A. Botanical dietary supplement use in peri- and postmenopausal women. Menopause 2003;10: 65–72.

2 Morse P F, Horrobin D F, Manku M S, Stewart J C, Allen R, Littlewood S, Wright S, Burton J, Gould D J, Holt P J. Meta-analysis of placebo-controlled studies of the efficacy of Epogam in the treatment of atopic eczema. Relationship between plasma essential fatty acid changes and clinical response. Br J Dermatol 1989;121:75–90

3 Whitaker D K, Cilliers J, De Beer C. Evening primrose oil (Epogam) in the treatment of chronic hand dermatitis: disappointing therapeutic results. Dermatology 1996;193:115–120

4 Berth-Jones J, Brown G. Placebo-controlled trial of essential fatty acid supplementation in atopic dermatitis. Lancet 1993;341:1557–1560

5 Hederos C A, Berg A. Epogam evening primrose oil treatment in atopic dermatitis and asthma. Arch Dis Child 1996;75:494–497

6 Budeiri D, Li Won Po D, Dornan J C. Is evening primrose oil of value in the treatment of premenstrual syndrome? Controlled Clin Trials 1996;17:60–68

7 Bassey E J, Littlewood J J, Rothwell M C, Pye D W. Lack of effect of supplementation with essential fatty acids on bone mineral density in healty pre- and postmenopausal women: two randomized controlled trials of Efacal v. calcium alone. Br J Nutr 2000;83:629–635

8 Ebden P, Bevan C, Banks J, Fennerty A, Walters E H. A study of evening primrose seed oil in atopic asthma. Prostagland Leukot Essent Fatty Acids 1989;35:69–72

9 Stenius-Aarniala B, Aro A, Hakulinen A, Ahola I, Seppala E, Vapaatalo H. Evening primrose oil and fish oil are ineffective as supplementary treatment of bronchial asthma. Ann Allergy 1989;62:534–537

10 Strong A M M, Hamill E. The effect of combined fish oil and evening primrose oil (Efamol Marine) on the remission phase of psoriasis: a 7-month double-blind randomized placebo-controlled trial. J Dermatol Treat 1993;4:33–36

11 Oliwiecki S, Burton J L. Evening primrose oil and marine oil in the treatment of psoriasis. Clin Exp Dermatol 1994;19:127–129

12 Lis-Balchin M. Parallel placebo-controlled clinical study of a mixture of herbs sold as a remedy for cellulite. Phytother Res 1999;13:627–629

13 Arnold L E, Kleykamp D, Votolato N A, Taylor W A, Kontras S B, Tobin K. Gamma-linolenic acid for attention-deficit hyperactivity disorder: placebo-controlled comparison to D-amphetamine. Biol Psychiatr 1989;25:222–228

14 Aman M G, Mitchell E A, Turbott S H. The effects of essential fatty acid supplementation by Efamol in hyperactive children. J Abnorm Child Psychol 1987;15:75–90

15 Bates D, Fawcett P R W, Shaw D A, Weightman D. Trial of polyunsaturated fatty acids in non-relapsing multiple sclerosis. BMJ 1977;2:932–933

16 Bates D, Fawcett P R W, Shaw D A, Weightman D. Polyunsaturated fatty acids in treatment of acute remitting multiple sclerosis. BMJ 1978;2: 404–405

17 Chenoy R, Hussain S, Tayob T, O'Brien P M S, Moss M Y, Morse P F. Effect of oral gamolenic acid from evening primrose oil on menopausal flushing. BMJ 1994;308:501–503

18 Joy C B, Mumby-Croft R, Joy L A. Polyunsaturated fatty acid supplementation (fish or evening primrose oil) for schizophrenia. The Cochrane Database of Systematic Reviews 2003, Issue 2. Art. No.: CD001257.

19 Haslett C, Douglas J G, Chalmers S R, Weighhill A, Munro J F. A double-blind evaluation of evening primrose oil as an antiobesity agent. Int J Obes 1983;7:549–553

20 Garcia C, Carter J, Chou A. Gamma linolenic acid causes weight loss and lower blood pressure in overweight patients with family history of obesity. Swed J Biol Med 1986;4:8–11

21 Behan P O, Behan W M H, Horrobin D. Effect of high doses of essential fatty acids on the postviral fatigue syndrome. Acta Neurol Scand 1990;82:209–216

22 Warren G, McKendrick M, Peet M. The role of essential fatty acids in chronic fatigue syndrome. Acta Neurol Scand 1999;99:112–116

23 Theander E, Horrobin DF, Jacobson-Lennart TH, Manthorpe R. Gammalinolenic acid treatment of fatigue associated with primary Sjögren's syndrome. Scand J Rheumatol 2002;31:72–79

24 Veale D J, Torley H I, Richards I M, O'Dowd A, Fitzsimons C, Belch J J, Sturrock R D. A double-blind placebo-controlled trial of Efamol Marine on skin and joint symptoms of psoriatic arthritis. Br J Rheumatol 1994;33:954–958

25 Brzeski M, Madhok R, Capell H A. Evening primrose oil in patients with rheumatoid arthritis and side effects of non-steroidal anti-inflammatory drugs. Br J Rheumatol 1991;30:370–372

26 Belch J J, Ansell D, Madhok R, O'Dowd A, Sturrock R D. Effects of altering dietary essential fatty acids on requirements for non-steroidal anti-inflammatory drugs in patients with rheumatoid arthritis: a double-blind placebo-controlled study. Ann Rheum Dis 1988;47:96–104

27 Gateley C A, Miers M, Mansel R E, Hughes L E. Drug treatments for mastalgia: 17 years experience in the Cardiff mastalgia clinic. J Roy Soc Med 1992;85:12–15

28 Gateley C A, Maddox P R, Pritchard G A, Sheridan W, Harrison B J, Pye J K, Webster D J, Hughes L E, Mansel R E. Plasma fatty acid profiles in benign breast disorders. Br J Surg 1992;79:407–409

29 Mansel R E, Harrison B J, Melhuish J, Sheridan W, Pye J K, Pritchard G, Maddox P R, Webster D J, Hughes L E. A randomized trial of dietary intervention with essential fatty acids in patients with categorised cysts. Ann NY Acad Sci 1990;586:288–294

30 Blommers J, de Lange-De Klerk E, Kuik D J, Bezemer P D, Meijer S. Evening primrose oil and fish oil for severe chronic mastalgia: a randomized, double-blind, controlled trial. Am J Obstet Gynecol 2002;187:1389–1394

31 Jamal G A, Carmichael H, Weir A I. Gamma-linolenic acid in diabetic neuropathy. Lancet 1986;1:1098

32 Keen H, Payan J, Allawi J, Walker J, Jamal G A, Weir A I, Henderson L M, Bissessar E A, Watkins P J, Sampson M. Treatment of diabetic neuropathy with gamma-linolenic acid. Diabetes Care 1993;16:8–15

33 Yoshimoto-Furuie K, Yoshimoto K, Tanaka T, Saima S, Kikuchi Y, Shay J, Horrobin D F, Echizen H. Effects of oral supplementation with evening primrose oil for six weeks on plasma essential fatty acids and uraemic skin symptoms in hemodialysis patients. Nephron 1999;81:151–159

FEVERFEW
(*Tanacetum parthenium*)

Source	Leaves.
Main constituents	Camphor, chrysanthenyl acetate and flavonoids. Parthenolide is thought to be the active principle.
Background	Feverfew is a perennial plant, native to Asia Minor. It is widely naturalised throughout much of Europe, North America and Canada. Its use as a herbal remedy goes back to ancient times when it was employed for many aches and pains, in particular for conditions associated with fevers and women's ailments. Today the extract of feverfew is predominantly used for the prevention of migraine attacks and to alleviate the accompanying symptoms.
Examples of traditional uses	Colds, fevers, general aches, headaches, rheumatism, women's ailments.
Pharmacologic action	Analgetic, anti-inflammatory, antithrombotic, cytotoxic, spasmolytic. It has been suggested that parthenolide exerts inhibiting

HERBAL AND NON-HERBAL MEDICINES

effects on serotonin release by human platelets in vitro. Other evidence suggests that chrysanthenyl acetate may be important. This constituent has been shown to inhibit prostaglandin synthesis in vitro and seems to possess analgesic properties.

Conditions frequently treated

Migraine, rheumatoid arthritis.

Clinical evidence

A Cochrane review assessed five double-blind RCTs (n = 343) of feverfew for preventing migraine.[1] While the two studies with high methodological quality showed no beneficial effects, three others were in favour of feverfew. Of the four trials with a sample size of 50 or above, two studies reported feverfew to be superior to placebo, while two did not. The results therefore do not convincingly establish that feverfew is efficacious for preventing migraine. For a combination preparation of 400 mg riboflavin, 300 mg magnesium and 100 mg feverfew daily there was no difference compared with placebo for the reduction in migraine attacks.[2] One double-blind RCT of feverfew as a treatment for rheumatoid arthritis found no relevant differences for clinical or laboratory variables compared with placebo, but reports some beneficial effects for grip strength.[3]

Dosage

50–140 mg of powdered or granulated dried leaf preparation daily in divided doses.

Risks

Contraindications
Pregnancy and lactation (see p 5), hypersensitivity to members of the *Asteraceae* family.

Precautions/warnings
Should not be used for longer than 4 months due to the lack of long-term toxicity data.

Adverse effects
Allergic reactions, contact dermatitis, mouth ulceration and soreness, gastrointestinal complaints, 'post-feverfew syndrome' including rebound of migraine symptoms, anxiety, dizziness, insomnia, muscle and joint stiffness.

Interactions
May potentiate the effects of anticoagulants.

Quality issues
The amount of active constituents may vary according to the origin of the plant and the plant parts used.

Risk–benefit assessment

The data indicate that there is insufficient evidence from rigorous clinical trials to convincingly suggest an effect of feverfew over and above placebo for preventing migraine. However, given that feverfew presents no major safety problems, the limited number of available options for preventing migraine and the severity of the condition, in many cases it is worth considering while carefully monitoring the patient. There are too few studies for any firm judgement to be made on its effectiveness in rheumatoid arthritis.

REFERENCES

1 Pittler M H, Ernst E. Feverfew for preventing migraine. The Cochrane Database of Systematic Reviews 2004, Issue 1. Art. No.: CD002286
2 Maizels M, Blumenfeld A, Burchette R. A combination of riboflavin, magnesium, and feverfew for migraine prophylaxis: a randomized trial. Headache 2004;44:885–890
3 Pattrick M, Heptinstall S, Doherty M. Feverfew in rheumatoid arthritis: a double-blind, placebo-controlled study. Ann Rheum Dis 1989;48: 547–549

GARLIC
(Allium sativum)

Source	Bulb and oil from bulb.
Main constituents	Alliin, diallyl disulfide, ajoens and many others; alliin is enzymatically converted to allicin which is thought to be one of the main active ingredients and is responsible for the characteristic, sulfur-like smell.
Background	For millennia, garlic has been used as a food and spice in many countries. It has also been used in most cultures for various medicinal purposes. Its extensive scientific investigation started relatively recently but today it is one of the best-researched (and best-selling) herbal remedies.
Examples of traditional uses	Garlic has been used both orally and topically for many purposes, most consistently perhaps to prevent and treat infections and as a way of maintaining general health.
Pharmacologic action	Antibacterial, antiviral, antifungal, antihypertensive, blood glucose lowering, antithrombotic, antimutagenic, antiplatelet. Its best-researched property is that of lowering total serum cholesterol levels; its main mechanism of action is probably the inhibition of hepatic cholesterol synthesis.
Conditions frequently treated	Hypercholesterolaemia, prevention of arteriosclerosis.
Clinical evidence	Numerous RCTs published in the late 1980s and early 1990s demonstrated a reduction of total cholesterol and low-density lipoprotein cholesterol. Several systematic reviews of these data therefore arrived at positive conclusions. Subsequently, however, several negative RCTs have emerged. An updated meta-analysis of all rigorous RCTs produced an overall result which was marginally positive when all RCTs were included (average reduction 0.41 mmol/l), but a

HERBAL AND NON-HERBAL MEDICINES

non-significant effect on total cholesterol when only the high-quality RCTs were analysed.[1] More recently, multiple meta-analyses found a small short-term benefit on lipid and platelet factors and insignificant effects on blood pressure and no effect on blood glucose.[2] The trial data since then generated mixed results: seven CCTs suggested no effects on lipid parameters,[3–9] two yielded small positive effects[10,11] and one trial found favourable effects in women and adverse effects in men.[12] A small RCT (n = 19) suggested that garlic intake might inhibit coronary calcification.[13]

Some interesting, though not compelling data (e.g.[14]) suggest that, due to its broad-ranging effects on cardiovascular risk factors, the regular intake of garlic might prevent or delay the development of arteriosclerosis. Epidemiological data indicate that the regular consumption of garlic might convey a protective effect for malignancies, in particular intestinal cancers.[15] This was confirmed in a small RCT (n = 37) suggesting both preventative and therapeutic effects of garlic on colorectal adenoma formation.[16] An RCT (n = 100) implies that high-dose garlic consumption reduces the frequency of tick bites in a tick-endemic area.[17] When tested as a mosquito repellent, oral garlic showed no difference to placebo.[18] A recent RCT (n = 146) suggests that volunteers taking garlic regularly for 12 weeks had less episodes of common cold and recovered more quickly than those receiving placebo.[19] Finally one CCT generated encouraging findings for garlic as a symptomatic treatment for rheumatoid arthritis.[20]

Dosage

Bulb: 4 g of fresh garlic daily.
Oil: 8 mg of garlic oil daily.
Extract: 600–900 mg of standardised extract (1.3% alliin content) daily in divided doses.

Risks

Contraindications
Pregnancy and lactation (see p 5), peptic ulcers, allergies to *Liliaceae* family.

Precautions/warnings
Patients with bleeding abnormalities; before major surgery garlic supplements should be discontinued.

Adverse effects
Breath and body odour are frequent; other effects are rare: allergic reactions, nausea, heartburn, flatulence, abdominal pain or fullness, anorexia, Ménière's disease, myocardial infarction, bleeding, small intestinal obstruction, oesophageal pain.[2]

Overdose
Nausea, vomiting, risk of bleeding.

Interactions
Can increase effects of anticoagulants, could theoretically enhance hypoglycaemic effects of antidiabetic medications.

Quality issues
Commercial products vary greatly in terms of concentration of active ingredients.

Risk–benefit assessment

Garlic probably does lower total cholesterol but only to a minor degree. It is worth considering it as an adjunct to dietary and lifestyle measures in selected patients with hypercholesterolaemia. The regular intake of fresh garlic with food probably has some protective effects against intestinal cancer.

REFERENCES

1 Stevinson C, Pittler M H, Ernst E. Garlic for treating hypercholesterolemia: a meta-analysis of randomized clinical trials. Ann Intern Med 2000;133:420–429

2 Ackermann R T, Mulrow C D, Ramirez G, Gardner C D, Morbidoni L, Lawrence V A. Garlic shows promise for improving some cardiovascular risk factors. Arch Intern Med 2001;161: 813–824

3 Satitvipawee P, Rawdaree P, Indrabhakti S, Ratanasuwan T, Getn-gern P, Viwatwongkasem C. No effect of garlic extract supplement on serum lipid levels in hypercholesterolemic subjects. J Med Assoc Thai 2003;86:750–757

4 Peleg A, Hershcoviei T, Lipa R, Anbar R, Redler M, Beigel Y. Effect of garlic on lipid profile and psychopathologic parameters in people with mild to moderate hypercholesterolemia. Isr Med Assoc J 2003;5:637–640

5 Ziaei S, Hantoshzadeh S, Rezasoltani P, Lamyian M. The effect of garlic tablet on plasma lipids and platelet aggregation in nulliparous pregnants at high risk of preeclampsia. Eur J Obstet Gynecol Reprod Biol 2001;99:201–206

6 Gardner C D, Chatterjee L M, Carlson J J. The effect of a garlic preparation on plasma lipid levels in moderately hypercholesterolemic adults. Atherosclerosis 2001;154:213–220

7 Byrne D J, Neil H A, Vallance D T, Winder AF. A pilot study of garlic consumption shows no significant effect on markers of oxidation or sub-fraction composition of low-density lipoprotein including lipoprotein (a) after allowance for non-compliance and the placebo effect. Clin Chim Acta 1999;285:21–33

8 Turner B, Molgaard C, Marckmann P. Effect of garlic (Allium sativum) powder tablets on serum lipids, blood pressure and arterial stiffness in normo-lipidaemic volunteers: a randomised, double-blind, placebo-controlled trial. Br J Nutr 2004;92:701–706

9 Tanamai J, Veeramanomai S, Indrakosas N. The efficacy of cholesterol-lowering action and side effects of garlic enteric coated tablets in man. J Med Assoc Thai 2004;87:1156–1161

10 Kannar D, Wattanapenpaiboon N, Savige G S, Wahlqvist M L. Hypocholesterolemic effect of an enteric-coated garlic supplement. J Am Coll Nutr 2001;20:225–231

11 Zhang X H, Lowe D, Giles P, Fell S, Board A R, Baughan J A, Connock M J, Maslin D J. A randomized trial of the effects of garlic oil on coronary heart disease risk factors in trained male runners. Blood Coagul Fibrinolysis 2001;12:67–74

12 Zhang X H, Lowe D, Giles P, Fell S, Connock M J, Maslin D J. Gender may affect the action of garlic oil on plasma cholesterol and glucose levels of normal subjects. J Nutr 2001;131:1471–1478

13 Budoff M J, Takasu J, Flores-Ferdinand R, Niihara Y, Lu B, Lau B H, Rosen R T, Amagase H. Inhibiting progression of coronary calcification using aged garlic extract in patients receiving statin therapy: a preliminary study. Prev Med 2004;39.985–991

14 Breithaupt-Grogler K, Ling M, Boudoulas H, Belz G G. Protective effects of chronic garlic intake on elastic properties of aorta in the elderly. Circulation 1997;96:2649–2655

15 Fleischauer A T, Poole C, Arab L. Garlic consumption and cancer prevention: meta-analyses of colorectal and stomach cancers. Am J Clin Nutr 2000;72:1047–1052

16 Tanaka S, Haruma K, Kunihiro M, Nagata S, Kitadai Y, Manabe N, Sumii M, Yoshihara M, Kajiyama G, Chayama K. Effects of aged garlic extract (AGE) on colorectal adenomas: a double-blinded study. Hiroshima J Med Sci 2004;53: 39–45

17 Stjernberg L, Berglund J. Garlic as insect repellent. JAMA 2000;284:831

18 Rajan T V, Hein M, Porte P, Wikel S. A double-blinded, placebo-controlled trial of garlic as a mosquito repellant: a preliminary study. Med Vet Entomol 2005;19:84–89

HERBAL AND NON-HERBAL MEDICINES

19   Josling P. Preventing the common cold with a garlic supplement: a double-blind, placebo-controlled survey. Adv Ther 2001;18:189–193

20   Denisov L N, Andrianova I V, Timofeeva S S. Garlic effectiveness in rheumatoid arthritis. Ter Arkh 1999;71:55–58

GINGER
(Zingiber officinale)

Source	Rhizome.
Main constituents	Niacin, non-pungent substances, non-volatile pungent principles, starch, triglycerides, vitamins and volatile oil.
Background	Ginger is a perennial plant native to southern Asia. It has been used as food and for medicinal purposes since ancient times, particularly to treat ailments such as stomach ache, diarrhoea and nausea. In the 16th century, ginger was introduced to the Caribbean and Central America by the Spanish and was later cultivated for export. German and European monographs are available and in 1997, the US Pharmacopeia approved ginger and powdered ginger monographs for inclusion in the National Formulary.
Examples of traditional uses	Diarrhoea, dyspepsia, gastrointestinal complaints, nausea, osteoarthritis, respiratory disorders, vomiting.
Pharmacologic action	Antiemetic, anti-inflammmatory, positive inotropic, carminative, promotes secretion of saliva and gastric juices, cholagogue, inhibition of platelet aggregation.
Conditions frequently treated	Dyspepsia, loss of appetite, prevention of motion sickness.
Clinical evidence	For treating nausea and vomiting in pregnancy a systematic review[1] identified six double-blind RCTs with a total of 675 participants. It concluded that ginger may be an effective treatment but more data are needed to confirm these findings. For postoperative nausea and vomiting a meta-analysis[2] identified a borderline non-significant effect and concluded that ginger is not a clinically relevant antiemetic.[3] Another systematic review identified trials for motion sickness, and chemotherapy-induced nausea.[4] For motion sickness, the earlier positive findings were corroborated in another trial.[5] For chemotherapy-induced nausea and vomiting, additional trials reported some positive effects when compared with standard antiemetic drugs,[6,7] but not in addition to metoclopramide.[8] Three double-blind RCTs tested whether ginger is effective for reducing pain associated with osteoarthritis of the knee.[9–11] All three trials reported beneficial effects compared with placebo. However, the three extracts used were from different plant genera.[12]

Dosage   1–4 g of powdered extract daily.

Risks   *Contraindications*
Pregnancy and lactation (see p 5). A clinical review found no scientific or medical evidence for the contraindication of ginger during pregnancy.[13] There is, however, a theoretical risk of congenital deformity in neonates. Allergy to members of the *Zingiberaceae* family.

Precautions/warnings
Children under 6 years of age; gallstones. Patients using anticoagulants, prior to surgery.

Adverse effects
Heartburn, belching, bloating, flatulence, nausea; mutagenic potential shown in vitro studies requires further systematic investigations.

Interactions
Increased effects of anticoagulants; may interfere with cardiac and antidiabetic therapy; may enhance the effects of central nervous system depressants.

Quality issues
The term ginger used in the studies might relate to different plant genera.[12] The principal components of ginger may vary greatly depending on the country of origin.

Risk–benefit assessment

For treating nausea and vomiting in pregnancy the evidence is promising but not fully convincing. However, due to the theoretical risk of congenital deformity in neonates it is contraindicated in this condition. For postoperative nausea and vomiting the evidence suggests that ginger is not a clinically relevant option. Encouraging findings exist for motion sickness, chemotherapy-induced nausea and vomiting. For osteoarthritis of the knee the evidence is not convincing due to the heterogeneity of the plant extracts used. Given the reported low frequency of risks involved, ginger is worthy of consideration for chemotherapy-induced nausea and vomiting and motion sickness.

HERBAL AND NON-HERBAL MEDICINES

REFERENCES

1 Borrelli F, Capasso R, Aviello G, Pittler M H, Izzo A A. Effectiveness and safety of ginger in the treatment of pregnancy-induced nausea and vomiting. Obstet Gynecol 2005;105:849–856

2 Morin A M, Betz O, Kranke P, Geldner G, Wulf H, Eberhart L H. Is ginger a relevant antiemetic for postoperative nausea and vomiting? Anasthesiol Intensivmed Notfallmed Schmerzther 2004;39: 281–285

3 Betz O, Kranke P, Geldner G, Wulf H, Eberhart L H. Is ginger a clinically relevant antiemetic?

A systematic review of randomized controlled trials Forsch Komplementärmed Klass Naturheilkd 2005;12:14–23

4 Ernst E, Pittler M H. Efficacy of ginger for nausea and vomiting: a systematic review of randomised clinical trials. Br J Anaesth 2000;84: 367–371

5 Lien H C, Sun W M, Chen Y H, Kim H, Hasler W, Owyang C. Effects of ginger on motion sickness and gastric slow-wave dysrhythmias induced by circular vection. Am J Physiol Gastrointest Liver Physiol 2003;284:G481–489.

6 Sontakke S, Thawani V, Naik M S. Ginger as an antiemetic in nausea and vomiting induced by chemotherapy: A randomized, cross-over, double-blind study. Indian J Pharmacol 2003;35:32–36

7 Manusirivithaya S, Sripramote M, Tangjitgamol S, Sheanakul C, Leelahakorn S, Thavaramara T, Tangcharoenpanich K. Antiemetic effect of ginger in gynecologic oncology patients receiving cisplatin. Int J Gynecol Cancer 2004;14:1063–1069

8 Visalyaputra S, Petchpaisit N, Somcharoen K, Choavaratana R. The efficacy of ginger root in the prevention of postoperative nauseaand vomiting after outpatient gynaecological laparoscopy. Anaesthesia 1998;53:506–510

9 Bliddal H, Rosetzky A, Schlichting P, Weidner MS, Andersen LA, Ibfelt H H, Christensen K, Jensen O N, Barslev J. A randomized, placebo-controlled, cross-over study of ginger extract and Ibuprofen in osteoarthritis. Osteoarthritis Cartilage 2000;8:9–12

10 Altman R D, Marcussen K C. Effects of a ginger extract on knee pain in patients with osteoarthritis. Arthritis Rheum 2001;44:2531–2538

11 Wigler I, Grotto I, Caspi D, Yaron M. The effects of Zintona E C (a ginger extract) on symptomatic gonarthritis. Osteoarthritis Cartilage 2003;11:783–789

12 Canter P. Ginger – do we know what we are talking about? Focus Altern Complement Ther 2004;9:184–185

13 Fulder S, Tenne M. Ginger as an anti-nausea remedy in pregnancy: the issue of safety. Herbalgram 1996;38:47–50

GINKGO
(Ginkgo biloba)

Source	Leaves.
Main constituents	Bilobalide, ginkgolides, flavonoids.

Background

The ginkgo tree, native to China, Korea and Japan is believed to be one of the most ancient trees on earth. It is the last remaining member of the *Ginkgoaceae* family, which has survived almost unchanged during the evolutionary timespan of about 200 million years and is often referred to as a 'living fossil'. Individual trees may live as long as 1000 years and grow up to a height of 40–50 m. The unique botany of *Ginkgo biloba* is accompanied by some equally unique chemistry. The structures of the main active principles, which are thought to be flavonoids and terpene trilactones, comprising bilobalide and ginkgolides, are complex. The tree is the only source and is cultivated, for instance, in the south of France and in south-eastern parts of the USA. It is one of the most extensively researched medicinal plants and is the top-selling herbal remedy in the USA.

Examples of traditional uses

Angina, asthma, hypertension, headache, schizophrenia, tinnitus.

Pharmacologic action

Increase of microcirculatory blood flow, inhibition of erythrocyte aggregation, platelet-activating factor antagonism, free radical scavenging.

Conditions frequently treated

Cognitive impairment, dementia, intermittent claudication, tinnitus.

Clinical evidence

A meta-analysis of *Ginkgo biloba* for treating peripheral arterial occlusive disease assessed eight double-blind RCTs and suggested a modest increase of painfree walking distance compared with placebo.[1] This conclusion is confirmed by another meta-analysis of all double-blind placebo-controlled RCTs, which assessed the effectiveness of *G. biloba* special extract EGb 761.[2] For cognitive impairment and dementia a Cochrane review cautiously concludes that overall there is promising evidence of improvement in cognition and function associated with *G. biloba*.[3] A delay in the loss of capacities needed to cope with the demands of daily living may be achieved.[4] For treating vertigo in elderly patients, a homeopathic preparation was not inferior to ginkgo.[5] Whether *G. biloba* is a smart drug and able to enhance cognitive function in healthy subjects was assessed in a systematic review of double-blind placebo-controlled RCTs which concluded that it cannot be recommended for this indication on the basis of the existing evidence.[6] Further double-blind placebo-controlled RCTs are available to confirm this conclusion,[7,8] but also trials to the contrary.[9-11] For treating tinnitus a Cochrane review concluded that the limited evidence did not demonstrate that *G. biloba* was effective.[12] There is no reliable evidence to address the question of *G. biloba* for tinnitus associated with cerebral insufficiency.[12] Another double-blind placebo-controlled RCT and meta-analysis confirm these findings.[13] Beneficial effects were reported in double-blind RCTs for treating sudden hearing loss.[14,15] For treating age-related macular degeneration a Cochrane review identified one published trial and concluded that the question as to whether people with age-related macular degeneration should take *G. biloba* extract to prevent progression of the disease has not been answered by research to date.[16] For preexisting visual field damage in normal tension glaucoma some positive effects have been reported.[17] *G. biloba* was also tested for preventing acute mountain sickness and was found to not reduce the incidence of this condition.[18-20] Single double-blind placebo-controlled RCTs suggest some positive effects of *G. biloba* in vitiligo,[21] Raynaud's disease,[22] and as an addition to haloperidol in treatment-resistant patients with schizophrenia,[23] whereas no effects were found for cocaine dependence,[24] winter depression[25] and antidepressant-induced sexual dysfunction.[26,27]

Dosage

Dementia and memory impairment: 120–240 mg of standardised leaf extract daily in divided doses.
Intermittent claudication, vertigo, tinnitus: 120–160 mg of standardised leaf extract daily in divided doses.

HERBAL AND NON-HERBAL MEDICINES

Risks

Contraindications

Pregnancy and lactation (see p 5), hypersensitivity to *G. biloba* containing preparations.

Precautions/warnings

Effects in children under 12 years are largely unknown.

Adverse effects

Gastrointestinal disturbances, diarrhoea, vomiting, allergic reactions, pruritus, headache, dizziness, epileptic seizures, Stevens-Johnson syndrome.

Overdose

Excessive ingestion of ginkgo seeds by children (more than 50 seeds) may cause seizures.

Interactions

Potentiation of anticoagulants is often mentioned but a systematic review of the evidence refuted the notion.[28] An additional RCT also found that ginkgo at recommended doses does not affect clotting status, the pharmacokinetics or pharmacodynamics of warfarin in healthy subjects.[29] May have additive effects on antihypertensive drugs, may have additive effects on drugs used in the management of vascular erectile dysfunction.

Quality issues

Evidence in the scientific literature mostly relates to EGb761 (Schwabe, Germany), standardised to 24% ginkgo flavonol glycosides and 6% terpene lactones (3.1% ginkgolide A, B, C and 2.9% bilobalide).

Risk–benefit assessment

The available evidence suggests that ginkgo extract is an effective treatment for peripheral arterial occlusive disease. In the light of its relative safety and the poor compliance with conventional treatment such as regular physical exercise and similarly modest effects of other conventional oral medications, gingko extract seems worthy of consideration. For treating cognitive impairment and dementia, the evidence suggests that ginkgo is effective. The mild nature and rare occurrence of adverse events render ginkgo a reasonable therapeutic option for patients with this condition. Encouraging data are available for sudden hearing loss. For all other indications the evidence is too weak for any firm judgment.

REFERENCES

1   Pittler M H, Ernst E. The efficacy of Ginkgo biloba extract for the treatment of intermittent claudication. A meta-analysis of randomized clinical trials. Am J Med 2000;108: 276–281

2   Horsch S, Walther C. Ginkgo biloba special extract EGb 761 in the treatment of peripheral arterial occlusive disease (PAOD) – A review based on randomized controlled studies. Int J Clin Pharmacol Ther 2004;42:63–72

3   Birks J, Grimley Evans J. Ginkgo biloba for cognitive impairment and dementia. The Cochrane Database of Systematic Reviews 2002, Issue 4. Art. No.: CD003120

4   Haan J, Horr R. Delay in progression of dependency and need of care of dementia patients treated with Ginkgo special extract EGb 761. Wien Med Wochenschr 2004;154:511–514

5   Issing W, Klein P, Weiser M. The homeopathic preparation Vertigoheel versus Ginkgo biloba in the treatment of vertigo in an elderly population: a double-blinded, randomized, controlled clinical trial. J Altern Complement Med 2005;11:155–160

6   Canter P H, Ernst E. Ginkgo biloba: a smart drug? A systematic review of controlled trials of the cognitive effects of ginkgo biloba extracts in healthy people. Psychopharmacol Bull 2002;36: 108–123

7   Solomon P R, Adams F, Silver A, Zimmer J, DeVeaux R. Ginkgo for memory enhancement: A randomized controlled trial. J Am Med Assoc 2002;288:835–840

8   Mattes R D, Pawlik M K. Effects of Ginkgo biloba on alertness and chemosensory function in healthy adults. Hum Psychopharmacol 2004;19: 81–90

9   Cieza A, Maier P Pöppel E. Effects of Ginkgo biloba on mental functioning in healthy volunteers. Arch Med Res 2003;34:373–381

10 Mix J A, Crews Jr W D. A double-blind placebo controlled randomized trial of Ginkgo biloba extract EGb 761 in a sample of cognitively intact older adults: Neuropsychological findings. Hum Psychopharmacol 2002;17:267–277

11 Hartley D E, Heinze L, Elsabagh S, File S E. Effects on cognition and mood in postmenopausal women of 1-week treatment with Ginkgo biloba. Pharmacol Biochem Behav 2003;75:711–720

12 Hilton M, Stuart E. Ginkgo biloba for tinnitus. The Cochrane Database of Systematic Reviews 2004, Issue 2. Art. No.: CD003852

13 Rejali D, Sivakumar A, Balaji N. Ginkgo biloba does not benefit patients with tinnitus: a randomized placebo-controlled double-blind trial and meta-analysis of randomized trials. Clin Otolaryngol 2004;29:226–231

14 Burschka M A, Hassan H A, Reineke T, van Bebber L, Caird D M, Mosges R. Effect of treatment with Ginkgo biloba extract EGb 761 (oral) on unilateral idiopathic sudden hearing loss in a prospective randomized double-blind study of 106 outpatients. Eur Arch Otorhinolaryngol 2001;258:213–219

15 Reisser C H, Weidauer H. Ginkgo biloba extract EGb 761 or pentoxifylline for the treatment of sudden deafness: a randomized, reference-controlled, double-blind study. Acta Otolaryngol 2001;121:579–584

16 Evans J R. Ginkgo biloba extract for age-related macular degeneration. Cochrane Database Syst Rev 1999, Issue 3. Art. No.: CD001775

17 Quaranta L, Bettelli S, Uva M G, Semeraro F, Turano R, Gandolfo E. Effect of Ginkgo biloba extract on preexisting visual field damage in normal tension glaucoma. Ophthalmology 2003;110:359–362

18 Gertsch J H, Seto T B, Mor J, Onopa J. Ginkgo biloba for the prevention of severe acute mountain sickness (AMS) starting one day before rapid ascent. High Alt Med Biol 2002;3:29–37

19 Gertsch J H, Basnyat B, Johnson E W, Onopa J, Holck P S. Randomised, double blind, placebo controlled comparison of ginkgo biloba and acetazolamide for prevention of acute mountain sickness among Himalayan trekkers: the prevention of high altitude illness trial (PHAIT). BMJ 2004,328.797–799

20 Chow T, Browne V, Heileson H L, Wallace D, Anholm J, Green S M. Ginkgo biloba and acetazolamide prophylaxis for acute mountain sickness: a randomized, placebo-controlled trial. Arch Intern Med 2005;165:296–301

21 Parsad D, Pandhi R, Juneja A. Effectiveness of oral Ginkgo biloba in treating limited, slowly spreading vitiligo. Clin Exp Dermatol 2003;28: 285–287

22 Muir A H, Robb R, McLaren M, Daly F, Belch J J. The use of Ginkgo biloba in Raynaud's disease: a double-blind placebo-controlled trial. Vasc Med 2002;7:265–267

23 Zhang X Y, Zhou D F, Zhang P Y, Wu G Y, Su J M, Cao L Y. A double-blind, placebo-controlled trial of extract of Ginkgo biloba added to haloperidol in treatment-resistant patients with schizophrenia. J Clin Psychiatry 2001;62:878–883

24 Kampman K, Majewska M D, Tourian K, Dackis C, Cornish J, Poole S, O'Brien C. A pilot trial of piracetam and ginkgo biloba for the treatment of cocaine dependence. Addict Behav 2003;28: 437–448

25 Lingaerde O, Foreland A R, Magnusson A. Can winter depression be prevented by Ginkgo biloba extract? A placebo-controlled trial. Acta Psychiatr Scand 1999;100:62–66

26 Kang B J, Lee S J, Kim M D, Cho M J. A placebo-controlled, double-blind trial of Ginkgo biloba for antidepressant-induced sexual dysfunction. Hum Psychopharmacol 2002;17:279–284

27 Wheatley D. Triple-blind, placebo-controlled trial of Ginkgo biloba in sexual dysfunction due to antidepressant drugs. Hum Psychopharmacol 2004;19:545–548

HERBAL AND NON-HERBAL MEDICINES

28 Savovic J, Wider B, Ernst E. Effects of Ginkgo biloba on blood coagulation parameters: a systematic review of randomised controlled trials. in press

29 Jiang X, Williams K M, Liauw W S, Ammit A J, Roufogalis B D, Duke C C, Day R O,

McLachlan A J. Effect of ginkgo and ginger on the pharmacokinetics and pharmacodynamics of warfarin in healthy subjects. Br J Clin Pharmacol 2005;59:425–432

GINSENG, ASIAN
(Panax ginseng)

Source	Roots.
Main constituents	Triterpene saponins known as ginsenosides or panaxosides.
Background	Asian ginseng is a perennial herb reaching a height of about 60–80 cm. It is native to the mountain forests of China and Korea. Today, however, it is rarely found in the wild. The common name ginseng is derived from the Chinese *gin* (man) and *seng* (essence) and stands for the ideogram 'crystallisation of the essence of the earth in the form of a man'. The genus name *Panax* is derived from the Greek *pan* (all) and *akos* (cure), which refers to the cure-all or *panacea* quality often attributed to the herb. Ginseng comprises a number of different species, which all belong to the same family, the *Araliaceae*. However, Korean, Japanese and American ginseng belong to the genus *Panax*, whereas Siberian ginseng belongs to the genus *Eleutherococcus*. It is widely available as an over-the-counter food supplement.
Examples of traditional uses	To reduce susceptibility to illness, promote health and longevity and as an aid during convalescence.
Pharmacologic action	Anti-inflammatory, antitumour, immunomodulatory, hypoglycaemic, smooth muscle relaxant and stimulatory.
Conditions frequently treated	Cancer, cardiovascular diseases, diabetes, immune function, sexual function and vitality.
Clinical evidence	A systematic review assessed the clinical evidence from all double-blind RCTs of *P. ginseng* for any indication.[1] The limited number of rigorous clinical trials which could be identified relate to physical performance, psychomotor performance, cognitive function, immunomodulation, type II diabetes mellitus, cancer and herpes simplex type II infections. The review concluded that the effectiveness of *P. ginseng* root extract is not established beyond reasonable doubt for any indication. This conclusion is corroborated by a more recent systematic review[2] and a double-blind

HERBAL AND NON-HERBAL MEDICINES

RCT.[3] *P. ginseng* might improve pulmonary function,[4] health related quality of life[5,6] and memory[7] but has shown no effect on mood and affect in healthy adults,[8] on glycaemic control[9] and on memory and concentration in post-menopausal women.[10] A systematic review of potential cancer-preventative effects concluded that the evidence is not conclusive as to its effects in humans.[11] In a double-blind RCT, *P. ginseng* was found to be superior to placebo for patients with erectile dysfunction on the International Index of Erectile Function.[12] A placebo-controlled RCT assessed 90 patients with erectile dysfunction and suggests beneficial effects for penile rigidity, girth, libido and patient satisfaction compared with Trazodone.[13] Another small (n = 15) double-blind RCT reports positive effects for psychomotor performance in young athletes.[14] A systematic review of the safety profile of *P. ginseng* concluded that monopreparations are rarely associated with adverse events or drug interactions. Documented cases are usually mild and transient. Combined preparations are more often associated with adverse events but causal attribution is usually not possible.[15] These findings are largely corroborated by another independent study.[16]

Dosage

Extract: 100 mg of standardised extract (4% total ginsenosides) two to three times daily.
Root: 0.5–2.0 g of dry root daily in divided doses.

Risks

Contraindications
Pregnancy and lactation (see p 5).

Precautions/warnings
Hypertension, cardiovascular disease, hypotension, diabetes, patients receiving steroid therapy.

Adverse effects
Insomnia, excitability, anxiety, diarrhoea, vaginal bleeding, nosebleeds, mastalgia, increased libido, manic symptoms, skin rash, Stevens–Johnson syndrome, anaphylaxis.

Overdose
'Ginseng abuse syndrome' (dose approximately 3 g daily) with symptoms including hypertension, sleeplessness, skin eruptions, morning diarrhoea, agitation. Doses of 15 g daily and over were associated with depersonalisation, confusion and depression.

Interactions
Monoamine oxidase inhibitors such as phenelzine, may reduce the effects of warfarin, increased effects of hypoglycaemics.

Quality issues
Evidence in the scientific literature mostly relates to G115 standardised ginseng extract (containing 100 mg of a 4% ginsenoside

HERBAL AND NON-
HERBAL MEDICINES

concentration from *Panax ginseng*) and G115S standardised ginseng extract (containing 100 mg of a 7% ginsenoside concentration from *Panax ginseng*). Considerable inconsistencies in terms of active ingredients in commercial preparations exist.

Risk–benefit assessment

The data from rigorous clinical trials suggest that the effectiveness of ginseng root extract from *P. ginseng* is not established beyond reasonable doubt for any indication. The possibility of serious adverse events exists and thus may outweigh any potentially beneficial effects. Therefore, recommendations for the use of *P. ginseng* as a therapeutic intervention cannot, at present, be given.

REFERENCES

1   Vogler B K, Pittler M H, Ernst E. The efficacy of ginseng. A systematic review of randomised clinical trials. Eur J Clin Pharmacol 1999;55:567–575

2   Ernst E. The risk–benefit profile of commonly used herbal therapies: Ginkgo, St. John's wort, ginseng, echinacea, saw palmetto, and kava. Ann Intern Med 2002;136:42–53

3   Engels H J, Fahlman M M, Wirth JC. Effects of ginseng on secretory IgA, performance, and recovery from interval exercise. Med Sci Sports Exerc 2003;35:690–696

4   Gross D, Shenkman Z, Bleiberg B, Dayan M, Gittelson M, Efrat R. Ginseng improves pulmonary functions and exercise capacity in patients with COPD. Monaldi Arch Chest Dis 2002;57:242–246

5   Ellis J M, Reddy P. Effects of Panax ginseng on quality of life. Ann Pharmacother 2002;36:375–379

6   Wiklund I K, Mattsson L A, Lindgren R, Limoni C. Effects of a standardized ginseng extract on quality of life and physiological parameters in symptomatic postmenopausal women: A double-blind, placebo-controlled trial. Int J Clin Pharmacol Res 1999;19:89–99

7   Kennedy D O, Haskell C F, Wesnes K A, Scholey A B. Improved cognitive performance in human volunteers following administration of guarana (Paullinia cupana) extract: comparison and interaction with Panax ginseng. Pharmacol Biochem Behav 2004;79:401–411

8   Cardinal B J, Engels H J. Ginseng does not enhance psychological well-being in healthy, young adults: results of a double-blind, placebo-controlled, randomized clinical trial. J Am Diet Assoc 2001;101:655–660

9   Sievenpiper J L, Arnason J T, Leiter L A, Vuksan V. Null and opposing effects of Asian ginseng (Panax ginseng C.A. Meyer) on acute glycemia: Results of two acute dose escalation studies. J Am Coll Nutr 2003;22:524–532

10 Hartley D E, Elsabagh S, File S E. Gincosan (a combination of Ginkgo biloba and Panax ginseng): the effects on mood and cognition of 6 and 12 weeks' treatment in post-menopausal women. Nutr Neurosci 2004;7:325–333

11 Shin H R, Kim J Y, Yun T K, Morgan G, Vainio H. The cancer-preventive potential of Panax ginseng: A review of human and experimental evidence. Cancer Causes Control 2000;11:565–576

12 Hong B, Ji Y H, Hong J H, Nam K Y, Ahn T Y. A double-blind crosover study evaluating the efficacy of Korean red ginseng in patients with erectile dysfunction: a preliminary report. J Urol 2002;168:2070–2073

13 Choi H K, Seong D H, Rha K H. Clinical efficacy of Korean red ginseng for erectile dysfunction. Int J Impot Res 1995;7:181–186

14 Ziemba A W, Chmura J, Kaciuba-Uscilko H, Nazar K, Wisnik P, Gawronski W. Ginseng treatment improves psychomotor performance in young athletes. Int J Sports Nutr 1999;9:371–377

15 Thompson Coon J, Ernst E. Panax ginseng: A systematic review of adverse effects and drug interactions. Drug Saf 2002;25:323–344

16 Carabin I G, Burdock G A, Chatzidakis C. Safety assessment of Panax ginseng. Int J Toxicol 2000;19:293–301

GINSENG, SIBERIAN
(Eleutherococcus senticosus)

Source	Root.
Main constituents	Eleutherosides (A–G), starch, vitamin A.
Background	Siberian ginseng is a slender shrub native to Siberia and northern China, which grows to a height of about 2–3 m. It belongs to the same family (*Araliaceae*) as Asian ginseng (*Panax ginseng*) but is of a different genus and therefore not considered a true ginseng. It was tested in the former Soviet Union during the 1960s as a substitute for ginseng. In pharmacological studies it was found to exert similar effects to *Panax ginseng* root.
Examples of traditional uses	Adaptogen to increase resistance against environmental stress, aid memory, counteract weakness and fatigue, improve general health and appetite, increase physical performance.
Pharmacologic action	Antioxidant, antiproliferative, hypoglycaemic, immunostimulatory, inhibition of platelet aggregation.
Conditions frequently treated	Boost vitality, cancer, cardiovascular diseases, exercise performance, immune function and sexual function.
Clinical evidence	A systematic review assessed all available double-blind RCTs of Siberian ginseng root extract for any indication.[1] This study identified three trials, which reported positive effects on psychomotor performance and cognitive function and herpes simplex type II infections.[2,3] One study administered 3.4 ml once daily for 6 weeks and reported no intergroup differences on measures of physical performance.[4] Overall, the systematic review concluded that the effectiveness of Siberian ginseng root extract is not established beyond reasonable doubt for any indication. This finding is independently corroborated for physical performance,[5,6] although some positive effects are reported for ergospirometric tests.[7] Some positive effects are also reported for heart rate after a stressful cognitive task[8] and social fuctioning.[9] No improvements in patients with chronic fatigue syndrome are reported compared with placebo.[10]
Dosage	100–200 mg of solid (20:1) extract daily in divided doses.
Risks	***Contraindications*** Pregnancy and lactation (see p 5), hypertension, children under the age of 12 years.

Precautions/warnings

Premenopausal women, fever, mania, schizophrenia, asthma, diabetes, cardiac disorders.

Adverse effects

Dizziness, drowsiness, anxiety, irritability, hypertension, pericardial pain, tachycardia, extrasystoles, insomnia, headaches, mastalgia, diarrhoea.

Overdose

'Ginseng abuse syndrome' (dose approximately 3 g daily) has been reported for Asian ginseng (*Panax ginseng*), which may be sold in combination preparations including Siberian ginseng *(Eleutherococcus senticosus)*. Symptoms include hypertension, sleeplessness, skin eruptions, morning diarrhoea, agitation. Doses of 15 g daily and over were associated with depersonalisation, confusion and depression.

Interactions

May increase the effects of anxiolytic, sedative, antihypoglycaemic and antihyperglycaemic agents, may increase serum digoxin levels, may interact with cardiac, hypo- and hypertensive and anticoagulant agents, may inhibit cytochrome P450 1A2 and P450 2C9.

Quality issues

Evidence in the scientific literature relates mostly to Elagen standardised ginseng extract from *Eleutherococcus senticosus* (eleutherosides B, E) and ESML *Eleutherococcus senticosus* Maxim L extract (including eleutherosides B, E and ethanol 30–34%).

Risk–benefit assessment

The available trial evidence suggests that the effectiveness of Siberian ginseng root extract for any indication is not established beyond reasonable doubt. Thus, considering the possibility of adverse effects, the use of Siberian ginseng as a therapeutic intervention cannot, at present, be recommended.

REFERENCES

1 Vogler B K, Pittler M H, Ernst E. The efficacy of ginseng. A systematic review of randomised clinical trials. Eur J Clin Pharmacol 1999;55:567–575

2 Winther K, Ranløv C, Rein E, Mehlsen J. Russian root (Siberian Ginseng) improves cognitive functions in middle-aged people, whereas Ginkgo biloba seems effective only in the elderly. J Neurol Sci 1997;150:S90

3 Williams M. Immuno-protection against herpes simplex type II infection by eleutherococcus root extract. Int J Alt Complement Med 1995;13:9–12

4 Dowling E A, Redondo D R, Branch J D, Jones S, McNabb G, Williams M H. Effect of Eleutherococcus senticosus on submaximal and maximal exercise performance. Med Sci Sports Exerc 1996;28:482–489

5 Bahrke M S, Morgan W P. Evaluation of the ergogenic properties of ginseng. Sports Med 2000;29:113–133

6 Eschbach L F, Webster M J, Boyd J C, McArthur P D, Evetovich T K. The effect of siberian ginseng (Eleutherococcus senticosus) on substrate utilization and performance. Int J Sport Nutr Exerc Metab 2000;10:444–451

7 Szolomicki J, Samochowiec L, Wojcicki J, Drozdzik M, Szolomicki S. The influence of active components of Eleutherococcus senticosus on cellular defence and physical fitness in man. Phytother Res 2000;14:30–35

8   Facchinetti F, Neri I, Tarabusi M.
    Eleutherococcus senticosus reduces
    cardiovascular stress response in healthy
    subjects: A randomized, placebo-controlled
    trial. Stress & Health 2002;18:11–17
9   Cicero A F, Derosa G, Brillante R, Bernardi R,
    Nascetti S, Gaddi A. Effects of Siberian
    ginseng (Eleutherococcus senticosus maxim.)
    on elderly quality of life: a randomized
    clinical trial. Arch Gerontol Geriatr Suppl
    2004;38:69–73
10 Hartz A J, Bentler S, Noyes R, Hoehns J,
    Logemann C, Sinift S, Butani Y, Wang W,
    Brake K, Ernst M, Kautzman H. Randomized
    controlled trial of Siberian ginseng for
    chronic fatigue. Psychol Med 2004;34:51–61

GLUCOSAMINE

Source

Glucosamine is an amino sugar that occurs naturally in cartilage. It is produced synthetically for the food supplements market.

Background

Glucosamine sulfate is the sulfate salt of 2-amino-2-deoxy-D-chitin glucopyranose which is a constituent of joint cartilage. It was therefore hypothesised that its oral supplementation might enhance cartilage repair. Glucosamine has since become a popular 'natural' treatment for arthritis.

Examples of traditional uses

Joint pain, osteoarthritis.

Pharmacologic action

Increased mucopolysaccharide and collagen production in fibroblasts in vitro, inhibition of enzymes which break down cartilage (e.g. elastase), similar actions to chondroitin (see p 381).

Conditions frequently treated

Osteoarthritis.

Clinical evidence

Numerous trials have investigated the effect of glucosamine in the treatment of osteoarthritis of the knee. Earlier systematic reviews concluded that glucosamine is superior to placebo[1,2] but results from more recent studies are no longer uniformly positive. A Cochrane review[3] assessed 20 studies including 2570 patients. Collectively, the 20 analysed RCTs found glucosamine to be superior to placebo with a 28% improvement in pain and a 21% improvement in function from baseline using the Lequesne index. WOMAC pain, function and stiffness outcomes did not reach statistical significance. When only the studies with adequate allocation concealment were analysed (n = 8), the results failed to show benefit of glucosamine for pain and WOMAC function.

Two RCTs investigated the effect of glucosamine in the treatment of temperomandibular joint disorders; one found glucosamine to be at least as effective as analgesic doses of ibuprofen on function and pain,[4] and one using a glucosamine/chondroitin combination was inconclusive.[5]

Effects of glucosamine in glycaemic control were investigated in two RCTs; one concluded that glucosamine supplementation did not cause glucose intolerance in healthy adults[6] and one found that glucosamine supplementation did not result in clinically significant alterations in glucose metabolism in elderly patients with type 2 diabetes mellitus.[7] Another RCT found poly-N-acetyl glucosamine patches to improve haemostasis at the arterial puncture site in patients undergoing cardiac catheterisation.[8]

Dosage

500 mg of glucosamine sulfate three times daily.

Risks

Contraindications
Pregnancy and lactation (see p 5).

Precautions/warnings
Avoid use in children under the age of 2 years, in patients with asthma, or shell fish allergies. Although initial concerns about use in diabetic patients based on in vitro and rat studies were not confirmed in human studies[4,5] it is advisable to monitor these patients closely.

Adverse effects
Mild gastrointestinal complaints including nausea, heartburn, diarrhoea, and constipation, drowsiness, dyspepsia, headache, rash.

Interactions
None known.

Quality issues
Both glucosamine sulfate and hydrochloride are used; it is unclear which is superior.

Risk–benefit assessment

There is some evidence from RCTs that glucosamine (sulfate) is superior to placebo in the treatment of osteoarthritis although more recent results are no longer unanimously positive and only show a benefit in Lequesne index. Best results have been reported for mild to moderate osteoarthritis of the knee. A number of studies also suggest that it is similarly effective as ibuprofen but longer treatment periods are needed (e.g. 4 weeks and longer) for a clinical benefit to become manifest. The size of the clinical effect is usually moderate. Glucosamine seems to be well tolerated for up to three years and no major safety problems are on record. Thus glucosamine can be recommended as an adjuvant therapy for osteoarthritis.

REFERENCES

1 Richy F, Bruyere O, Ethgen O, Cucherat M, Henrotin Y, Reginster J Y. Structural and symptomatic efficacy of glucosamine and chondroitin in knee osteoarthritis: a comprehensive meta-analysis. Arch Intern Med 2003;163:1514–1522

2 McAlindon T E, LaValley M P, Gulin J P, Felson D T. Glucosamine and chondroitin for treatment of osteoarthritis: a systematic quality assessment and meta-analysis. JAMA 2000;283:1469–1475

3 Towheed T E, Maxwell L, Anastassiades T P, Shea B, Houpt J, Robinson V, Hochberg M C, Wells G. Glucosamine therapy for treating osteoarthritis. The Cochrane Database of Systematic Reviews 2005, Issue 2. Art. No.: CD002946

4 Thie N M, Prasad N G, Major P W. Evaluation of glucosamine sulfate compared to ibuprofen for the treatment of temporomandibular joint osteoarthritis: a randomized double blind

controlled 3 month clinical trial. J Rheumatol 2001;28:1347–1355

5 Nguyen P, Mohamed S E, Gardiner D, Salinas T. A randomized double-blind clinical trial of the effect of chondroitin sulfate and glucosamine hydrochloride on temporomandibular joint disorders: a pilot study. Cranio 2001;19:130–139

6 Tannis A J, Barban J, Conquer J A. Effect of glucosamine supplementation on fasting and non-fasting plasma glucose and serum insulin concentrations in healthy individuals. Osteoarthritis Cartilage 2004;12:506–511

7 Monauni T, Zenti M G, Cretti A, Daniels M C, Targher G, Caruso B, Caputo M, McClain D, Del Prato S, Giaccari A, Muggeo M, Bonora E, Bonadonna R C. Effects of glucosamine infusion on insulin secretion and insulin action in humans. Diabetes 2000;49:926–935

8 Najjar S F, Healey N A, Healey C M, McGarry T, Khan B, Thatte H S, Khuri S F. Evaluation of poly-N-acetyl glucosamine as a hemostatic agent in patients undergoing cardiac catheterization: a double-blind, randomized study. J Trauma 2004;57(1 Suppl):S38–S41

GRAPE
(Vitis vinifera)

Source — Fruits, skin, seeds and leafs.

Main constituents — Flavonoids, fruit acids, polyphenols (oligomeric proanthocyanidins, procyanidins), tannins, tocopherols.

Background — A mounting body of (mostly epidemiological) evidence suggests that wine has a protective effect on arteriosclerotic diseases. The effect is thought to be due to polyphenols which are highly concentrated in grapeseeds. The 'French paradox', i.e. the fact that, in spite of high levels of saturated fat consumption, the cardiovascular morbidity and mortality are relatively low in France, has been explained by the regular intake of red wine.[1] Others have suggested, however, that the cardioprotective effects are not specific to red wine but relate to regular, moderate alcohol consumption (e.g.[2,3]). Nevertheless, grapeseed extracts are being promoted for their alleged health effects.

Examples of traditional uses — *Seeds and leafs:* vascular or circulatory disorders. *Fruit:* coronary heart disease.

Pharmacologic action — Antioxidant, antimutagenic, anti-inflammatory, astringent, laxative, vasorelaxant.

Conditions frequently treated — Cancer, prevention of arteriosclerotic diseases.

Clinical evidence — A meta-analysis of 13 studies involving 209 418 participants found an inverse association between light to moderate wine consumption and vascular risk up to a daily intake of 150 ml of wine. A similar, although smaller association was also apparent in beer consumption studies.[3] A meta-analysis of prospective

HERBAL AND NON-HERBAL MEDICINES

cohort studies assessing the association of dietary flavonol intake with the subsequent risk of coronary heart disease mortality indicated that high dietary intake of flavonols from (amongst others) red wine may be associated with a reduced risk from coronary heart disease mortality.[4]

A double-blind RCT compared grape seed extract with chromium polynicotinate, a combination of the two, and placebo in the treatment of hypercholesterolaemic patients. It found that the combination of grape seed extract and chromium polynicotinate decreased total cholesterol and low-density lipoprotein levels compared with baseline.[5] Moderate alcohol compared with grape juice intake increased serum low-density lipoprotein cholesterol levels and stimulated cellular cholesterol efflux in postmenopausal women.[6] An RCT of the effect of moderate alcohol consumption of red wine on lipoprotein metabolism showed an increase compared with red grape juice in overall low-density lipoprotein cholesterol in postmenopausal women and a reduction of the plasma low-density lipoprotein cholesterol level in premenopausal women using oral contraceptives.[7] An RCT investigating the effects of grape seed extract in heavy smokers reported no effects on total, low-density lipoprotein and low-density lipoprotein cholesterol but some preliminary evidence for oxidative stress.[8] A small RCT (n = 15) found no effects of grape skin extract on markers of oxidative status but reduced plasma vitamin C and plasma 2-aminoadipic saemialdehyde residues.[9]

The effect of grape seed extract on 24 h energy intake in humans was investigated in a placebo-controlled double-blind RCT which reported a decreased energy intake in a subgroup of normal to overweight subjects but no effect on any other eating patterns.[10] An RCT (n = 40) investigating the effects of moderate consumption of white wine on the effectiveness of an energy-restricted diet in overweight and obese subjects found a diet with 10% of energy derived from white wine as effective as an isocaloric diet with 10% of energy derived from grape juice.[11]

Daily moderate amounts of red wine and red grape juice had no effect on the immune system of healthy men (n = 24).[12]

A placebo-controlled double-blind RCT found grape seed extract not to be beneficial in the treatment of seasonal allergic rhinitis[13] and a controlled crossover trial reported no support for the use of aromatherapy with the oils of lavender, thyme and grape seed to decrease agitation in severely demented patients.[14]

One placebo-controlled RCT found an extract of the leaf of red vine to be effective in mild chronic venous insufficiency compared with baseline.[15]

Dosage

Seed: 40–80 mg of extract once daily.
Leaf: 360–720 mg of red vine leaf extract daily.

Risks

Contraindications
Pregnancy and lactation (see p 5), allergies to grapes.

Precautions/warnings
None known.

Adverse effects
Dry itchy scalp, headache, dizziness and nausea with grape seed.

Overdose
Excessive consumption of grapes might cause diarrhoea due to laxative effects.

Interactions
Theoretically increases the risk of bleeding when used with anti-coagulants or antiplatelet drugs.[16] A significant interaction between grape seed and vitamin C for effects on blood pressure has been reported.[17]

Quality issues
Use extracts with standardised polyphenol content.

Risk–benefit assessment
Mainly cohort studies report an association between moderate alcohol consumption and reduced cardiovascular risk. It is however not clear whether grape seeds or moderate alcohol consumption in general are responsible for the effects; our understanding of grape seed extract is therefore not sufficient to make any recommendations. The results for red vine leaf in mild to moderate chronic venous insufficiency are encouraging but further data are required.

REFERENCES

1 Renaud S C, Gueguen R, Siest G, Salamon R. Wine, beer and mortality in middle-age men from Eastern France. Arch Intern Med 1999;159:1865–1870

2 Rimm E B, Williams P, Fosher K, Griqui M, Stampfer M J. Moderate alcohol intake and lower risk of coronary heart disease: a meta-analysis of effects on lipids and haemostatic factors. BMJ 1999;319:1523–1528

3 de Gaetano G, Di Castelnuovo A, Rotondo S, Iacoviello L, Donati M B. A meta-analysis of studies on wine and beer and cardiovascular disease. Pathophysiol Haemost Thromb 2002;32:353–355

4 Huxley R R, Neil H A. The relation between dietary flavonol intake and coronary heart disease mortality: a meta-analysis of prospective cohort studies. Eur J Clin Nutr 2003; 57:904–908

5 Preuss H G, Wallerstedt D, Talpur N, Tutuncuoglu S O, Echard B, Myers A, Bui M, Bagchi D. Effects of niacin-bound chromium and grape seed proanthocyanidin extract on the lipid profile of hypercholesterolemic subjects: a pilot study. J Med 2000;31:227–246

6 Sierksma A, Vermunt S H, Lankhuizen I M, van der Gaag M S, Scheek L M, Grobbee D E, van Tol A, Hendriks H F. Effect of moderate alcohol consumption on parameters of reverse cholesterol transport in postmenopausal women. Alcohol Clin Exp Res 2004;28:662–666

7 van der Gaag M S, Sierksma A, Schaafsma G, van Tol A, Geelhoed-Mieras T, Bakker M, Hendriks H F. Moderate alcohol consumption and changes in postprandial lipoproteins of premenopausal and postmenopausal women: a diet-controlled, randomized intervention study. J Womens Health Gend Based Med 2000;9:607–616

8 Vigna G B, Costantini F, Aldini G, Carini M, Catapano A, Schena F, Tangerini A, Zanca R, Bombardelli E, Morazzoni P, Mezzetti A, Fellin R, Maffei Facino R. Effect of a standardized grape seed extract on low-density lipoprotein susceptibility to oxidation in heavy smokers. Metabolism 2003;52:1250–1257

9 Young J F, Dragsted L O, Daneshvar B, Lauridsen S T, Hansen M, Sandstrom B. The effect of grape-skin extract on oxidative status. Br J Nutr 2000;84:505–513

10 Vogels N, Nijs I M T, Westerterp-Plantenga MS. The effect of grape-seed extract on 24 h energy intake in humans. Eur J Clin Nutr 2004;58:667–673

11 Flechtner-Mors M, Biesalski H K, Jenkinson CP, Adler G, Ditschuneit H H. Effects of moderate consumption of white wine on weight loss in overweight and obese subjects. Int J Obes Relat Metab Disord 2004;28:1420–1426

12 Watzl B, Bub A, Pretzer G, Roser S, Barth S W, Rechkemmer G. Daily moderate amounts of red wine or alcohol have no effect on the immune system of healthy men. Eur J Clin Nutr 2004;58:40–45

13 Bernstein D I, Bernstein C K, Deng C, Murphy K J, Bernstein I L, Bernstein J A, Shukla R. Evaluation of the clinical efficacy and safety of grapeseed extract in the treatment of fall seasonal allergic rhinitis: a pilot study. Ann Allergy Asthma Immunol 2002;88:272–278

14 Snow L A, Hovanec L, Brandt J. A controlled trial of aromatherapy for agitation in nursing home patients with dementia. J Altern Complement Med 2004;10:431–437

15 Kiesewetter H, Koscielny J, Kalus U, Vix J M, Peil H, Petrini O, van Toor B S, de Mey C. Efficacy of orally administered extract of red vine leaf AS 195 (folia vitis viniferae) in chronic venous insufficiency (stages I-II). A randomized, double-blind, placebo-controlled trial. Arzneimittelforschung 2000;50:109–117

16 Keevil J G, Osman H E, Reed J D, Folts J D. Grape juice, but not orange juice or grapefruit juice, inhibits human platelet aggregation. J Nutr 2000;130:53–56

17 Ward N C, Hodgson J M, Croft K D, Burke V, Beilin L J, Puddey I B. The combination of vitamin C and grape-seed polyphenols increases blood pressure: a randomized, double-blind, placebo-controlled trial. J Hypertens 2005;23: 427–434

GREEN TEA
(Camellia sinensis)

Source	Leaves.
Main constituents	Caffeine, polyphenols (e.g. epigallocatechin and epigallocatechin-3-gallate).
Background	The tea plant is native to East Asia. Tea has been used as a refreshing beverage for millennia. Black, oolong and green teas are made from the same plant and differ according to the curing method of the leaves. Green tea has more powerful medicinal effects which have recently become the subject of intense research.
Examples of traditional uses	As a beverage and stimulant.
Pharmacologic action	Antibacterial, antimutagenic, anticarcinogenic, antioxidant, antiangiogenic, cholesterol-lowering, inhibition of cell proliferation and tumour promotion and lipid-peroxidation as well as stimulation of the central nervous system.[1]
Conditions frequently treated	Adjuvant treatment for AIDS, prevention of cancer, cardiovascular diseases and tumour progression.
Clinical evidence	A systematic review of its anticancer effects was based mostly on epidemiological data and included 31 human studies. Its conclusions were cautiously positive.[2] When 21 epidemiological investiga-

tions were submitted to a systematic review, protective effects were found on adematous polyps and chronic atrophic gastritis; no clear evidence emerged that green tea protects against stomach or intestinal cancer.[3] Recent epidemiological data suggest a role of green tea in the prevention of both breast[4] and ovarian cancer.[5] Other epidemiological studies showed strong inverse associations of tea intake with aortic arteriosclerosis[6] and cardiovascular risk factors.[7,8]

A small CCT with 83 asymptomatic carriers of the human T-cell lymphotropic virus type 1, which is causally associated with adult T-cell leukaemia, showed that 5 months intake of a green tea extract reduced the virus load.[9] Fifty-one patients with cervical human papilloma virus infections were either treated with oral green tea extracts plus green tea ointment or left untreated for 12 weeks. The response rate (69 vs 10%) favoured green tea.[10]

Forty-seven patients with gingivitis were randomised to receive green tea extract or placebo for 21 days. The inflammation was significantly more reduced in the experimental group.[11] Similar results emerged from a small CCT which also suggested the effect to be related to the antibacterial activity of green tea.[12] A large (n = 240) RCT showed that 12 weeks of green tea extract normalised the lipid pattern in hypercholesterolaemia men.[13] However, a small (n = 13) RCT failed to demonstrate that 1000 ml of green tea consumed daily for 4 weeks inhibits in vivo lipid peroxidation.[14] Another RCT tested the effect of green tea versus placebo in 104 overweight volunteers. The results did not suggest a positive effect on body weight.[15] However, the consumption of green tea seems to lead to a sympathetic activation of thermogenesis[16] and energy expenditure.[17] The notion that green tea might be an effective adjuvant for treating AIDS is so far only hypothetical.[18]

Dosage

Tea: 6–10 cups daily.
Capsules: Three capsules of standardised extract daily in divided doses.

Risks

Contraindications
Pregnancy and lactation (see p 5), known allergy.

Precautions/warnings
None known.

Adverse effects
Gastrointestinal complaints, insomnia.

Interactions
None known.

Quality issues
Standardised extracts or infusion should be used.

Risk–benefit assessment

According to epidemiological data, green tea might be an effective preventive agent for cancer and cardiovascular disease. RCTs and CCTs suggest that green tea may reduce the inflammation in gingivitis and normalise blood lipids. There are few serious safety concerns. A risk–benefit assessment therefore arrives at a cautiously positive conclusion.

REFERENCES

1 Koo M W L, Cho C H. Pharmacological effects of green tea on the gastrointestinal system. Eur J Pharmacol 2004;500:177–185

2 Bushman J L. Green tea and cancer in humans: a review of the literature. Nutr Cancer 1998;31:151–159

3 Borrelli F, Capasso R, Russo A, Ernst E. Systematic review: green tea and gastrointestinal cancer risk. Aliment Pharmacol Ther 2004;19:497–510

4 Wu A H, Yu M C, Tseng C C, Hankin J, Pike M C. Green tea and risk of breast cancer in Asian Americans. Int J Cancer 2003;106:574–579

5 Zhang M, Binns C W, Lee A H. Tea consumption and ovarian cancer risk: a case-control study in China. Cancer Epidemiol Biomarkers Prev 2002;11:713–718

6 Geleijnse J M, Launer L J, Hofman A, Pols H A P, Witterman J C M. Tea flavonoids may protect against atherosclerosis. Arch Intern Med 1999;159:2170–2174

7 Imai K, Nakachi K. Cross sectional study of effects of drinking green tea on cardiovascular and liver diseases. Br Med J 1995;310:693–695

8 Trevisanato S I, Kim Y-I. Tea and health. Nutr Rev 2000;58:1–10

9 Sonoda J, Koriyama C, Yamamoto S, Kozako T, Li H C, Lema C, Yashiki S, Fujiyoshi T, Yoshinaga M, Nagata Y, Akiba S, Takezaki T, Yamada K, Sonoda S. HTLV-1 provirus load blood lymphocytes of HTLV-1 carriers is diminished by green tea drinking. Cancer Sci 2004;95:596–601

10 Ahn W S, Yoo J, Huh S W, Kim C K, Lee J M, Namkoong S E, Bae S M, Lee I P. Protective effects of green tea extracts (polyphenon E and EGCG) on human cervical lesions. Eur J Cancer Prev 2003;12:383–390

11 Krahwinkel T, Willershausen B. The effect of sugar-free green tea chew candies on the degree of inflammation of the gingiva. Eur J Med Res 2000;5:463–467

12 Hirasawa M, Takada K, Maimura M, Otake S. Improvement of periodontal status by green tea catechin using a local delivery system: a clinical pilot study. J Periodontal Res 2002;37:433–438

13 Maron D J, Lu G P, Cai N S, Wu Z G, Li Y H, Chen H, Zhu J Q, Jin X J, Wouters B C, Zhao J. Cholesterol-lowering effect of a theaflavin-enriched green tea extract: a randomized controlled trial. Arch Intern Med 2003;163: 1448–1453

14 Hodgson J M, Croft K D, Mori T A, Burke V, Beilin L J, Puddey I B. Regular ingestion of tea does not inhibit in vivo lipid peroxidation in humans. J Nutr 2002;132:55–58

15 Kovacs E, Lejeune M, Nijs I, Weterterp-Plantenga MS. Effects of green tea on weight maintenance after body-weight loss. Br J Nutr 2004;91:431–437

16 Dulloo AG, Duret C, Rohrer D, Girardier L, Mensi N, Fathi M, Chantre P, Vandermander J. Efficacy of a green tea extract rich in catechin polyphenols and caffeine in increasing 24-h energy expenditure and fat oxidation in humans. Am J Clin Nutr 1999;70:1040–1045

17 Komatsu T, Nakamori M, Komatsu K, Hosoda K, Okamura M, Toyama K, Ishikura Y, Sakai T, Kunii D, Yamamoto S. Oolong tea increases energy metabolism in Japanese females. J Med Invest 2003;50:170–175

18 McCarthy M F. Natural antimutagenic agents may prolong efficacy of human immunodeficiency virus drug therapy. Med Hypotheses 1997;48:215–220

GUAR GUM
(*Cyamopsis tetragonolobus*)

Source   Seeds.

Main constituents   Galactomannan, lipids, proteins, saponins.

Background   Guar gum is a non-absorbable dietary fibre derived from the seeds of the Indian cluster bean (*Cyamopsis tetragonolobus* L). It is obtained from the grinding of the seed albumen and is a white to yellowish powder. *Cyamopsis tetragonolobus* is cultivated mainly in India and Pakistan during the months of July to December. It is also grown in Australia, South Africa and the USA and is widely used by the food industry as a thickening agent.

Examples of traditional uses   Diabetes, hyperlipidaemia, weight reduction.

Pharmacologic action   Antihyperglycaemic, laxative, lipid lowering.

Conditions frequently treated   Constipation, diabetes, diarrhoea, hypercholesterolaemia, obesity.

Clinical evidence   Guar gum has been the subject of a large number of RCTs. A Cochrane review assessed the effects for treating cholestasis of pregnancy.[1] It identified one trial, which assessed guar gum versus placebo and reported no differences in pruritus and bile salts. A meta analysis of RCTs assessing its hypolipidaemic effects concluded that guar gum reduces total and low-density lipoprotein cholesterol levels by a relatively small amount.[2] These findings are supported by a further RCT.[3] It has also been suggested as a treatment to reduce body weight. A meta-analysis,[4] and a subsequently published RCT,[5] however, concluded that the evidence does not support the use of guar gum for this indication. Several relatively small double-blind RCTs suggested beneficial effects of guar gum on blood glucose levels in healthy subjects[6–8] and type II diabetic patients.[9–12] RCTs also reported positive evidence for type I diabetes,[13] uncomplicated duodenal ulcer,[14] dumping syndrome,[15] irritable bowel syndrome,[16] acute childhood diarrhoea,[17,18] diarrhoea in septic patients,[19] and postprandial blood pressure.[20,21]

Dosage   15–30 g of flour or granulated guar gum daily in divided doses.

Risks   ***Contraindications***
Pregnancy and lactation (see p 5), intestinal obstruction, oesophageal disease.

HERBAL AND NON-HERBAL MEDICINES

Precautions/warnings

Should be taken with adequate amounts of fluid.

Adverse effects

Flatulence, diarrhoea and abdominal distension, nausea, hypo-glycaemic symptoms.

Interactions

May potentiate the effects of antiglycaemic drugs, reduce absorption of acetaminophen (paracetamol), nitrofurantoin, digoxin and penicillin; may slow the absorption of oral contra-ceptives.

Quality issues

Composition and purity of the extract may vary.

Risk–benefit assessment

Guar gum is beneficial for lowering total serum cholesterol and low-density lipoprotein cholesterol levels. The effect, however, is small and the possibility of adverse effects and drug interactions exists, which may outweigh its modest benefits. The data for blood glucose levels in type II diabetic patients and for postprandial blood pressure are encouraging but more data are still required. For all other indications the available evidence is not compelling.

REFERENCES

1 Burrows R F, Clavisi O, Burrows E. Interventions for treating cholestasis in pregnancy. The Cochrane Database of Systematic Reviews 2001, Issue 4. Art. No.: CD000493

2 Brown L, Rosner B, Willet W W, Sacks F M. Cholesterol-lowering effects of dietary fiber: a meta-analysis. Am J Clin Nutr 1999;69:30–42

3 Tai E S, Fok A C, Chu R, Tan C E. A study to assess the effect of dietary supplementastion with a soluble fibre (Minolest) on lipid levels in normal subjects with hypercholesterolaemia. Ann Acad Med Singapore 1999;28:209–213

4 Pittler M H, Ernst E. Guar gum for body weight reduction. Meta-analysis of randomized trials. Am J Med 2001;110:724–730

5 Kovacs E M R, Westerterp-Plantenga M S, Saris W H M, Melanson K J, Goossens I, Geurten P, Brouns F. Associations between spontaneous meal initiations and blood glucose dynamics in overweight men in negative energy balance. Br J Nutr 2002;87:39–45

6 Kovacs E M R, Westerterp-Plantenga M S, Saris W H M, Melanson K J, Goossens I, Geurten P, Brouns F. The effect of guar gum addition to a semisolid meal on appetite related to blood glucose, in dieting men. Eur J Clin Nutr 2002;56:771–777

7 Sierra M, Garcia J J, Fernández N, Diez M J, Calle A P, Sahagún A M. Effects of ispaghula husk and guar gum on postprandial glucose and insulin concentrations in healthy subjects. Eur J Clin Nutr 2001;55:235–243

8 Wolf B W, Wolever T M S, Lai C S, Bolognesi C, Radmard R, Maharry K S, Garleb K A, Hertzler S R, Firkins J L. Effects of a beverage containing an enzymatically induced-viscosity dietary fiber, with or without fructose, on the postprandial glycemic response to a high glycemic index food in humans. Eur J Clin Nutr 2003;57: 1120–1127

9 Fuessl H S, Williams G, Adrian T E, Bloom S R. Guar sprinkled on food: effect on glycaemic control, plasma lipids and gut hormones in non-insulin-dependent diabetic patients. Diabet Med 1987;4:463–468

10 Uusitupa M, Tuomilehto J, Karttunen P, Wolf E. Long term effects of guar gum on metabolic control, serum cholesterol and blood pressure levels in type 2 (non-insulin-dependent) diabetic patients with high blood pressure. Ann Clin Res 1984;16(suppl 43):126–131

11 Uusitupa M, Siitonen O, Savolainen K, Silvasti M, Penttilä I, Parviainen M. Metabolic and nutritional effects of long-term use of guar gum in the treatment of noninsulin-

dependent diabetes of poor metabolic control. Am J Clin Nutr 1989;49:345–351

12 Uusitupa M, Södervik H, Sivasti M, Karttunen P. Effects of a gel forming dietary fiber, guar gum, on the absorption of glibenclamide and metabolic control and serum lipids in patients with non-insulin dependent (type 2) diabetes. Int J Clin Pharmacol Ther Toxicol 1990; 28:153–157

13 Ebeling P, Yki-Järvinen H, Aro A, Helve E, Sinisalo M, Koivisto V A. Glucose and lipid metabolism and insulin sensitivity in type 1 diabetes: the effect of guar gum. Am J Clin Nutr 1988;48:98–103

14 Harju E J, Larmi T K. Effect of guar gum added to the diet of patients with duodenal ulcer. J Parenteral Enteral Nutr 1985;9:496–500

15 Harju E J, Larmi T K. Efficacy of guar gum in preventing the dumping syndrome. J Parenteral Enteral Nutr 1983;7:470–472

16 Parisi G C, Zilli M, Miani M P, Carrara M, Bottona E, Verdianelli G, Battaglia G, Desideri S, Faedo A, Marzolino C, Tonon A, Ermani M, Leandro G. High-fiber diet supplementation in patients with irritable bowel syndrome (IBS): a multicenter, randomized, open trial comparison between wheat bran diet and partially hydrolyzed

guar gum (PHGG). Dig Dis Sci 2002;47:1697–1704

17 Alam N H, Meier R, Schneider H, Sarker SA, Bardhan P K, Mahalanabis D, Fuchs G J, Gyr N. Partially hydrolyzed guar gum-supplemented oral rehydration solution in the treatment of acute diarrhea in children. J Pediatr Gastroenterol Nutr 2000;31:503–507

18 Alam N H, Meier R, Sarker S A, Bardhan P K, Schneider H, Gyr N. Partially hydrolysed guar gum supplemented comminuted chicken diet in persistent diarrhoea: a randomised controlled trial. Arch Dis Child 2005;90:195–199

19 Spapen H, Diltoer M, Van Malderen C, Opdenacker G, Suys E, Huyghens L. Soluble fiber reduces the incidence of diarrhea in septic patients receiving total enteral nutrition: A prospective, double-blind, randomized, and controlled trial. Clin Nutr 2001;20:301–305

20 Jones K L, MacIntosh C, Su Y C, Wells E, Chapman I M, Tonkin A, Horowitz M. Guar gum reduces postprandial hypotension in older people. J Am Geriatr Soc 2001;49:162–167

21 Russo A, Stevens J E, Wilson T, Wells F, Tonkin A, Horowitz M, Jones K L. Guar attenuates fall in postprandial blood pressure and slows gastric emptying of oral glucose in type 2 diabetes. Dig Dis Sci 2003;48: 1221–1229

HAWTHORN
(*Crataegus* spp)

Source	Flowers, leaves and berries. *Crataegus* species found in hawthorn preparations include mainly *C. laevigata* and *C. monogyna*.
Main constituents	Catechin, epicatechin, flavonoids (quercetin, hyperoside, vitexin, rutin), procyanidins.
Background	About 300 *Crataegus* species exist which are native to temperate regions of North America, Asia and Europe. *Crataegus* has been praised for its heart-strengthening properties since the first century. Systematic investigation of this plant started in the early part of the 20th century. Today it is a popular herbal cardiac medication particularly in Germany.
Examples of traditional uses	For 'strengthening' the heart and other cardiovascular conditions.
Pharmacologic actions	Dilation of coronary arteries, positive inotropic, decrease of atrio-ventricular conduction time and increase of refractory period, cardioprotective, anti-arrhythmic, hypotensive, beta-blocking

HERBAL AND NON-HERBAL MEDICINES

and ACE-inhibiting activity, antioxidant, central nervous system depressant. The mechanism of action is similar to digitalis.

Conditions frequently treated

Congestive heart failure (New York Heart Association (NYHA) stages I and II).

Clinical evidence

In a meta-analysis,[1] eight double-blind placebo-controlled RCTs of patients with chronic heart failure stage I to III NYHA provided data, which were suitable for statistical pooling. In all of these RCTs monoextract of hawthorn leaves and flowers were used. For maximal workload an effect was found in favour of hawthorn extract (n = 310). The pressure-heart rate product showed a beneficial decrease in favour of hawthorn (n = 329). Symptoms such as dyspnoea and fatigue improved. These findings are largely corroborated in two double-blind RCTs testing the effects of fresh Crataegus berries.[2,3] One RCT compared 900 mg hawthorn extract with 37.5 mg Captopril per day in 132 patients with NYHA II heart failure.[4] The results suggested that the regimens were similarly effective in increasing work capacity. Hawthorn extract has also been tested in patients with mild hypertension[5] and in combination with camphor in orthostatic hypotension[6] with mixed results. A double-blind RCT of *Crataegus curvisepala* Lind. suggested some positive effects in primary mild hypertension.[7] Another double-blind RCT tested a combination preparation of *Crataegus oxyxantha* and *Eschscholtzia californica* and found beneficial effects for patients with mild to moderate anxiety for the total score on the Hamilton anxiety scale.[8] An interaction study[9] and two large post-marketing surveillance studies reported excellent tolerability.[10,11]

Dosage

900 mg standardised (2.2% flavonoids or 18.75% oligomeric procyanidines) extract daily.

Risks

Contraindications
Pregnancy and lactation (see p 5), allergy to plants from the *Rosaceae* family.

Precautions/warnings
Sedation, hypotension or arrhythmias with high doses; hawthorn should only be used under medical supervision.

Adverse effects
Nausea, dizziness, vertigo, fatigue, sweating, palpitations, tachycardia, gastrointestinal complaints.

Overdose
Respiratory failure.

Interactions
Additive effects with antihypertensive drugs, nitrates, cardiac glycosides and central nervous system depressants.

Quality issues
Only standardised products should be used.

Risk–benefit assessment

The data for chronic heart failure (NYHA I–II) suggest that there is benefit over placebo from hawthorn extract as an adjunctive treatment for chronic heart failure. Its safety profile is encouraging. There is also some preliminary evidence to show that the effect size is similar to that of conventional drugs. It can therefore be cautiously recommended for this indication in patients who insist on a herbal alternative to effective synthetic drugs. However, due to the nature of the condition, close medical supervision seems essential. Hawthorn cannot be recommended for NYHA stage III and IV. For other indications the evidence from rigorous clinical trials is not sufficient for any firm recommendations.

REFERENCES

1 Pittler M H, Schmidt K, Ernst E. Hawthorn extract for treating chronic heart failure. Meta-analysis of randomized trials. Am J Med 2003;114:665–674

2 Degenring F H, Suter A, Weber M, Saller R. A randomised double blind placebo controlled clinical trial of a standardised extract of fresh Crataegus berries (Crataegisan) in the treatment of patients with congestive heart failure NYHA II. Phytomedicine 2003;10:363–369

3 Rietbrock N, Hamel M, Hempel B, Mitrovic V, Schmidt T, Wolf G K. Wirksamkeit eines standardisierten Extraktes aus frischen Crataegus-Beeren auf Belastungstoleranz und Lebensqualität bei Patienten mit Herzinsuffizienz (NYHA II). Arzneimittelforschung 2001;51:793–798

4 Tauchert M, Ploch M, Hübner W D. Wirksamkeit des Weißdorn-Extraktes LI 132 im Vergleich mit Captopril – Multizentrische Doppelblindstudie bei 132 Patienten mit Herzinsuffizienz im Stadium II nach NYHA. Münch Med Wschr 1994;136(Suppl 136/I Feb):27–32

5 Walker A F, Marakis G, Morris A P, Robinson P A. Promising hypotensive effect of hawthorn extract: a randomized double-blind pilot study of mild, essential hypertension. Phytother Res 2002;16:48–54

6 Belz G G, Butzer R, Gaus W, Loew D. Camphor-Crataegus berry extract combination dose-dependently reduces tilt induced fall in blood pressure in orthostatic hypotension. Phytomedicine 2002; 9:581–588

7 Asgary S, Naderi G H, Sadeghi M, Kelishadi R, Amiri M. Antihypertensive effect of Iranian Crataegus curvisepala Lind.: a randomized, double-blind study. Drugs Exp Clin Res 2004;30:221–225

8 Hanus M, Lafon J, Mathieu M. Double-blind, randomised, placebo-controlled study to evaluate the efficacy and safety of a fixed combination containing two plant extracts (Crataegus oxyacantha and Eschscholtzia californica) and magnesium in mild-to-moderate anxiety disorders. Curr Med Res Opin 2004;20:63–71

9 Tankanow R, Tamer H R, Streetman D S, Smith S G, Welton J L, Annesley T, Aaronson K D, Bleske B E. Interaction study between digoxin and a preparation of hawthorn (Crataegus oxyacantha). J Clin Pharmacol 2003;43:637–642

10 Schmidt U, Albrecht M, Podzuweit H, Ploch M, Maisenbacher J. Hochdosierte Crataegus-Therapie bei herzinsuffizienten Patienten NYHA-Stadium I und II. Zeitschrift für Phytotherapie 1998;19:22–30

11 Tauchert M, Gildor A, Lipinski J. Einsatz des hochdosierten Crataegusextraktes WS 1442 in der Therapie der Herzinsuffizienz Stadium. Herz 1999;24:465–474

HOP
(Humulus lupulus)

Source	Female flowering parts (strobiles).
Main constituents	Chalcones, flavonoids, oleo-resin (e.g. alpha-bitter acids including humulone, beta-bitter acids including lupulone), tannins, volatile oils.
Background	A climbing perennial herb belonging to the *Cannabaceae* family, hop is found in marshy areas throughout Asia, the United States and Europe. As well as being crucial to the brewing industry, hop has a long history of use as a sedative. This potential use was first identified from observations that hop-pickers became easily fatigued, possibly from inhaling the volatile oil from the plants. Hop pillows were widely used in traditional folk medicine.
Examples of traditional uses	Excitability, indigestion, insomnia, neuralgia restlessness.
Pharmacologic action	Sedative, antimicrobial.
Conditions frequently treated	Insomnia, nervous tension, restlessness.
Clinical evidence	There are no controlled trials of hops as a monopreparation. The effects on sleep have been assessed in combination products with valerian (see p 468).[1-6] Although these trials have suggested possible hypnotic effects, only one trial[3] demonstrated its effectiveness: in an equivalence trial a hops/valerian combination was found to be equally effective as benzodiazepine after 2 weeks of therapy but without producing the hangover effect experienced by benzodiazepine patients. The activity of hops on its own remains unclear since it has not been separately tested. One double-blind crossover study[4] comparing a hops/valerian combination with valerian on its own, and placebo found it to be similar to placebo and less effective than the valerian monotherapy.
Dosage	*Dried extract:* 0.5–1 g of dried extract three times daily. *Liquid extract:* 0.5–1 ml of liquid extract (1:1 in 45% alcohol) three times daily; 300–400 mg hops extract combined with 240–300 mg valerian taken once before bedtime.
Risks	***Contraindications*** Pregnancy and lactation (see p 5), depression.

Precautions/warnings
May have oestrogenic agonist or antagonist properties, with unknown effects on hormone sensitive conditions such as certain types of cancer, or endometriosis; disruption to menstrual cycle is considered possible. Might potentially increase blood sugar levels in diabetic patients.

Adverse effects
Allergic dermatitis, respiratory allergy and anaphylaxis have been reported following inhalation or external contact with the herb or oil.

Overdose
No information is available for humans. In animals, large parenteral doses resulted in a soporific effect followed by death and chronic administration resulted in weight loss before death.

Interactions
Theoretical interactions exist for central nervous system depressants, antipsychotics, hormonal agents and any drugs metabolised by the cytochrome P-450 system (e.g. warfarin, anticonvulsants, digoxin, theophylline, HIV protease inhibitors). Also alcohol, although a study of a hop/valerian combination reported no potentiation of alcohol.

Quality issues
Some active constituents break down during storage.

Risk–benefit assessment

There is insufficient clinical data to demonstrate that hop has any specific therapeutic effects. Conclusive safety information is also lacking, but some risks have been identified. Therefore its use as a monopreparation cannot be recommended due to insufficient evidence on the risk–benefit ratio.

HERBAL AND NON-HERBAL MEDICINES

REFERENCE
1 Schellenberg R, Sauer S, Abourashed E A, Koetter U, Brattström A. The fixed combination of valerian and hops (Ze91019) acts via a central adenosine mechanism. Planta Med 2004;70:594–597

2 Vonderheid-Guth B, Todorova A, Brattström A, Dimpfel W. Pharmacodynamic effects of valerian and hops extract combination (Ze 91019) on the quantitative-topographical EEG in healthy volunteers. Eur J Med Res 2000,5.139–144

3 Schmitz M, Jäckel M. Vergleichsstudie zur Untersuchung der Lebensqualität von Patienten mit exogenen Schlafstörungen (vorübergehenden Ein-und Durchschlafstörungen) unter Therapie mit einem Hopfen-Baldrian-Präparat und einem Benzodiazepin-Präparat. Wien Med Wochenschr 1998;148:291–298

4 Leathwood P D, Chauffard F, Heck E, Munoz-Box R. Aqueous extract of valerian root (Valeriana officinalis L.) improves sleep quality in man. Pharmacol Biochem Behav 1982;17:65–71

5 Gerhard U, Linnenbrink N, Georghiadou C, Hobi V. [Vigilance-decreasing effects of 2 plant-derived sedatives] Schweiz Rundsch Med Prax 1996;85:473–481

6 Müller-Limmroth W, Ehrenstein W. Untersuchungen über die Wirkung von Seda-Kneipp auf den Schlaf schlafgestörter Menschen. Med Klin 1977;72:1119–1125

HORSE CHESTNUT
(*Aesculus hippocastanum*)

Source	Seeds.
Main constituents	Fatty acids, flavonoids, quinones, saponins, sterols, tannins, and triterpene.
Background	The horse chestnut tree is native to south-east Europe and was allegedly first introduced to northern Europe in the mid 16th century by the botanist Charles de l'Écluse, from seeds brought from Constantinople. Today the tree is widely distributed all over the world. The genus name *Aesculus* derives from the Latin *esca* meaning 'food' and the Latin *hippocastanum* is reported to derive from the practice of feeding the seeds to horses to treat respiratory ailments.
Examples of traditional uses	Diarrhoea, haemorrhoids, malaria, respiratory diseases, varicose veins.
Pharmacologic action	Antiexudative, anti-inflammatory and immunomodulatory activity. Escin, the principal active component of horse chestnut seed extract (HCSE), constricts veins and reduces the permeability of venous capillaries in vitro. It has been shown to inhibit the activity of elastase and hyaluronidase, both involved in enzymatic proteoglycan degradation. Studies have shown increased levels of leukocytes in affected limbs and suggested a possible subsequent activation with release of such enzymes. Other studies reported an increased serum activity of proteoglycan hydrolases in patients with chronic venous insufficiency which were reduced with HCSE.
Conditions frequently treated	Haematoma, symptoms (pain, fatigue, pruritus, oedema) or trophic changes associated with chronic venous insufficiency.
Clinical evidence	A systematic review and meta-analysis,[1] assessed the efficacy and safety of oral (HCSE) monopreparations and concluded that the evidence suggests that HCSE is an efficacious and safe short-term treatment for chronic venous insufficiency. Sixteen RCTs were included; all except one were conducted double-blind. Leg pain was assessed in seven placebo-controlled trials (n = 595). Six studies (n = 543) reported a reduction of leg pain on various measurement scales in patients treated with HCSE compared with placebo. Leg volume was assessed in six placebo-controlled trials (n = 472). All of these studies used water displacement plethysmography to measure this outcome. Meta-analysis of five trials reporting adequate data (n = 289) suggested a reduction of 56.3 ml in favour of HCSE compared with placebo. One trial (n = 240)

indicated that HCSE may be as effective as compression stockings at reducing leg volume.[2] These results are corroborated by an earlier, independent meta-analysis.[3] For its topical use and for other indications there seems to be no evidence from rigorous clinical trials.

Dosage

Internal use: extract standardised to 100–150 mg escin daily in divided doses.
External use: apply several times daily.

Risks

Contraindications
Pregnancy and lactation (see p 5), bleeding disorders, allergy to any of its constituents.

Precautions/warnings
Open wounds, weeping eczema (external use), intravenous administration.

Adverse effects
Pruritus, nausea, gastrointestinal complaints, bleeding, dizziness, headache, nephropathy, allergic reactions.

Interactions
Increased effects of aspirin and other anticoagulants, antihyperglycaemics.

Quality issues
Preparations are generally standardised to 50–75 mg escin per capsule. Quality of the extracts may vary between preparations.

Risk–benefit assessment

The available evidence suggests that HCSE is effective for treating patients with chronic venous insufficiency. Given the nature and frequency of the reported adverse events and the relatively poor compliance with conventional treatments such as compression therapy, HCSE is worthy of consideration when treating patients with chronic venous insufficiency.

HERBAL AND NON-HERBAL MEDICINES

REFERENCES

1 Pittler M H, Ernst E. Horse chestnut seed extract for chronic venous insufficiency. The Cochrane Database of Systematic Reviews 2004, Issue 2. Art. No.: CD003230
2 Diehm C, Trampisch H J, Lange S, Schmidt C. Comparison of leg compression stocking and oral horse-chestnut seed extract therapy in patients with chronic venous insufficiency. Lancet 1996;347:292–294
3 Siebert U, Brach M, Sroczynski G, Berla K. Efficacy, routine effectiveness, and safety of horsechestnut seed extract in the treatment of chronic venous insufficiency. A meta-analysis of randomized controlled trials and large observational studies. Int Angiol 2002;21:305–315

KAVA KAVA
(Piper methysticum)

Source	Rhizome.
Main constituents	Dihydrokavain, dihydromethysticin, kavain, methysticin, yangonin.
Background	Native to the islands of the South Pacific, kava, the beverage prepared from the rhizome of *P. methysticum* has long been used for medicinal and recreational purposes. The name kava derives from the Polynesian word *awa* or *kava* meaning bitter and refers to the characteristic taste of the beverage. At the beginning of the 19th century the knowledge of kava as a medicinal plant led to its usage as a treatment particularly for venereal diseases. At the beginning of the 20th century scientists isolated a number of compounds which were called kavapyrones and are thought to be the active principle of kava.
Examples of traditional uses	Chronic cystitis, gonorrhoea, muscle relaxation, sleep induction, syphilis, weight reduction.
Pharmacologic action	Anxiolytic, sedative, anesthetic, muscle relaxant. Studies suggest that kavapyrones, the pharmacologically active components, act on the central nervous system. Kavapyrones are thought to mediate effects on gamma-aminobutyric acid receptors, particularly in the hippocampus and amygdala complex. Central nervous effects of kavain and kava extract have also been demonstrated in studies on human volunteers using EEG measurements.
Conditions frequently treated	Anxiety, insomnia.
Clinical evidence	A systematic review and meta-analysis[1] assessed a total of 11 randomised, double-blind trials of kava for anxiety. The meta-analysis of six studies (n = 345) using the total score on the Hamilton Anxiety scale as a common outcome measure suggests a reduction in patients receiving kava extract compared with patients receiving placebo. It concluded that kava extract appears to be an effective symptomatic treatment option for anxiety, which is corroborated by another systematic review.[2] Comparative studies indicate no difference between conventional medication and kavain or kava extract.[3–5] A rigorous trial also concluded that kava can additionally facilitate cognitive functioning and increase positive affectivity related to exhilaration.[6] For the treatment of insomnia, only limited evidence exists. The suggested mechanism of action and data from animal experiments, however, support the notion that the extract may be helpful for this condition. One RCT reported improved quality of sleep after a single dose of 300 mg kava extract.[7] A number of cases of suspected kava

hepatotoxicity have been reported worldwide,[8] which triggered the banning of kava in many countries. However, factors exist which complicate causal attribution. Further data particularly on the long-term safety profile of kava are required.

Dosage

300 mg of standardised extract (210 mg kavapyrones) daily in divided doses.

Risks

Contraindications

Pregnancy and lactation (see p 5), endogenous depression, allergy, liver conditions, Parkinson's disease.

Precautions/warnings

Avoid long-term use. The extract can cause visual disturbances and may affect reaction time. Care must be taken when driving or operating machinery.

Adverse effects

Stomach complaints, tremor, headache, drowsiness, restlessness, dyskinesia, mydriasis, allergic skin reactions, kava dermopathy, dermatomyositis, liver damage.

Interactions

Potentiation of drugs acting on the central nervous system such as alcohol, benzodiazepines, barbiturates and anesthetics. May potentiate the effects of hepatotoxic agents. May reduce the effects of levodopa.

Quality issues

The extract is generally standardised to kavapyrone content. The quality of the extracts may vary between preparations.

Risk–benefit assessment

The available evidence suggests that kava extract is superior to placebo for treating patients with anxiety disorders. Some suggestions exist that it may be as effective as conventional anxiolytic drug treatment. It may be beneficial for the treatment of insomnia in some patients, but the evidence is as yet insufficient. Due to the safety concerns, if kava is taken it should be short term and under close medical observation.

HERBAL AND NON-HERBAL MEDICINES

REFERENCES

1 Pittler M H, Ernst E. Kava extract for treating anxiety. The Cochrane Database of Systematic Reviews 2003, Issue 1. Art. No.: CD003383

2 Cairney S, Maruff P, Clough A R. The neurobehavioral effects of kava. Aust NZ J Psychiatry 2002;36:657–662

3 Lindenberg D, Pitule-Schödel H. D,L-Kavain im Vergleich zu Oxazepam bei Angstzuständen. Fortschr Med 1990;108:49–50

4 Woelk H, Kapoula O, Lehrl S, Schröter K, Weinholz P. Behandlung von Angst-Patienten. Z Allg Med 1993;69:271–277

5 Boerner R J, Sommer H, Berger W, Kuhn U, Schmidt U, Mannel M. Kava-Kava extract LI150 is as effective as opipramole and buspirone in generalized anxiety disorder – an 8-week randomized double-blind multi-centre trial in 129 outpatients. Phytomedicine 2003;10(Suppl 4):38–49

6 Thompson R, Ruch W, Hasenöhrl R U. Enhanced cognitive performance and cheerful mood by standardized extracts of Piper methysticum (kava-kava). Hum Psychopharmacol 2004;19:243–250

7 Emser W, Bartylla K. Verbesserung der Schlafqualität. Zur Wirkung von Kava-Extrakt WS1490 auf das Schlafmuster bei Gesunden. TW Neurologie Psychiatrie 1991;5:636–642

8 Pittler M H, Ernst E. Systematic review: hepatotoxic events associated with herbal medicinal products. Aliment Pharmacol Ther 2003;18:451–471

KOMBUCHA
(Fungus japonicus)

Source	A variable range of yeast-bacteria-fungal aggregates surrounded by a semi-permeable membrane.
Main constituents	Acetic acid, alcohol, B vitamins, chondroitin-sulphate, glucoronic acid, hyalronic acid, heparin, lactic acid, mukoitin sulfate, usnic acid, sugar.
Background	Kombucha has been used in China since 220 BCE. Later it became popular particularly in Russia, continental Europe and the USA. Contrary to what the name 'kombucha mushroom' implies, it is not a mushroom but a symbiot.
Examples of traditional uses	Aging, anorexia, arthritis, general tonic, memory loss.
Pharmacologic action	No specific pharmacological actions have been identified in humans. Animal studies suggest antioxidant, immunomodulating[1] and hepato-protective properties.[2]
Conditions frequently treated	Aging, AIDS, anorexia, arthritis, atherosclerosis, cancer, constipation, diabetes, gout, haemorrhoids, hair growth, headache, hypertension, increase of vitality, indigestion.
Clinical evidence	A systematic review found no clinical trials (controlled or uncontrolled) or case series testing the efficacy of kombucha in humans.[3] The conclusion was that kombucha cannot be recommended for therapeutic use.
Dosage	*Orally:* as a tea several times per day. *Topically:* several times per day.
Risks	*Contraindications* Patients on disufiram as kombucha tea can contain alcohol. Pregnancy and lactation (see p 5). *Precautions/warnings* Can leach lead and other toxic chemicals from its container.[4]

Adverse effects

Gastrointestinal problems, yeast infections, allergic reactions, jaundice, nausea, vomiting, headache, lead poisoning, infections with contaminating bacteria, e.g. anthrax.[5]

Interactions

None known.

Quality issues

Kombucha is a non-standardised product; therefore its constituents will vary considerably from batch to batch.

Risk–benefit assessment

There are no well-documented benefits in human patients and a range of risks have been noted, some of which are serious. A risk–benefit assessment must therefore come to negative conclusions.

REFERENCES

1 Dipti P, Yogesh B, Kain AK, Pauline T, Anju B, Sairam M, Singh B, Mongia S S, Kumar G, Ilavazhagan G, Devengra K, Selvamurthy W. Lead induced oxidative stress: beneficial effects of Kombucha tea. Biomed Environ Sci 2003;16:276–282

2 Pauline T, Dipti P, Anju P, Kavimani S, Sharma S K, Kain A K, Sarada S K, Sairam M, Ilavazhagan G, Devengra K, Selvamurthy W. Studies on toxicity, anti-stress and hepato-protective properties of Kombucha tea. Biomed Environ Sci 2001;14:207–213

3 Ernst E. Kombucha: a systematic review of the clinical evidence. Forsch Komplementärmed Klass Naturheilkd 2003;10:85–87

4 Phan T G, Estell J, Duggin G, Beer I, Smith D, Ferson M J. Lead poisoning from drinking Kombucha tea brewed in a ceramic pot. Med J Aust 1998;169:644–646

5 Kombucha tea monograph. Natural Medicines Comprehensive Database, www. Naturaldatabase.com, accessed 05/10/2004

HERBAL AND NON-HERBAL MEDICINES

LAVENDER
(*Lavendula angustifolia*)

Source

Flowering tops.

Main constituents

Camphor, cineole, flavonoids, hydroxycoumarins, limonene, perillyl alcohol, tannins, triterpens, volatile oil (linalyl acetate, linalool).

Background

The name lavender is derived from the Latin *lavare* (to wash). Native to the Mediterranean and common in southern Europe, lavender is widely cultivated in domestic gardens and for use in perfumes and toiletries. It has been used for centuries to treat various ailments.

Examples of traditional uses

Appetite stimulant, bruises, burns, cuts, functional abdominal complaints, insomnia, migraines, neuralgia.

Pharmacologic action	Astringent, sedative, anticonvulsant, antioxidant, lipid lowering.
Conditions frequently treated	Headaches, insomnia.
Clinical evidence	The evidence from trials of lavender on mood is weak. The only double-blind RCT[1] of a monopreparation of lavender tincture concluded that it was less effective than imipramine in the treatment of 45 patients with mild to moderate depression but imipramine plus lavender was more effective than imipramine alone. No positive effects of aromatherapy with lavender on mood were found in 90 healthy undergraduate women[2] or on resistive behaviour in individuals with dementia.[3] Small trials report delayed changes in autonomic activity associated with the addition of lavender essential oil to a footbath,[4] and reduced stress after exposure to a lavender odorant,[5] increased relaxation and less depressed mood following lavender oil aromatherapy;[6] as well as modest positive effects on agitated behaviour in patients with severe dementia after aromatherapy with lavender oil[7] and on psychological well-being after lavender baths;[8] an RCT (n = 144) found a significant decrement in performance of working memory, impaired reaction time and reduced alertness after lavender aromatherapy.[9]
	One RCT of acupoint stimulation followed by acupressure with aromatic lavender oil suggests that this treatment is effective for short-term low back pain relief.[10] No direct analgesic effect was found by an RCT for lavender aromatherapy in experimentally induced pain[11] and one RCT found no long-term benefit of aromatherapy massage with lavender oil on pain, anxiety or QoL in 42 cancer patients.[12] A large RCT (n = 635) of postnatal perineal discomfort found no difference between lavender essential oil, synthetic lavender oil and an inert substance added to a bath.[13] A small RCT found no effect of lavender oil aromatherapy on recovery from exercise compared with no intervention.[14] A small controlled trial comparing two odour therapies, lavender and lemon, and two music therapies, found lavender and preferred music to reduce pain after but not during dressing change of vascular wounds.[15]
Dosage	*Tea:* 1–2 teaspoons of dried flowers in 150 ml of hot water (lavender tea); *Drops:* 2–4 drops in 2–3 cups of boiling water for aromatherapy inhalation.
Risks	***Contraindications*** Pregnancy and lactation (see p 5). ***Precautions/warnings*** The essential oil should be regarded as potentially poisonous if taken internally.

Adverse effects

Nausea, vomiting, headache and chills have been reported following inhalation or absorption through the skin. Contact allergy and phototoxicity are also possible.

Overdose

Nausea, vomiting, anorexia have been reported after large doses of lavender. Large doses are also reported to exert 'narcotic-like' effects.

Interactions

Theoretically could potentiate effects of central nervous system depressants.

Quality issues

Standardised preparations of the herb are rare, but lavender oil is often an ingredient in external rubs and massage oils and the essential oil is widely available.

Risk–benefit assessment

Although some trials suggest that lavender has relaxing effects, the evidence from clinical trials does not show that it has specific therapeutic effects. In recommended doses lavender is generally considered well tolerated with minimal adverse events. No positive effects have been reported for the treatment of pain with lavender on its own and no conclusive evidence exists for any other condition.

REFERENCES

1 Akhondzadeh S, Kashani L, Fotouhi A, Jarvandi S, Mobaseri M, Moin M, Khani M, Jamshidi A II, Baghalian K, Taghizadeh M. Comparison of Lavandula angustifolia Mill. tincture and imipramine in the treatment of mild to moderate depression: a double-blind, randomized trial. Prog Neuropsychopharmacol Biol Psychiatry 2003;27:123–127

2 Campenni C E, Crawley E J, Meier M E. Role of suggestion in odor-induced mood change. Psychol Rep 2004;94:1127–1136

3 Gray S G, Clair A A. Influence of aromatherapy on medication administration to residential-care residents with dementia and behavioral challenges. Am J Alzheimers Dis Other Demen 2002;17:169–174

4 Saeki Y. The effect of foot-bath with or without the essential oil of lavender on the autonomic nervous system: a randomised trial. Compl Ther Med 2000;8:2–7

5 Motomura N, Sakurai A, Yotsuya Y. Reduction of mental stress with lavender odorant. Percept Mot Skills 2001;93:713–718

6 Diego M A, Jones N A, Field T, Hernandez-Reif M, Schanberg S, Kuhn C, McAdam V, Galamaga R, Galamaga M. Aromatherapy positively affects mood, EEG patterns of alertness and math computations. Int J Neurosci 1998;96:217–224

7 Holmes C, Hopkins V, Hensford C, MacLaughlin V, Wilkinson D, Rosenvinge H. Lavender oil as a treatment for agitated behaviour in severe dementia: a placebo controlled study. Int J Geriatr Psychiatry 2002;17:305–308

8 Morris N. The effects of lavender (Lavendula angustifolium) baths on psychological well-being: two exploratory randomised control trials. Complement Ther Med 2002;10:223–228

9 Moss M, Cook J, Wesnes K, Duckett P. Aromas of rosemary and lavender essential oils differentially affect cognition and mood in healthy adults. Int J Neurosci 2003;113:15–38

10 Yip Y B, Tse S H. The effectiveness of relaxation acupoint stimulation and acupressure with aromatic lavender essential oil for non-specific low back pain in Hong Kong: a randomised controlled trial. Complement Ther Med 2004;12:28–37

11 Soden K, Vincent K, Craske S, Lucas C, Ashley S. A randomized controlled trial of aromatherapy massage in a hospice setting. Palliat Med 2004;18:87–92

HERBAL AND NON-HERBAL MEDICINES

12 Gedney J J, Glover T L, Fillingim R B. Sensory and affective pain discrimination after inhalation of essential oils. Psychosom Med 2004;66:599–606

13 Dale A, Cornwell S. The role of lavender oil in relieving perineal discomfort following childbirth: a blind randomised clinical trial. J Adv Nurs 1994;19:89–96

14 Romine I J, Bush A M, Geist C R. Lavender aromatherapy in recovery from exercise. Percept Mot Skills 1999;88:756–758

15 Kane F M, Brodie E E, Coull A, Coyne L, Howd A, Milne A, Niven C C, Robbins R. The analgesic effect of odour and music upon dressing change. Br J Nurs 2004;13:S4–12

MELATONIN

Source

Melatonin is produced endogenously mainly by the pineal gland. Commercially available melatonin is usually produced synthetically.

Background

Melatonin is a neurohormone synthesised from tryptophan. Release is stimulated by darkness and suppressed by light. Melatonin is involved in the regulation of bodily rhythms such as temperature and sleep. Serum concentrations increase 10–50-fold 1–2 hours before bedtime, reaching a peak at about midnight. Melatonin has a half-life of about 20–50 minutes.

Examples of traditional uses

None.

Pharmacologic action

Synchronising hormone secretion, sedative, antioxidative, immune stimulating, antiproliferative, anti-inflammatory, hypotensive.

Conditions frequently treated

Insomnia, jet lag.

Clinical evidence

A Cochrane review reported that eight out of ten trials found that melatonin taken close to the target bedtime at the destination decreased jet-lag from flights crossing five or more time zones. It concluded that melatonin is effective for preventing or reducing jet-lag and that occasional short-term use appears to be safe.[1] For elderly patients (65 to 79 years) with insomnia, a systematic review identified six double-blind RCTs and concluded that there is sufficient evidence to suggest that low doses of melatonin (0.5 mg to 6 mg) improve initial sleep quality.[2] This conclusion is supported by further double-blind RCTs reporting beneficial effects in asthmatic patients with sleep disturbances,[3] in medically ill patients with insomnia,[4] in patients with delayed sleep phase syndrome[5] and sleep disorders in DSM-IV diagnosed dementia,[6] although for patients with Alzheimer type dementia additional trials report mixed results.[7,8] For patients with chronic schizophrenia,[9] seasonal affective disorder[10] and unselected neuropsychiatric sleep disorders and reduced REM sleep duration[11] melatonin was also found to be beneficial. For chronic fatigue syndrome[12] no beneficial effects are reported and for primary insomnia the results are mixed.[13,14] For shift work disorder, RCTs with negative outcomes[15,16] have contradicted earlier findings.[17,18] In children with neurodevelopmental disabilities and sleep impairment, a systematic review of RCTs suggests that the clinical trial data are too limited for any firm conclusion.[19] For chronic sleep-onset insomnia in children, RCTs show beneficial results,[20,21] and in children with epilepsy receiving valproate it also seems to improve sleep.[22] In two RCTs assessing cancer patients it is reported that melatonin might enhance the efficacy of chemotherapy.[23,24] No evidence of a dose effect between 5 mg and 10 mg melatonin was shown in children with sleep disorders associated with tuberous sclerosis complex.[25]

No effect over placebo is reported for the relief of menopausal symptoms[26] but some positive results are reported for pituitary and thyroid function in perimenopausal and menopausal women.[27] Other single RCTs reporting encouraging results were identified for cluster headache,[28] hypertension,[29] diffuse or androgenic alopecia,[30] tardive dyskinesia,[31] benign prostatic hyperplasia,[32] whiplash syndrome,[33] as an adjunct to antiepileptic therapy,[34] and for premedication of adult patients.[35] Melatonin does not seem to impair psychomotor performance,[36] not reduce the use of benzodiazepines in the elderly[37] and not have any additional positive effects in motor restless behaviour in dementia.[38] No toxicological effects were noted in a double-blind placebo-controlled RCT which assessed 10 mg melatonin for 28 days.[39]

Dosage

Insomnia: 0.3–10 mg (0.3–1 mg initially) 1 to 2 hours before bedtime.
Jet lag: 5 mg 22–2400 hrs local time on arrival for 4 days.

Risks

Contraindications
Pregnancy and lactation (see p 5), prepubertal children, autoimmune disease, hepatic insufficiency, cerebrovascular or neurologic disorders, patients taking immunosuppressants or corticosteroids.

Precautions/warnings
Impairment of psychomotor vigilance. Driving or operating machinery should be avoided for 4–5 hours following melatonin administration. Melatonin may be pro-atherosclerotic.

Adverse effects
Abdominal cramps, fatigue, dizziness, headache, irritability. Hangover effects are unlikely, due to the short half-life.

Overdose
Large doses (1200 mg) have been associated with depression.

HERBAL AND NON-HERBAL MEDICINES

Interactions

May potentiate the effects of benzodiazepines and antihypertensive drugs. May reduce the effects of warfarin and antihyperglycaemic drugs.

Quality issues

Most commercial melatonin is produced synthetically. Extracts from animal preparations should not be used due to possible contaminants. Melatonin is available for sale over the counter in the USA, but not in the UK or Germany.

Risk–benefit assessment

The evidence suggests that melatonin is effective in preventing or reducing jet-lag. It seems to improve sleep quality in elderly patients with insomnia, which is supported by evidence in a number of other conditions including sleep-onset insomnia in children. Encouraging results are reported for melatonin to enhance the efficacy of chemotherapy. The short-term safety profile seems to be favourable and therefore it can be recommended for symptoms of jet lag and for improving sleep quality. For all other indication the evidence is too limited for any firm recommendations.

REFERENCES

1 Herxheimer A, Petrie K J. Melatonin for the prevention and treatment of jet lag. The Cochrane Database of Systematic Reviews 2002, Issue 2. Art. No.: CD001520

2 Olde-Rikkert M G, Rigaud A S. Melatonin in elderly patients with insomnia. A systematic review. Z Gerontol Geriatr 2001;34:491–497

3 Campos F L, da Silva-Junior F P, de Bruin V M, de Bruin P F. Melatonin improves sleep in asthma: a randomized, double-blind, placebo-controlled study. Am J Respir Crit Care Med 2004;170:947–951

4 Andrade C, Srihari B S, Reddy K P, Chandramma L. Melatonin in medically ill patients with insomnia: a double-blind, placebo-controlled study. J Clin Psychiatry 2001;62:41–45

5 Kayumov L, Brown G, Jindal R, Buttoo K, Shapiro C M. A randomized double-blind, placebo-controlled, crossover study of the effect of exogenous melatonin on delayed sleep phase syndrome. Psychosom Med 2001;63:40–48

6 Serfaty M, Kennell-Webb S, Warner J, Blizard R, Raven P. Double-blind randomised placebo controlled trial of low dose melatonin for sleep disorders in dementia. Int J Geriatr Psychiatry 2002;17:1120–1127

7 Singer C, Tractenberg R E, Kaye J, Schafer K, Gamst A, Grundman M, Thomas R, Thal L J, Alzheimer's Disease Cooperative Study. A multicenter, placebo-controlled trial of melatonin for sleep disturbance in Alzheimer's disease. Sleep 2003;26:893–901

8 Asayama K, Yamadera H, Ito T, Suzuki H, Kudo Y, Endo S. Double blind study of melatonin effects on the sleep-wake rhythm, cognitive and non-cognitive functions in Alzheimer type dementia. J Nippon Med Sch 2003;70:334–341

9 Shamir E, Laudon M, Barak Y, Anis Y, Rotenberg V, Elizur A, Zisapel N. Melatonin improves sleep quality of patients with chronic schizophrenia. J Clin Psychiatry 2000;61:373–377

10 Leppamaki S, Partonen T, Vakkuri O, Lonnqvist J, Partinen M, Laudon M. Effect of controlled-release melatonin on sleep quality, mood, and quality of life in subjects with seasonal or weather-associated changes in mood and behaviour. Eur Neuropsychopharmacol 2003;13:137–145

11 Kunz D, Mahlberg R, Muller C, Tilmann A, Bes F. Melatonin in patients with reduced REM sleep duration: two randomized controlled trials. J Clin Endocrinol Metab 2004;89:128–134

12 Williams G, Waterhouse J, Mugarza J, Minors D, Hayden K. Therapy of circadian rhythm disorders in chronic fatigue syndrome: no

symptomatic improvement with melatonin or phototherapy. Eur J Clin Invest 2002;32:831–837

13 Almeida Montes L G, Ontiveros Uribe M P, Cortes Sotres J, Heinze Martin G. Treatment of primary insomnia with melatonin: a double-blind, placebo-controlled, crossover study. J Psychiatry Neurosci 2003;28:191–196

14 Zemlan F P, Mulchahey J J, Scharf M B, Mayleben D W, Rosenberg R, Lankford A. The efficacy and safety of the melatonin agonist beta-methyl-6-chloromelatonin in primary insomnia: a randomized, placebo-controlled, crossover clinical trial. J Clin Psychiatry 2005;66:384–390

15 Wright S W, Lawrence L M, Wrenn K D, Haynes M L, Welch L W, Schlack H M. Randomized clinical trial of melatonin after night-shift work: efficacy and neuropsychologic effects. Ann Emerg Med 1998;32:334–340

16 James M, Tremea M O, Jones J S, Krohmer J R. Can melatonin improve adaption to night shift? Am J Emerg Med 1998;16:367–370

17 Folkard S, Arendt J, Clark M. Can melatonin improve shift workers' tolerance of the night shift? Some preliminary findings. Chronobiol Int 1993;10:315–320

18 Dawson D, Encel N, Lushington K. Improving adaptation to simulated night shift: timed exposure to bright light versus daytime melatonin administration. Sleep 1995;18:11–21

19 Phillips L, Appleton R E. Systematic review of melatonin treatment in children with neurodevelopmental disabilities and sleep impairment. Dev Med Child Neurol 2004;46:771–775

20 Smits M G, van Stel H F, van der Heijden K, Meijer A M, Coenen A M, Kerkhof G A. Melatonin improves health status and sleep in children with idiopathic chronic sleep-onset insomnia: a randomized placebo controlled trial. J Am Acad Child Adolesc Psychiatry 2003;42:1286–1293

21 Smits M G, Nagtegaal E E, van der Heijden J, Coenen A M, Kerkhof G A. Melatonin for chronic sleep onset insomnia in children: a randomized placebo-controlled trial. J Child Neurol 2001;16:86–92

22 Gupta M, Aneja S, Kohli K. Add-on melatonin improves sleep behavior in children with epilepsy: randomized, double-blind, placebo-controlled trial. J Child Neurol 2005;20:112–115

23 Lissoni P, Chilelli M, Villa S, Cerizza L, Tancini G. Five years survival in metastatic non-small cell lung cancer patients treated with chemotherapy alone or chemotherapy and melatonin: a randomized trial. J Pineal Res 2003;35:12–15

24 Cerea G, Vaghi M, Ardizzoia A, Villa S, Bucovec R, Mengo S, Gardani G, Tancini G, Lissoni P. Biomodulation of cancer chemotherapy for metastatic colorectal cancer: a randomized study of weekly low-dose irinotecan alone versus irinotecan plus the oncostatic pineal hormone melatonin in metastatic colorectal cancer patients progressing on 5-fluorouracil-containing combinations. Anticancer Res 2003;23:1951–1954

25 Hancock E, O'Callaghan F, Osborne J P. Effect of melatonin dosage on sleep disorder in tuberous sclerosis complex. J Child Neurol 2005;20:78–80

26 Secreto G, Chiechi L M, Amadori A, Miceli R, Venturelli E, Valerio T, Marubini E. Soy isoflavones and melatonin for the relief of climacteric symptoms: a multicenter, double-blind, randomized study. Maturitas 2004;47:11–20

27 Bellipanni G, Bianchi P, Pierpaoli W, Bulian D, Ilyia E. Effects of melatonin in perimenopausal and menopausal women: a randomized and placebo controlled study. Exp Gerontol 2001;36:297–310

28 Leone M, D'Amico D, Moschiano F, Fraschini F, Bussone G. Melatonin versus placebo in the prophylaxis of cluster headache: a double-blind pilot study with parallel groups. Cephalalgia 1996;16:494–496

29 Scheer F A, Van Montfrans G A, van Someren E J, Mairuhu G, Buijs R M. Daily nighttime melatonin reduces blood pressure in male patients with essential hypertension. Hypertension 2004;43:192–197

30 Fischer T W, Burmeister G, Schmidt H W, Elsner P. Melatonin increases anagen hair rate in women with androgenetic alopecia or diffuse alopecia: results of a pilot randomized controlled trial. Br J Dermatol 2004;150:341–345

31 Shamir E, Barak Y, Shalman I, Laudon M, Zisapel N, Tarrasch R, Elizur A, Weizman R. Melatonin treatment for tardive dyskinesia: a double-blind, placebo-controlled, crossover study. Arch Gen Psychiatry 2001;58:1049–1052

32 Drake M J, Mills I W, Noble J G. Melatonin pharmacotherapy for nocturia in men with benign prostatic enlargement. J Urol 2004;171:1199–1202

HERBAL AND NON-HERBAL MEDICINES

33 Van Wieringen S, Jansen T, Smits M G, Nagtegaal J E, Coenen A M L. Melatonin for chronic whiplash syndrome with delayed melatonin onset: Randomised, placebo-controlled trial. Clin Drug Invest 2001;21:813–820

34 Gupta M, Aneja S, Kohli K. Add-on melatonin improves quality of life in epileptic children on valproate monotherapy: a randomized, double-blind, placebo-controlled trial. Epilepsy Behav 2004;5:316–321

35 Naguib M, Samarkandi A H. The comparative dose-response effects of melatonin and midazolam for premedication of adult patients: a double-blinded, placebo-controlled study. Anesth Analg 2000;91:473–479

36 Paul M A, Gray G, Kenny G, Pigeau R A. Impact of melatonin, zaleplon, zopiclone, and temazepam on psychomotor performance. Aviat Space Environ Med 2003;74:1263–1270

37 Cardinali D P, Gvozdenovich E, Kaplan MR, Fainstein I, Shifis H A, Perez Lloret S, Albornoz L, Negri A. A double blind-placebo controlled study on melatonin efficacy to reduce anxiolytic benzodiazepine use in the elderly. Neuro Endocrinol Lett 2002;23:55–60

38 Haffmans P M, Sival R C, Lucius S A, Cats Q, van Gelder L. Bright light therapy and melatonin in motor restless behaviour in dementia: a placebo-controlled study. Int J Geriatr Psychiatry 2001;16:106–110

39 Seabra M L, Bignotto M, Pinto L R Jr, Tufik S. Randomized, double-blind clinical trial, controlled with placebo, of the toxicology of chronic melatonin treatment. J Pineal Res 2000;29:193–200

MILK THISTLE
(Silybum marianum)

Source	Seeds.
Main constituents	Silymarin which is composed of the flavoligans silybin, silychristin and silydianin.
Background	Milk thistle belongs to the *Compositae* (*Asteraceae*) family. Its common name stems from the legend that the white veins in the plant leaves come from a drop of the Virgin Mary's milk. Milk thistle is native to the Mediterranean but also grows in North and South America.
Examples of traditional uses	Antidote after mushroom poisoning, 'liver cleansing' agent, psoriasis, tonic for nursing mothers.
Pharmacologic action	Alters the membrane structure of liver cells so that toxins are hindered from entering hepatocytes, increases their regenerative capacity, competes with binding sites for liver toxins, antioxidant, free radical scavenger and possibly cholesterol-lowering agent.
Conditions frequently treated	Liver diseases, in particular hepatitis and (alcoholic) cirrhosis.
Clinical evidence	A Cochrane review[1] assessed the effects of milk thistle in patients with alcoholic liver disease and/or viral liver diseases (hepatitis B and hepatitis C). Thirteen RCTs involving 915 patients were included. Milk thistle versus placebo or no intervention had no significant effect on mortality, complications of liver disease or

liver histology. Liver-related mortality was reduced by milk thistle in all trials but not in high quality trials. Milk thistle was not associated with an increased risk of adverse events.

Dosage

160–480 mg of standardised extract (70–80% silymarin) three times daily.

Risks

Contraindications
Pregnancy and lactation (see p 5).

Precautions/warnings
Intake for an extended duration. Caution in patients with diabetes or taking hypoglycaemic agents.

Adverse effects
Mild gastrointestinal complaints, diarrhoea, pruritus, headache, rare cases of anaphylaxis.

Interactions
Theoretically, improvement of liver function could increase metabolism of some medications which are metabolised in the liver. There is preliminary evidence that milk thistle might inhibit cytochrome P450 (CYP2C9 and CYP3A4).

Quality issues
Products are generally standardised to 70–80% silymarin content.

Risk–benefit assessment

Overall the current evidence from RCTs does not demonstrate significant effects of milk thistle on mortality or complications of liver diseases in patients with alcoholic and/or hepatitis B or C liver diseases. Although low-quality trials report some beneficial effects and no serious risks exist there is no high-quality evidence to support the use of milk thistle in these liver diseases.

REFERENCE

1 Rambaldi A, Jacobs B, Iaquinto G, Gluud C. Milk thistle for alcoholic and/or hepatitis B or C virus liver diseases. Cochrane Database Syst Rev 2005; Issue 2. Art. No.: CD003620

HERBAL AND NON-HERBAL MEDICINES

MISTLETOE
(Viscum album)

Source	Leaves, branches and berries.
Main constituents	Alkaloids, amines, choline, flavonoids, histamine, mistletoe lectins, phoratoxins and viscotoxins, tannins, and terpenoids.
Background	*Viscum album* (and related species such as *Viscum abietis* and *Viscum austriacum* which are native to Europe and Asia) is a semiparasitic plant that lives in tree species such as oak, pine, elm and apple. The medicinal use of mistletoe goes back to early Celtic times. Rudolf Steiner (1861–1925), the founder of anthroposophy, believed the parasitic nature of mistletoe was similar to the nature of malignant growth and thus hypothesised that mistletoe could be used therapeutically for cancer. Based on anecdotal reports of cancer improvement, mistletoe became a popular anthroposophical 'cancer cure' in Europe and its use has now spread to the USA and beyond. Anthroposophical products are usually fermented while phytotherapeutic preparations are conventional extracts. In addition, a pure mistletoe lectin product has recently become available.
Example of traditional uses	Because of its toxicity, mistletoe has relatively few traditional uses; they include depression, epilepsy, hypertension and insomnia.
Pharmacologic actions	Cytotoxic, immunomodulatory.
Conditions frequently treated	All types of cancer. The treatment is promoted both for reducing tumour burden and for increasing quality of life in palliative cancer care. The immunomodulatory effect is also invoked for promoting mistletoe as a treatment for AIDS.
Clinical evidence	Several clinical studies have indicated improvements in immune function, quality of life and survival rate of cancer patients[1] yet the evidence is far from uniform. An independent and authoritative systematic review[2] included 11 CCTs (bronchial carcinoma, colorectal carcinoma, breast cancer, gastric cancer and ovarian cancer). All except one (the most rigorous) of these studies yielded results or trends in favour of mistletoe. Because of the methodological weaknesses of these trials, the authors conclude that 'Mistletoe preparations cannot be recommended in the treatment of cancer patients except in clinical trials'.[2] When the data of prospective, non-randomised and randomised matched pair studies of 10 226 mixed cancer patients were pooled, it was noted that survival time was longer for all types of cancer treated with adjuvant mistletoe extract compared with no such treatment.[3] Similarly, a systematic review of 16 RCTs, two quasi-randomised

and five non-randomised studies arrived at a positive conclusion. Twelve of these trials showed significant results but all studies suffered from methodological shortcomings.[4] A systematic review confined only to RCTs included ten such studies and demonstrated considerable flaws in most of them. While the weaker studies tended to generate positive results, the rigorous ones failed to do so.[5] The methodologically best RCT included 477 patients with resected head and neck cancers receiving either standard treatment alone or with additional subcutaneous mistletoe injections. After an average follow-up period of 4 years there were no intergroup differences in disease-free survival or any other outcomes.[6] More recently, several RCTs have emerged. An RCT with 272 breast cancer patients receiving injections of 10, 30 or 70 mg mistletoe lectin per mL or placebo for 15 weeks showed benefits for the group treated with 30 mg/ml.[7] Another RCT included 133 patients with various cancers treated with the mistletoe extract Helixor or with Lentinan. The results suggest that the former reduces the adverse effects of chemotherapy thus improving quality of life.[8]

Mistletoe extracts have also been tested for conditions other than cancer. Promising data emerged from an RCT with 48 healthy volunteers; the frequency and duration of common colds were marginally reduced compared with placebo over a 12-week period.[9] Finally, a non-randomised, open crossover study generated encouraging results for hepatitis C patients; there was no effect on viral load but the frequency and intensity of clinical signs and symptoms improved.[10]

Dosage

Leaf: 2–6 g of dried leaves orally three times daily.
Liquid extract: 1–3 ml (1:1 solution in 25% alcohol) three times daily.
Tincture: 0.5 ml (1:5 solution in 45% alcohol) three times daily.
Solutions for injection: as instructed by the manufacturer.

Risks

Contraindications
Pregnancy and lactation (see p 5).

Precautions/warnings
Patients should be monitored for dehydration and electrolyte imbalances and warned about the toxicity of mistletoe; cancer patients should be advised not to discontinue their conventional therapies.

Adverse effects
Bradycardia, dehydration, delirium, diarrhoea, gastroenteritis, hallucinations, hepatitis, hypo- and hypertension, fever, leukocytosis, mydriasis, myosis, nausea, seizures, vomiting. Several fatalities have been reported. Local reactions at the site of injection are common. Serious adverse effects seem, however, rare.[11]

Overdose
Adverse effects as above.

Interactions
Can enhance or potentiate effects of antihypertensive drugs, cardiac depressants and central nervous system depressants.

Quality issues
Only standardised preparations with standardised lectin content should be used.

Risk–benefit assessment

The evidence regarding mistletoe preparations is full of contradictions. The methodologically best studies suggest that it is not useful for cancer, neither in terms of tumour burden nor quality of life. Mistletoe injections are associated with considerable risks. Thus, on the basis of the data currently available, they should not be used as a sole cancer treatment and used only with caution as an adjunctive cancer therapy. Whether mistletoe is effective for the treatment or prevention of any other conditions awaits independent confirmation of the scant evidence available to date.

REFERENCES

1 Kaegi E. Unconventional therapies for cancer: 3. Iscador. Canad Med Assoc J 1998;158: 1157–1159

2 Kleijnen J, Knipschild P. Mistletoe treatment for cancer. Review of controlled trials in humans. Phytomedicine 1994;1:255–260

3 Grossarth-Maticek R, Kiene H, Baumgartner S M, Ziegler R. Use of Iscador, an extract of European mistletoe (Viscum album), in cancer treatment: prospective nonrandomized and randomized matched-pair studies nested within a cohort study. Altern Ther Health Med 2001;7:57–66, 68–72, 74–76

4 Kienle G S, Berrino F, Büssing A, Portalupi E, Rosenzweig S, Kiene H. Mistletoe in cancer – a systematic review on controlled clinical trials. Eur J Med Res 2003;8:109–119

5 Ernst E, Schmidt K, Steuer-Vogt M K. Mistletoe for cancer? A systematic review of randomized clinical trials. Int J Cancer 2003;107:262–267

6 Steuer-Vogt M K, Bonkowsky V, Ambrosch P, Scholz M, Neiss A, Strutz J, Hennig M, Lenarz T, Arnold W.. The effect of an adjuvant mistletoe treatment programme in resected neck cancer patients. Eur J Cancer 2001;37:23–31

7 Semiglasov V F, Stepula V V, Dudov A, Lehmacher W, Mengs U. The standardized mistletoe extract PS76A2 improves QoL in patients with breast cancer receiving adjuvant CMF chemotherapy: a randomized, placebo-controlled, double-blind, multicentre clinical trial. Anticancer Res 2004;24:1293–1302

8 Piao B K, Want Y X, Xie G R, Mansmann U, Natthes H, Beuth J, Lin H S. Impact of complementary mistletoe extract treatment on quality of life in breast, overain and non-small cell lung cancer patients. A prospective randomized controlled clinical trial. Anticancer Res 2004;24:303–309

9 Huber R, Klein R, Lüdtke R, Werner M. Frequency of common cold in healthy subjects during exposure to a lectin-rich and a lectin-poor mistletoe preparation in a randomized, double-blind, placebo-controlled study. Forsch Komplementärmed Klass Naturheilkd 2001;8:354–358

10 Huber R, Lüdtke R, Klassen M, Müller-Buscher G, Wolff-Vorbeck G, Scheer R. Effects of a misltetoe preparation with defined lectin content on chronic hepatitis C: an individually controlled cohort study. Eur J Med Res 2001;6:399–405

11 Bock P R, Friedel W E, Hanisch J, Karasmann M, Schneider B. Efficacy and safety of long-term complementary treatment with standardized European mistletoe extract (Viscum album L.) in addition to the conventional adjuvant oncologic therapy in patients with primary non-metastasized mammary carcinoma. Results of a multi-center, comparative, epidemiological cohort study in Germany and Switzerland. Arzneimittelforsch 2004;54:456–466

NETTLE
(*Urtica dioica*)

Source	Leaves and roots.
Main constituents	*Leaf*: minerals, flavonoids, sterols, tannins, vitamins. *Root*: coumarin, fatty acids, lectins, lignans, polysaccharides, sterols, tannins, terpenes.
Background	Stinging nettle is a perennial herb, which grows throughout much of the temperate zones of both hemispheres. The genus name *Urtica* derives from the Latin verb *urere* ('to burn'), while the species name *dioica* ('two houses') refers to the flowers bearing male and female on separate plants. Nettle is considered a weed and causes a characteristic itching rash upon contact with the skin. It has enjoyed a long history of medicinal use for a number of conditions such asthma and disorders of the spleen.
Examples of traditional uses	Asthma, bleeding conditions, infantile and psychogenic eczema, kidney disorders, muscle relaxant during childbirth, rheumatism. In culinary practice, young stinging nettle is eaten as a cooked vegetable.
Pharmacologic action	Diuretic, analgesic, antihypertensive, immunostimulatory and anti-inflammatory.
Conditions frequently treated	*Leaf*: kidney gravel, lower urinary tract infections, musculoskeletal pain. *Root*: micturition disorders in benign prostatic hyperplasia.
Clinical evidence	A number of RCTs have investigated nettle root extract for the treatment of benign prostatic hyperplasia (BPH).[1-4] These trials report improvements in symptom scores and urinary flow compared with placebo. Evidence from a double-blind RCT[5] suggests intergroup differences in favour of nettle root extract on the International Prostate Symptom Score, but no effect on maximum urinary flow. A combination preparation of nettle root extract and saw palmetto fruit extract has also been suggested as an effective intervention for patients with BPH (e.g.[6,7]). Other evidence from double-blind RCTs investigating combination preparations of nettle with extract of *Pygeum africanum* shows mixed results in patients with BPH.[8,9] Stinging nettle herb has also been the subject of RCTs reporting positive effects in patients with allergic rhinitis[10] and acute arthritis.[11] One RCT investigated the effects of stinging nettle leaves for osteoarthritic pain of the base of the thumb or index finger and reported beneficial effects for pain and disability scores compared with deadnettle (*Laminum album*).[12]

HERBAL AND NON-HERBAL MEDICINES

Dosage

Leaf: 0.6–2.1 g of dry extract daily in divided doses.
Root: 0.7–1.3 g of dry extract daily in divided doses.

Risks

Contraindications
Pregnancy and lactation (see p 5).

Precautions/warnings
Children under the age of 2 years.

Adverse effects
Gastrointestinal complaints, diarrhoea, allergic reactions, urticaria, pruritus, oedema, decreased urine volume.

Interactions
May potentiate the effects of diuretic, antihypertensive, antihyperglycaemic, central nervous system depressant agents. Might decrease the effects of anticoagulant drugs.

Risk–benefit assessment

The evidence of nettle root extract monopreparations for BPH is encouraging but not compelling. The available data on the nature and frequency of its adverse effects, however, indicate that it may be worthy of consideration. This is supported by the evidence on combination preparations with saw palmetto. There is little evidence of the efficacy of nettle root extract for any other condition. For nettle leaf, encouraging findings are emerging for its use in arthritis yet the evidence is not sufficiently strong to allow any firm recommendation.

REFERENCES

1 Engelmann U, Boos G, Kres H. Therapie der benignen Prostatahyperplasie mit Bazoton Liquidum. Urologe B 1996;36:287–291

2 Fischer M, Wilbert D. Wirkprüfung eines Phytopharmakons zur Behandlung der benignen Prostatahyperplasie. In: Rutishauser G (ed) Benigne Prostatahyperplasie III. München: Zuckerschwerdt; 1992, p 79

3 Dathe G, Schmid H. Phytotherapie der benignen Prostatahyperplasie (BPH). Doppelblindstudie mit Extraktum Radicis Urticae (ERU). Urologe B 1987;27:223–226

4 Vontobel H P, Herzog R, Rutishauser G, Kres H. Ergebnisse einer Doppelblindstudie über die Wirksamkeit von ERU-Kapseln in der konservativen Behandlung der benignen Prostatahyperplasie. Urologe A 1985;24:49–51

5 Schneider T, Rübben H. Stinging nettle root extract (Bazoton-uno) in long term treatment of benign prostatic syndrome (BPS). Results of a randomized, double-blind, placebo controlled multicenter study after 12 months. Der Urologe A 2004;43:302–306

6 Bondarenko B, Walther C, Funk P, Schläfke S, Engelmann U. Long-term efficacy and safety of PRO 160/120 (a combination of Sabal and Urtica extract) in patients with lower urinary tract symptoms (LUTS). Phytomedicine 2003; 10(Suppl4):53–55

7 Sökeland-J. Combined sabal and urtica extract compared with finasteride in men with benign prostatic hyperplasia: analysis of prostate volume and therapeutic outcome. BJU-Int 2000;86:439–442

8 Krzeski T, Kazon M, Borkowski A, Witeska A, Kuczera J. Combined extract of Urtica dioica and Pygeum africanum in the treatment of benign prostatic hyperplasia: double-blind comparison of two doses. Clin Therapeut 1993;15:1011–1020

9 Melo É A, Bertero E B, Rios L A S, Mattos Jr D. Evaluating the efficiency of a combination of Pygeum africanum and stinging nettle (Urtica dioica) extracts in treating benign prostatic hyperplasia (BPH): Double-blind,

randomized, placebo controlled trial. Int Braz J Urol 2002; 28:418–425

10 Mittman P. Randomized, double-blind study of freeze-dried Urtica dioica in the treatment of allergic rhinitis. Planta Med 1990;56:44–47

11 Chrubasik S, Enderlein W, Bauer R, Grabner W. Evidence of antirheumatic effectiveness of Herba Urticae dioicae in acute arthritis. A pilot study. Phytomedicine 1997;4:105–108

12 Randall C. Randall H, Dobbs F, Hutton C, Sanders H. Randomised controlled trial of nettle sting for treatment of base-of-thumb pain. J Roy Soc Med 2000;93:305–309

PASSION FLOWER
(Passiflora incarnata)

Source	Aerial parts, particularly leaves.
Main constituents	Alkaloids, coumarin derivatives, fatty acids, flavonoids, maltol.
Background	A member of the *Passifloraceae* family, passion flower is a perennial vine native to the southern USA, Central and South America. Its Latin name is connected to Christ, *passio* meaning suffering and *incarnata* meaning incarnate, with its flowered fringe thought to represent the crown of thorns and its five anthers representing the five stigmata. Historically, it has been used as a sedative at least as far back as the Aztecs.
Examples of traditional uses	Gastrointestinal spasms, generalised seizures, hysteria, insomnia, nervous restlessness, neuralgia.
Pharmacologic action	Sedative, hypnotic, anxiolytic, antispasmolytic.
Conditions frequently treated	Agitation, generalised anxiety disorder, insomnia, irritability, tension.
Clinical evidence	One RCT shows that passionflower liquid extract in combination with clonidine seems to be better than clonidine alone when used for reducing opiate withdrawal symptoms such as anxiety, irritability, insomnia and agitation.[1] There is some evidence from an RCT by the same author that passion flower liquid extract can be comparable to oxazepam for treating symptoms of generalised anxiety disorders in some patients.[2] Two RCTs of herbal combinations including passion flower extract reported reduced anxiety in patients with adjustment disorder with anxious mood[3] and sedative effects in healthy volunteers.[4] Also, in combination with hawthorn, improvements were demonstrated in the physical exercise capacity of patients (n = 40) with dyspnoea in a double-blind, placebo-controlled RCT.[5] The role of passion flower in these effects is however unknown.

HERBAL AND NON-HERBAL MEDICINES

Dosage

Above ground parts: 0.25–2 g of the dried above ground parts, three times daily.
Liquid extract: 0.5–1 ml (1:1 in 25% alcohol) three times daily.
Tincture: 0.5–1 ml (1:8 in 45% alcohol) three times daily.

Risks

Contraindications
Pregnancy and lactation (see p 5)

Precautions/warnings
Ability to drive or operate machinery may be impaired.

Adverse effects
Dizziness, confusion, ataxia, nausea, vomiting, drowsiness, ventricular tachycardia and vasculitis have been reported.

Overdose
Excessive doses may cause sedation.

Interactions
Theoretically potentiation of drugs with sedative properties and anticoagulant/antiplatelet potential is possible.

Quality issues
Passion flower is often combined with other herbs in commercial preparations for insomnia. Its active principles have not been identified, although flavonoids are generally used for standardisation.

Risk–benefit assessment

Although some evidence exists supporting the effectiveness of passion flower extract in combination with other herbs for anxiety, irritability, insomnia and agitation, there is little clinical data to support the medicinal use of monopreparations of passion flower. Information on its safety is also lacking. Its use as a monopreparation cannot therefore be recommended due to insufficient evidence on the risk–benefit ratio.

REFERENCES

1 Akhondzadeh S, Kashani L, Mobaseri M, Hosseini S H, Nikzad S, Khani M. Passionflower in the treatment of opiates withdrawal: a double-blind randomized controlled trial. J Clin Pharm Ther 2001;25:369–373

2 Akhondzadeh S, Naghavi H R, Shayeganpour A, Shayeganpour A, Rashidi H, Khani M. Passionflower in the treatment of generalized anxiety: a pilot double-blind randomized controlled trial with oxazepam. J Clin Pharm Ther 2001;26:363–367

3 Boutin R N, Bouhrtol T, Guitton B, Broutin E. A combination of plant extracts in the treatment of outpatients with adjustment disorder with anxious mood: controlled study versus placebo. Fundament Clin Pharmacol 1997;11:127–132

4 Gerhard U, Hobi V, Kocher R, Konig C. Acute sedative effect of a herbal relaxation tablet as compared to that of bromazepam. Schweiz Rundsch Med Prax 1991;80:1481–1486

5 Von Eiff M, Brunner H, Haegeli A, Kreuter U, Martina B, Meier B, Schaffner W. Hawthorne/passion flower extract and improvement in physical exercise capacity of patients with dyspnoea class II of the NYHA functional classification. Acta Ther 1994;20:47–66

PEPPERMINT
(Mentha x piperita)

Source	Leaves and oil.
Main constituents	*Leaf*: caffeic, chlorogenic and rosmarinic acids, hesperidin, luteolin, rutin, volatile oil. *Oil*: cineol, isomenthone, limonene, menthofuran, menthol, menthone, menthyl acetate.
Background	Peppermint is a perennial herb that grows to a height of about 1 m. It grows along stream banks and moist wastelands throughout much of Europe and North America and is characterised by its smell and its square stem, which is typical for members of the mint family. It is a natural hybrid of water mint (*Mentha aquatica*) and spearmint (*Mentha spicata*). Its genus name, *Mentha*, is derived from the Greek mythical nymph *Mintha*, who metamorphosed into this plant. Peppermint is mainly cultivated for its fragrant oil, which is obtained through steam distillation of the fresh aerial parts of the plant. The leading producer of peppermint oil is the USA.
Examples of traditional uses	*Leaf*: complaints of the gallbladder and bile duct, flatulence, gastrointestinal disorders. *Oil*: common cold, headache, inflammation of the oral mucosa, irritable bowel syndrome, myalgia, neuralgia.
Pharmacologic action	Antispasmodic, antimicrobial, antiseptic, carminative, cholagogue, cooling. The principal active constituent of peppermint oil is thought to be menthol, a cyclic monoterpene with calcium channel-blocking activity.
Conditions frequently treated	*Leaf*: complaints of the gastrointestinal tract. *Oil*: common cold, headache, irritable bowel syndrome, myalgia.
Clinical evidence	For irritable bowel syndrome an earlier systematic review and meta-analysis suggested that, although the majority of RCTs report beneficial effects, methodological limitations prevent firm conclusions.[1] This was corroborated by a further independent systematic review.[2] For children with recurrent abdominal pain, a systematic review found evidence of effectiveness.[3] For treating non-ulcer dyspepsia, a systematic review identified nine RCTs of combination preparations containing peppermint and caraway and concluded that they seem to have effects of at least a similar magnitude as conventional therapies and encouraging safety profiles.[4] Antispasmodic effects for intraluminally administered peppermint oil have been reported during upper endoscopy.[5] RCTs from the same research group suggested positive effects of externally applied peppermint oil in healthy volunteers and for

patients with tension-type headache.[6–8] Single RCTs suggested peppermint tea as a possible adjuvant treatment for urinary tract infection[9] and no difference for aromatherapy with peppermint oil compared with placebo for postoperative nausea.[10]

Dosage

Leaf: 3–6 g as infusion daily.
0.8–1.8 g of dry extract daily in divided doses.
Essential oil: 0.6–1.2 ml in enteric-coated capsules daily.
3–4 drops three times daily in hot water internally (as inhalant).
Apply as needed externally.

Risks

Contraindications
Pregnancy and lactation (see p 5), children under the age of 12 years, obstruction of the bile duct, cholecystitis, allergy to any constituent of peppermint.

Precautions/warnings
Individuals with glucose-6 phosphate dehydrogenase deficiency, gallstones, hiatal hernia.

Adverse effects
Allergic reactions, skin irritation, contact dermatitis, laryngeal or bronchial spasm, mouth ulceration, eye irritation, heartburn, belching, perianal burning, gastrointestinal complaints, headache, dizziness, pruritus.

Overdose
The fatal dose of menthol in humans is estimated to be 1 g per kg body weight.

Interactions
Might increase levels of drugs metabolised by CYP3A4.

Risk–benefit assessment

Although RCTs of peppermint oil for irritable bowel syndrome report positive effects, the evidence is not convincing. The possibility of adverse effects exists. For functional dyspepsia there seems to be good evidence of effectiveness for combination preparations of peppermint/caraway oil. Considering their safety profile it seems that peppermint/caraway oil preparations can be recommended for functional dyspepsia. For all other indications, the evidence is as yet not established beyond reasonable doubt.

REFERENCES

1   Pittler M H, Ernst E. Peppermint oil for irritable bowel syndrome: a critical review and meta-analysis. Am J Gastroenterol 1998;93:1131–1135

2   Jailwala J, Imperiale T F, Kroenke K. Pharmacologic treatment of the irritable bowel syndrome: A systematic review of randomized, controlled trials. Ann Intern Med 2000;133:136–147

3   Weydert J A, Ball T M, Davis M F. Systematic review of treatments for recurrent abdominal pain. Pediatrics 2003;111:e1–e11

4   Thompson Coon J, Ernst E. Systematic review: herbal medicinal products for non-ulcer dyspepsia. Aliment Pharmacol Ther 2002:16: 1689–1699

5   Hiki N, Kurosaka H, Tatsutomi Y, Shimoyama S, Tsuji E, Kojima J, Shimizu N, Ono H,

Hirooka T, Noguchi C, Mafune K I, Kaminishi M.Peppermint oil reduces gastric spasm during upper endoscopy: A randomized, double-blind, double-dummy controlled trial. Gastrointest Endosc 2003;57:475–482

6 Göbel H, Schmidt G, Soyka D. Effect of peppermint and eucalyptus oil preparations on neurophysiological and experimental algesimetric headache parameters. Cephalalgia 1994;14:228–234

7 Göbel H, Fresenius J, Heinze A, Dworschak M, Soyka D. Effectiveness of peppermint oil and paracetamol in the treatment of tension type headache. Nervenarzt 1996;67:672–681

8 Göbel H, Heinze A, Dworschak M, Heinze-Kuhn K, Stolze H. Oleum menthae piperitae in the acute therapy of migraine and tension-type headache. Z Phytother 2004;25:129–139

9 Ebbinghaus K D. A 'tea' containing various plant products as adjuvant to chemotherapy of urinary tract infections. Therapiewoche 1985;35:2041–2051

10 Anderson L A, Gross J B. Aromatherapy with peppermint, isopropyl alcohol or placebo is equally effective in relieving postoperative nausea. J Perianesth Nurs 2004;19:29–35

PHYTOESTROGENS

Source	Plants, fruits, vegetables, grains.
Main constituents	Coumestans, isoflavones, lignans.
Background	Phytoestrogens are plant-derived compounds with weak oestrogen-like activities. It has been suggested that the high consumption of dietary phytoestrogens of Asian populations is associated with a low incidence of hormone-related disease. Certain foods such as red clover- or soy-derived products are known to have high levels of phytoestrogens. One of the most important phytoestrogens is the isoflavone genistein. Human exposure to genistein occurs through normal dietary intake and through the intake of genistein or other isoflavone extracts as dietary supplements.
Pharmacologic action	Oestrogenic, antioestrogenic, proliferative, antiproliferative, antioxidative, anti-inflammatory.
Conditions frequently treated	Breast cancer, osteoporosis and vasomotor symptoms in menopausal women, prevention of heart disease.
Clinical evidence	A meta-analysis of all available data on red clover (*Trifolium pratense*) isoflavones concluded that there is evidence of a small beneficial effect for treating hot flushes in menopausal women,[1] which is in contrast to other findings.[2] There is little evidence, at present, to support the use of red clover isoflavones in any other aspect of women's health. This is supported by a systematic review, which concluded that, based on data up to 1999, there is insufficient evidence to recommend the use of phytoestrogens in place of traditional oestrogen replacement therapy.[3] Additional RCTs of soy phytoestrogens report mixed results for menopausal

symptoms in postmenopausal women[4,5] and no alleviation of hot flushes and menopausal symptoms in breast cancer patients.[6–8] This notion is, however, in disagreement with other evidence.[9,10] Positive evidence is available for the phytoestrogen genistein for treating hot flushes,[11] the preparation melbrosia[12] and for a preparation of *Pueraria mirifica* in post- and perimenopausal women.[13] A meta-analysis of 38 controlled trials reported that consumption of soy protein rather than animal protein decreased serum concentrations of total cholesterol, low-density lipoprotein cholesterol and triglycerides.[14] Additional evidence from placebo-controlled RCTs could not confirm these results for postmenopausal women,[15–18] whereas other studies have produced mixed results.[19,20] Positive data are available for flaxseed derived phytoestrogens for improving lipid profiles,[21–23] whereas for red clover the data are negative.[24] For bone resorption and bone mineral density positive effects were reported in peri- and postmenopausal women,[25–28] but not for markers of bone turnover in adolescent males.[29] An RCT reported that compared with sunflower seed, consumption of flaxseed for 6 weeks reduced the rate of bone resorption in postmenopausal women.[30] Ipriflavone, a synthetic isoflavone, has also been shown to prevent postmenopausal bone loss (e.g.[31]). Beneficial effects of phytoestrogens have also been reported for memory enhancement,[32] menstrual migraine,[33] type 2 diabetes,[34] vaginal cell maturation,[35] pregnancy rate in in vitro fertilisation-embryo transfer cycles[36] and on the risk of prostate cancer development and progression.[37] *Pueraria lobata* showed some beneficial effects on cognitive function in postmenopausal women.[38]

Dosage

40–100 mg of isoflavones daily.

Risks

Contraindications
None known for phytoestrogens consumed as part of diet. Concentrated isoflavone supplements should not be taken during pregnancy or lactation (see p 5), by children or those with hormone-dependent tumours.

Precautions/warnings
May affect the menstrual cycle. Possible proliferative effects on the endometrium.[39]

Adverse effects
Flatulence. For red clover, the limited evidence indicates no serious safety concerns associated with short-term use. No long-term safety data are available.

Overdose
Effects of large quantities of phytoestrogens, as consumed by infants fed soy milk or individuals taking concentrated supple-

ments, are not known. Impairments to the reproductive system are considered possible, but have not been reported. Overdoses have been linked with endometrial cancer in one case.[40]

Interactions
None known.

Quality issues
Soy products may be genetically modified.

Risk–benefit assessment

The available evidence suggests that phytoestrogens from red clover extracts have a small beneficial effect for treating hot flushes in menopausal women. Phytoestrogens seem to have small beneficial effects on lipid profiles. Positive effects have also been reported for bone loss in postmenopausal women. Other than epidemiological studies, no long-term safety data are available, but few risks have been reported during short-term use. Therefore, the risk–benefit balance may be favourable for these indications. However, there is insufficient evidence to recommend the use of phytoestrogens as an alternative to oestrogen replacement therapy.

REFERENCES

1 Thompson Coon J, Pittler M H, Ernst E. Systematic review and meta-analysis of Trifolium pratense (red clover) isoflavones for treating vasomotor symptoms in menopausal women. (in press)

2 Krebs E E, Ensrud K E, MacDonald R, Wilt T J. Phytoestrogens for treatment of menopausal symptoms: a systematic review. Obstet Gynecol 2004;104:824–836

3 Glazier M G, Bowman M A. A review of the evidence for the use of phytoestrogens as a replacement for traditional estrogen replacement therapy. Arch Intern Med 2001;161:1161–1172

4 Kotsopoulos D, Dalais F S, Liang Y L, McGrath B P, Teede H J. The effects of soy protein containing phytoestrogens on menopausal symptoms in postmenopausal women. Climacteric 2000;3:161–167

5 Colacurci N, Zarcone R, Borrelli A, De Franciscis P, Fortunato N, Cirillo M, Fornaro F. Effects of soy isoflavones on menopausal neurovegetative symptoms. Minerva Ginecol 2004;56:407–412

6 Quella S K, Loprinzi C L, Barton D L, Knost J A, Sloan J A, LaVasseur B I, Swan D, Krupp K R, Miller K D, Novotny P J. Evaluation of soy phytoestrogens for the treatment of hot flashes in breast cancer survivors: A North Central Cancer Treatment Group Trial. J Clin Oncol 2000;18:1068–1074

7 Van Patten C L, Olivotto I A, Chambers G K, Gelmon K A, Hislop T G, Templeton E, Wattie A, Prior J C. Effect of soy phytoestrogens on hot flashes in postmenopausal women with breast cancer: a randomized, controlled clinical trial. J Clin Oncol 2002;20:1449–1455

8 Nikander E, Kilkkinen A, Metsa-Heikkila M, Adlercreutz H, Pietinen P, Tiitinen A, Ylikorkala O. A randomized placebo-controlled crossover trial with phytoestrogens in treatment of menopause in breast cancer patients. Obstet Gynecol 2003;101:1213–1220

9 Ingram D, Sanders K, Kolybaba M, Lopez D. Case-control study of phytoestrogens and breast cancer. Lancet 1997;350:990–994

10 Scambia G, Mango D, Signorile PG, Anselmi Angeli R A, Palena C, Gallo D, Bombardelli E, Morazzoni P, Riva A, Mancuso S. Clinical effects of a standardized soy extract in postmenopausal women: a pilot study. Menopause 2000;7:105–111

11 Crisafulli A, Marini H, Bitto A, Altavilla D, Squadrito G, Romeo A, Adamo E B, Marini R, D'Anna R, Corrado F, Bartolone S, Frisina N, Squadrito F. Effects of genistein on hot flushes in early postmenopausal women: a randomized, double-blind EPT- and placebo controlled study. Menopause 2004;11:400–404

12 Kolarov G, Nalbanski B, Kamenov Z, Orbetsova M, Georgiev S, Nikolov A, Marinov B. Possibilities for an individualized approach

to the treatment of climacteric symptoms with phytoestrogens. Akush Ginekol (Sofiia) 2001;40:18–21

13 Lamlertkittikul S, Chandeying V. Efficacy and safety of Pueraria mirifica (Kwao Kruea Khao) for the treatment of vasomotor symptoms in perimenopausal women: Phase II Study. J Med Assoc Thai 2004;87:33–40

14 Anderson J W, Johnstone B M, Cook-Newell M E. Meta-analysis of the effects of soy protein intake on serum lipids. New Engl J Med 1995;333:276–282

15 Lissin L W, Oka R, Lakshmi S, Cooke JP. Isoflavones improve vascular reactivity in post-menopausal women with hypercholesterolemia. Vasc Med 2004;9:26–30

16 Carranza-Lira S, Barahona O F, Ramos D, Herrera J, Olivares-Segura A, Cardoso G, Posadas-Romero C. Changes in symptoms, lipid and hormone levels after the administration of a cream with phytoestrogens in the Climacteric – preliminary report. Int J Fertil Womens Med 2001;46:296–299

17 Simons L A, von Konigsmark M, Simons J, Celermajer D S. Phytoestrogens do not influence lipoprotein levels or endothelial function in healthy, postmenopausal women. Am J Cardiol 2000;85:1297–1301

18 Dewell A, Hollenbeck CB, Bruce B. The effects of soy-derived phytoestrogens on serum lipids and lipoproteins in moderately hypercholesterolemic postmenopausal women. J Clin Endocrinol Metab 2002;87:118–121

19 Washburn S, Burke G L, Morgan T, Anthony M. Effect of soy protein supplementation on serum lipoproteins, blood pressure, and menopausal symptoms in perimenopausal women. Menopause 1999;6:7–13

20 Teede H J, Dalais F S, Kotsopoulos D, Liang Y L, Davis S, McGrath B P. Dietary soy has both beneficial and potentially adverse cardiovascular effects: a placebo-controlled study in men and postmenopausal women. J Clin Endocrinol Metab 2001;86:3053–3060

21 Lucas E A, Wild R D, Hammond L J, Khalil D A, Juma S, Daggy B P, Stoecker B J, Arjmandi B H. Flaxseed improves lipid profile without altering biomarkers of bone metabolism in postmenopausal women. J Clin Endocrinol Metab 2002;87:1527–1532

22 Lemay A, Dodin S, Kadri N, Jacques H, Forest J C. Flaxseed dietary supplement versus hormone replacement therapy in hypercholesterolemic menopausal women. Obstet Gynecol 2002;100:495–504

23 Dodin S, Lemay A, Jacques H, Legare F, Forest J C, Masse B. The effects of flaxseed dietary supplement on lipid profile, bone mineral density, and symptoms in menopausal women: a randomized, double-blind, wheat germ placebo-controlled clinical trial. J Clin Endocrinol Metab 2005;90:1390–1397

24 Howes J B, Sullivan D, Lai N, Nestel P, Pomeroy S, West L, Eden J A, Howes L G. The effects of dietary supplementation with isoflavones from red clover on the lipoprotein profiles of post menopausal women with mild to moderate hypercholesterolaemia. Atherosclerosis 2000;152:143–147

25 Potter S M, Baum J A, Teng H, Stillman R J, Shay N F, Erdman J W. Soy protein and isoflavones: their effects on blood lipids and bone density in postmenopausal women. Am J Clin Nutr 1998;68:1375–1379

26 Morabito N, Crisafulli A, Vergara C, Gaudio A, Lasco A, Frisina N, D'Anna R, Corrado F, Pizzoleo M A, Cincotta M, Altavilla D, Ientile R, Squadrito F. Effects of genistein and hormone-replacement therapy on bone loss in early postmenopausal women: a randomized double-blind placebo-controlled study. J Bone Miner Res 2002;17:1904–1912

27 Nikander E, Metsa-Heikkila M, Ylikorkala O, Tiitinen A. Effects of phytoestrogens on bone turnover in postmenopausal women with a history of breast cancer. J Clin Endocrinol Metab 2004;89:1207–1212

28 Atkinson C, Compston J E, Day N E, Dowsett M, Bingham S A. The effects of phytoestrogen isoflavones on bone density in women: a double-blind, randomized, placebo-controlled trial. Am J Clin Nutr 2004;79:326–333

29 Jones G, Dwyer T, Hynes K, Dalais F S, Parameswaran V, Greenaway TM. A randomized controlled trial of phytoestrogen supplementation, growth and bone turnover in adolescent males. Eur J Clin Nutr 2003;57:324–327

30 Arjmandi B H, Juma S, Lucas E A, Wei L, Venkatesh S, Khan D A. Flaxseed supplementation positively influences bone metabolism in postmenopausal women. J Am Nutraceutical Assoc 1998;1:27–32

31 Gennari C, Agnusdei D, Crepaldi G, Isaia G, Mazzuoli G, Ortolani S, Bufalino L, Passeri M. Effect of ipriflavone – a synthetic derivative of natural isoflavones – on bone mass loss in the early years after menopause. Menopause 1998;5:9–15

32 File S E, Jarrett N, Fluck E, Duffy R, Casey K, Wiseman H. Eating soya improves human

memory. Psychopharmacology (Berl) 2001;157:430–436

33 Burke B E, Olson R D, Cusack B J. Randomized, controlled trial of phytoestrogen in the prophylactic treatment of menstrual migraine. Biomed Pharmacother 2002;56:283–288

34 Jayagopal V, Albertazzi P, Kilpatrick E S, Howarth E M, Jennings P E, Hepburn D A, Atkin SL. Beneficial effects of soy phytoestrogen intake in postmenopausal women with type 2 diabetes. Diabetes Care 2002;25:1709–1714

35 Chiechi L M, Putignano G, Guerra V, Schiavelli M P, Cisternino A M, Carriero C. The effect of a soy rich diet on the vaginal epithelium in postmenopause: a randomized double blind trial. Maturitas 2003;45:241–246

36 Unfer V, Casini M L, Gerli S, Costabile L, Mignosa M, Di Renzo GC. Phytoestrogens may improve the pregnancy rate in in vitro

fertilization-embryo transfer cycles: a prospective, controlled, randomized trial. Fertil Steril 2004;82:1509–1513

37 Dalais F S, Meliala A, Wattanapenpaiboon N, Frydenberg M, Suter D A, Thomson W K, Wahlqvist M L. Effects of a diet rich in phytoestrogens on prostate-specific antigen and sex hormones in men diagnosed with prostate cancer. Urology 2004;64:510–515

38 Woo J, Lau E, Ho S C, Cheng F, Chan C, Chan A S, Haines C J, Chan T Y, Li M, Sham A. Comparison of Pueraria lobata with hormone replacement therapy in treating the adverse health consequences of menopause. Menopause 2003;10:352–361

39 Arici A, Bukulmez O. Phyto-oestrogens and the endometrium. Lancet 2004;364:2081–2082

40 Johnson E B, Muto M G, Yanushpolsky E H, Mutter G L. Phytoestrogen supplementation and endometrial cancer. Obstet Gynecol 2001;98: 947–950

PROPOLIS

Source Beehives.

Main constituents Flavonoids, hydroxycinammic acids.

Background Propolis is a resinous material made by bees, produced by combining resin from the buds of various trees, particularly *Populus* species, with other substances such as salivary secretions and bee wax. It has antimicrobial properties and the bees primarily use it to apply a thin layer on the internal walls of their hives, in particular the brood chambers. Propolis is responsible for the relatively low rate of bacterial contamination and moulds in the hive or other cavities that are inhabited by bees. The material is also used to disinfect incoming bees at the entrance to the hive. This is reflected by the meaning of the term propolis, which is derived from the Greek *pro* ('before') and *polis* ('town').

Examples of traditional uses Acne, common cold, dermatitis, duodenal ulcers, gastric disturbances, laryngitis, wound healing.

Pharmacologic action Antibacterial, antifungal, antiviral, anti-inflammatory, antioxidant, cytotoxic.

Conditions frequently treated A constituent of mouthwash liquids.

HERBAL AND NON-HERBAL MEDICINES

Clinical evidence

A non-randomised, double-blind, placebo-controlled trial assessed the effects of a mouthrinse containing propolis (n = 100).[1] It reported some positive effects on the Silness & Löe plaque index after 4 weeks of treatment. Another small (n = 6) double-blind, placebo controlled crossover trial[2] reported beneficial intergroup differences on the Silness & Löe plaque index in favour of a mouthwash containing propolis. It is unclear whether the patients in this trials were randomised. In a double-blind RCT (n = 42) patients were instructed to rinse twice daily with 10% propolis in ethanol for 5 days. There were no differences on the Silness & Löe plaque index compared with placebo.[3] Toothpaste containing propolis was tested in a non-randomised, double-blind trial (n = 103) which reported no beneficial effects on caries and plaque formation compared with placebo toothpaste.[4] Double-blind, placebo-controlled RCTs exist for ulcerative colitis and Crohn's disease[5], reporting negative results, and acute uterine cervicitis[6], herpes labialis recurrences (cold sores),[7] and respiratory tract infections[8] reporting positive results. Beneficial effects for rheumatic disorders are reported in a non-randomised, single-blind, placebo-controlled trial (n = 190).[9] A multicentre RCT which assessed propolis for genital herpes[10] found some antiviral activity, corroborating the results of another study,[11] and concluded that propolis appeared to be more effective than acyclovir and placebo in healing lesions and reducing local symptoms.

Dosage

Mouthwash: apply once or twice daily.

Risks

Contraindications
Allergy to bee stings.

Precautions/warnings
Other allergic predispositions.

Adverse effects
Allergic reactions, contact dermatitis, hyperkeratotic dermatitis, vesicular dermatitis, itching, swelling, mucositis, stomatitis.

Interactions
None known.

Quality issues
Depending on the plant sources and the geographic origin, the chemical composition will vary. An accepted method of standardisation for propolis preparations is lacking.

Risk–benefit assessment

A coherent body of evidence is lacking from rigorous clinical studies of propolis to make firm recommendations for any condition. Some positive findings exist for cold sores, respiratory tract infections, uterine cervicitis and genital herpes. Whether it has beneficial effects as a constituent in mouthwashes is unclear. Propolis seems relatively safe although allergic reactions have been reported. In the light of the costs involved and the availability of other conventional treatment approaches, these might be preferred.

REFERENCES

1 Schmidt H, Hampel C-M, Schmidt G, Riess E, Rödel C. Doppelblindversuch über den Einflua eines propolishaltigen Mundwassers auf die entzündete und gesunde Gingiva. Stomatol der DDR 1980;30:491–497

2 Koo H, Cury J A, Rosalen P L, Ambrosano G M B, Ikegaki M, Park Y K. Effect of a mouthrinse containing selected propolis on 3-day dental plaque accumulation and polysaccharide formation. Caries-Res 2002;36:445–448

3 Murray M C, Worthington H V, Blinkhorn A S. A study to investigate the effect of a propolis-containing mouthrinse on the inhibition of de novo plaque formation. J Clin Periodontol 1997;24:796–798

4 Poppe B, Michaelis H. Ergebnisse einer zweimal jährlich kontrollierten Mundhygieneaktion mit propolishaltiger Zahnpasta (Doppelblindstudie). Stomatol der DDR 1986;36:195–203

5 Danø A P, Hylander Møller E, Jarnum S. Effekten af naturstoffet propolis ved colitis ulcerosa og Crohn's sygdom. Ugeskr Læg 1979;141:1888–1890

6 Santana Pérez E, Lugones Botell M, Pérez Stuart O, Castillo Brito B. Parasitisimo vaginal y cervicitis aguda: tratamiento local con propoleo. Informe preliminar. Rev Cubana Enfermer 1995;11:51–56

7 Hoheisel O. The effects of Herstat (3% propolis ointment ACF) application in cold sores: A double-blind placebo-controlled clinical trial. J Clin Res 2001;4:65–75

8 Cohen H A, Varsano I, Kahan E, Sarrell E M, Uziel Y. Effectiveness of an herbal preparation containing echinacea, propolis, and vitamin C in preventing respiratory tract infections in children: a randomized, double-blind, placebo-controlled, multicenter study. Arch Pediatr Adolesc Med 2004;158:217–221

9 Béla S, Sándor S, Béla L, György M, Ede S. Local treatment of rheumatic disorders by propolis. Orvosi Hetilap 1996;137:1365–1370

10 Vynograd N, Vynograd I, Sosnowski Z. A comparative multi-centre study of the efficacy of propolis, acyclovir and placebo in the treatment of genital herpes (HSV). Phytomedicine 2000;7:1–6

11 Szmeja Z, Sosnowski Z. Therapeutic value of flavonoid in rhinovirus infections. Otolaryngol Pol 1989;43:180–184

HERBAL AND NON-HERBAL MEDICINES

RED CLOVER
(*Trifolium pratense*)

Source	Flower heads.
Main constituents	Carbohydrates, coumarins, flavonoids, isoflavonoids, saponins, volatile oil.
Background	A member of the *Leguminosae* family, red clover is native to most of Europe and naturalised in the USA. It has a long history in agriculture and religion and was considered a charm against witchcraft in the Middle Ages. It has been used by traditional Chinese physicians and Russian folk healers for various medicinal purposes.
Examples of traditional uses	Cancer, chronic skin disease, tuberculosis, whooping cough.

Pharmacologic action	Oestrogenic.
Conditions frequently treated	Cough, eczema, menopausal symptoms, psoriasis.
Clinical evidence	A systematic review included 11 RCTs.[1] Five studies tested the effects of red clover isoflavones on vasomotor symptoms in menopausal women and were suitable for inclusion in a meta-analysis. Its results indicated a small reduction in hot flush frequency in women receiving active treatment (40–80 mg/day) compared with those receiving placebo. Data were limited regarding effects on postmenopausal osteoporosis, cyclical mastalgia and protection against breast and endometrial cancers. Similar findings emerged from other systematic reviews which, however, included only four or five RCTs.[2–4] A further RCT (n = 177) suggested that regular intake of red clover extract for 1 year is more effective than placebo in attenuating bone loss in postmenopausal women.[5] Preliminary data suggest positive effects on cardiovascular risk factors such as lipid pattern, blood pressure and arterial stiffness.[6–8]
Dosage	*Dried extract:* 500 mg daily standardised to 40 mg isoflavones. *Liquid extract:* 1.5–3 ml (1:1 in 25% alcohol) three times daily.
Risks	*Contraindications* Pregnancy and lactation (see p 5), infants.
	Precautions/warnings Bleeding disorders, coagulation disorders, one long-term trial found no effect on mammographic breast density but other authors are cautious regarding hormone sensitive cancers.[5]
	Adverse effects Breast tenderness, menstruation changes, weight gain, allergic reactions, myalgia, headache, nausea, vaginal spotting.[9]
	Interactions Theoretically red clover may interfere with anticoagulants, hormonal therapies and tamoxifen. Red clover may inhibit the cytochrome P450 system and could thus increase blood levels of drugs metabolised by it.[10]
	Quality issues Red clover may appear in products combined with other herbs.
Risk–benefit assessment	There is reasonably strong evidence of a small effect in the short-term treatment of vasomotor symptoms in menopausal women. Long-term effects are largely unknown. No serious adverse effects of short-term use are on record. Therefore short-term treatment of hot flushes with red clover can be recommended.

HERBAL AND NON-HERBAL MEDICINES

REFERENCES

1 Thompson Coon J, Pittler M H, Ernst E. The role of red clover (Trifolium pratense) isoflavones in women's reproductive health: a systematic review and meta-analysis of randomized trials. (in press)

2 Hsu I P, Chia S L, Lin C T, Jou H J. The effect of isoflavones from red clover on hot flushes in menopausal women – a systematic review of randomized, placebo-controlled trials. Nutr Sci J 2004;29:184–190

3 Krebs E E, Ensrud K E, MacDonald R, Wilt T J. Phytoestrogens for treatment of menopausal symptoms: a systematic review. Obstet Gynecol 2004;104:824–836

4 Kashani L, Bathaei F S, Ojaghi M, Bathaei M, Akondzadeh S. A systematic review of herbal medical products for the treatment of menopausal symptoms. J Med Plants 2004;3: 1–13

5 Atkinson C, Compston J E, Day N E, Dowsett M, Bingham S A. The effects of phytoestrogen isoflavones on bone density in women: a double-blind, randomized, placebo-controlled trial. Am J Clin Nutr 2004;79:326–333

6 Campbell M J, Woodside J V, Honour J W, Morton M S, Leathem A J. Effect of red clover derived isoflavone supplementation on insulin-like growth factor, lipid and antioxidant status in healthy female volunteers: a pilot study. Eur J Clin-Nutr 2004;58:173–179

7 Teede H J, McGrath B P, DeSilva L, Cehun M, Fassoulakis A, Nestel P J. Isoflavones reduce arterial stiffness: a placebo-controlled study in men and postmenopausal women. Arterioscler Thromb Vasc Biol 2003;23:1066–1071

8 Howes J B, Tran D, Brillante D, Howes L G. Effects of dietary supplementation with isoflavones from red clover on ambulatory blood pressure and endothelial function in postmenopausal type 2 diabetes. Diabetes Obes Metab 2003;5:325–232

9 Atkinson C, Oosthuizen W, Scollen S, Loktionov A, Day N E, Bingham S A. Modest protective effects of isoflavones from a red clover-derived dietary supplement on cardiovascular disease risk factors in perimenopausal women, and evidence of an interaction with ApoE genotype in 49–65 year old women. J Nutr 2004;6.170–179

10 Red clover monograph. Natural Medicines Comprehensive Database. *www.naturaldatabase.com*, accessed 05/10/04

SAW PALMETTO
(Serenoa repens)

Source	Fruits
Main constituents	Fatty acids, flavonoids, phytosterols, and polysaccharides.
Background	Saw palmetto is a dwarf palm native to the coastal regions of the southern states in North America, particularly South Carolina and Florida. In traditional medicine it was used as an extract for conditions such as bladder or urethral irritations. The fruits of saw palmetto were also employed as a tonic in cases of consumption or bronchitis. Today, commercially available preparations contain the lipophilic fraction, extracted with hexane or liquid carbon dioxide. It is a popular herbal remedy, and it is frequently used for the urinary symptoms of benign prostatic hyperplasia.
Examples of traditional uses	Cystitis, dysentery, hirsutism, increase of sexual vigor, testicular atrophy.
Pharmacologic action	Inhibition of 5-alpha-reductase, inhibitory effects on the binding of dihydrotestosterone to androgen receptors in the prostate, anti-inflammatory, antiproliferative, prolactin inhibition.

HERBAL AND NON-HERBAL MEDICINES

Conditions frequently treated	Benign prostatic hyperplasia.
Dosage	320 mg of liposterolic extract daily in divided doses.
Clinical evidence	A Cochrane review assessed 21 RCTs lasting 4 to 48 weeks of saw palmetto for treating benign prostatic hyperplasia.[1] It concluded that saw palmetto provides mild to moderate improvement in urinary symptoms and flow measures compared with placebo. Compared with finasteride, saw palmetto produces similar improvements of urinary symptoms and flow measures, with fewer adverse events. These conclusions are corroborated by another meta-analysis of 14 RCTs of a single saw palmetto monopreparation. It concluded that the meta-analysis of all available published trials of Permixon for treating men with benign prostatic hyperplasia showed an improvement in peak flow rate and reduction in nocturia above placebo, and a 5-point reduction in the International Prostate Symptom Score.[2] These results are also confirmed by additional evidence from double-blind RCTs;[3-6] although one further double-blind RCT did not report differences compared with placebo.[7] Double-blind RCTs also report beneficial effects of saw palmetto for androgenic alopecia[8,9] and an open RCT reported no appreciable improvement in patients with category III prostatitis or chronic pelvic pain syndrome over a 1-year treatment period.[10]

Risks

Contraindications
Pregnancy and lactation (see p 5).

Precautions/warnings
Allergy or hypersensitivity to saw palmetto or any of its constituents, may increase bleeding time.

Adverse effects
Gastrointestinal complaints, bleeding, haemorrhage, dizziness, headache, constipation, diarrhoea, dysuria, decreased libido.

Interactions
May interact with hormone replacement therapy, oral contraceptives. May increase the effects of antiandrogenic drugs, and decrease the effects of androgenic drugs. Appears to pose a minimal risk for cytochrome P450-mediated herb–drug interactions in humans.[11]

Quality issues
The quality of the extracts may vary between preparations.

Risk–benefit assessment

There is good evidence for the effectiveness of saw palmetto for benign prostatic hyperplasia. It seems to improve the symptoms and objective signs of benign prostatic hyperplasia to the same extent as finasteride. The encouraging safety profile of saw palmetto extract renders it an attractive option for patients with this condition. Data from long-term clinical studies are, as yet, not available. There are some encouraging data for androgenic alopecia.

REFERENCES

1 Wilt T, Ishani A, MacDonald R. Serenoa repens for benign prostatic hyperplasia. The Cochrane Database of Systematic Reviews 2002, Issue 3. Art. No.: CD001423

2 Boyle P, Robertson C, Lowe F, Roehrborn C. Updated meta-analysis of clinical trials of Serenoa repens extract in the treatment of symptomatic benign prostatic hyperplasia. BJU Int 2004;93:751–756

3 Mohanty N K, Jha R J, Dutt C. Randomized double-blind controlled clinical trial of Serenoa repens versus placebo in the management of patients with symptomatic grade I to grade II benign prostatic hyperplasia. Indian J Urol 1999;16:26–31

4 Stepanov V N, Siniakova L A, Sarrazin B, Raynaud J P. Efficacy and tolerability of the lipidosterolic extract of Serenoa repens in benign prostatic hyperplasia. A double-blind comparison of two dosage regimens. Adv Ther 1999;16:231–241

5 Giannakopoulos X, Baltogiannis D, Giannakis D, Tasos A, Sofikitis N, Charalabopoulos K, Evangelou A. The lipidosterolic extract of Serenoa repens in the treatment of benign prostatic hyperplasia: a comparison of two dosage regimens. Adv Ther 2002;19: 285–296

6 Debruyne F, Boyle P, Calais da Silva F, Gillenwater J G, Hamdy F C, Perrin P, Teillac P, Vela Navarrete R, Raynaud JP, Schulman C. Evaluation of the clinical benefit of Permixon and tamsulosin in severe BPH patients – PERMAL study subset analysis. Prog-Urol 2004;14:326–331

7 Willetts K E, Clements M S, Champion S, Ehsman S, Eden J A. Serenoa repens extract for benign prostate hyperplasia: a randomized controlled trial. BJU Int 2003;92:267–270

8 Morganti P, Fabrizi G, James D, Bruno C. Effect of gelatine-cystine and Serenoa repens extract on free radicals levels and hair growth. J Appl Cosmetol 1998;16:57–64

9 Prager N, Bickett K, French N, Marcovici G. A randomized, double-blind, placebo-controlled trial to determine the effectiveness of botanically derived inhibitors of 5-alpha-reductase in the treatment of androgenetic alopecia. J Altern Complement Med 2002;8:143–152

10 Kaplan S A, Volpe M A, Te A E. A prospective, 1-year trial using saw palmetto versus finasteride in the treatment of category III prostatitis/chronic pelvic pain syndrome. J Urol 2004;171:284–288

11 Gurley B J, Gardner S F, Hubbard M A, Williams D K, Gentry W B, Carrier J, Khan I A, Edwards D J, Shah A. In vivo assessment of botanical supplementation on human cytochrome P450 phenotypes: Citrus aurantium, Echinacea purpurea, milk thistle, and saw palmetto. Clin Pharmacol Ther 2004;76:428–440

SHARK CARTILAGE

Source	Cartilage from the fin of the hammerhead shark (*Sphyrna lewini*) and the spiny dogfish shark (*Squalus acanthias*).
Main constituents	Sphyrastatin 1 and 2 (glycoproteins).
Background	Based on the assumption that sharks never get cancer, it was hypothesised that shark cartilage might have anticancer properties in humans. Due to much publicity and clever marketing, shark cartilage became a popular food supplement in the 1990s. The debate over whether or not shark cartilage is associated with health benefits has developed into an ongoing, at times emotional controversy.[1-3]
Examples of traditional uses	None.
Pharmacologic action	Antiangiogenic (starving tumours of essential nutrients) effects have been well documented in various test models and constitute the postulated mechanism of action. However, it seems debatable whether this is applicable to oral administration in humans because large macromolecules like sphyrastatins are not usually absorbed in sufficiently large quantities by the intestinal tract.
Conditions frequently treated	Cancer, arthritis.
Clinical evidence	Early reports that shark cartilage cured cancer, prolonged patients' lives or improved their quality of life were based on anecdotes or uncontrolled studies.[4] One such trial reported that ten out of 20 patients experienced a partial or complete response after 8 weeks of therapy with shark cartilage.[2] One RCT found no difference in overall survival or quality of life between patients receiving standard care plus a shark cartilage product versus standard care plus placebo.[5] No rigorous studies for other indications exist. The debate continues about the bioavailability of the large glycoproteins from shark cartilage taken orally. A Canadian company developed and patented a purified fraction of shark cartilage which has much more potent antiangiogenic properties. It has generated promising results in refractory renal cell carcinoma[6] and now has FDA orphan drug status. As a purified drug it no longer falls under the umbrella of a natural dietary supplement and is therefore excluded from this discussion.

Dosage

Depending on the purity of the supplement, 500–4500 mg daily in divided doses.

Risk

Contraindications
Pregnancy, lactation due to insufficient information.

Precautions/warnings
Liver diseases.

Adverse effects
Hepatitis, taste disturbances, nausea, vomiting, dyspepsia, constipation, hypotension, dizziness, hyperglycaemia, hypoglycaemia, hypercalcaemia, altered consciousness, decreased motor strength, decreased sensation, erythema, peripheral oedema, generalised weakness and fatigue.[7]

Interactions
None known.

Quality issues
Large variations in the purity of commercially available preparations exist.

Risk–benefit assessment

According to the most reliable evidence to date, shark cartilage is not an effective cure for cancer. Serious safety concerns have been repeatedly voiced (e.g.[4,8]). For all other alleged indications there is a total absence of reliable clinical data. Its use should be discouraged unless data to the contrary emerge.

REFERENCES

1 Lane I W, Comac L. Sharks don't get cancer. How shark cartilage can save your life. New York: Avery, 1992
2 Mathews J. Media feeds frenzy over shark cartilage as a cancer treatment. J Natl Cancer Inst 1993;85:1190–1191
3 Folkman J. What is the evidence that tumors are angiogenesis dependent? J Natl Cancer Inst 1990;82:2–4
4 Miller D R. Phase I/II trial of the safety and efficacy of shark cartilage in the treatment of advanced cancer. J Clin Oncol 1998;16: 3649–3655
5 Loprinzi C L, Levitt R, Barton D L; North Central Cancer Treatment Group. Evaluation of shark cartilage in patients with advanced cancer: a North Central Cancer Treatment Group trial. Cancer 2005;104:176–182
6 Batist G, Patenaude F, Champagne P, Croteau D, Levinton C, Hariton C, Escudier B, Dupont E. Neovastat (AE-941) in refractory renal cell carcinoma patients: report of a phase II trial with two dose levels. Ann Oncol 2002;13:1259–1263
7 Shark cartilage monograph. Natural Medicines Comprehensive Database, www.naturaldatabase.com accessed 05/10/2004
8 Hunt T J, Conelly J F. Shark cartilage for cancer treatment. Am J Health-Syst Pharm 1995;52:1756–1760

ST JOHN'S WORT
(Hypericum perforatum)

Source	Aerial parts.
Main constituents	Flavonoids, naphthodianthrones (e.g. hypericin, pseudohypericin), phloroglucinols (e.g. adhyperforin, hyperforin), tannins, volatile oils, xanthones.
Background	A member of the *Hypericaceae* family, St John's wort is a herbaceous, yellow-flowered perennial growing on woodland, heathland and roadsides. It is native to most of Europe, Asia and northern Africa and naturalised in the USA and Australia. The Latin name *Hypericum* derives from the two Greek words *hyper* and *eikon* meaning 'over' and 'icon', as in 'over an apparition', referring to the belief that it had the power to ward off evil spirits. The common name St John's wort is thought to derive from associations with St John the Baptist – the flowers tend to bloom around the time of his feast day (June 24th) and the red pigments in the buds and flowers were associated with his blood. St John's wort has been used for medicinal purposes since the classical period.
Examples of traditional uses	Diuretic, melancholy, pain relief, wound healing and many others as diverse as bedwetting in children, insanity, malaria and snake bites.
Pharmacologic actions	Antiretroviral, antidepressant. The mechanism is unclear but possibilities include inhibition of reuptake of serotonin, noradrenaline glutamate and dopamine, modulation of interleukin-6 activity and gamma-aminobutyric acid receptor binding; suggestions that monoamine oxidase inhibition is responsible have been disproved.[1]
Conditions frequently treated	Depression, low mood.
Clinical evidence	The efficacy of St John's wort in treating mild to moderate depressive disorders has been demonstrated in numerous double-blind, placebo-controlled RCTs and confirmed by many meta-analyses (e.g.[2]). Numerous comparative RCTs (e.g.[2-11]) indicated that it may be as effective as conventional antidepressants, including trials with severely depressed patients (e.g.[12,13]). However, recent RCT data were mixed: two placebo-controlled RCTs generated ambiguous or negative results,[14,15] while others produced positive findings.[16-18] When these new data were included in a meta-analysis, the risk ratio decreased from 1.97 to 1.73, but was still positive.[19] Linde et al demonstrated that smaller trials tend to generate more positive results than larger trials.[20]

Further studies suggest that St John's wort may be effective for seasonal affective disorder,[21,22] and for somatoform disorders[23] |

but ineffective for social phobia[24] or premenstrual syndrome.[25] An RCT suggests that St John's wort cream is effective for atopic dermatitis.[26]

Dosage

300–900 mg of standardised dried extract (0.3% hypericin content) daily in divided doses.

Risks

Contraindications
Pregnancy and lactation (see p 5).

Precautions/warnings
Photosensitisation is possible, particularly in fair-skinned individuals.

Adverse effects
Most common reports are of gastrointestinal symptoms, allergic reactions, fatigue and anxiety. Several cases of mania and one of subacute toxic neuropathy have been reported.[27] The RCT data, however, suggest that adverse events of St John's wort are similar to placebo.[28–30]

Overdose
No cases have been reported in humans, so consequences are unknown. Data from animal and preclinical studies suggest that the usual therapeutic doses are about 2–3 times below the level of phototoxicity.

Interactions
Concomitant use with serotonin reuptake inhibitors has resulted in cases of serotonin syndrome.[27] Breakthrough bleeding has been reported for combined oral contraceptives. Acute rejection in transplant patients has been reported for cyclosporins.[31] Other reports show reduced plasma levels of medications metabolised by hepatic cytochrome P450 microsomal oxidase enzymes (e.g. warfarin, anticonvulsants, digoxin, theophylline, HIV protease inhibitors).[32]

Quality issues
Until the active constituents are established beyond doubt, the whole extract must be considered necessary for a therapeutic effect. Hypericin is used as a marker substance in most standardised preparations although some products are standardised to hyperforin.

Risk–benefit assessment

The totality of the evidence suggests that St John's wort is better than placebo and as effective as conventional antidepressants for treating mild to moderate depression, and all analyses agree that it is associated with fewer adverse effects. Unquestionably, St John's wort interacts with a wide range of other drugs. It can be recommended for mildly or moderately depressed patients as a monotherapy. For severe depression and other conditions the evidence is insufficient.

HERBAL AND NON-HERBAL MEDICINES

REFERENCES

1 Di Carlo G, Borrelli F, Ernst E, Izzo A. St John's wort: Prozac from the plant kingdom. Trends Pharmacol Sci 2001;22:292–297

2 Linde K, Mulrow C, Berner M, Egger M. St John's Wort for depression. Cochrane Database of Systematic Reviews, 2005. Issue 2. Art No.: CD000448

3 Harrer G, Schmidt U, Kuhn U, Biller A. Comparison of equivalence between the St. John's wort extract LoHyp-57 and fluoxetine. Drug Res 1999;49:289–296

4 Philipp M, Kohnen R, Hiller K O. Hypericum extract versus imipramine or placebo in patients with moderate depression: randomised multicentre study of treatment for eight weeks. BMJ 1999;319:1534–1538

5 Schrader E. Equivalence of St. John's wort extract (Ze 117) and fluoxetine: a randomized, controlled study in mild-moderate depression. Int Clin Psychopharm 2000;15:61–68

6 Woelk H. Comparison of St. John's wort and imipramine for treating depression: randomised controlled trial. BMJ 2000;421:536–539

7 Friede M, Henneicke von Zepelin H H, Freudenstein J. Differential therapy of mild to moderate depressive episodes (ICD-10 F 32.0; F 32.1) with St John's wort. Pharmacopsychiatry 2001;34:S38–41

8 Behnke K, Jensen S, Graubaum H J, Gruenwald J. Hypericum perforatum versus fluoxetine in the treatment of mild to moderate depression. Adv Ther 2002;19:43–52

9 van Gurp G, Meterissian G B, Haiek L N, McCusker J, Bellavance F. St John's wort or sertraline? Randomized controlled trial in primary care. Can Fam Physician 2002;48:905–912

10 Bjerkenstedt L, Edman G V, Alken R G, Mannel M. Hypericum extract LI 160 and fluoxetine in mild to moderate depression: a randomized, placebo-controlled multi-center study in outpatients. Eur Arch Psychiatry Clin Neurosci 2005;255:40–47

11 Gastpar M, Singer A, Zeller K. Efficacy and tolerability of hypericum extract STW3 in long-term treatment with a once-daily dosage in comparison with sertraline. Pharmacopsychiatry 2005;38:78–86

12 Vorbach E U, Arnoldt K H, Hubner W D. Efficacy and tolerability of St. John's wort extract LI 160 versus imipramine in patients with severe depressive episodes according to ICD-10. Pharmacopsychiatr 1997;30(suppl):81–85

13 Szegedi A, Kohnen R, Dienel A, Kieser M. Acute treatment of moderate to severe depression with hypericum extract WS 5570 (St John's wort): randomised controlled double blind non-inferiority trial versus paroxetine. BMJ 2005;330:503

14 Shelton R C, Keller M B, Gelenberg A, Dunner D L, Hirschfield R, Thase M E, Russell J, Lydiard R B, Crits-Cristoph P, Gallop R, Todd L, Hellerstein D, Goodnick P, Keitner G, Stahl SM, Halbreich U. Effectiveness of St John's wort in major depression: a randomized controlled trial. JAMA 2001;285:1978–1986

15 Hypericum Depression Trial Study Group. Effectiveness of St John's wort in major depression: a randomized controlled trial. JAMA 2002;287:1807–1814

16 Kalb R, Trautmann-Sponsel R D, Kieser M. Efficacy and tolerability of hypericum extract WS 5572 versus placebo in mildly to moderately depressed patients. A randomized double-blind multicenter clinical trial. Pharmacopsychiatry 2001;34:96–103

17 Lecrubier Y, Clerc G, Didi R, Kieser M. Efficacy of St John's wort extract WS 5570 in major depression: a double-blind, placebo-controlled trial. Am J Psychiatry 2002;159:1361–1366

18 Uebelhack R, Gruenwald J, Graubaum H J, Busch R. Efficacy and tolerability of Hypericum extract STW 3-VI in patients with moderate depression: a double-blind, randomized placebo-controlled clinical trial. Adv Ther 2004;21:265–275

19 Werneke U, Horn O, Taylor D M. How effective is St John's wort? The evidence revisited. J Clin Psychiatry 2004;65:611–617

20 Linde K, Mulrow C, Berner M, Egger M. St John's Wort for depression. Cochrane Database of Systematic Reviews, 2005. Issue 2. Art No.: CD000448

21 Wheatley D. Hypericum in seasonal affective disorder (SAD). Cur Med Res Opin 1999;15:33–37

22 Kasper S. Treatment of seasonal affective disorder (SAD) with Hypericum extract. Pharmacopsychiatr 1997;30:89–93

23 Volz H P, Murck H, Kasper S, Möller H J. St John's wort extract (LI 160) in somatoform disorders: results of a placebo-controlled trial. Psychopharmacology (Berl) 2002;164:294–300

24 Kobak K A, Taylor L V, Warner G, Futterer R. St. John's wort versus placebo in social

phobia: results from a placebo-controlled pilot study. J Clin Psychopharmacol 2005;25:51–58

25 Hicks S M, Walker A F, Gallagher J, Middleton R W, Wright J. The significance of 'nonsignificance' in randomized controlled studies: a discussion inspired by a double-blinded study on St. John's wort (Hypericum perforatum L.) for premenstrual symptoms. J Altern Complement Med 2004; 10:925–932

26 Schempp C M, Windeck T, Hezel S, Simon J C. Topical treatment of atopic dermatitis with St John's wort cream – a randomized, placebo-controlled, double blind half-side comparison radiation. Phytomedicine 2003;10:31–37

27 Stevinson C, Ernst E. Safety of hypericum in patients with depression. CNS Drugs 1999;11: 125–132

28 Trautmann-Sponsel R D, Dienel A. Safety of Hypericum extract in mildly to moderately depressed outpatients: a review based on data from three randomized, placebo-controlled trials. J Affect Disord 2004;82:303–307

29 Knuppel L, Linde K. Adverse effects of St. John's Wort: a systematic review. J Clin Psychiatry 2004;65:1470–1479

30 Linde K, Knuppel L. Large-scale observational studies of hypericum extracts in patients with depressive disorders – a systematic review. Phytomedicine 2005;12:148–157

31 Ernst E. St John's wort supplements endanger the success of organ transplantation. Arch Surg 2002;137:316–319

32 Mills E, Montori V M, Wu P, Gallicano K, Clarke M, Guyatt G. Interaction of St John's wort with conventional drugs: systematic review of clinical trials. BMJ 2004;329:27–30

TEA TREE
(Melaleuca alternifolia)

Source	Essential oil from leaves and branches.
Main constituents	Cineole, terpenes (pinene, terpinene, symene) and numerous other compounds.
Background	A member of the myrtle family (*Myrtaceae*), the tea tree is native to the coastal areas of Australia. Apparently, early European settlers made a tea from its leaves and thus the name was derived. Tea tree oil has become immensely popular as a topical antiseptic agent. Today it is included in many cosmetic products
Examples of traditional uses	Australian aborigines used it for burns, cuts and insect bites. It is sometimes advocated for eczema, lice infestation and psoriasis. Most of its present usage is for its antimicrobial action.
Pharmacologic action	Antifungal, antibacterial, antiviral.
Conditions frequently treated	Skin infections and associated conditions.
Clinical evidence	A systematic review of four RCTs[1] generated some evidence that tea tree oil may be effective in treating non-inflamed acne, tinea pedis and onychomycosis. More recent RCTs confirm the effectiveness of topical tea tree oil preparations for toenail onychomycosis,[2] interdigital tinea pedis,[3] dandruff (a yeast infection

HERBAL AND NON-HERBAL MEDICINES

of the scalp),[4] oral candidiasis of AIDS-patients,[5] chronic gingivitis[6] as well as a decolonisation agent for methicillin-resistant *Staphylococcus aureaus*.[7,8] A systematic review of two RCTs (n = 30 and 224) found little evidence that tea tree oil is helpful in infections with methicillin-resistant *Staphylococcus aureus*.[9] Finally, a systematic review generated encouraging results for tea tree oil in the treatment of fungal infections.[10]

Dosage

5–100% tea tree oil preparations applied several times daily.

Risks

Contraindications
Pregnancy and lactation (see p 5), allergy to tea tree oil.

Precautions/warnings
Not for internal use; not for external use on mucous membranes.

Adverse effects
Allergic reactions (frequent), mild skin irritation, toxic when taken orally.

Interactions
None known.

Quality issues
According to a 1995 Australian standard, tea tree oil should contain at least 30% terpinen-4-ol and less than 15% cineole.

Risk–benefit assessment

There are few risks associated with the proper use of tea tree oil. In vitro experiments demonstrate its antimicrobial activity and clinical evidence suggests effectiveness predominantly for fungal infections of the skin and mucous membranes. For such conditions the balance of evidence seems to favour tea tree oil.

REFERENCES

1 Ernst E. Huntley A. Tea tree oil: a systematic review of randomised clinical trials. Forsch Komplementärmed Klass Naturheilkd 2000;7:17–20.

2 Syed T A, Qureshi Z A, Ali S M, Ahmad S, Ahmad S A. Treatment of toenail onychomycosis with 2% butenafine and 5% Melaleuca alternifolia (tea tree) oil in cream. Trop Med Int Health 1999;4:284–287

3 Satchell A C, Saurajen A, Bell C, Barnetson R. Treatment of interdigital tinea pedis with 25% and 50% tea tree oil solution: a randomized, placebo-controlled, blinded study. Australas J Dermatol 2002;43:175–178

4 Satchell A C, Saurajen A, Bell C, Barnetson R. Treatment of dandruff with 5% tea tree oil shampoo. J Am Acad Dermatol 2002;47:852–855

5 Vazquez J A, Zawawi A A. Efficacy of alcohol-based and alcohol-free melaleuca oral solution for the treatment of fluconazole-refractory oropharyngeal candidiasis in patients with AIDS. HIV Clin Trials 2002;3:379–385

6 Soukoulis S, Hirsch R. The effects of a tea tree oil-containing gel on plaque and chronic gingivitis. Aust Dent J 2004;49:78–83

7 Caelli M, Porteous J, Carson CF, Heller R, Riley T V. Tea tree oil as an alternative topical decolonization agent for methicillin-resistant Staphylococcus aureus. J Hosp Infect 2000;46:236–237

8 Dryden M S, Dailly S, Crouch M. A randomized, controlled trial of tea tree topical preparations versus a standard topical regimen for the clearance of MRSA

colonization. J Shop Infect 2004;56:283–286

9   Flaxman D, Griffiths P. Is tea tree oil effective at eradicating MRSA colonization? A review. Br J Community Nurs 2005;10:123–126

10 Martin K W, Ernst E. Herbal medicines for treatment of fungal infections: a systematic review of controlled clinical trials. Mycoses 2004;47:97–92

THYME
(Thymus vulgaris)

Source	Leaves and flowers.
Main constituents	Camphene, eugenol, flavonoids, phenols (thymol, carvacrol), rosmarinic acid.
Background	*Thymus vulgaris* is of the same genus as mint. It is native to Italy and Spain and is cultivated throughout the world. Thyme has been used for culinary and medicinal purposes for millennia. Many subspecies exist; *Thymus vulgaris* and *Thymus zygis* are used interchangeably for medicinal purposes.
Examples of traditional uses	Dental hygiene, disinfection of skin and mucous membranes, dyspepsia, upper respiratory tract infections, (whooping) cough.
Pharmacologic actions	Antimicrobial, antibacterial, antiseptic, carminative, expectorant, antitussive, diaphoretic, antimutagenic, spasmolytic, antiflatulent, astringent, antihelminthic, antioxidant and anti-inflammatory.
Conditions frequently treated	Bronchitis, cough and upper respiratory tract infections; dental antiseptic.
Clinical evidence	No compelling trial evidence exists for thyme taken on its own. Encouraging data have been reported for chronic bronchitis treated by thyme in combination with other herbs in large (n > 3000) comparative clinical trials (e.g.[1]). Thyme oil applied topically in combination with other essential oils seemed to improve hair growth in patients with alopecia areata in one RCT.[2] A small RCT evaluating the effects of aromatherapy massage with essential oils including thyme in a group of children with atopic eczema showed no improvement between the treatment and control group.[3] Taking thyme oil in combination with evening primrose oil, fish oils, and vitamin E is reported to improve movement disorders in children with dyspraxia.[4]
Dosage	1–2 g of extract daily in divided doses.
Risks	***Contraindications*** Pregnancy and lactation (see p 5), gastritis, enterocolitis, allergy to *Labiatae* family, chronic heart failure.

Precautions/warnings
Patients with gastrointestinal problems, thyroid disorders. Avoid oral ingestion or non-diluted application.

Adverse effects
Nausea, vomiting, diarrhoea, headache, dizziness, respiratory distress, bradycardia, dermatitis (topical use).

Overdose
Effects on humans are not known but loss of reflexes has been reported in animal studies.

Interactions
None known.

Quality issues
Use standardised extracts with 0.6–1.2% volatile oil and 0.5% phenol content.

Risk–benefit assessment

Lack of data regarding thyme as a monotherapy prevents a conclusive evaluation. For combination products containing thyme, large comparative trials have suggested superiority when compared with synthetic medications for bronchitis. Promising results exist for thyme-containing products in the treatment of alopecia areata and dyspraxia. The specific role of thyme in the combination products is, however, unclear.

REFERENCES

1 Ernst E, März R, Sieder C. A controlled multi-centre study of herbal versus synthetic secretolytic drugs for acute bronchitis. Phytomedicine 1997;4:287–293
2 Hay I C, Jamieson M, Ormerod A D. Randomized trial of aromatherapy. Successful treatment for alopecia areata. Arch Dermatol 1998;134: 1349–1352
3 Anderson C, Lis-Balchin M, Kirk-Smith M. Evaluation of massage with essential oils on childhood atopic eczema. Phytother Res 2000;14:452–456
4 Stordy B J. Dark adaptation, motor skills, docosahexaenoic acid, and dyslexia. Am J Clin Nutr 2000;71:323S–326S

VALERIAN
(*Valeriana officinalis, Valeriana edulis*)

Source

Rhizome.

Main constituents

Alkaloids, amino acids (gamma-aminobutyric acid), iridoids/valepotriates, phenylpropanoids, sesquiterpenoids volatile oils.

Background

Valeriana officinalis is one of over 200 members of the *Valerianaceae* family. A herbaceous perennial, it is native to most of Europe and Asia and grows in damp swampy areas. The name *Valeriana* derives from the Latin word *valere* meaning well-being. Its use as a medicinal herb dates back to Hippocrates' time. *Valeriana edulis* is widely used in South America for insomnia and anxiety.

Examples of traditional uses	Digestive problems, flatulence, urinary tract disorders.
Pharmacologic action	Sedative, anxiolytic. Mechanisms are unclear, but gamma-aminobutyric acid receptors may be involved.
Conditions frequently treated	Anxiety, insomnia.
Clinical evidence	The hypnotic effects of valerian have been investigated in several double-blind placebo-controlled RCTs. Improvements following single doses have been reported (e.g.[1]) as well as with repeated administration (e.g.[2]). A systematic review of the subject concluded that the evidence was promising but not conclusive, due to inconsistent results and methodological limitations.[3] RCTs published subsequently found valerian to be as effective as oxazepam in enhancing the sleep quality of insomniacs after 4 weeks.[4] A sizeable (n = 202) RCT with patients suffering from insomnia confirmed that valerian extract (600 mg/day) is at least as effective as oxazepam (10 mg/day) in increasing sleep quality when taken for 6 weeks.[5] Recent placebo-controlled RCTs generated mixed results: two small studies suggested efficacy in enhancing sleep,[6,7] while a series of 42 n = 1 trials failed to show such effects in any individual patient with insomnia or for the group as a whole.[8] One comparison between *Valeriana officinalis* and *Valeriana edulis* concluded that both have equal hypnotic activity.[9] A further crossover RCT (n = 16) conducted under sleep laboratory conditions tested 300 mg vs 600 mg valerian extract vs placebo.[10] No EEG or psychometric changes were noted suggestive of sleep-promoting actions.

In addition to single herb preparations, several combination products are on the market. Promising data has emerged for valerian/hops,[11] valerian/lemonbalm,[12] and valerian/kava combinations.[13] Valerian has also been tested for indications other than insomnia. Encouraging data from RCTs or CCTs is available for valerian as a symptomatic treatment for situational anxiety,[14] of generalised anxiety disorder,[15] for reducing mental stress under experimental conditions,[16] and as an aid during benzodiazepine withdrawal.[17]

Dosage	400–900 mg of extract 30–60 minutes before bedtime.
Risks	***Contraindications*** Pregnancy and lactation (see p 5), known allergy, hepatic impairment. ***Precautions/warnings*** Care should be taken if driving or operating machinery when taking valerian. Long-term risks are under-researched.

Adverse effects

Headache and gastrointestinal symptoms are occasionally reported. Morning hangover reported occasionally although RCTs investigating safety factors have found no impairment of reaction time or alertness the morning after intake. Hepatotoxicity has been reported from herbal preparations in which valerian was combined with other herbs, including skullcap. The trial data suggest that adverse effects of valerian are less frequent than those of benzodiazepines.[4,5]

Overdose

Symptoms of tachycardia, nausea, vomiting, dilated pupils, drowsiness, confusion, visual hallucinations, blurred vision, cardiac disturbance, excitability, headache, hypersensitivity reactions and insomnia have been reported following acute overdoses, with full recoveries made in all cases.

Interactions

Potentiation of the effects of sedatives, hypnotics or other central nervous system depressants is possible at high doses.[18] RCTs have shown no potentiation of alcohol.

Quality issues

Composition and purity of extracts vary greatly. Standardised extracts often use valepotriates as the marker substance although valerenic acid is considered more reliable due to its stability. Aqueous extracts are devoid of valepotriates.

Risk–benefit assessment

Even though the evidence is not entirely uniform, the majority of the sound clinical trials suggest efficacy for insomnia. For that indication, valerian may offer advantages over benzodiazepines. It is unclear whether herbal combinations have advantages over single valerian extracts. Indications other than insomnia require further study. The risks of short-term valerian monotherapy seem to be acceptable. Therefore valerian can be recommended as a short-term solution to insomnia.

REFERENCES

1 Leathwood P D, Chauffard F, Heck E, Munoz-Box R. Aqueous extract of valerian root (Valeriana officinalis L) improves sleep quality in man. Pharmacol Biochem Behav 1982;17:65–71

2 Vorbach E U, Gortelmeyer R, Bruning J. Therapie von Insomnien: Wirksamkeit und Verträglichkeit eines Baldrianpräparats. Psychopharmakotherapie 1996;3:109–115

3 Stevinson C, Ernst E. Valerian for insomnia: systematic review of randomized placebo-controlled trials. Sleep Med 2000;1:91–99

4 Dorn M. Baldrian versus oxazepam: efficacy and tolerability in non-organic and non-psychiatric insomniacs: a randomized, double-blind, clinical comparative study. Forsch Komplementärmed Klass Naturheilkd 2000;7:79–84

5 Ziegler G, Ploch M, Miettinen-Baumann A, Collet W. Efficacy and tolerablity of valerian extract LI 156 compared with oxzaepam in the treatment of non-organic insomnia: a randomized, double-blind, comparative clinical study. Eur J Med Res 2002;7:480–486

6 Donath F, Quispe S, Diefenbach K, Maurer A, Fietze I, Roots I. Critical evaluation of the effect of valerian extract on sleep structure and sleep quality. Pharmacopsychiatry 2000;33:47–53

7 Francis A J P, Dempster R J W. Effect of valerian, Valeriana edulis, on sleep difficulties in

children with intellectual deficits: randomised trial. Phytomedicine 2002;9:273–279

8   Coxeter P D, Schluter P J, Eastwood H. Valerian does not appear to reduce symptoms for patients with chronic insomnia in general practice using a series of randomised n-of-1 trials. Complement Ther Med 2003;11:215–222

9   Herrera Arellano A, Luna Villegas G, Cuevas Uriostegui M L. Polysomnographic evaluation of the hypnotic effect of Valeriana edulis standardized extract in patients suffering from insomnia. Planta Med 2001;67:695–699

10   Diaper A, Hindmarch I. A double-blind, placebo-controlled investigation of the effects of two doses of a valerian preparation on the sleep, cognitive and psychomotor function of sleep-disturbed older adults. Phytother Res 2004;18:831–836

11   Vonderheid Guth B, Todorova A, Brattström A. Pharmacodynamic effects of valerian and hops extract combination (Ze 91019) on the quantitative-topographical EEG in healthy volunteers. Eur J Med Res 2000;5:139–144

12   Cerny A, Schmid K. Tolerability and efficacy of valerian/lemon balm in healthy volunteers (a double-blind, placebo-controlled, multicentre study). Fitoterapia 1999;70:221–228

13   Wheatley D. Stress-induced insomnia treated with kava and valerian: singly and in combination. Human Psychopharmacology 2001;4:353–356

14   Kohnen R, Oswald W D. The effects of valerian, propranolol and their combination on activation, performance and mood of healthy volunteers under social stress conditions. Pharmacopsychiatry 1988;21:447–448

15   Andreatini R, Sartori V A, Seabra M L, Leite J R. Effect of valepotriates (valerian extract) in generalized anxiety disorder: a randomized placebo-controlled pilot study. Phytother Res 2002;16:650–654

16   Cropley M, Cave Z, Ellis J, Middleton R W. Effect of kava and valerian on human physiological and psychological responses to mental stress assessed under laboratory conditions. Phytother Res 2002;16:23–27

17   Poyares D R, Guilleminault C, Ohayon M M, Tufik S. Can valerian improve the sleep of insomniacs after benzodiazepine withdrawal? Prog Neuropsychopharmacol Biol Psychiatry 2002;26:539–545

18   Donovan J L, DeVane C L, Chavin K D, Wang J S, Gibson B B, Gefroh H A, Markowitz J S. Multiple night-time doses of valerian (Valeriana officinalis) had minimal effects on CYP3A4 activity and no effect on CYP2D6 activity in healthy volunteers. Drug Metab Dispos 2004;32:1333–1336

WILLOW
(*Salix* spp)

Source	Bark.
Main constituents	Derivatives of salicin, mainly salicortin, tannins, tremulacin.
Background	Willow bark has been used as a remedy for inflammatory joint diseases and gout since 50 BCE. It was later rediscovered as a remedy against fever and pain. Salicin was isolated as an active compound and eventually the compound was synthesised by Löwing, a German chemist working for Bayer. As he had used extracts from plants of the genus *Spirea*, he called the substance spiric acid, which appears in the brand name aspirin (acetylsalicylic acid).
Examples of traditional uses	Fever, pain, rheumatic complaints.
Pharmacologic action	Salicin is metabolised to salicylic acid which has antipyretic and analgesic effects.

Conditions frequently treated

Common cold, headache, rheumatic diseases.

Clinical evidence

Few CCTs have been carried out with willow bark preparations. A systematic review identified one RCT of willow bark extract for treating osteoarthritis.[1] This double-blind RCT (n = 78) reports a difference compared with placebo in favour of willow bark extract for the WOMAC pain dimension.[2] A double-blind RCT including 82 patients with chronic arthritic pain over a treatment period of 2 months confirmed these findings,[3] whereas another RCT including 127 patients with osteoarthritis did not.[4] An RCT in 210 patients with lower back pain, using placebo and willow bark dry extracts equivalent to 120 mg of salicin daily and 240 mg of salicin daily respectively, showed positive results.[5] When willow bark extract, equivalent to a daily dose of 240 mg salicin, was compared with 12.5 mg of the COX-2 inhibitor rofecoxib (n = 228) for low back pain, there was no difference as measured on a modified Arhus index, its pain component and the total pain index.[6]

Dosage

120–240 mg of total salicin daily in divided doses.

Risks

Contraindications
Pregnancy and lactation (see p 5), patients with salicylate intolerance.

Precautions/warnings
Patients on anticoagulation treatment. Although there are data indicating that willow bark has no effect on coagulation time[7] and affects platelet aggregation to a far lesser extent than acetyl-salicylate.[8] Patients on this kind of pharmacologic therapy should use willow bark extracts only under careful supervision.

Adverse effects
Anaphylactic reactions, gastrointestinal complaints, skin rashes.

Interactions
Additive effects on anticoagulants and other salicylate-containing drugs.

Quality issues
Preparations standardised to salicin should be used.

Risk–benefit assessment

Although the evidence is limited, the data suggest that, overall, willow bark extracts are efficacious in chronic pain. Whether they are as useful as aspirin (or other NSAIDs) is doubtful. However, the adverse effects profile appears to be more favourable. Therefore willow bark extracts may be worthy of consideration for patients with mild pain who insist on a herbal remedy.

REFERENCES

1 Long L, Soeken K, Ernst E. Herbal medicines for the treatment of osteoarthritis: A systematic review. Rheumatology 2001;40:779–793

2 Schmid B, Lüdtke R, Selbmann H K, Kötter I, Tschirdewahn B, Schaffner W, Heide L. Efficacy and tolerability of a standardized willow bark extract in patients with osteoarthritis: randomized placebo-controlled, double blind clinical trial. Phytother Res 2001;15:344–350

3 Mills S Y, Jacoby R K, Chacksfield M, Willoughby M. Effect of a proprietary herbal medicine on the relief of chronic arthritic pain: a double-blind study. Br J Rheumatol 1996;35:874–878

4 Biegert C, Wagner I, Ludtke R, Kotter I, Lohmuller C, Gunaydin I, Taxis K, Heide L. Efficacy and safety of willow bark extract in the treatment of osteoarthritis and rheumatoid arthritis: results of 2 randomized double-blind controlled trials. J Rheumatol 2004;31:2121–2130

5 Chrubasik S, Eisenberg E, Balan E, Weinberger T, Luzzati R, Conradt C. Treatment of low back pain exacerbations with willow bark extract: a randomised double-blind study. Am J Med 2000;109:9–14

6 Chrubasik S, Künzel O, Model A, Conradt C, Black A. Treatment of low back pain with a herbal or synthetic anti-rheumatic: A randomized controlled study. Willow bark extract for low back pain. Rheumatology 2001;40:1388–1393

7 Krivoy N, Pavlotzky F, Eisenberg E, Chrubasik J, Chrubasik S, Brook G. Salix cortex (willow bark dry extract) effect on platelet aggregation. Drug Monit 1999;21:202

8 Krivoy N, Pavlotzky E, Chrubasik S, Eisenberg E, Brook G.. Effect of salicis cortex extract on human platelet aggregation. Planta Med 2001;67:209–212

YOHIMBE
(Pausinystalia johimbe)

Source	Bark.
Main constituents	Indole alkaloids of which 10–15% are yohimbine.
Background	Yohimbe is a tall evergreen tree, which is native to Central Africa. The ground bark is traditionally used as an aphrodisiac, particularly for male erectile dysfunction. Interestingly, It is also used as an alternative to anabolic steroids for enhancing athletic performance. Yohimbine is the main active constituent of yohimbe bark extract and also present in other plants such as the Indian snakeroot (*Rauwolfia serpentina*) and quebracho (*Aspidosperma quebracho-blanco*). Most clinical studies relate to the effects of this isolated constituent of yohimbe bark.
Examples of traditional uses	As an aphrodisiac, hypotension, obesity, pruritus, skin diseases.
Pharmacologic action	Alpha-2-adrenoceptor blockade. Causes a rise in sympathetic drive by increasing noradrenaline release and firing rate of noradrenergic nuclei in the central nervous system.
Conditions frequently treated	Erectile dysfunction.

HERBAL AND NON-HERBAL MEDICINES

Clinical evidence

No evidence from rigorous clinical trials for yohimbe bark extracts was located. The main active constituent, yohimbine, was assessed in a systematic review and meta-analysis for treating erectile dysfunction.[1] This study, which included seven double-blind RCTs concluded that yohimbine is superior to placebo for the treatment of erectile dysfunction of organic or non-organic causes. This is corroborated by a double-blind RCT for a combination of L-arginine and yohimbine.[2] For female sexual arousal disorder, beneficial effects are also reported for a combination of L-arginine and yohimbine in postmenopausal women[3] whereas yohimbine was not different from placebo in sexual dysfunction in premenaupausal women.[4] For treating overweight or obesity, a systematic review identified three double-blind RCTs, which found conflicting results.[5] Another double-blind RCT suggests that yohimbine has no beneficial effects for the treatment of orthostatic hypotension in patients with Parkinson's disease.[6] Other single RCTs report positive effects for dry mouth in patients receiving psychotropic drugs,[7] for treating withdrawal symptoms due to drug abuse[8] and as an addition to fluoxetine in major depressive disorder.[9]

Dosage

16–18 mg of yohimbine hydrochloride daily in divided doses.

Risks

Contraindications
Pregnancy and lactation (see p 5), children, known allergy to yohimbe, psychiatric conditions, use of phenothiazine containing agents, sympathomimetic agents.

Precautions/warnings
Children, individuals with chronic inflammation of the prostate or the reproductive organs, anxiety disorders, hypertension, cardiac, renal or hepatic diseases.

Adverse effects
Nervous excitation, tremor, irritability, sleeplessness, anxiety, hypertension, hypotension, tachycardia, bronchospasm, gastrointestinal complaints, skin flushing, rash, mydriasis.

Overdose
Doses of 20–30 mg yohimbine hydrochloride daily may cause increased heart rate and raised blood pressure.

Interactions
Increased effects of antidepressants, central nervous system stimulants, phenothiazines and other $alpha_2$-adrenoceptor blocking agents, reduced effects of antihypertensive drugs, benzodiazepines; interaction with sildenafil is theoretically possible.

Quality issues

Yohimbine hydrochloride preparations may contain other drugs including strychnine and methyltestosterone. Commercial yohimbe products may contain no yohimbine.

Risk–benefit assessment

There is little evidence for the effectiveness and safety of yohimbe bark extract. The evidence relates mostly to its isolated main constituent yohimbine, which has beneficial effects in the treatment of erectile dysfunction of various causes. This has obvious advantages over invasive interventions and is relatively safer. Comparative studies with other oral medications such as sildenafil, which has been shown to be effective for this condition, are not available yet. There is no compelling evidence from rigorous clinical trials on yohimbine for treating other conditions.

REFERENCES

1 Ernst E, Pittler M H. Yohimbine for erectile dysfunction: a systematic review and meta-analysis. J Urol 1998;159:433–436
2 Lebret T, Herve J M, Gorny P, Worcel M, Botto H. Efficacy and safety of a novel combination of L-arginine glutamate and yohimbine hydrochloride: a new oral therapy for erectile dysfunction. Eur Urol 2002;41:608–613
3 Meston C M, Worcel M. The effects of yohimbine plus L-arginine glutamate on sexual arousal in postmenopausal women with sexual arousal disorder. Arch Sex Behav 2002;31:323–332
4 Michelson D, Kociban K, Tamura R, Morrison M F. Mirtazapine, yohimbine or olanzapine augmentation therapy for serotonin reuptake-associated female sexual dysfunction: a randomized, placebo controlled trial. J Psychiatr Res 2002;36:147–152
5 Pittler M H, Ernst E. Dietary supplements for body-weight reduction: a systematic review. Am J Clin Nutr 2004;79:529–536
6 Senard J M, Rascol O, Raskol A, Montastruc J L. Lack of yohimbine effect on ambulatory blood pressure recording: a double blind cross-over trial in Parkinsonians with orthostatic hypotension. Fundament Clin Pharmacol 1993;7:465–470
7 Bagheri H, Schmitt L, Berlan M, Montastruc J L. A comparative study of the effects of yohimbine and anetholtrithioneon salivary secretion in depressed patients treated with psychotropic drugs. Eur J Clin Pharmacol 1997;52:339–342
8 Hameedi F A, Woods S W, Rosen M I, Pearsall H R, Kosten T R. Dose dependent effects of yohimbine on methadone maintained patients. Am J Drug Alcohol Abuse 1997;23:327–333
9 Sanacora G, Berman R M, Cappiello A, Oren D A, Kugaya A, Liu N, Gueorguieva R, Fasula D, Charney D S. Addition of the alpha2-antagonist yohimbine to fluoxetine: effects on rate of antidepressant response. Neuropsychopharmacology 2004;29:1166–1171

HERBAL AND NON-HERBAL MEDICINES

Table 4.1   **Other medicinal herbs which have been tested for effectiveness or are used frequently**

Name*	Pharmacologic action**	Conditions frequently treated**	Safety concerns**
African plum (*Pygeum africanum*)	Antiproliferative effects on fibroblasts, antihormonal	Benign prostatic hyperplasia, inflammation, kidney disease, etc	Nausea, abdominal pain
Angelica (*Angelica archangelica*)	Smooth muscle relaxant	Loss of appetite, abdominal discomfort, flatulence	Photosensitisation
Anise (*Pimpinella anisum*)	Expectorant, anti-spasmodic, antibacterial	Dyspepsia, catarrh	Allergic reactions
Arnica (*Arnica montana*)	Anti-inflammatory, antimicrobial	Sprains and bruises (topical)	Oral: should only be taken in homeopathic doses because of toxicity Topical: allergies, dermatitis
Asparagus (*Asparagus officinalis*)	Diuretic	Urinary tract inflammation, prevention of kidney stones	Allergic reactions
Baizhu (*Atractylodis macrocephalus*)	Digestive, diuretic	Anorexia, diarrhoea	None known
Balloon flower (*Platycodon grandiflorum*)	Expectorant, antitussive, anti-inflammatory	Upper respiratory tract infections	None known
Banxia (*Pinellia ternata*)	Expectorant, antiemetic	Asthma, cough	Could cause abortion in pregnant women
Beimu (*Fritillaria cirrhosa*)	Antitussive, mucolytic, expectorant	Inflammation of respiratory tract	None known
Black seed oil (*Nigella sativa*)	Antihistamine, immuno-protectant, cytotoxic	Gastrointestinal and respi-ratory conditions, cancer	Allergic reactions, hepa-totoxicity
Blueberry (*Vaccinium angustifolium*)	Antioxidative	Diabetes mellitus, cancer prevention	None known
Borage (*Borago officinalis*)	Anti-inflammatory	Arthritis	Contains hepatotoxic pyrrolizidine alkaloids
Boxwood (*Buxus sempervirens*)	Inhibition of viral replication	AIDS, arthritis	Diarrhoea, cramps, paralysis, death
Brindal berry (*Garcinia cambogia*)	Purgative, enzyme inhibitor	Dysentery, against weight loss	None known
Brucca amarissima	Antimicrobial	Amebic dysentery, malaria	Anaphylaxis
Buckwheat (*Fagopyrum esculentum*)	Improves capillary tone	Venous and arterial diseases	Phototoxic
Butcher's broom (*Ruscus aculeatus*)	Diuretic, anti-inflammatory	Chronic venous insufficiency	Gastrointestinal discom-fort, nausea

TABLE 4.1 OTHER MEDICINAL HERBS **477**

Name*	Pharmacologic action**	Conditions frequently treated**	Safety concerns**
Butterbur (*Petasites hybridus*)	Antispasmodic, anti-inflammatory	Pain, gastrointestinal disorders, headaches, cough, anxiety, fever, allergies	Hepatoxic (pyrrolizidine alkaloid)
Caiapo, Mexican Scammony Root (*Ipomoea batatas*)	Purgative, laxative	Constipation	Vomiting, intestinal colic
Calendula (*Calendula officinalis*)	Anti-inflammatory, immune stimulating, antimicrobial	Wound healing, gastric ulcers, postmastectomy, lymphedema	None known
Caraway (*Carum carvi*)	Antispasmodic, antimicrobial	Dyspepsia, flatulence	None known
Cardamom (*Elettaria cardamomum*)	Cholagogue, virustatic	Dyspepsia	Precaution: do not use in cases of gallstones
Cascara (*Rhamnus purshiana*)	Increases mobility of colon	Constipation	Fresh bark is toxic and must be stored before use, not for use in inflammatory bowel diseases, gastrointestinal cramps
Cat's claw (*Uncaria tomentosa*)	Vasodilatory, anti-inflammatory	Diverticulitis, peptic ulcers, colitis, gastritis, haemorrhoids, parasitosis	Headache, dizziness, vomiting
Chinese club moss (*Huperzia serrata*)	Acetylcholinesterase inhibitor	Alzheimer's disease, fever, menorrhagia	Dizziness, nausea, sweating
Chinese goldthread (*Loptis chinensis*)	Antimicrobial	Diarrhoea, conjunctivitis, leishmaniasis, malaria	Gastrointestinal symptoms
Chinese rhubarb (*Rheum officinale*)	Stimulant of colonic activity, increases paracellular permeability	Constipation	Abdominal cramps, diarrhoea, fluid loss (overdose)
Chorella (*Chlorella pyrenoidosa*)	Source of vitamin B_{12}, immune stimulant	Cancer prevention, prevention of infections	Inhibits anticoagulant activity
Cinnamon (*Cinnamonum verum*)	Carminative, antimicrobial	Loss of appetite, dyspepsia	Allergies
Cloves (*Syzygium aromaticum*)	Antiseptic, antimicrobial, anesthetic, antispasmodic	Skin or mucosa inflammation and pain (topical)	Skin or mucosa irritation
Comfrey (*Symphytum officinale*)	Anti-inflammatory	Bruises and sprains (topical)	Herb contains pyrrolizidine alkaloids which are hepatotoxic, therefore not for internal use

table continues

Name*	Pharmacologic action**	Conditions frequently treated**	Safety concerns**
Danshen (*Salvia miltiorrhiza*)	Anticoagulant, vasodilatation	Circulatory problems, menstrual problems, chronic hepatitis, etc	Pruritus, gastrointestinal problems, reduction of appetite, bleeding
Diahuang (*Rehmannia glutinosa*)	Antipyretic, antirheumatic, diuretic	Rheumatic pain	None known
Dong quai= Chinese angelica (*Angelica sinensis*)	Vasodilatation, quinidine-like, alters uterine activity	Gynecological disorders, circulation conditions	Bleeding, photosensitivity, interaction with anticoagulants
Eucalyptus (*Eucalyptus globulus*)	Expectorant, secretolytic, antiseptic	Inflammation of respiratory tract	Nausea, vomiting, diarrhoea
Fennel (*Foeniculum vulgare*)	Antispasmodic, secretolytic	Dyspepsia, flatulence	Allergies
Fenugreek (*Trigonella foenum-graecum*)	Cholagogue, anti-inflammatory, galactagogue	Diabetes mellitus, hypercholesterolaemia	Minor gastrointestinal symptoms, allergic reactions
Flaxseed oil (*Linum usitatissimum*)	Anti-inflammatory, anticoagulant	Constipation, arthritis, cancer, anxiety	Bleeding
French maritime pine (*Pinus pinaster*)	Reduction of capillary permeability, enzyme inhibition, antioxidant	Venous conitions, allergies, hypertension, muscle soreness, etc	None known
Gentian (*Gentiana lutea*)	Digestive stimulant	Loss of appetite, flatulence	Headache
Geranium (*Pelargonium* spp)	Antibacterial, antifungal, astringent	Diarrhoea	Dermatitis
Giant fennel (*Asa foetida*)	Hypocholesterolaemic, cytotoxic	Bronchitis, asthma, pertussis, hysteria, gastritis, convulsions	May increase effects of anticoagulants
Glucomannan (*Amorphophallus konjac*)	Bilk forming agent	Constipation, weight loss, control of blood glucose and lipids	Intestinal obstruction
Goldenseal (*Hydrastis canadensis*)	Oxytocic, laxative, anti-inflammatory, vasoconstrictive	Wound healing, herpes labialis	Digestive problems, hypertension, hallucinations
Gotu kola (*Centella asiatica*)	Stimulation of collagen synthesis, anti-inflammatory	Wound healing (topical), leprosy, venous conditions, memory improvement, increasing longevity etc	Allergic reactions, can elevate blood glucose
Guggul (*Commiphora mukul*)	Inhibition of hepatic cholesterol synthesis, antioxidant	Arthritis, acne, weight loss	Increase of anticoagulation, headache, nausea
Hibiscus (*Hibiscus sabdariffa*)	Laxative, diuretic, anti-spasmodic, antibacterial	Loss of appetite, colds, constipation	None known

TABLE 4.1 OTHER MEDICINAL HERBS **479**

Name*	Pharmacologic action**	Conditions frequently treated**	Safety concerns**
Iceland moss (*Cetraria islandica*)	Antimicrobial, immunostimulant	Loss of appetite, dry cough, irritation of mucous membranes	None known
Indian Frankincense (*Boswellia serrata*)	Anti-inflammatory	Arthritis, ulcerative colitis, cancer, etc	None known
Indian gooseberry (*Phyllanthus embilica*)	Antimicrobial, anti-mutagenic, antioxidant	Hypercholesterolaemia, diabetes, dyspepsia, eye problems, etc	None known
Ivy (*Hedera helix*)	Expectorant, antispasmodic, antimicrobial, analgesic	Chronic respiratory inflammation	Contact dermatitis
Juniper (*Juniperus communis*)	Diuretic, carminative, antirheumatic	Dyspepsia	Kidney damage (prolonged use or overdose)
Kamala (*Mullotus philippinensis*)	Purgative, anthelmintic	Tape worm infestation	None known
Kudzu (*Pueraria lobata*)	Inhibition of alcohol dehydrogenanse	Alcohol hangover, alcoholism, myalgia, dysentery, fever, etc	Increase of anticoagulation
Lemon balm (*Melissa officinalis*)	Sedative, spasmolytic, antimicrobial	Insomnia, herpes labialis (external use)	No serious safety concerns known
Liquorice (*Glycyrrhiza glabra*)	Expectorant, secretolytic, antispasmodic, anti-inflammatory, adrenocortico-trophic, aldosterone-like effects	Gastric, ulcers, catarrhs, cancer prevention, detoxification, anti-inflammatory, antioxidation	Adverse effects consistent with adrenocorticotrophic actions
Ma huang (*Ephedra sinica*)	Sympathomimetic, ephedrine-like effects	Weight loss, bronchospasm, asthma, bronchitis	Hypertension, myocardial infarction, stroke, seizures, abused as a stimulant (e.g. herbal 'ecstasy')
Marshmallow (*Althaea officinalis*)	Demulcent	Dry cough	None known
Maté (*Ilex paraguariensis*)	Laxative, diuretic, analgetic	Stimulant, pain, constipation	Increased risk of oesophagus and other cancers, hypertension
Milk vetch (*Astragalus polygonum, A. membranaceus*)	Antioxidant, immune-stimulant	Common cold, cancer	None known
Myrrh (*Commiphora molmol*)	Astringent	Skin or mucosa inflammation	None known

HERBAL AND NON-HERBAL MEDICINES

table continues

Name*	Pharmacologic action**	Conditions frequently treated**	Safety concerns**
Nux vomica (*Strychnos nux-vomica*)	Centrally acting neurotoxin	Impotence, gastrointestinal, cardiovascular, nervous conditions, etc	Convulsion, death
Olive leaf (*Olea europea*)	Antispasmodic, hypotensive, antiarrhythmic, hypoglycaemic, etc	Infections, meningitis, hypertension, diabetes, etc	Allergy
Onion (*Allium cepa*)	Antimicrobial, diuretic, glucose lowering, general tonic	Arteriosclerosis, loss of appetite, wound healing (topical)	Allergic reactions
Pineapple (*Ananas comosus*)	Platelet inhibition, anti-inflammatory, fibrinolytic	Sprains, bruises and post-traumatic oedema	Could prolong bleeding time, diarrhoea
Pomegranate (*Punica granatum*)	Astringent, abortive, antioxidant	Diarrhoea, haemorrhoids, intestinal worms	Allergic reactions, heightened arousal, paralysis
Poplar=American aspen (*Populus alba*)	Salicylates exert anti-inflammatory effects	Rheumatic conditions	Renal dysfunction, GI symptoms, interaction with anticoagulants
Poria Mushroom (*Polyporus*)	Anti-inflammatory, immunosuppressive, antiemetic	Amnesia, anxiety, dizziness, dysuria, oedema, diarrhoea, etc	None known
Psyllium (*Plantago ovata=Isphagula*)	Bulk-forming laxative	Constipation	Allergic reactions including anaphylaxis
Pumpkin (*Curcurbita pepo*)	Antiandrogenic, anti-inflammatory	Benign prostatic hyperplasia	None known
Qianghuo (*Notopterygium incisum*)	Analgesic	Rheumatic pain, common cold	None known
Raspberry leaf (*Rubus idaeus*)	Astringent, vasoconstrictive, anti-inflammatory, oestrogenic	Gastrointestinal, cardiovascular and respiratory problems, fever, diabetes	Could interfere with oestrogen sensitive conditions, e.g. breast cancer, endometriosis
Red pepper (*Capsicum frutescens*)	Stimulates digestion, applied topically it releases substance P	Flatulence, colic, diarrhoea, improves blood circulation, seasickness, etc	Numerous drug interactions are conceivable
Reishi (*Ganoderma lucidum*)	Immune stimulation, anticoagulant, antitumour	Hypercholesterolaemia, hypertension, viral infections, cancer, asthma, etc	Dryness of mucosa, gastrointestinal problems, bleeding
Rye grass pollen (*Secale cereale*)	Relaxes smooth muscle, anti-inflammatory	Benign prostatic hyperplasia	None known

TABLE 4.1 OTHER MEDICINAL HERBS **481**

Name*	Pharmacologic action**	Conditions frequently treated**	Safety concerns**
Saffron (Crocus sativus)	Increases oxygen diffusion, stimulates gastric secretion	Asthma, insomnia, cough, arteriosclerosis	May have abortifacient effects
Sage (Salvia officinalis)	Antimicrobial, antisecretory	Dyspepsia, persistent perspiration	Epileptiform convulsions (prolonged use)
Sarsaparilla (Smilax)	Tonic, anti-inflammatory, hepatoprotective	Psoriasis, leprosy, appetite stimulant	Renal damage, interaction with hypnotics and digitalis
Shegan (Belamcanda sinensis)	Antiphlogistic, expectorant	Asthma, cough, pain	None known
Sweet orange (Citrus aurantium)	Anti-inflammatory, antibiotic, antioxidant	Coughs, colds, anorexia, tonic, dyspepsia	Intestinal colic, convulsions (children)
Turmeric (Curcuma longa)	Choleritic, anti-inflammatory, antioxidant, antimutagenic	Functional gallbladder problems	None known
Wheat grass (Agropyron repens)	Antibacterial, anticoagulant	Diabetes, wound healing, detoxification, cancer	Bleeding
White peony (Paeonia lactiflora)	Antispasmodic, anti-inflammatory, analgesic, abortifacient, anticoagulant	Pain (e.g. menstrual)	Could increase action of anticoagulants
Wild yam (Dioscorea villosa)	Oestrogenic	Menopause, osteoporosis, tonic	Vomiting, interference with oestrogen sensitive conditions
Witch hazel (Hamamelis virginiana)	Astringent, anti-inflammatory	Minor skin injuries, haemorrhoids, varicose veins (external use)	None known
Wuweizu (Schisandra chinensis)	Anti-inflammatory, antihepatotoxic	Liver protection, asthma	None known
Xixin (Asarum heterotropoides)	Analgesic, antitussive, sedative	Common cold, headache, other pains	None known
Yarrow (Achillea millefolium)	Choleretic, antibacterial, astringent, antispasmodic, diaphoretic, antipyretic, diuretic, spasmodic	Loss of appetite, dyspepsia, a range of conditions, e.g. fever, common cold, amenorrhoea, dysentery, etc	Allergic reactions, dermatitis, sedation
Yuxingcao (Houttuynia cordata)	Diuretic, anti-inflammatory	Inflammation of respiratory tract, acute dysentery, acute urinary tract infections	None known
Zelan (Lycopus lucidus)	Activation of blood circulation, diuretic	Menstrual disorders, postpartum pain	None known

*English or Chinese common name, Latin name **Examples only

Table 4.2 **Other non-plant based medicines which have been tested for effectiveness or are used frequently**

Name	Description	Pharmacologic action	Conditions frequently treated	Safety concerns
Acidophilus	*Lactobacillus acidophilus* is a bacterium which is commercially prepared for oral consumption (probiotic)	Digestive aid, production of B-complex vitamins and a 'healthy' bacterial flora in the gastrointestinal tract	Gastrointestinal problems, prevention of infections, after antibiotic treatments	None known
Agar	Aqueous extract from the cell wall of red marine algae	Promotion of faecal bulk	Constipation	Bowel obstruction, decrease of intestinal absorption of minerals
Arginine	Essential amino acid, substrate for nitric oxide synthase	Vasodilatation, reduction of monocyte adhesion	Chronic heart failure, angina pectoris, hypertension, peripheral vascular disease	Interactions with many other drugs are conceivable
Bee pollen	Flower pollen and nectar, mixed with digestive enzymes from honeybees	Antioxidative	Allergic conditions including asthma, impotence, prevention of cancer and cardiovascular disease	Allergic reactions including anaphylaxis
Beta-glucan extracts	Primary component of call walls of bacteria, fungi, yeast, algae, etc	Antimicrobial, antitumour, immuno-stimulant	Hypercholesterol-aemia, diabetes, cancer, AIDS	Might interfere with immuno-suppression
Carnitine	Quaternary amine, constituent of muscle cells	Participation in cellular energy production and removal of toxins, cholinergic antagonist, membrane stabiliser	Numerous chronic conditions including cardiovascular disease and Alzheimer's disease	None known
Chromium	Essential trace element	Is part of complex caked glucose tolerance factor	Diabetes, hypercholesterolaemia, weight loss	Cognitive motor dysfunction, anaemia, thrombocytopenia
Creatine	Amino acid found in red meat, milk and fish. Also synthesised by the kidneys, liver and pancreas	Maintaining high levels of adenosine triphosphate (main energy source for muscle contraction)	Enhancement of physical performance, cramps	Dehydration, gastrointestinal discomfort, muscle cramps

TABLE 4.2 OTHER NON-PLANT BASED MEDICINES **483**

Name	Description	Pharmacologic action	Conditions frequently treated	Safety concerns
Dehydro-epiandrosterone (DHEA)	Precursor of steroid hormones found in some plants (e.g. yam)	Raising levels of androgens and oestrogens; assumed anti-aging effects	Prevention of cancer, cardio-vascular disease, osteoporosis	Hirsutism, insomnia, irritability, interactions with steroid hormones
Docosahexaenic acid (DHA)	Essential fatty acid	Anti-inflammatory anticoagulant	Arthritis, circulatory disorders, neuro-logical problems	Might enhance effects of anticoagulants
Eicosapentaenic acid (EPA)	Essential fatty acid	Anti-inflammatory anticoagulant	Arthritis, circulatory disorders, neuro-logical problems	Might enhance effects of anticoagulants
Fish oil	Oil from fatty fish such as salmon or mackerel	Anti-inflammatory, anticoagulant	Arthritis, circulatory disorders	Vitamin D hypervitaminosis
Gamma-hydroxybutyric acid	Substance occurring naturally in the brain	Anesthetic, central nervous system suppressant	Insomnia	Headache, dizziness, confusion, hallucinations
Glutamine	Amino acid abundantly available in the body	Immune stimulant, essential for amino acid homeostasis	Chemotherapy-induced mucositis, depression, anxiety, insomnia	None known
Green-lipped mussel (*Perna canaliculus*)	Rich source of omega-3 fatty acids	Anti-inflammatory	Arthritis	Bleeding
Hydrazine sulfate	Organic compound used in industry	Blocks glyconeogenesis	Cancer	Nausea, dizziness, neuropathy, confusion, seizures
Kelp	Product derived from marine brown algae; used in Japanese folk medicine	Anticarcinogenic	Cancer prevention, obesity, rheumatism	Acne, thrombo-cytopenia, bleeding, hypotension, arsenic poi-soning, interactions with antico-agulants possible
Laetrile	Substance from apricot kernels	Cytotoxic	Cancer	Vomiting, dyspnoea, palpitations, convulsions, death

table continues

Name	Description	Pharmacologic action	Conditions frequently treated	Safety concerns
Nicotinamide adenine dinucleotide (NADH)	Essential intermediate on the process that generates energy from glucose	Hydrogen donor in respiratory chain	Improved cognitive function, depression, Parkinson's disease, tonic	None known
Octacosanol	28-carbon long-chain alcohol isolated from vegetable waxes	Enhancement of intramuscular lipolysis		Irritability, orthostatic hypotension
Pyruvate	2-oxo-propanoate	Reduction of free radical production	Weight loss, tonic, cancer	None known
Red yeast rice (*Monascus purpureus*)	Fermentation product of yeast and rice used in traditional Chinese medicine	Reduction of hepatic cholesterol synthesis (contains lorastatin)	Hypercholesterolaemia	As lorastatin
Royal jelly	Secretion of worker bees that is fed to the queen bee	Antimicrobial, antitumour	Impotence, baldness, menopause, prevention of cancer and cardiovascular disease	Allergies including anaphylaxis
S-adenosyl-L-methionine (SAMe),	Naturally occurring substance present in all parts of the body involved in the synthesis, activation and metabolism of hormones, neurotransmitters etc	Analgesic, anti-inflammatory, stimulation of cartilage growth	Depression, heart disease, fibromyalgia, arthritis, Alzheimer's disease, etc	Flatulence, diarrhoea, nausea, headache
Selenium	Essential trace element	Antioxidant	AIDS, prevention of cancer, cardiovascular disease, arthritis	Nausea, irritability, weight loss
Thymus extract	Extracts from bovine thymus cells usually for injection	Stimulation of immune system	Cancer, AIDS	Allergic reactions, infection

TABLE 4.3 PRODUCTS REQUIRING THERAPEUTIC MONITORING **485**

Table 4.3
Herbal medicinal products and other food supplements for which therapeutic monitoring is advised

Name	Recommended tests
Aloe vera (Aloe barbadensis)	Renal function, electrolytes
Andrographis (Andrographis paniculata)	Blood glucose
Angelica (Angelica sinensis)	Coagulation
Basil (Basilicum)	Blood glucose
Bayberry (Myrica cerifera)	Liver function
Bearberry (Arctostaphylos uva ursi)	Renal function, electrolytes
Betony (Stachys officinalis)	Liver function
Black haw (Viburnum prunifolium)	Coagulation
Black root (Veronicastrum virginicum)	Liver function
Blue cohosh (Actaea racemosa)	Blood glucose
Boneset (Eupatorium perfoliatum)	Liver function
Borage (Borago officinalis)	Liver function
Buchu (Barosma betulina)	Liver function
Cascara sagrada (Rhamnus purshiana)	Renal function, electrolytes
Castor bean (Ricinus communis)	Renal function, electrolytes
Cat's claw (Uncaria tomentosa)	Coagulation
Chaparral (Larrea tridentata)	Liver function
Condurango (Marsedenia condurango)	Liver function
Cowslip (Primula veris)	Liver function
Cucumber (Cucumis sativus)	Renal function, electrolytes
Dandelion (Taraxacum officinale)	Blood glucose
Fenugreek (Trigonella foenum-graecum)	Coagulation, blood glucose
Garlic (Allium sativum)	Full blood count
Ginger (Zingiber officinalis)	Coagulation
Gingko (Ginkgo biloba)	Coagulation
Ginseng, Asian (Panax ginseng)	Blood glucose
Gotu kola (Centella asiatica)	Blood glucose
Horse chestnut (Aesculus hippocastanum)	Coagulation
Jaborandi tree (Pilocarpus Jaborandi)	Liver function
Kava (Piper methysticum)	Full blood count, liver function
Kelp (Neveocystis luetkeaua)	Coagulation
Kelpware (Fucus vesiculosus)	Renal function, electrolytes, coagulation, blood glucose
Khella (Ammi visnaga)	Liver function
Lovage (Levisticum officinale)	Renal function, electrolytes
Lungwort (Pulmonaria officinalis)	Coagulation
Marshmallow (Althaea officinalis)	Blood glucose
Mayapple (Podophyllum peltatum)	Full blood count, liver function, renal function, electrolytes
Myrrh (Commiphora myrrha)	Blood glucose
Myrtle (Myrtus communis)	Blood glucose
Pau d'arco (Tabebuia impetiginosa)	Coagulation
Pennyroyal oil (Mentha pulegium)	Liver function, renal function, electrolytes
Pomegranate (Punica granatum)	Liver function
Poplar (Populus alba)	Liver function, coagulation
Ragwort (Senecio aureus)	Liver function
Red clover (Trifolium pratense)	Coagulation
Rhatany (Krameria triandra)	Liver function
Sage (Salvia officinalis)	Blood glucose
Sarsaparilla (Smilax aristochiifolia)	Renal function, electrolytes

HERBAL AND NON-HERBAL MEDICINES

table continues

Name	Recommended tests
Skullcap (*Scutellaria lateriflora*)	Liver function
Soapwort *(Saponaria officinalis)*	Liver function, renal function, electrolytes
Sorrel (*Rumex acetosella*)	Liver function, renal function, electrolytes
Squaw vine (*Michella repens*)	Liver function
St John's wort (*Hypericum perforatum*)	Coagulation, concomitant drug levels
Tonka bean (*Dipteryx odorata*)	Liver function, coagulation
Turmeric (*Curcuma longa*)	Coagulation
Valerian (*Valeriana officinalis*)	Liver function
Willow (*Salix alba*)	Liver function, renal function, electrolytes, coagulation
Wintergreen (*Gaultheria procumbens*)	Coagulation
Wormwood *(Artemisia absinthium)*	Renal function, electrolytes
Yellow dock *(Rumex crispus)*	Renal function, electrolytes

SOURCE

Fetrow C W, Avila J R. Complementary and alternative medicine. Springhouse, PA: Springhouse; 1999

TABLE 4.4 INTERACTIONS WITH HEART MEDICATIONS **487**

Table 4.4 **Herbal medicinal products and other food supplements with the potential to interact with heart medications**

Name	Direction of effect	Concomitant medication
Adonis (*Acacia senegal*)	⇧	Cardiac glycosides, beta-blockers, Ca1 channel blockers,
Agrimony (*Agrimonia eupateria*)	⇧	Antihypertensives, cardiac glycosides
Aloe vera (*Aloe barbadensis*)	⇧	Cardiac glycosides, antiarrhythmics
Angelica (*Angelica sinensis*)	⇧	Ca1 channel blockers,
Anise seed (*Pimpinella anisum*)	⇧	Antihypertensives
Arnica (*Arnica montana*)	⇩	Antihypertensives
Asafoetida (*Ferula asafoetida*)	⇧	Antihypertensives
Astralagus (*Astralagus* spp)	⇧	Antiarrhythmics
Bayberry (*Myrica cerifera*)	⇧	Antihypertensives, Ca1 channel blockers, nitrates
Bearberry (*Arctostaphylos uva ursi*)	⇧	Cardiac glycosides
Betony (*Stachys officinalis*)	⇧	Antihypertensives
Black cohosh (*Actaea racemosa*)	⇧	Antihypertensives
Blue cohosh (*Caulophyllum thalictroides*)	⇩	Antihypertensives, Ca1 channel blockers, nitrates
Boldo (*Peumus boldus*)	⇧	Cardiac glycosides
Broom (*Cytisus scoparius*)	⇧	Beta-blockers, cardiac glycosides, Ca1 channel blockers
Buchu (*Barosma betulina*)	⇧	Cardiac glycosides
Buckthorn (*Rhamnus catharticus*)	⇧	Cardiac glycosides, antiarrhythmics
Cascara (*Rhamnus purshiana*)	⇧	Cardiac glycosides
Castor bean (*Ricinus communis*)	⇧	Cardiac glycosides
Cat's claw (*Uncaria tomentosa*)	⇧	Antihypertensives
Chaparral (*Larrea tridentata*)	⇧	Cardiac glycosides
Chaste tree (*Vitex agnus castus*)	⇧	Beta-blockers, antihypertensives
Chilli pepper (*Capsicum* spp.)	⇧	Antihypertensives
Coltsfoot (*Tussilago farfara*)	⇩	Antihypertensives
Cowslip (*Primula veris*)	⇧	Antihypertensives
Dandelion (*Taraxacum officinale*)	⇧	Antihypertensives
Devil's claw (*Hapargophytum procumbens*)	⇧	Antihypertensives, antiarrhythmics
Ephedra (*Ephedra sinica*)	⇩	Antihypertensives, antiarrhythmics
Evening primrose (*Oenothera biennis*)	⇧	Antihypertensives
Figwort (*Scrophularia nodosa*)	⇧	Beta-blockers, cardiac glycosides, Ca1 channel blockers
Frangula (*Rhamnus frangula*)	⇧	Cardiac glycosides
Fumitory (*Fumaria officinalis*)	⇧	Antihypertensives, beta-blockers, cardiac glycosides, Ca1 channel blockers
Garlic (*Allium sativum*)	⇧	Antihypertensives
Ginger (*Zingiber officinalis*)	⇧	Antihypertensives
Ginseng (*Eleutherococcus senticosus*)	⇧	Antihypertensives, cardiac glycosides
Goldenseal (*Hydrastis canadensis*)	⇧	Antihypertensives Ca1 channel blockers, cardiac glycosides
Guarana (*Paullinia cupana*)	⇧	Cardiac glycosides
Hawthorn (*Crataegus laevigata*)	⇧	Cardiac glycosides, nitrates, antiarrhythmics, antihypertensives
Horsetail (*Equisetum arvense*)	⇧	Cardiac glycosides
Indian snakeroot (*Rauwolfia serpentina*)	⇧	Antihypertensives
Irish moss (*Chondrus crispus*)	⇧	Antihypertensives

table continues

Name	Direction of effect	Concomitant medication
Juniper (*Juniperus* spp.)	⇧	Antiarrhythmics, antihypertensives, cardiac glycosides
Kelp (*Neveocystis luetkeaua*)	⇧	Antihypertensives
Khat (*Catha edulis*)	⇧	Antihypertensives, antiarrhythmics, beta-blockers
Khella (*Ammi visnaga*)	⇧	Antihypertensives, Ca I channel blockers
Licorice (*Glycyrrhiza glabra*)	⇧	Antihypertensives, cardiac glycosides
Lily-of-the-valley (*Convallaria majalis*)	⇧	Cardiac glycosides, beta-blockers, Ca I channel blockers
Lungwort (*Pulmonaria officinalis*)	⇧	Cardiac glycosides
Mistletoe (*Viscum album*)	⇧	Antihypertensives, cardiac glycosides
Motherwort (*Leonurus cardiaca*)	⇩	Beta-blockers, cardiac glycosides
Myrrh (*Commiphora myrrha*)	⇩	Antihypertensives
Nettle (*Urtica dioica*)	⇧	Antihypertensives
Night-blooming Cereus (*Selenicereus grandiflorus*)	⇧	Cardiac glycosides, ACE inhibitors, antiarrhythmics, Ca I channel blockers, beta-blockers
Oleander (*Nerium oleander*)	⇧	Cardiac glycosides
Pansy (*Viola tricolor*)	⇧	Antihypertensives
Papaya (*Papaya carica*)	⇧	Antihypertensives, cardiac glycosides
Parsley (*Petroselinum sativum*)	⇧	Antihypertensives
Peppermint (*Mentha x piperita*)	⇧	Cardiac glycosides, antihypertensives
Pill-bearing spurge (*Euphorbia pilulifera*)	⇧	ACE inhibitors
Pineapple (*Ananas comosus*)	⇩	ACE inhibitors
Pleurisy root (*Asclepias tuberosa*)	⇧	Cardiac glycosides
Psyllium (*Plantago ovata*)	⇧	Cardiac glycosides
Queen Anne's lace (*Daucus carota*)	⇧	Antihypertensives, cardiac glycosides
Ragwort (*Senecio aureus*)	⇧	Antihypertensives, cardiac glycosides
Red clover (*Trifolium pratense*)	⇧	Cardiac glycosides
Rhubarb (*Rheum officinale*)	⇧	Cardiac glycosides, antiarrhythmics,
Rue (*Ruta graveolens*)	⇧	Cardiac glycosides, antihypertensives
Sarsaparilla (*Smilax aristochiifolia*)	⇧	Cardiac glycosides
Senna (*Cassia senna*)	⇧	Cardiac glycosides, Ca I channel blockers, antiarrhythmics
Shepherd's purse (*Capsella bursa pastoris*)	⇧	Antihypertensives, beta-blockers, cardiac glycosides, Ca I channel blockers
Squaw vine (*Michella repens*)	⇧	Cardiac glycosides
Squill (*Urginea maritima*)	⇧	Cardiac glycosides, antiarrhythmic, Ca I channel blockers, beta-blockers
St John's wort (*Hypericum perforatum*)	⇩	Cardiac glycosides
Stephania (*Stephania tetranda*)	⇧	Ca I channel blockers
Strophantus (*Strophanthus kombé*)	⇧	Cardiac glycosides
Yarrow (*Achillea millefolium*)	⇧	Antihypertensives

⇧ increase in effect
⇩ decrease in effect

SOURCES

Braun L, Cohen M. Herbs and nutritional supplements. Sydney: Elsevier; 2005
Ernst E. Herb–drug interactions – an update. Perfusion 2003;16:175–194

TABLE 4.5 INTERACTIONS WITH ANTICOAGULANTS **489**

Table 4.5
Herbal medicinal products and other food supplements with the potential to interact with anticoagulants

Name	Direction
Agrimony (*Agrimonia eupateria*)	⇩
Alfalfa (*Medicago sativa*)	⇧
Andrographis (*Andrographis paniculata*)	⇧
Angelica (*Angelica sinensis*)	⇧
Anise seed (*Pimpinella anisum*)	⇧
Arnica (*Arnica montana*)	⇩
Asafoetida (*Ferula asafoetida*)	⇧
Bilberry (*Vaccinium myrtillus*)	⇧
Black haw (*Viburnum prunifollum*)	⇧
Bogbean (*Menyanthes trifoliata*)	⇧
Bromelain (*Ananas comosus*)	⇧
Buchu (*Barosma betulina*)	⇧
Cat's claw (*Uncaria tomentosa*)	⇧
Chamomile (*Chamomilla recutita*)	⇧
Chilli pepper (*Capsicum* spp.)	⇧
Cinchona (*Cinchona* spp.)	⇧
Cloves (*Syzgium aromaticum*)	⇧
Cordyceps (*Cordyceps sinensis*)	⇧
Cumin (*Cuminum cyminum*)	⇧
Danshen (*Salvia miltiorrhiza*)	⇧
Devil's claw (*Hapargophytum procumbens*)	⇧
Evening primrose (*Oenothera biennis*)	⇧
Fenugreek (*Trigonella foenum-graecum*)	⇧
Feverfew (*Tanacetum parthenium*)	⇧
Garlic (*Allium sativum*)	⇧
Ginger (*Zingiber officinalis*)	⇧
Ginkgo (*Ginkgo biloba*)	⇧
Ginseng, Asian (*Panax ginseng*)	⇧
Goldenseal (*Hydrastis canadensis*)	⇩
Grape seed (*Vitis vinifera*)	⇧
Green tea (*Camellia sinensis*)	⇩
Guarana (*Paullinia cupana*)	⇧
Horse chestnut (*Aesculus hippocastanum*)	⇧
Horseradish (*Armoracia rusticana*)	⇧
Irish moss (*Chondrus crispus*)	⇧
Kelp (*Neveocystis luetkeaua*)	⇧
Khella (*Ammi visnaga*)	⇧
Licorice (*Glycyrrhiza glabra*)	⇧
Lovage (*Levisticum officinale*)	⇧
Lungwort (*Pulmonaria officinalis*)	⇧
Meadowsweet (*Filipendula ulmaria*)	⇧
Mistletoe (*Viscum album*)	⇧
Mugwort (*Artemesia vulgaris*)	⇧
Papaya (*Papaya carica*)	⇧
Pau d'arco (*Tabebuia impetiginosa*)	⇧
Pill-bearing spurge (*Euphorbia pilulifera*)	⇧
Pineapple (*Ananas comosus*)	⇧
Poplar (*Populus alba*)	⇧
Prickly ash (*Zanthoxylum americanum*)	⇧
Red clover (*Trifolium pratense*)	⇧
Reishi (*Ganoderma lucidum*)	⇧
Roman chamomile (*Chamaemelum nobile*)	⇧
Safflower (*Carthamus tinctorius*)	⇧
Sage (*Salvia officinalis*)	⇧

table continues

Name	Direction
Senega (*Polygala senega*)	⇧
Shitake mushroom (*Lentinula edodes*)	⇧
St John's wort (*Hypericum perforatum*)	⇩
Sweet clover (*Melilotus officinale*)	⇧
Sweet woodruffe (*Gallium odoratum*)	⇧
Tonka bean (*Dipteryx odorata*)	⇧
Turmeric (*Curcuma longa*)	⇧
Vervain (*Verbena officinalis*)	⇧
Willow (*Salix alba*)	⇧
Wintergreen (*Gaultheria procumbens*)	⇧
Woodruff (*Asperula odorata*)	⇧
Yarrow (*Achillea millefolium*)	⇧

⇧ increase in anticoagulation
⇩ decrease in anticoagulation

SOURCES

Braun L, Cohen M. Herbs and nutritional supplements. Sydney: Elsevier; 2005
Ernst E. Herb–drug interactions – an update. Perfusion 2003;16:175–194

TABLE 4.6 INTERACTIONS WITH ANTIDIABETIC MEDICATIONS **491**

Table 4.6
Herbal medicinal products and other food supplements with the potential to interact with antidiabetic medications

Name	Direction
Aceitilla (*Bidens pilosa*)	⇧
Agrimony (*Agrimonia eupateria*)	⇧
Alfalfa (*Medicago sativa*)	⇧
Aloe vera (*Aloe barbadensis*)	⇧
Andrographis (*Andrographis paniculata*)	⇧
Basil (*Basilicum*)	⇧
Bilberry (*Vaccinium myrtillus*)	⇧
Bitter lemon (*Momordica charantia*)	⇧
Blackberry (*Rubus fruticosus*)	⇧
Broom (*Cytisus scoparius*)	⇩
Buchu (*Barosma betulina*)	⇧
Bugleweed (*Lycopus virginicus*)	⇧
Burdock (*Arctium lappa*)	⇧
Celandine (*Chelidonium majus*)	⇧
Coriander (*Coriandrum sativum*)	⇧
Cumin (*Cuminum cyminum*)	⇧
Damiana (*Turnera diffusa*)	⇧
Dandelion (*Taraxacum officinale*)	⇧
Danshen (*Salvia miltiorrhiza*)	⇧
Devil's claw (*Hapargophytum procumbens*)	⇧
Fenugreek (*Trigonella foenum – graecum*)	⇧
Ginseng, Asian (*Panax ginseng*)	⇧
Siberian ginseng (*Eleutherococcus senticosus*)	⇧
Goldenseal (*Hydrastis canadensis*)	⇧
Gotu kola (*Centella asiatica*)	⇩
Green tea (*Camellia sinensis*)	⇧
Guar gum (*Cyamopsis tetragonolobus*)	⇧
Horehound (*Marrubium vulgare*)	⇧
Horse chestnut (*Aesculus hippocastanum*)	⇧
Juniper (*Juniperus* spp.)	⇧
Long pepper (*Piper longum*)	⇧
Lupine (*Lupinus albus*)	⇧
Madagascar periwinkle (*Catharanthus roseus*)	⇧
Maitake mushroom (*Grifola frondosa*)	⇧
Milk thistle (*Silybum marianum*)	⇧
Myrrh (*Commiphora molmol*)	⇧
Myrtle (*Myrtus communis*)	⇧
Neem (*Azadirachta indica*)	⇧
Night-blooming cereus (*Selenicereus grandiflorus*)	⇧
Onion (*Allium cepa*)	⇧
Pansy (*Viola tricolor*)	⇧
Raspberry (*Rubus idaeus*)	⇧
Roman chamomile (*Chamaemelum nobile*)	⇧
Rosemary (*Rosmarinus officinalis*)	⇧
Sage (*Salvia officinalis*)	⇩
St John's wort (*Hypericum perforatum*)	⇩

⇧ increase in antidiabetic effect
⇩ decrease in antidiabetic effect

SOURCES

Braun L, Cohen M. Herbs and nutritional supplements. Sydney: Elsevier; 2005
Ernst E. Herb–drug interactions – an update. Perfusion 2003;16:175–194

HERBAL AND NON-HERBAL MEDICINES

Table 4.7
Herbal medicinal products with the potential to interact with oral contraceptives

Name	Direction
Angelica (*Angelica sinensis*)	⇑
Chaste tree (*Vitex agnus-castus*)	⇑
Guar gum (*Cyamopsis tetragonolobus*)	⇓
Herbal laxatives (e.g. *Aloe vera*, senna)	⇓
Hops (*Humulus lupulus*)	⇑
Pokeweed (*Phytolacca americana*)	⇓
Red clover (*Trifolium pratense*)	⇑
Rue (*Ruta graveolens*)	⇑
St John's wort (*Hypericum perforatum*)	⇓

⇑ increase in drug plasma levels
⇓ decrease in drug plasma levels

SOURCES

Braun L, Cohen M. Herbs and nutritional supplements. Sydney: Elsevier, 2005
Ernst E. Herb–drug interactions – an update. Perfusion 2003;16:175–194

General topics

Diagnostic methods

Edzard Ernst

It is frequently forgotten that much of CAM involves diagnostic methods which are not used in conventional practice. Some of these techniques are specific to one type of practice, e.g. tongue diagnosis in TCM, others are used by several types of practitioners, e.g. kinesiology. All of these approaches have one thing in common: they are woefully under-researched. Thus there is considerable uncertainty regarding their validity. The issue is, of course, complicated by the fact that some traditional medical systems also have their own diagnostic categories.

Ideally, a diagnostic method should be reproducible, sensitive and specific. Reproducibility means that, firstly, if one patient is tested several times by the same person, the result should be very similar each time (intra-rater reproducibility). Secondly, if several people test the same patient or sample repeatedly the results should all be within an equally narrow range (inter-rater reproducibility). Sensitivity of a test describes the requirement that, if the parameter or quality captured by any given diagnostic technique (e.g. pain) changes in the patient, the test results should reflect this change adequately. Specificity of a diagnostic method expresses the need that, ideally, a test should be specific, for example to a certain condition or a range of related conditions. For instance, a 'positive reading' for hypertension (i.e. an elevated blood pressure reading) is specific to that condition and does not indicate diabetes or urinary tract infection.

The dangers associated with invalid diagnostic methods are considerable. Such tests can lead either to false positive or false negative results. 'False positive' describes a test indicating a condition that is actually absent in the patient tested. In such cases a practitioner may diagnose a 'condition' which does not afflict the patient concerned, e.g. a traditional Chinese medicine (TCM) practitioner may diagnose an 'energy blockage' in an entirely healthy person. This can have a range of adverse effects. For instance, it could unnecessarily worry that 'patient' and even make her ill as a consequence. It would almost certainly also cause the 'patient' to spend money unnecessarily on the treatment aimed at normalising a non-existing abnormality.

False negative diagnoses are potentially much more harmful. If an invalid test suggests the absence of a condition in a patient who is, in fact, afflicted by it, this patient's access to effective therapy would be delayed, hindered or stopped. For instance, if a patient with an early but diagnosable cancer is given the 'all clear' by her TCM practitioner, she would lose valuable time for early treatment. In extreme cases, such negative diagnoses can contribute to unnecessary deaths of patients.

There are probably hundreds of diagnostic methods unique to CAM.[1,2] A systematic evaluation of these techniques would be highly desirable but, at present, seems rather impossible. For the vast majority, no scientific data on reliability, sensitivity or specificity are available. Where at least some information exists, this has been summarised in Table 5.1.1.[3-48] Overall the conclusions drawn from these studies tend to be negative.[29,49,50] With a few exceptions for which preliminary results are encouraging, 'no complementary or alternative diagnostic procedure can be recommended'.[49]

Table 5.1.1   **Studies of diagnostic methods predominantly used in CAM**

Name of method	Related methods (or synonyms)	Description	Comments/Results
Acupuncture	n.a.	Traditional acupuncturists diagnosed patients with back pain	High diagnostic agreement in terms of TCM diagnoses existed in five of seven acupuncturists[3]
Ayurveda	n.a.	Ayurvedic therapists diagnosed patients with specific conditions	Preliminary data suggest both reasonable and insufficient agreement between practitioners[4,5]
Bioresonance	Mora	Electromagnetic waves from the body are received by an electronic device which 'normalises' them and sends them back to the patient	Bioresonance is diagnosis and treatment in one. Several assessments exist and the rigorous ones usually conclude that it is not useful for diagnosis nor treatment[6]
Chiropractic	X-ray diagnostic for malalignment or contra-indication Manual diagnostic techniques	A range of techniques, not all are specific to chiropractic	Several assessments exist, results are mixed but frequently indicate poor reliability[7-17]
Constitutional diagnosis	None	Several traditional medical systems evaluate the 'constitution' of patients	Preliminary findings showed no specificity of constitutional diagnostic methods[18]
Iridology	None	Irregularities in the iris are thought to reflect abnormalities of specific organs/functions	A systematic review concluded that rigorous assessments demonstrated iridology to be not a valid technique[19,20]
Kinesiology	Applied kinesiology	Aspects of muscle function are tested manually and linked to function of organs or organ systems	The technique has been assessed repeatedly, usually with negative results[21]

GENERAL TOPICS

table continues

Name of method	Related methods (or synonyms)	Description	Comments/Results
Kirlian photography	None	High frequency electrical currents are applied to the body and the resulting images of the discharges are linked to human health	Reliability of method is low[27,28]
Laboratory tests	None	Blood, hair, saliva, stool or other samples are assessed with a range of optical, chemical or other methods. Results are interpreted as indicators for diseases such as cancer	This is an extremely heterogeneous category. By and large 'alternative' laboratory tests are not of proven value[29,30]
Manual therapy	Massage, chiropractic, osteopathy	Manual therapists use their hands to feel the state of the musculoskeletal system and draw conclusions about human health	Palpation techniques have poor reproducibility[31–33]
Pulse diagnosis	None	In TCM, 12 different of the radial pulse qualities are palpated and related to the function of inner organs	Reliability of method is generally poor[34–36]
Radionics	Dowsing, pendulum, devining	Technique utilising a motor automatism in conjunction with mechanical or electronic instruments to obtain information	Results of testing dowsing for medical diagnosis were 'wholly negative'[37]
Reflexology	None	Palpation of the sole of the foot provides information about the function of inner organs	Several assessments have been performed, most results fail to show validity of method[38–41]
Tongue diagnosis	None	In TCM, the colour, texture, shape and structure of the tongue are visually assessed and linked to human health	Results of scientific evaluations are inconclusive[42,43]
Traditional Chinese medicine	None	How consistent are TCM practitioners at making the same diagnosis	Reproducibility is poor[44–46]
Vega-Test	Electroacupuncture	Electromagnetic properties of acupuncture points are measured and linked to specific medical conditions and their treatments	Several assessments are available most results fail to show validity of the method[47–49]

n.a. = not applicable

REFERENCES

1 Barrett S. Dubious diagnostic tests. Quackwatch Database. Online. Available at *www.quackwatch.org*, accessed 15 June 2005

2 Renckens C N M. A comparison between alternative pseudodiagnoses and regularly accepted fashionable diseases: an analysis prompted by the Dutch epidemic of obstetric 'pelvic instability'. Sci Rev Altern Med 2002;6:91–96

3 Sherman K J, Cherkin D C, Hogeboom C J. The diagnosis and treatment of patients with chronic low-back pain by traditional Chinese medical acupuncturists. J Altern Complement Med 2001;7:641–650

4 Prlic H M, Lehman A J, Cibere J, Sodhi V, Varma S, Sukumaran T, Esdaile J M. Agreement among Ayurvedic practitioners in the identification and treatment of three cases of inflammatory arthritis. Clin Exp Rheumatol 2003;21:747–752

5 Falkenbach A, Oberguggenberger R. Ayurveda in ankylosing spondylitis and low back pain. Ann Rheum Dis 2003;62:276–277

6 Kofler H, Ulmer H, Mechtler E, Falk M, Fritsch P O. Bioresonanz bei Pollinose. Allergologie 1996;19:114–122

7 Assendelft W J J, Bouter L M, Knipschild P G, Wilmink J T. Reliability of lumbar spine radiography reading by chiropractors. Spine 1997;22:1235–1241

8 de Zoete A, Assendelft W J, Algra P R, Oberman W R, Vanderschueren G M, Bezemer P D. Reliability and validity of lumbosacral spine radiograph reading by chiropractors, chiropractic radiologists, and medical radiologists. Spine 2002;27:1926–1933

9 Leboeuf C. The reliability of specific sacro occipital techniques and diagnostic tests. J Manip Physiol Ther 1991;14:512–517

10 Panzer D M. The reliability of lumbar motion palpation. J Manip Physiol Ther 1992;15:518–524

11 Nilsson N, Christensen H W, Hartvigsen J. The inter-examiner reliability of measuring passive cervical range of motion, revisited. J Manip Physiol Ther 1996;19:302–305

12 Hubka M J, Phelen S P. Interexaminer reliability of palpation for cervical spine tenderness. J Manip Physiol Ther 1994;17:591–596

13 Hestboek L, Leboeuf-Yde C. Are chiropractic tests for the lumbo-pelvic spine reliable and valid? A systematic critical literature review. J Manip Physiol Ther 2000;23:258–275

14 Leboeuf-Yde C, Ohm Kyvik K. Is it possible to differentiate people with or without low back pain on the basis of tests of lumbo-pelvic dysfunction? J Manip Physiol Ther 2000;23:160–167

15 French S D, Green S, Forbes A. Reliability of chiropractic methods commonly used to detect manipulable lesions in patients with chronic low back pain. J Manip Physiol Ther 2000;23:231–237

16 Pollard H, Lakay B, Tucker F, Watson B, Bablis P. Interexaminer reliability of the deltoid and psoas muscle test. J Manipulative Physiol Ther 2005;28:52–56

17 Humphreys B K, Delahaye M, Peterson C K. An investigation into the validity of cervical spine motion palpation using subjects with congenital block vertebrae as a 'gold standard'. BMC Musculoskelet Disord 2004;5:19

18 Hoffmann C, Rosenberger A, Troeger W, Stange R, Buehring M. Validation of questionnaires from several medical fields regarding the constitution of patients. Forsch Komplementärmed Klass Naturheilkd 2002;9:37–44

19 Ernst E. Iridology: not useful and potentially harmful. Arch Ophthalmol 2000;118:120–121

20 Worrall R, Cannon W, Eastwood M, Steinberg D. Iridology: diagnostic validity in orthopedic trauma. Sci Rev Altern Med 2002;6:63–67

21 Garrow J S. Kinesiology and food allergy. BMJ 1988;298:1573–1574

22 Haas M, Peterson D, Hoyer D, Ross G. Muscle testing response to provocative vertebral challenge and spinal manipulation. A randomized controlled trial of construct validity. J Manip Physiol Ther 1994;17:141–148

23 Lüdtke R, Seeber N, Kinz B, Ring J. Health kinesiology is neither reliable nor valid. Focus Altern Complement Ther 2000;5:95

24 Pothmann R, von Frankenberg S, Hoicke C, Weingarten H, Lüdtke R. Evaluation der klinisch angewandten Kinesiologie bei Nahrungsmittel-Unverträglichkeiten im Kindesalter. Forsch Komplementärmed Klass Naturheilkd 2001;8:336–344

25 Moncayo R, Moncayo H, Ulmer H, Kainz H. New diagnostic and therapeutic approach to thyroid-associated orbitopathy based on applied kinesiology and homeopathic therapy. J Altern Complement Med 2004;10:643–650

26 Teuber S S, Porch-Curren C. Unproved diagnostic and therapeutic approaches to food allergy and intolerance. Curr Opin Allergy Clin Immunol 2003;3:217–221

27 Treugut H, Corner C, Lüdtke R, Mandel P. Kirlian-Fotografie: Reliabilität der

energetischen Terminalpunktdiagnose (ETD) nach Mandal bei gesunden Probanden. Forsch Komplementärmed 1997;4:210–217

28 Treugut H, Koppen M, Nickolay B, Fua R, Schmid P. Kirlian-Fotografie: Zufälliges oder Personen-spezifisches Entladungsmuster? Forsch Komplementärmed Klass Naturheilkund 2000;7: 12–16

29 Ernst E, Hentschel C H. Diagnostic methods in complementary medicine. Which craft is witchcraft? Int J Risk Safety Med 1995;7:55–63

30 Seidel S, Kreutzer R, Smith D, McNeel S, Gilliss D. Assessment of commercial laboratories performing hair mineral analysis. JAMA 2001;285: 67–72

31 Anonymous. Palpatory accuracy: time to reflect. J Bodywork Move Ther 2001;5:223–226

32 Lehmann B, Ningel K, Kopp S, Schellberg H, Smolenski U C, Strauss B. Manualmedizinische Funktionsbeurteilung innerhalb einer interdisziplinären Diagnostik bei Patienten mit craniomanibulärer Dysfunktion (CMS). Phys Med Rehab Kuror 2001;11:145

33 Schöps P, Pfingsten M, Siebert U. Reliability of manual medical examination techniques of the cervical spine. Study of quality assurance in manual diagnosis [Article in German] Z Orthop Ihre Grenzgeb 2000;138:2–7

34 Vincent CA. Acupuncture research: why do it? Complement Med Res 1992;6:21–24

35 King E, Cobbin D, Ryan D. The reliable measurement of radial pulse: gender differences in pulse profiles. Acupunct Med 2002;20:160–167

36 Walsh S, Cobbin D, Bateman K, Zaslawski C. Feeling the pulse. Eur J Orient Med 2001;3:25–31

37 McCarney R, Fisher P, Spink F, Flint G, van Haselen R. Can homeopaths detect homeopathic medicines by dowsing? A randomized, double-blind, placebo-controlled trial. J R Soc Med 2002;95:189–191

38 Baerheim A, Algory R, Skogedal K R, Stephansen R, Sandvik H. Fottene – et diagnostic hjelpemiddel? Tidsskr Nor Laegeforen 1998;5:753–765

39 Sudmeier I, Bodner G, Egger I, Mur E, Ulmer H, Herold M. Änderung der Nierendurchblutung durch organasoziierte Reflexzonentherapie am Fuss gemessen mit farbkodierter Doppler-Sonographie. Forsch Komplementärmed 1999;6:129–134

40 White A R, Williamson J, Hart A, Ernst E. A Blinded investigation into the accuracy of reflexology charts. Complement Ther Med 2000;8:166–172

41 Raz I, Rosengarten Y, Carasso R. Correlation study between conventional medical diagnosis and the diagnosis by reflexology (non conventional) [Article in Hebrew] Harefuah 2003;142:600–605, 646

42 Fuzhonf M, Weiying Z. Observation on the analysis of nailfold microcirculation and tongue picture in 150 cases of cardio-cerebral angiopathy. Proceedings of the 2nd Asian Congress on Microcirculation, Beijing, August 1995

43 Pang B, Zhang D, Li N, Wang K. Computerized tongue diagnosis based on Bayesian networks. IEEE Trans Biomed Eng 2004;51:1803–1810

44 Zhang G G, Bausell B, Lao L, Handwerger B, Berman B M. Assessing the consistency of traditional Chinese medical diagnosis: an integrative approach. Altern Ther Health Med 2003;9:66–71

45 Sung J J, Leung W K, Ching J Y, Lao L, Zhang G, Wu J C, Liang S M, Xie H, Ho Y P, Chan L S, Berman B, Chan F K. Agreements among traditional Chinese medicine practitioners in the diagnosis and treatment of irritable bowel syndrome. Aliment Pharmacol Ther 2004;20:1205–1210

46 Krop J, Lewith G T, Gziut W, Radutescuc A. A double-blind, randomized controlled investigation of electrodermal testing in the diagnosis of allergies. J Alt Complement Med 1997;3:241–248

47 Gloerfeld H. Elektroakupunktur nach Voll. Unpublished MD thesis, University of Marburg, 1987

48 Lewith G T, Kenyon J N, Broomfield J, Prescott P, Goddard J, Holgate S T. Is electrodermal testing as effective as skin prick tests for diagnosing allergies? A double blind, randomised block design study. BMJ 2001;322:131–134

49 Niggemann B, Gruber C. Unproven diagnostic procedures in IgE-mediated allergic diseases. Allergy 2004;59:806–808

50 Senna G, Gani F, Leo G, Schiappoli M. Alternative tests in the diagnosis of food allergies. Recenti Prog Med 2002;93:327–334

Prevalence of complementary and alternative medicine use

Max H Pittler

The understanding of what precisely constitutes CAM differs considerably between countries. Different historical developments and traditions have meant that therapies such as herbal medicine, hydrotherapy and massage are firmly established in mainstream medicine in many European countries, while they are often classified as CAM outside Europe. In addition, some treatments such as the 'cure' (German *Kur*), which includes aspects of hydrotherapy and is considered a mainstream medical approach, are specific to some European countries. Regardless of these national differences and their implications for research, there is evidence for a substantial increase in the use and demand for CAM. To define requirements for the scientific investigation, education and regulation of CAM, information on the level of use among the general population and specific patient populations is of considerable importance. Although inconsistencies abound in many surveys it is possible to derive estimates and eventually outline the development of CAM over time.

Table 5.2.1 **One-year prevalence of CAM in general population samples**[1]

Country and reference	Year of publication	Year of sampling	Sample n	Prevalence %
Australia[2]	1996	1993	Random 3004	48.5
Canada[3]	1997	1995	Representative 17 626	15
Finland[4]	1993	1982	Random 1618	23
France[5]	1990	1985	Representative 1000	49
Germany[6]	2004	2002	Representative 1750	62.3
Hungary[7]	2002	1999	Not reported 2357	13
Israel[8]	2004	2000	Representative 2505	10
Italy[9]	2002	1997–99	Representative 70 898	15.6
Japan[10]	2002	2001	Random 1000	76
United Kingdom[11]	2004	2001	Representative 1794	10
United States[12]	2004	2002	Representative 31 044	62 (incl prayer)

REFERENCES

1 Harris P, Rees R. The prevalence of complementary and alternative medicine use among the general population: a systematic review of the literature. Complement Ther Med 2000;8:88–96

2 MacLennan A H, Wilson D H, Taylor A W. Prevalence and cost of alternative medicine in Australia. Lancet 1996;347:569–573

3 Millar W J. Use of alternative health care practitioners by Canadians. Can J Public Health 1997;88:154–158

4 Vaskilampi T, Merilainen P, Sinkkonen S. The use of alternative treatments in the Finnish adult population. In: G T Lewith, D Aldridge (eds). Clinical research methodology for compelemtnary therapies. London: Hodder & Stoughton; 2004:204–229

5 Bouchayer F. Alternative medicines: a general approach to the French situation. Complement Med Res 1990;4:4–8

6 Härtel U, Volger E. Use and acceptance of classical natural and alternative medicine in Germany–findings of a representative population-based survey. Forsch Komplementarmed Klass Naturheilkd 2004;11:327–334

7 Buda L, Lampek K, Tahin T. Correlations of alternative medicine, health status and health care in Hungary. Orv Hetil 2002;143:891–896

8 Shmueli A, Shuval J. Use of complementary and alternative medicine in Israel: 2000 vs. 1993. Isr Med Assoc J 2004;6:3–8

9 Menniti-Ippolito F, Gargiulo L, Bologna E, Forcella E, Raschetti R. Use of unconventional medicine in Italy: a nation-wide survey. Eur J Clin Pharmacol 2002;58:61–64

10 Yamashita H, Tsukayama H, Sugishita C. Popularity of complementary and alternative medicine in Japan: a telephone survey. Complement Ther Med 2002;10:84–93

11 Thomas K, Coleman P. Use of complementary or alternative medicine in a general population in Great Britain. Results from the National Omnibus survey. J Public Health (Oxf) 2004;26:152–157

12 Barnes P M, Powell-Griner E, McFann K, Nahin R L. Complementary and alternative medicine use among adults: United States, 2002. Adv Data 2004;343:1–19

Why patients use complementary and alternative medicine

Clare Stevinson, Edzard Ernst

Investigations of the use of complementary and alternative medicine (CAM) generally address three points:

- the extent to which it is used (prevalence)
- the people who use it (patient characteristics)
- the reasons for using it (motives).

Some forms of CAM have a long history but, given the fast progress in orthodox medicine, might have been expected to have gradually fallen into obscurity. However, the indications are that the reverse is true.

The popularity of CAM

CAM is used by a sizable proportion of both adult and paediatric populations in a number of countries.[1,2] The most authoritative estimates of prevalence exist for the United States (75% during 2002),[3] Australia (49% in 1993)[4] and the United Kingdom (20% in 1998).[5] The data from the USA and UK demonstrate an increase in use during the last decade[6-8] and it is reasonable to assume that elsewhere the rise is similar. Other surveys demonstrate that CAM use can be substantially higher in patient populations than in samples of the general public.[9]

Compared with non-users, CAM users are more likely to be female,[4-6,10,11] better educated,[4,6,12,13] have higher incomes[4,6,12,13] and suffer from chronic (mainly musculoskeletal) conditions.[4,10,12]

Given the growing popularity of CAM and the fact that the majority of this use is based on 'out-of-pocket' expenditure,[6] the issue of why people use it is both relevant and intriguing. Although the question itself is a simple one, the answer is undoubtedly complex. In fact, there are probably as many different sets of reasons as there are users. One important and consistent finding is that the majority of CAM use does not occur instead of orthodox medical care, but in addition to it.[14,15] Patients report using orthodox medicine for some complaints and CAM for others or, in particular cases, they may choose to use CAM alongside conventional treatment. A number of explanations have been proposed.

Explanations for CAM use

Furnham[16] summarised the main hypotheses relating to why people use CAM (Box 5.3.1). Some he described as 'push' factors. These include dissatisfaction with or outright rejection of orthodox medicine through prior negative experiences or a general anti-establishment attitude. For these reasons, patients are 'pushed' away from conventional treatment in search of alternatives. Other factors 'pull' or attract patients towards CAM. These include compatibility between the philosophy of certain therapies and patients' own beliefs and a greater sense of control over one's own treatment.

Three of these hypotheses were tested by Astin in a preliminary attempt to develop explanatory models that account for the increasing use of CAM.[17] He predicted that dissatisfaction with conventional care, need for personal control over treatment and philosophical congruence with own beliefs would distinguish CAM users from non-users. A total of 1035 US residents were surveyed about their use of CAM, health status, values and attitudes to conventional medicine and the results were subjected to multiple logistic regression analyses. These indicated that only philosophical congruence was predictive of CAM use. Rather than being 'pushed' towards alternatives to conventional medi-

Box 5.3.1
Possible factors
contributing to CAM
use

Push factors

- Dissatisfaction with orthodox medicine
  - ineffective
  - adverse effects
  - poor communication with doctor
  - insufficient time with doctor
  - waiting lists
- Rejection of orthodox medicine
  - anti-science or anti-establishment attitude
- Desperation
- Cost of private orthodox medical care

Pull factors

- Philosophical congruence
  - spiritual dimension
  - emphasis on holism
  - active role of patient
  - explanation intuitively acceptable
  - natural treatments
- Personal control over treatment
- Good relationship with therapist
  - on equal terms
  - time for discussion
  - allows for emotional factors
- Accessible
- Increased well-being

cine due to disillusionment, participants were 'pulled' towards CAM because it is seen as more compatible with their values, worldview, spiritual/religious philosophy or beliefs about health and illness. Borrowing from Ray[18] the notion of 'value subcultures', Astin found that those respondents who could be identified as 'cultural creatives' were more likely to be users of CAM. These individuals tend to be at the cutting edge of cultural change and innovation in society. They are identifiable by their interests in environmentalism, feminism, globalism, esoteric forms of spirituality, self-actualisation, altruism and self-expression and a love of the foreign and exotic. This subgroup represents almost one quarter of the US adult population.[18]

The persuasive appeal of CAM

Perhaps the most obvious reason for trying CAM is that, persuaded for instance by the media,[19] or by past experience, many consumers are convinced that CAM is effective[20-23] and improves psychosocial functioning.[24] Kaptchuk and Eisenberg[25] suggest that certain fundamental premises of most forms of CAM contribute to its persuasive appeal. One of these is the perceived association of CAM with nature. It is inextricably linked with certain terminology: natural rather than artificial; pure versus synthetic; and organic as opposed to processed.[26] Natural is often somewhat naively equated with safe.[27] This relationship is not restricted to plant-based medicines but the metaphor of nature pervades most other forms of CAM. Another fundamental component of CAM is vitalism. The enhancement or balancing of 'life forces', 'qi', 'psychic energy', etc is central to many forms of CAM. For patients, there is intuitive appeal in this non-invasive notion of healing from within. The science of CAM is a further important aspect in its attraction. Many therapies have long intellectual traditions and sophisticated philosophies, with training involving many years of study of complex systems and concepts. This contributes to the credibility and authority of the scientific label. The science of CAM is less dependent on the principles of objectivity and clinical experimentation than positivist science. The approach tends to be person centred, relying on observation, self-knowledge and human awareness. The language is one of unity and holism in contrast to the distant, reductionist terminology of normative science.[28] Human experience, rather than being marginalised, is the central element of CAM science. A fourth element in the appeal of CAM is spirituality. This bridges the gap between the domain of medical science, with its search for truth and strict causality, and the domain of religion, with its moral freedom and self-chosen values. CAM offers a satisfying unification of the physical and spiritual.[29]

Underlying motives

Other proposed explanations for use of CAM refer to underlying reasons rather than deliberate patient motives. One of these is that CAM users are essentially neurotic so are drawn towards the touching/talking approach of many therapies. While levels of

GENERAL TOPICS

neurosis are reported to be high in patients visiting CAM therapists[30] and higher than those visiting a general practitioner (GP),[31] this may be nothing more than a reflection of the nature of the conditions being treated. CAM practitioners often see patients with chronic or incurable disorders in whom the incidence of neurosis is likely to be high. However, a study of 480 US breast cancer patients found an association between poorer mental health and depression and use of CAM following surgery,[32] suggesting that those with greater psychosocial stress may be more likely to turn to CAM. Significant associations have also been found between CAM use and specific domains of personality, coping strategies and social support.[33]

Another suggestion is that patients with a better understanding of the workings of the human body are attracted to CAM therapists because diagnosis and treatment involve more discussion and explanation than offered by orthodox medical practitioners. Again, although one study did show that patients visiting CAM therapists had greater knowledge of human biology than those visiting a GP,[34] this does not prove a causal relationship. It is possible that CAM therapists attempt to educate their patients on biological or physiological processes, making enhanced knowledge a consequence rather than a cause of their choice. Furthermore, better understanding of the human body may simply be a reflection of the higher levels of education that have been consistently reported for CAM users.

The limitations of survey data

There are numerous limitations to the use of surveys in attempting to understand what motivates patients to use CAM.[31,34] First, a comparison of patients visiting a CAM therapist with those visiting a GP is not necessarily the same as a comparison of people who do and do not use CAM. The patients visiting the GP on the day of the survey may be equally likely to consult a CAM therapist another day for a different complaint, and vice versa. Without knowing the purpose of the visit, an examination of patient variables is meaningless. Only a comparison of patients consulting different practitioners for the same condition would provide relevant information.

Second, this approach only tackles explanations for use of CAM practitioners rather than CAM use in general. These may well be two separate questions. People who purchase a homeopathic or herbal product off the shelf may have very different motives from those who consult a homeopath or herbalist. Similarly, the act of learning a relaxation technique or self-massage from a book is not necessarily the same as visiting a therapist to learn these techniques. Many people who self-treat with CAM may not even contemplate visiting a CAM therapist. It seems reasonable to suggest that these represent different forms of CAM usage and different motives may underlie them. This draws attention to the wider problem of referring to CAM in such general terms. The term encompasses a vast number of very different therapies and approaches, and it is possible that motives for using them are highly therapy-specific. Reasons for participating in yoga, for example, may not be readily generalisable to mega-vitamin supplementation. Understanding of why people use CAM would probably be enhanced by separate investigations of different modalities.

A third weakness of many surveys is their indirect approach to identifying patient motives. Although attempting to address the question of why patients use CAM, they actually contribute more to the issue of who uses it. Rather than directly asking patients about their reasons for using CAM, there is a tendency to examine patient characteristics, beliefs and attitudes and from them make assumptions about motives.[35,36] Just because a survey finds that patients visiting a CAM therapist display scepticism about conventional treatments according to questionnaire items[31] does not necessarily mean that they chose to consult the CAM therapist due to disenchantment with orthodox medicine. As well as the assumption that measuring attitudes necessarily reveals motives, there are problems regarding causality. Do patients visit a CAM therapist because of particular attitudes or beliefs or do they hold those attitudes or beliefs as a result of visiting the therapist? More valid answers could be derived from directly questioning patients about their motives for using CAM.

Direct investigations of patient motives

Examples of attempts to address the question directly was a qualitative study in the USA of 22 patients self-medicating with the herb St John's wort for depression[37] and a postal survey of 11 600 US patients suffering from multiple sclerosis.[38] The themes emerging from these investigations were:

- Incorporating mind, body and spirit
- Desire to take control of own health
- Desire for an effective treatment
- Perception that their condition was not serious and did not require medical treatment
- Belief that CAM is safe while drugs are dangerous
- Perception of CAM as an effective and easily accessible option, compared with lack of confidence in, and barriers to, orthodox medical care
- Following doctor's advice.

Another study that directly addressed patient motives was conducted with patients suffering from inflammatory bowel disease in Canada.[39] Questionnaire data from 134 patients revealed that adverse effects and ineffectiveness of orthodox treatments were the main reasons for trying CAM. Follow-up interviews confirmed the importance of adverse effects in decisions to try CAM, along with an attempt to improve their quality of life and have a greater control over their own treatment. A questionnaire study of 442 Norwegian patients with atopic dermatitis and psoriasis[40] also found that ineffectiveness and side effects of their conventional treatment were among the main reasons for considering CAM. However, the strongest motivation was a keenness to try all available options. This particular reason was also cited the most in a survey of 211 general practice patients from Austria, Germany and England who were asked why they thought people used CAM.[41] Using CAM as a 'last hope' was also one of the most common answers in this study.

Patients who turned to CAM as a last resort could be clearly differentiated from those who embraced CAM for its compatibility with their own beliefs in a UK-based study.[42] Interview and questionnaire data from 38 patients attending a CAM centre revealed two discrete patient types. Those who sought CAM as a last resort because no conventional treatments had proved effective for their complaint had similar scores to the general population on locus of control. Furthermore, they maintained faith in the principles of orthodox medicine and displayed little initial commitment to the values or philosophies of CAM. The other type of patient chose CAM because it matched his or her own beliefs about health and illness. These individuals showed a greater internal locus of control and scepticism about orthodox methods, as well as commitment to CAM.

These notions were partly confirmed by an interview study of 46 Hawaiian breast cancer patients.[43] These patients expected to be helped by the therapy of their choice in terms of both quality of life and tumour burden. Gaining control, being proactive and trying everything to become healthy were prominent motivators. Similarly, the reasons given for CAM use by elderly US cardiac patients were to gain better control over their condition, receive effective therapy and better care, experience fewer adverse effects and have lower costs.[44] A strong theme from a study of young people with inflammatory bowel disease was the hope to receive benefit from using CAM.[45]

The role of the therapeutic relationship

Sixty-eight percent of patients reported a better relationship with the CAM practitioner than with their own GP and this finding was not related to their commitment to CAM.[42] The specific reasons given for this were that practitioners were more friendly and personal, treated the relationship more like a partnership and provided more time for the consultation. Satisfaction with the therapeutic encounter was also greater with CAM practitioners than GPs in a survey of arthritis sufferers in the UK,[46] although 'friendliness' was rated higher in GPs. Again, satisfaction with the time spent on the patient was higher with CAM practitioners, as it also was in a Spanish study of CAM use by patients with somatoform disorder.[47] The duration of CAM consultations is invariably longer than with orthodox medicine. A comparison of physicians using homeopathy with those practising conventional medicine reported that the former spent more than twice as long on patient consultations.[48] As well as leading to greater satisfaction with patients, this may be one of the key factors in the success of CAM. A clinical trial of homeopathy for premenstrual syndrome reported a response rate of 47% in a pre-treatment placebo wash-out phase,[49] which the authors suggested may have been due largely to the depth and intimacy of the homeopathic interview.

Shopping for health

Rather than replacing orthodox medical care CAM usually serves as a substitute in some particular situations and as an adjunct in others, while being disregarded when not considered appropriate for the condition in question. This has led to CAM use being described as 'shopping for health'.[16] Rather than being specifically 'pushed' or 'pulled' towards CAM, patients simply perceive it as one of a range of treatment options available to them and exercise their freedom of choice and discriminating power accordingly. The desire to try all available options may be for some an attempt to leave no stone unturned as they become increasingly desperate for an effective treatment. However, for others it may simply reflect opportunism, a desire for experimentation or what is aptly expressed in an advertising slogan for cosmetics 'because you are worth it'. The finding that CAM use is associated with higher levels of income may support the concept of CAM as a commodity for those that can afford it. Intriguingly, a strong positive correlation was reported between sale data of BMW cars (a possible measure of affluence) and use of herbal remedies in the USA and the UK.[50]

Barriers to CAM

'Shopping for health' is not a particularly new concept. A UK study of CAM users in 1989 concluded that interviewees had an eclectic approach to healthcare which could be described as 'consumerist'.[51] In modern, consumer-orientated societies this seems entirely reasonable and perhaps it is more pertinent to ask why people don't use CAM. One study of 90 fibromyalgia patients in the UK actually addressed this question.[52] Those that did not make any use of CAM cited two reasons: lack of information and expense. A qualitative study involving 36 Canadian breast cancer patients[53] also investigated why some individuals chose not to use CAM. The main reasons were lack of information, scepticism about efficacy and fear of therapies being harmful. Some patients who wanted to use CAM did not actually do so because they encountered certain barriers. These mainly related to the cost of therapies, lack of access and lack of time to devote to the therapy. A survey of 411 breast cancer survivors confirmed these findings.[54] Cost and lack of information were the most common barriers stated, with fear of harm, lack of time and lack of access also cited. Only a small percentage reported fear of their physician's disapproval as a barrier. Studies of US patients suggested intriguing reasons for abandoning, or not using CAM[55,38] (Box 5.3.2).

Box 5.3.2
Reasons for not using
or abandoning CAM

Not using CAM
• Never considered it
• Not enough information
• Too expensive
• Satisfied with conventional treatment
• No belief in its effectiveness
• Doctor advised against it
• Religious/moral reasons
• Not available
• Too embarrassing
Terminating CAM use
• Not helpful
• No longer affordable
• Experienced adverse effects
• Doctor advised against it

Directions for future research

CAM generates more surveys than any other medical field. A Medline search informs us that one CAM survey is currently being published every 1.5 days! Yet most survey data are of very limited value. Perhaps it is time to redirect CAM's 'obsession' with surveys towards research aimed at generating data which translate into important improvements in healthcare.

CAM use in the general population is influenced more by philosophical attraction than negative attitudes to orthodox medicine or desire for personal control of health.[17] However, individual studies in specific populations suggest that these other factors are nevertheless important for patients. Differences in motivation are likely to exist for using CAM between particular patient groups depending on the nature and severity of their condition and the existence of effective conventional treatments. Differences between individual therapies and between patients of different nationalities are also probable. Finally, differences in time are conceivable; the reasons of yesterday may be less important tomorrow. Greater insights could be generated by exploring the reasons for not using CAM and reasons for abandoning conventional medicine in favour of CAM. Differentiating between those never using CAM and those no longer using CAM might also be relevant. Despite the interest in examining dissatisfaction with orthodox medicine, disillusionment with CAM remains under-researched.

REFERENCES

1 Harris P, Rees R. The prevalence of complementary and alternative medicine use among the general population: a systematic review of the literature. Complement Ther Med 2000;8:88–96

2 Ernst E. Prevalence of complementary/ alternative medicine for children; a systematic review. Eur J Pediatr 1999;158:7–11

3 Barnes P, Powell-Griner E, McFann K, Nahin R. CDC Advance Data Report #343.

Complementary and alternative medicine use among adults: United States, 2002. May 27, 2004;XI:1-4

4   MacLennan A H, Wilson D H, Taylor A W. Prevalence and cost of alternative medicine in Australia. Lancet 1996;347:569-573

5   Ernst E, White A. The BBC survey of complementary medicine use in the UK. Complement Ther Med 2000;8:32-36

6   Eisenberg D M, Davis R B, Ettner S L, Appel S, Wilkey S, Van Rompay M, Kessler R C. Trends in alternative medicine use in the United States, 1990-1997: results of a follow-up national survey. JAMA 1998;280:1569-1575

7   Emslie M J, Campbell M K, Walker K A. Changes in public awareness of, attitudes to, and use of complementary therapy in North East Scotland: surveys in 1993 and 1999. Complement Ther Med 2002;10:148-153

8   Thomas K J, Coleman P, Nicholl J P. Trends in access to complementary or alternative medicines via primary care in England: 1995-2001 results from a follow-up national survey. Fam Pract 2003;20:575-577

9   Rhee S M, Garg V K, Hershey C O. Use of complementary and alternative medicines by ambulatory patients. Arch Intern Med 2004;164:1004-1009

10 Bullock M L, Pheley A M, Kiresuk T J, Lenz S K, Culliton P. Characteristics and complaints of patients seeking therapy at a hospital-based alternative medicine clinic. J Alt Complement Med 1997;3:31-37

11 Al-Windi A, Elmfeldt D, Svardsudd K. The relationship between age, gender, well-being and symptoms, and the use of pharmaceuticals, herbal medicines and self-care products in a Swedish municipality. Eur J Clin Pharmacol 2000;56:311-317

12 Blais R, Maiga A, Aboubacar A. How different are users and non-users of alternative medicine? Can J Pub Health 1997;88:159-162

13 Bruno J J, Ellis J J. Herbal use among US elderly: 2002 National Health Interview Survey. Ann Pharmacother 2005;39:643-648.

14 Kranz R, Rosenmund A. Über die Motivation zur Verwendung komplementärmedizinischer Heil-methoden. Schweiz Med Wochenschr 1998;128: 616-622

15 Druss B G, Rosenheck R A. Association between use of unconventional therapies and conventional medical services. JAMA 1999;282:651-656

16 Furnham A. Why do people choose and use complementary therapies? In: Ernst E (ed)

Complementary medicine: an objective appraisal. Oxford: Butterworth Heinemann, 1996

17 Astin J. Why patients use alternative medicine. Results of a national survey. JAMA 1998;279:1548-1553

18 Ray P H. The emerging culture. American Demographics 1997; February (available at *www.demographics.com*)

19 Passalacqua R, Caminiti C, Salvagni S, Barni S, Beretta G D, Carlini P, Contu A, Di Costanzo F, Toscano L, Campione F. Effects of media information on cancer patients' opinions, feelings, decision-making process and physician-patient communication. Cancer 2004;100:1077-1084

20 Harnack L J, Rydell S A, Stang J. Prevalence of use of herbal products by adults in the Minneapolis/St Paul, Minn, Metropolitan area. Mayo Clin Proc 2001;76:688-694

21 Tough S C, Johnston D W, Verhoef M J, Arthur K, Bryant H. Complementary and alternative medicine use among colorectal cancer patients in Alberta, Canada. Altern Ther 2002;8:54-64

22 Ernst E, White A. The BBC survey of complementary medicine use in the UK. Complement Ther Med 2000;8:32-36

23 Hartel U, Volger E. [Use and acceptance of classical natural and alternative medicine in Germany-findings of a representative population-based survey] Forsch Komplementärmed Klass Naturheilkd 2004;11:327-334

24 Jacobs J W G, Kraaimaat F W, Bijlsma J W J. Why do patients with rheumatoid arthritis use alternative treatments? Clin Rheumatol 2001;20:192-196

25 Kaptchuk T J, Eisenberg D M. The persuasive appeal of alternative medicine. Ann Intern Med 1998;129:1061-1065

26 Clement Y N, Williams A F, Aranda D, Chase R, Watson N, Mohammed R, Stubbs O, Williamson D. Medicinal herb use among asthmatic patients attending a specialty care facility in Trinidad. BMC Complement Altern Med 2005;5:3

27 Giveon S M, Liberman N, Klang S, Kahan E. Are people who use "natural drugs" aware of their potentially harmful side effects and reporting to family physician? Patient Educ Couns 2004;53:5-11

28 Richardson J. What patients expect from complementary therapy: a qualitative study. Am J Public Health. 2004;94:1049-1053

29 Feldman R H, Laura R. The use of complementary and alternative medicine

practices among Australian university students. Complement Health Pract Rev 2004;9:173–179

30 Davidson J, Rampes H, Eisen M, Fisher P, Smith R, Malik M. Psychiatric disorders in primary care patients receiving complementary medicine. Compr Psychiatr 1998;39:16–20

31 Furnham A, Smith C. Choosing alternative medicine: a comparison of the beliefs of patients visiting a general practitioner and a homoeopath. Soc Sci Med 1988;26:685–689

32 Burstein H J, Gelber S, Guadagnoli E, Weeks J C. Use of alternative medicine by women with early-stage breast cancer. New Engl J Med 1999;340:1733–1739

33 Honda K, Jacobson J S. Use of complementary and alternative medicine among United States adults: the influences of personality, coping strategies, and social support. Prevent Med 2005;40:46–53

34 Furnham A, Forey J. The attitudes, behaviours and beliefs of patients of conventional versus complementary (alternative) medicine. J Clin Psychol 1994;50:458–469

35 Hentschel C, Kohnen R, Hauser G, Lindner M, Hahn E G, Ernst E. Complementary medicine today: patient decision for physician or magician? A comparative study of patients deciding in favour of alternative therapies. Eur J Phys Med Rehab 1996;6:144–150

36 Mitzdorf U, Beck K, Horton-Hausknecht J, Weidenhammer W, Kindermann A, Takacs M, Astor G, Melchart D. Why do patients seek treatments in hospitals of complementary medicine? J Alt Complement Med 1999;5:463–473

37 Wagner P J, Jester D, LeClair B, Taylor T, Woodward L, Lambert J. Taking the edge off: why patients choose St. John's wort. J Fam Pract 1999;48:615–619

38 Nayak S, Matheis R J, Schoenberger N E, Shiflett S C. Use of unconventional therapies by individuals with multiple sclerosis. Clin Rehabil 2003;17:181–191

39 Hilsden R J, Scott C M, Verhoef M J. Complementary medicine use by patients with inflammatory bowel disease. Am J Gastroenterol 1998;93:697–701

40 Jensen P. Alternative therapy for atopic dermatitis and psoriasis: patient-reported motivation, information source and effect. Acta Derm Venereol 1990;70:425–428

41 Ernst E, Willoughby M, Weihmayr T. Nine possible reasons for choosing complementary medicine. Perfusion 1995;8:356–359

42 Finnigan M D. The Centre for the Study of Complementary Medicine: an attempt to understand its popularity through psychological, demographic and operational criteria. Complement Med Res 1991;5:83–88

43 Maskarinec G, Shumay D M. Choosing complementary treatments as a sign of active participation: a qualitative study among breast cancer patients. J Cancer Integr Med 2004;2:65–76

44 Ai A L, Bolling S F. The use of complementary and alternative therapies among middle-aged and older cardiac patients. Am J Med Qual 2002;17:21–27

45 Heuschkel R, Afzal N, Wuerth A, Zurakowski D, Leichtner A, Tolia V, Bousvaros A. Complementary medicine use in children and young adults with inflammatory bowel disease. Am J Gastroenterol 2002;97:382–388

46 Resch K L, Hill S, Ernst E. Use of complementary therapies by individuals with 'arthritis'. Clin Rheumatol 1997;16:391–395

47 Garcia-Campayo J, Sanz-Carrillo C. The use of alternative medicines by somatoform disorder patients in Spain. Br J Gen Pract 2000; 50:487–488

48 Jacobs J, Chapman E H, Crothers D. Patient characteristics and practice patterns of physicians using homeopathy. Arch Fam Med 1998;7: 537–540

49 Chapman E H, Angelica J, Spitalny G, Strauss M. Results of a study of the homeopathic treatment of PMS. J Am Inst Homeopath 1994;87:14–21

50 Ernst E, Furnham A. BMWs and complementary/alternative medicine. Focus Altern Complement Ther 2000;5:253–254

51 Sharma U M. Alternative choices of healing in North Staffordshire. Complement Med Res 1989; 3:1–4

52 Dimmock S, Troughton P R, Bird H A. Factors predisposing to the resort of complementary therapies in patients with fibromyalgia. Clin Rheumatol 1996;15:478–482

53 Boon H, Brown J B, Gavin A, Kennard M A, Stewart M. Breast cancer survivors' perceptions of complementary/alternative medicine (CAM): making the decision to use or not to use. Qual Health Res 1999; 9:639–653

54 Boon H, Stewart M, Kennard M A, Gray R, Sawka C, Brown J B, McWilliam C, Gavin A, Baron R A, Aaron D, Haines-Kamka T. Use of complementary/alternative medicine by breast cancer survivors in Ontario: prevalence and perceptions. J Clin Oncol 2000;18:2515–2521

55 Lewis D, Paterson M, Beckerman S, Sandilands C. Attitudes towards integration of complementary and alternative medicine with hospital-based care. J Altern Complement Med 2001;7:681–688

Legal and ethical issues regarding evidence-based complementary, alternative, and integrative medical therapies

Michael H. Cohen

Introduction

The literature regarding legal and ethical issues concerning CAM therapies is becoming ever more robust. Yet, as such therapies increasingly penetrate conventional healthcare, physicians and other healthcare providers may still find themselves providing (or being asked to provide) care at the borderland of medicine, ethics, public policy and law.[1] The questions are of international concern[2,3] and are changing a historical stance in which many physicians and patients shunned a dialogue concerning use and potential applicability of CAM therapies in mainstream healthcare. Indeed, within the USA, the Institute of Medicine at the National Academy of Sciences has released a Report on Complementary and Alternative Medicine,[4] calling for comprehensive care in which patients and physicians engage in shared decision-making concerning potential inclusion of evidence-based CAM therapeutic options.

Thus, discussions about CAM are enriching the physician-patient encounter, educating various stakeholders in the healthcare arena about the role of nutrition, herbal medicine, mind-body interactions and other phenomena in mainstream care and contributing to a greater foundation of world medical knowledge. Such dialogue is also leading physicians to reconsider their moral, ethical and legal obligation to be aware of the best available evidence emerging from CAM, to present such evidence to the patient in meaningful terms and to confront therapeutic issues and choices from a more comprehensive, unified perspective on health and the possibility for human healing.[5] This chapter explores and outlines the regulatory boundaries of such an obligation and related legal issues.

Background of the regulatory structure

In the USA, the law governing integration of CAM into conventional medical care is based on general health law, although the law provides no official definition of 'CAM.' Rather, a body of legislative codes and judicial decision-making at the federal, state and even municipal levels is emerging which, taken as a whole, creates the basic regulatory framework for physician integration of CAM.[6]

GENERAL TOPICS

Thus, some of the legal doctrines traditionally applied in healthcare law remain applicable, with some modification, to the practice and integration of CAM; for example, as discussed below, basic principles of malpractice and requirements of informed consent should theoretically apply across the board, whether a therapy is labelled 'conventional' or 'CAM.' Other legal rules, such as the potential liability associated with physician referrals to CAM providers who lack independent state licensure (e.g. massage therapists in states such as California), may require some fine tuning.[7] One reason the law in this field is relatively nascent is that regulatory structures governing CAM emerged out of the sectarian rivalries, destructive competition and attempts at medical monopolisation during the late 19th and early 20th centuries.[8] Legal authority typically follows consensus medical opinion in setting the parameters of healthcare law; thus, legal authority to date has mirrored the historical perspective of majority interests in biomedicine in treating patient use of CAM as deviant, suspect or marginal.[9]

It was only in the late 20th century, for example, that decisions by US courts (and/or in some cases, legislation) gave tangible recognition to allegations that the American Medical Association and other groups had engaged in a conspiracy to preserve a professional monopoly;[10] recognised a strong consumer autonomy interest in the selection and purchase of dietary supplements;[11] allowed physicians a defence to malpractice when patients knowingly, voluntarily and intelligently made a decision to utilise a CAM therapy over conventional care;[12] and otherwise affirmed the rights of CAM providers to practise and patients' rights to make autonomous therapeutic choices outside biomedicine. Similarly, it was only during this period that the National Institutes of Health elevated a nascent Office of Alternative Medicine to a National Center for Complementary and Alternative Medicine and, concomitantly, federal and state statutes and bills aimed at increasing consumer access to CAM.[13] Today, new and emerging government institutions, professional organisations, scientific publications, decision makers in legislatures and agencies (and public attitudes) are creating a complex and shifting medical and legal environment governing the integration of CAM into conventional care.[14-16] In this rapidly changing environment, three of the key regulatory areas that particularly highlight scientific considerations of evidence-based practice are licensing, professional discipline, and malpractice and informed consent.

Regulation through professional licensure

The requirements for professional practice vary by complementary and alternative modality and practitioner internationally. In the USA, professional licensure generally is governed by state law pursuant to the Tenth Amendment to the US Constitution, which leaves states free to regulate matters of health, safety and welfare affecting their citizens. Each state has enacted a medical licensing statute that prohibits the unlicensed practice of medicine. Typically, such statutes define such practice as including one or more of the following:

- diagnosing, preventing, treating and curing disease
- holding oneself out to the public as able to perform the above
- intending to receive a gift, fee or compensation for the above
- attaching such titles as MD to one's name
- maintaining an office for reception, examination and treatment
- performing surgery
- using, administering or prescribing drugs or medicinal preparations.[17]

In most states, therefore, CAM providers who lack licensure could be viewed as 'diagnosing' and 'treating' patients and thus as practising medicine unlawfully. Courts have interpreted medical practice acts broadly where state legislatures have failed to create separate licensure for providers such as midwives, naturopaths, homeopaths, hypnotherapists, faith healers, providers of colonic irrigation, nutritionists, iridologists and even those offering ear piercing, tattooing and massage.[18]

An example is *Stetina v State*, which involved a non-medical provider of healthcare lacking independent licensure.[19] The defendant, Stetina, was a nutritionist who practised iridology. An undercover investigator visited Stetina and she prescribed colonic irrigation and various nutritional remedies. On appeal from an injunction barring her from practice, Stetina argued that her conduct, which aimed at helping individuals follow proper nutritional advice, was outside the purview of the Medical Practice Act and that in any event, most physicians did not address nutrition and thus her practice was complementary. The Indiana Court of Appeals disagreed and held that Stetina was practising medicine without a licence.

Historically, unlicensed providers have had little success arguing that the prohibition in medical licensing statutes against unlicensed medical practice exempts a non-medical, holistic healing practice. Their typical remedy is to lobby state legislatures for licensure or, more infrequently, to lobby for an exemption from the medical licensing statute.

Because licensure is controlled by state legislatures, physician views of the scientific evidence favouring or disfavouring use of a particular CAM modality have had less and less influence over who can legally practise. Legislatures will take consensus medical views of safety and efficacy into account but social, political and larger policy considerations typically dictate the outcome. Frequently: 'Legislative recognition trumps medical recognition'.[20]

Although legislatures can decide which providers they wish to license and how broadly to define the legislatively authorised scope of practice for such providers, physicians in the USA will be liable for malpractice if, among other things, they refer patients to a 'known incompetent'.[21] The fact that the CAM provider to whom the physician has referred a patient is licensed by the state will not necessarily protect the physician from liability. The physician still has an obligation to exercise reasonable care in selecting the provider, to determine that the referral is clinically justifiable and to ascertain that the provider is offering therapies within legally authorised practice boundaries and is only utilising therapies accepted as safe within the provider's own profession.[22]

Regulation through professional discipline

Professional discipline similarly is governed by state law in the USA, and provisions for discipline typically are written into licensing statutes; sometimes statutes will delegate to the licensing board the power to establish rules for professional discipline. Most disciplinary provisions prohibit physicians from engaging in 'unprofessional conduct'. Generally, unprofessional conduct (or 'professional misconduct') includes such acts as obtaining the license fraudulently, practising the profession fraudulently, beyond its authorised scope, with gross incompetence or with gross negligence, practising while impaired by alcohol or drugs or while convicted of a crime, permitting or aiding an unlicensed person to perform activities requiring a license or failing to comply with relevant rules and regulations.[23] In many states, unprofessional conduct also includes such acts as 'any departure from, or the failure to conform to, the standards of acceptable and prevailing medical practice ... irrespective of whether or not a patient is injured thereby'.[24] The breadth of such statutory language has left physicians who use CAM therapies vulnerable to medical board disciplinary action in some states – even if the physicians have provided necessary, conventional medical care, and have not injured any patient through the inclusion of CAM therapies.

In *re Guess*,[25] for example, involved a licensed physician practising family medicine who administered homeopathic remedies to his patients when conventional treatment failed. The Board of Medical Examiners of North Carolina charged Guess with 'unprofessional conduct', alleging that his use of homeopathic medicines departed from community standards. There was no evidence that Guess's homeopathic treatments had harmed patients and, in fact, patients testified that homeopathy had helped them after biomedicine had failed to provide relief. The North Carolina Supreme Court, after a series of appeals, nonetheless affirmed the revocation of Guess's licensure.

As *Guess* suggests, although the licensee may appeal, a court will not reverse the medical board decision to revoke licensure, unless there is no rational basis for the exercise of discretion complained of or the action is arbitrary and capricious. These are fairly high standards of review. The consequence is that relatively few medical board decisions result in published judicial opinions overturning the decision.[26]

Proponents of greater freedom for healthcare consumers have responded by lobbying state legislatures to enact statutes protecting physicians from professional discipline merely for offering patients CAM. In many states, such legislative efforts have succeeded. For example, New York's legislation addresses 'concerns regarding the treatment of non-conventional physicians in the professional medical conduct process by recognising the role of legitimate non-conventional medical treatments in the practice of medicine' and 'secures the rights and freedoms of patients to choose their own medical treatments'.[27] The bill permits the 'physician's use of whatever medical care, conventional or non-conventional, which effectively treats human disease, pain, injury, deformity, or physical condition'.[28]

Similarly, North Carolina's legislation amends the disciplinary provisions of its medical licensing act to provide that: 'The Board shall not revoke the license of or deny a license to a person solely because of that person's practice of a therapy that is experimental, nontraditional, or that departs from acceptable and prevailing medical practices unless, by competent evidence, the Board can establish that the treatment has a safety risk greater than the prevailing treatment or that the treatment is generally not effective.'[29]

In similar fashion, Oklahoma's bill states: 'The Board shall not revoke the license of a person otherwise qualified to practise allopathic medicine within the meaning of this act solely because the person's practice of a therapy is experimental or nontraditional'.[30] These statutes legislatively expand patient access to CAM by safeguarding physicians against professional disciplinary proceedings based solely on medical board antipathy to complementary and alternative therapies.

In an effort to encompass some of the balance between paternalism and autonomy suggested by such legislation, the US Federation of State Medical Boards (FSMB) has issued its own model guidelines for physician inclusion of CAM therapies.[31] These guidelines suggest that medical boards contemplating physician discipline should look at the extent to which inclusion of CAM therapies is supported by the evidence.

If, for example, a physician ignores necessary conventional care and instead offers the patient an ineffective CAM therapy, hoping for a cure based solely on anecdotal evidence, a medical board would likely be justified, under the standards of the guidelines, in concluding that the physician engaged in professional misconduct. Because of the failure to follow community standards of care and even minimal professionally agreed norms regarding levels of proof justifying the selection of a therapy, the board's determination well might be upheld in court, state 'medical freedom' legislation notwithstanding. If, on the other hand, the physician continued to monitor the patient conventionally and utilised due care in selecting and delivering a therapy that

GENERAL TOPICS

had reasonable clinical evidence of safety and/or promise of efficacy, a conclusion of professional misconduct would be less likely. Thorough documentation, reasonable reliance on best scientific evidence justifying a therapy and continued conventional monitoring will help protect the physician against undue medical board action. In short, at least as far as professional discipline is concerned, physicians' legal and ethical obligations are more likely to coincide with a narrower range of scientifically acceptable options and less likely to follow broader legislative or populist notions.

Regulation through malpractice and the informed consent obligation

Malpractice typically is defined as unskilful practice that fails to conform to a standard of care in the profession and results in patient injury. The definition can be problematic for physicians integrating complementary and alternative treatments. Courts may look to a lack of general medical acceptance of specific modalities or to a lack of Food and Drug Administration approval as indicative of failure to follow the standard of care. Further, courts may tend to locate the cause of patient injury in the CAM treatment, since the treatment differs from the medical norm and may have an unknown or inadequately explained mechanism of action. In general, physicians can recommend CAM therapies supported by evidence of safety and efficacy with little, if any, risk of malpractice liability; while if either evidence of safety or efficacy are questionable, the liability risk rises proportionate with the extent of possible danger or inefficacy.[32]

A number of medical malpractice defenses might be adapted to physician inclusion of CAM in treatment protocols. Most promising are the respectable minority defense and assumption of risk. The first protects physicians if their conduct conforms to that adopted by a respectable minority within the profession; the second enables patients to knowingly, intelligently and voluntarily assume the risk of treatments outside the medical model and provides that if they do, physicians will have a viable defense to malpractice.[33] If the CAM practice in question is evidence based and thus thoroughly justified by the literature, a good case can be made that the physician is following a respectable minority within medicine in offering the therapy.

An important case supporting the assumption of risk defense is *Schneider v Revici*.[34] Here the patient learned that a lump had been found in her breast, refused a biopsy and consulted a physician for nutritional and other alternative methods of cancer treatment. Although the physician advised surgery, he acceded to the patient's request for treatment upon her signing a consent form by which she assumed the risk that the non-conventional cancer therapy would not cure her condition. The Second Circuit held that express assumption of risk by virtue of the unambiguous consent form could be a complete defense to the patient's malpractice claim. The court stated: 'We see no reason why a patient should not be allowed to make an informed decision to go outside currently approved medical methods in search of an unconventional treatment. While a patient should be encouraged to exercise care for his own safety, we believe that an informed decision to avoid surgery and conventional chemotherapy is within the patient's right to determine what shall be done with his own body.'[35]

As CAM increasingly enters mainstream healthcare, such therapies will begin to be considered to fall within provision of informed patient decisions, thus reducing the risk that physicians will incur malpractice liability merely for providing such therapies. Physicians still will have to use due care, however, in the selection and execution of such therapies.[36]

A second basis for the imposition of malpractice liability is inadequate informed consent. The informed consent obligation requires the physician to disclose to the patient, among other things, the risks and benefits of a recommended therapy and all reasonable and feasible options.

In assessing whether a specific failure to disclose has violated the informed consent obligation, many US courts look to whether the reasonable patient would find the information material to a decision to undergo or forego treatment. In other words, if the reasonable patient would have decided to forego a conventional therapy (for example, chemotherapy) in favour of a CAM therapy (for example, an herbal or nutritional protocol), the physician's failure to disclose the possibility of such an alternative could violate the informed consent obligation and hence constitute malpractice.[37] Other US courts judge materiality by the reasonable physician standard: non-disclosure violates informed consent only if the reasonable physician would have disclosed the information in question.

The reasonable physician standard should be guided by scientific rules regarding best evidence, whereas such rules of evidence are less significant if courts use the reasonable patient standard.[38] In other words, because best evidence rules are relevant to the physician and less important to the patient, such rules will control the physician's decision to disclose where the physician's reasonable judgement and not the patient's, governs the legal obligation of informed consent.

Evolution of law

Many physicians are beginning to recognise that health and disease correlate with not only biochemical and physiological influences but also nutritional, environmental, social, mind–body and spiritual factors. The question is whether legal and regulatory structures will evolve to support this broader, more inclusive system of healthcare by recognising the many legitimate facets of the person's search for wholeness. Internationally, there is a crucial need to provide leadership in legal and regulatory developments to serve hospitals, academic medical centres, educational institutions

GENERAL TOPICS

and federal, state and local governments who are creating law and setting policy. Indeed, few healthcare institutions to date have sufficiently grappled with the relevant issues to establish sound institutional policies to guide their own clinicians.[39] The need for leadership also exists in specialty medical professions, such as paediatrics.[40]

Developments in law parallel paradigmatic shifts in healthcare; regulatory goals adjust to meet the changing social consciousness.[41] While rules of best evidence are established by science, their application in clinical settings can be moulded by legal, ethical, administrative, and institutional considerations, refined by physician–patient dialogue and broadened by transcultural perspectives on the nature of healing. The more evidence-based practices open to the challenges raised by policy decisions involving CAM therapies, the more that shared perspectives may contribute to new views of learning, being, consciousness and health.

REFERENCES

1 Cohen M H. Healing at the borderland of medicine and religion: regulating potential abuse of authority by spiritual healers. J Law Relig 2002–2003;18:373–426

2 Cohen M H. Legal and ethical issues in complementary medicine: a U.S. perspective. Med J Aust 2004;181:168–169

3 Ernst E, Cohen M H, Stone J. Ethical problems arising in evidence-based complementary and alternative medicine. J Med Ethics 2004;30:156–159

4 Institute of Medicine. Complementary and Alternative Medicine in the U.S. Washington, DC: National Academies Press; 2005

5 Kemper K, Cohen M H. Ethics in complementary medicine: new light on old principles. Contemporary Pediatrics 2004;21:61–72

6 Cohen M H. The emerging field of law and complementary and alternative medicine Orange County Lawyer 2000;30:42

7 Cohen M H. Beyond complementary medicine: legal and ethical perspectives on health care and human evolution. Ann Arbor: University of Michigan Press; 2000, pp 55–58

8 Cohen M H. Complementary and alternative medicine: legal boundaries and regulatory perspectives. Baltimore: Johns Hopkins University Press; 1998, pp 15–23

9 Ibid, p 23 (citing cases)

10 Wilk v American Medical Association, 719 F.2d 207 (7th Cir. 1983), *cert. denied*, 467 U.S 1210 (1984), *on remand*. 671 F. Supp. 1465 (N.D. Ill. 1987), *aff'd*, 895 F.2d 352 (7th Cir.1990)

11 Pearson v Shalala, 164 F.3d 650 (D.C. Cir. 1999), *reh'g en banc denied*, 172 F.3d 72 (D.C. Cir. 1999)

12 Schneider v Revici, 817 F.2d 987 (2d Cir. 1987)

13 See, e.g., Dietary Supplement Health and Education Act of 1994, Pub. L. No. 103–417, 108 *Stat.* 4325, 21 *U.S.C.* §§ 301 et seq. (1994); proposed Access to Medical Treatment Act, H.R. 746, § 3(a) (Feb. 19, 1997); S. 578, 105th Cong., 1st Sess. (Apr. 18, 1997)

14 Cohen M H, Ruggie M. Integrating complementary and alternative medical therapies in conventional medical settings: legal quandaries and potential policy models. Cinn L Rev 2004;72:671–729

15 Cohen M H, Ruggie M. Overcoming legal and social barriers to integrative medicine. Medical Law Intl 2004;6:339–393

16 Cohen M H. Negotiating integrative medicine: a framework for provider-patient conversations. Negotiation J 2004;30:409–433

17 See ref 8, pp 26–29

18 See id. at 29–31 (citing cases)

19 513 N.E.2d 1234 (Ind. Ct. App. 1987)

20 Eisenberg D M, Cohen M H, Hrbek A, Grayzel J, van Rompay M I, Cooper, R A. Credentialing complementary and alternative medical providers. Ann Intern Med 2002;137:965–973.

21 See ref 6, p 50

22 Id., 57; Cohen M H. Malpractice considerations affecting the clinical integration of complementary and alternative medicine. Current Practice of Medicine 1999;87:2

23 See, e.g., New York Educ. L. § 6509

24 In re Guess, 393 S.E.2d 833 (N.C. 1990) (quoting N.C. Gen. Stat. § 90–14(a)(6)), *cert. denied*, Guess v. North Carolina Bd. of Medical Examiners, 498 U.S. 1047 (1991), *later proceeding*, Guess v. Board of Medical Examiners, 967 F.2d 998 (4th Cir. 1992)

25 See Guess, 393 S.E.2d at 833

26 See ref 8, p 88

27 NY State Assembly Mem. in Support of Legislation (Bill No. 5411-C (Assembly), 3636-C (Senate) (1994)

28 New York Educ. L. § 6527(4)(e)

29 N.C. Gen. Stat. § 90 14(a)(G)

30 Okla. Stat. Ann. tit 59, § 509.1(d)

31 Federation of State Medical Boards. Model Guidelines for Physician Use of Complementary and Alternative Therapies in Medical Practice, 2002. Online. Available: www.fsmb.org 22 April 2005

32 Cohen M H, Eisenberg D M. Potential physician malpractice liability associated with complementary/integrative medical therapies. Ann Intern Med 2002;136:596–603

33 See ref 8, pp 56–65

34 817 F.2d 987 (2d Cir. 1987)

35 Id. at 992

36 See ref 6, p 30

37 See ref 6, p 43

38 Ernst E, Cohen M H. Informed consent in complementary and alternative medicine. Arch Intern Med 2001;161:2288–2292

39 Cohen M H, Hrbek A, Davis R, Schachter S, Kemper K J, Boyer E W, Eisenberg D M. Emerging credentialing practices, malpractice liability policies, and guidelines governing complementary and alternative medical practices and dietary supplements recommendations: a descriptive study of 19 integrative health care centers in the U.S. Arch Intern Med 2005;165:289–295

40 Cohen M H, Kemper K J. Complementary therapies in pediatrics: A Legal Perspective. Pediatrics 2005;115:774–780

41 Cohen M H. Future medicine: ethical dilemmas, regulatory challenges, and therapeutic pathways to health and human healing in human transformation. Ann Arbor: University of Michigan Press; 2003

Safety issues in complementary and alternative medicine

Edzard Ernst

Throughout this book we have placed much emphasis on safety issues. In particular, we have alerted the reader to the risks associated with specific therapies and we have attempted to evaluate the risk–benefit profile of CAM treatments in comparison with that of conventional options. Direct toxicity, interactions, contraindications, etc. have therefore been given a prominent place.

More general aspects of safety issues related to CAM have, however, been somewhat neglected. The following discussion is aimed at filling this gap.

Problems with unregulated food supplements

In many countries, herbal medicinal products (HMPs) are marketed as food supplements. Rigorous regulation comparable to the pharmaceutical sector therefore does not apply. In particular, the necessity for a manufacturer to demonstrate safety and quality of the marketed product is far less. In Europe this situation will change through the EU Traditional Use Directive but for the near future unlicensed HMPs will remain on most national markets.[1,2]

A particular concern has been the quality of unlicensed HMPs. Table 5.5.1 shows some of the contaminants that have been found in HMPs which have obvious safety implications. Contamination of Asian and other HMPs with heavy metal and

Table 5.5.1
Contaminants that have been found in herbal medicines

Type of contaminant	Examples
Microorganisms	*Staphylococcus aureus, Escherichia coli* (certain strains), *Salmonella, Shigella, Pseudomonas aeruginosa*
Microbial toxins	Bacterial endotoxins, aflatoxins
Pesticides, herbicides	Chlorinated pesticides (e.g. DDT, DDE, HCH-isomers, HCB, aldrin, dieldrin, heptachlor), organic phosphates, carbamate insecticides and herbicides, dithiocarbamate fungicides, triazin herbicides
Fumigation agents	Ethylene oxide, methyl bromide, phosphine
Radioactivity	Cs-134, Cs-137, Ru-103, I-131, Sr-90
Heavy metals	Lead, cadmium, mercury, arsenic

other toxins is a continuous issue in many parts of the world.[3-7] Adulteration of HMPs with non-declared herbs or conventional drugs is a further problem with unregulated HMPs of dubious quality. It pertains in particular to Asian HMPs[8] and is a problem that is regularly reported from many regions (e.g.[9]). For instance, when 2609 Chinese herbal medicines were collected and analysed in Taiwan, 24% of them were shown to be adulterated with synthetic drugs like acetaminophen, hydrochlorothiazide, indomethacin, phenobarbital, theophylline and corticosteroids.[10]

Underdosing is another problem with HMPs. Whenever herbal food supplements from the US market are analysed by independent experts, the findings reveal that in a substantial proportion of them, the active ingredient content differs marginally from label claims (e.g. [11]). When 880 HMPs were purchased in the USA, 37% of them proved to be not consistent with the information on the label or the label information was insufficient.[12]

Problems caused by conventional providers of healthcare

Numerous studies show that patients fail to inform their physician of their CAM use.[13-15] This is not merely the fault of patients but can also be seen as a failure of doctors who tend to omit asking about CAM use or documenting CAM use in patients' records.[16-18] It is self-evident that such behaviour can increase the risk of CAM use.

Problems caused by unregulated providers of CAM

In most countries, CAM providers are predominantly non-medically qualified practitioners. Most of these are probably adequately trained to do what they do. However, in the absence of adequate regulations, some providers will not adhere to adequate standards of clinical practice. There is little systematic research into the question how frequently this causes health problems. Preliminary data suggest that there is sufficient reason for concern.[19] This can have obvious safety implications.

With depressing regularity we hear of cases where CAM providers have delayed or hindered access to potentially life-saving conventional treatment (e.g.[20,21]). The best-researched example in this respect is probably the advice of some CAM providers against any type of immunisation.[22,23] Similar problems relate to CAM providers not screening for contraindications to treatment. If, for instance, a bleeding abnormality or advanced osteoporosis are contraindications against chiropractic manipulation, how will the average chiropractor reliably exclude such abnormalities before treating a new patient?

Changing or omitting prescribed treatments might be another problem. There is preliminary evidence that a significant proportion of CAM providers are doing this,[24] which could obviously be associated with important risks. Recent survey data demonstrate that 3% of non-medically trained acupuncturists in the UK advise their patients to alter prescribed treatments.[25]

GENERAL TOPICS

Some CAM providers could also be unable to adequately diagnose medical problems while patients are in their care. For instance, one could imagine a patient being treated for headache which reveals increasingly clearer signs of a sinister underlying cause. If these signs are missed, valuable time for adequate, perhaps life-saving treatment could be lost.

Another problem could be the use of diagnostic techniques which are either in themselves not risk free or invalid. An example for the first scenario is the overt overuse of X-ray diagnosis by some chiropractors.[26] An example of the second scenario is the use of iridology which would lead to false-negative or false-positive diagnosis.[27]

A similar problem is the quality of the advice provided to consumers by health food stores or other outlets of CAM. Surveys have repeatedly shown that such recommendations can border on the irresponsible.[28,29] Worryingly, many websites on CAM also issue information which, if followed, has the potential to harm patients.[30]

A further risk associated with CAM might lie in the plethora of lay books on CAM now available in every high street bookstore. Preliminary evidence[31] suggests that this lay literature has the potential to put the health of the reader at risk if the advice from these books is adhered to by seriously ill individuals. Similarly, we have shown that a significant proportion of the UK daily press reports about CAM in a much more favourable tone than about mainstream medicine.[32] This could lead to distrust in the latter, unjustified trust in the former or both and thus put the health of CAM users at risk.

These concerns relate to the (lack of) competence or responsibility of CAM providers, sales people or authors. The only acceptable way to eliminate such concerns is to adequately train and regulate these professions.

Problems with users of CAM

The attitudes of the consumer towards CAM may constitute risks which are independent of CAM providers. For instance, when users of HMPs were interviewed about their behaviour vis à vis an adverse effect of a herbal versus a synthetic 'over-the-counter' drug, the results suggested that about one quarter would consult their doctor for a serious adverse effect of conventional medication while less than 1% would do the same in relation to a herbal remedy.[33] Other studies suggest that the majority of CAM users employ CAM with insufficient information.[34] Consumers want and need guidance on CAM. Survey data suggest that they foremost want information on the effectiveness and safety of treatments, and that they would prefer it in a brochure rather than from a website.[35] It is thus very disappointing that even government-sponsored guides for CAM users fail to provide such information.[36]

Conclusion

CAM is associated with complex safety concerns which are often difficult to quantify or resolve. Awareness and vigilance are, however, invariably a valuable first step towards minimising the risks to our patients.

REFERENCES

1   Dawson W. Herbal medicines and the EU Directive. J Roy Coll Physicians Edinb 2005;35:25–27

2   De Smet P A G M. Herbal medicine in Europe – relaxing regulatory standards. N Engl J Med 2005;352:1176–1178

3   Caldas E D, Machado L L. Cadmium, mercury and lead in medicinal herbs in Brazil. Food Chem Toxicol 2004;42:599–603

4   Schilling U, Mück R, Heidemann E. Bleiintoxikation durch Einnahme ayurvedischer Arzneimittel. Med Klin 2004;99:476–480

5   Saper R B, Kales S N, Paquin J, Burns M J, Eisenberg D M, Davis R B, Phillips R S. Heavy metal content of Ayurvedic herbal medicine products. JAMA 2004;292:2868–2873

6   Araujo J, Beelen A P, Lewis M D. Lead poisoning associated with Ayurvedic medications – five States, 2000–2003. MMWR 2004;53:582–584

7   Raman P, Patino L C, Nair M G. Evaluation of metal and microbial contamination in botanical supplements. J Agric Food Chem 2004;52.7822–7827

8   Ernst E. Toxic heavy metals and undeclared drugs in Asian herbal medicines. Trends Pharmacol Sci 2002;23:136–139

9   Woolterton E. Several Chinese herbal products may contain toxic aristolochic acid. CMAJ 2004;171:449

10 Huang W T, Wen K C, Hsiao M L. Adulteration by synthetic therapeutic substances of traditional Chinese medicines in Taiwan. J Clin Pharmacol 1997;37:334–350

11 Gurely B J, Gardner S T, Hubbord M A. Content versus label claims in ephedra-containing dietary supplements. An J Health Syst Pharm 2000;57:1–7

12 Garrard J, Harms S, Eberly L E, Matiak A. Variations in product choices of frequently purchased herbs. Arch Intern Med 2003;163:2290–2295

13 Crowe S, Lyons B. Herbal medicine use by children presenting for ambulatory anesthesia and surgery. Pediatric Anesthesia 2004;14:916–919

14 Tan M, Uzun O, Akçay F. Trends in complementary and alternative medicine in Eastern Turkey. J Altern Complement Med 2004;10:861–865

15 Kim S, Hohrmann J L, Clark S, Munoz K N, Braun J E, Doshi A, Radeos M S, Camargo C A. A multicenter study of complementary and alternative medicine usage among ED patients. Acad Emerg Med 2005;12:377–380

16 Kales H C, Blow F C, Welsh D E, Mellow A M. Herbal products and other supplements: use by elderly veterans with depression and dementia and their caregivers. J Geriatr Psychiatry Neurol 2004;17:25–31

17 Cockayne N L, Duguid M, Shenfield G M. Health professionals rarely record history of complementary and alternative medicines. Br J Clin Pharmacol 2004;59:254–258

18 Glintborg B, Andersen S E, Spang-Hanssen E, Dalhoff K. Disregarded use of herbal medical products and dietary supplements among surgical and medical patients as estimated by home inspection and interview. Pharmacoepidemiol Drug Saf 2004;www.interscience.wiley.com. DOI: 10.1002/pds.1049

19 Schmidt K. The World Wide Web as a medical information source for Internet users – benefits and boundaries. Focus Altern Complement Ther 2004;9:187–189

20 Coppes M J, Anderson R A, Egeler R M, Wolff J E A. Alternative therapies for the treatment of childhood cancer. New Engl J Med 1998;339:846

21 Oneschuk D, Brucra E. The potential dangers of complementary therapy use in a patient with cancer. J Palliat Care 1999;15:49–52

22 Ernst E. Attitude against immunisation within some branches of complementary medicine. Eur J Pediatr 1997;156:513–515

23 Schmidt K, Ernst E. Letter to the editor. Aspects of MMR. BMJ 2002;325:597

24 Moody G A, Eaden J A, Bhakta P, Sher K, Mayberry J F. The role of complementary medicine in European and Asian patients

with inflammatory bowel disease. Public Health 1998;112:269–271

25 MacPherson H, Scullion A, Thomas K J, Walters S. Patient report of adverse events associated with acupuncture treatment: a prospective national survey. Qual Saf Health Care 2004;13:349–355

26 Ernst E. Chiropractors' use of X-rays. Br J Radiol 1998;71:249–251

27 Ernst E. Iridology – not useful and potentially harmful. Arch Ophthalmol 2000;118:120–121

28 Mills E, Singh R, Ross C, Ernst E, Wilson K. Impact of federal safety advisories on health food store advice. J Gen Intern Med 2004;19: 269–272

29 Buckner K D, Chavez M L, Raney E C, Stoehr J D. Health food stores' recommendations for nausea and migraines during pregnancy. Ann Pharmacother 2005;39:274–279

30 Schmidt K, Ernst E. Assessing websites on complementary and alternative medicine for cancer. Ann Oncol 2004;15:733–742

31 Ernst E, Armstrong N C. Lay books on complementary/alternative medicine: a risk factor for good health? Int J Risk Safety Med 1998;11:209–215

32 Ernst E, Weihmayr T. UK and German media differ over complementary medicine. BMJ 2000;321:707

33 Barnes J, Mills S, Abbot N C, Willoughby M, Ernst E. Different standards for reporting ADRs to herbal remedies. Br J Clin Pharmacol 1998;45:496–500

34 Hyodo I, Amano N, Eguchi K, Narabayashi M, Imanishi J, Hirai M, Nakano T, Takashima S. Nationwide survey on complementary and alternative medicine in cancer patients in Japan. J Clin Oncol 2005;23:2645–2654

35 Kuo G M, Hawley S T, Weiss L T, Balkrishnan R, Volk R J. Factors associated with herbal use among urban multiethnic primary care patients: a cross-sectional survey. BMC Complement Altern Med 2004;4:18

36 The Prince of Wales's Foundation for Integrated Health. Complementary Health Care: a guide for patients. London: The Prince of Wales's Foundation for Integrated Health; 2005. Online. Available: *http://www.fihealth.org.uk/fs_publications.html* 10 May 2005.

Cost evaluation of CAM

Edzard Ernst

Even though estimates vary considerably as to the money spent on CAM, most experts agree that CAM is not cheap. Table 5.6.1 summarises recent survey data and highlights the heterogeneity of the information derived from such sources.[1-14]

Table 5.6.1 **Recent estimates of costs associated with CAM-use in defined populations**

First author and reference	Country	Cost included	Comment
Ernst[1]	UK	CAM users spent an average of £163 per year on CAM. This extrapolates to £1.6 billion per year for CAM use in the UK	Cost data were available only for 11% of the sample
Thomas[2]	UK	Out of pocket expenditure for acupuncture, chiropractic, homeopathy, hypnotherapy, herbalism, osteopathy was £450 million (£108 per user) / year	About 10% of the cost was paid for by the NHS
Harris[3]	UK	Out of pocket cost for CAM practitioners and products spent by cancer patients was £648/patient/year	Large sample from Wales (which might not be representative for all of the UK)
Ramsey[4]	USA	Older patients with osteoarthritis spent US$1127 per year on CAM	They spent a similar amount US$1148 for orthodox therapies
Patterson[5]	USA	Cancer patients spent an average of US$68 per year on CAM	356 patients with colon, breast or prostate cancer; range of expenditure was large (4–14 659)
Wasner[6]	Germany	Patients with amyotrophic lateral sclerosis spent an average of €4000/year on CAM	Small sample (n = 92); most of the costs were reimbursed by insurance schemes
Marstedt[7]	Germany	Cost of physicians' 20 928 CAM interventions paid by one health insurer was DM 6 million	Amount for CAM is ~1/7 of total medical cost
Schäfer[8]	Germany	Allergy patients spent an average of €205 for a complete series of CAM treatments	Different treatments had different average costs: bioresonance = €409, acupuncture = €363, homeopathy €192, autologous blood therapy €77

First author and reference	Country	Cost included	Comment
McKenzie[9]	Canada	Elderly Canadians spent an average of CAN$226 per year on vitamins, minerals and herbals	Small sample (n = 128)
Shenfield[10]	Australia	Asthmatic children spent on average AU$120 per year on CAM. Those who consulted CAM providers spent AU$480 per year	Small sample (n = 174)
Yamashita[11]	Japan	A random sample of the population (n = 1000) spent Yen 19080 per person annually on CAM	Costs were ~50% of costs for orthodox healthcare
Chrystal[12]	New Zealand	Cancer patients spent an average of NZ$102 on CAM (including visits and travel)	Small sample (n = 200), patients suffered from various types of cancer
Nielsen[13]	Denmark	88% of medical patients spent less than DKK 500/month; 55% less than DKK 100 and 12% spent more than DKK 500 per month	No group average supplied
Pucci[14]	Italy	Out of pocket expenditure for CAM by outpatients with multiple sclerosis was €483/patient/year	Small sample (n = 109)

A US analysis of insurance claims demonstrated that 'billed amounts for alternative services were about 2% of the overall medical bills for cancer patients'.[15] Studies from several countries suggest that CAM use is associated with higher rates of consultations in conventional medicine.[16–19] This implies that CAM use is unlikely to contribute to any overall cost savings. In other settings, however, CAM seems to be employed as a substitute for medical care.[20–22] Furthermore, it has been suggested that CAM use may save money on the costs of conventional drugs.[23] Much of the future of CAM will depend on the question whether it saves money or causes extra expenditure. Yet CAM researchers have been slow to face the challenge of conducting rigorous cost analyses.

This is perhaps understandable – such projects can be exceedingly complex and usually expensive (Table 5.6.2). Considering the fact that, in most countries, CAM has been paid for privately by its users,[1,2,24,25] there may not be a strong incentive by governments to change this situation. Thus cost evaluations are difficult to fund through official channels. A further important complication is that the results of cost-evaluation studies, even if performed to a high standard, may not be transferable from one healthcare system to another.

Table 5.6.2 **Types of cost evaluation**

Type of study	Description	Example
Cost analysis	Compares cost of alternative treatments without reference to benefits	
Cost–effectiveness analysis	Compares costs of two or more alternative treatments and their outcomes in natural units	Cost of chemotherapy vs surgery per life saved
Cost–benefit analysis	Compares costs of two or more treatments and outcomes in financial terms	Chiropractic vs GP care treatment costs and cost of working days lost
Cost–utility analysis	Compares costs of two or more treatments and outcomes measured in terms of quality adjusted life years (QALYs) gained	Cost of usual care vs usual care and acupuncture for migraine with quality of life measure as outcome
Cost minimisation analysis	Compares costs of two or more treatments which are known to have equivalent outcomes	Cost of two surgical procedures with similar success rate, complications and recurrences

NB: these definitions are used inconsistently and cost effectiveness and cost utility often used synonymously

Examples of recent studies

Notwithstanding such formidable obstacles, several informative studies have recently emerged (Table 5.6.3).[26–33] This list serves as a reminder that cost-evaluations typically address distinctly different research questions and use a range of research tools. It is therefore not surprising that their results fail to generate a

Table 5.6.3 **Examples of recent cost evaluations**

First author and reference	Country	Research question	Main result
Kominski[26]	USA	Comparison of total outpatient costs of various approaches for treating back pain	Chiropractic care was 52% more expensive than medical care
UK BEAM trial[27]	UK	Assess cost-effectiveness of adding spinal manipulation, exercise classes, or manipulation followed by exercise to best care for back pain	Spinal manipulation is a cost-effective addition
Wonderling[28]	UK	Evaluate cost-effectiveness of acupuncture for chronic headache	Total 1 year costs were higher for acupuncture compared to standard care but mean health gain was greater with acupuncture. One QALY equaled £9180
Williams[29]	UK	Assessment of cost-utility of primary care osteopathy for subacute back pain	Osteopathy plus usual GP care was more expensive but also more effective than GP care alone

table continues

GENERAL TOPICS

First author and reference	Country	Research question	Main result
Phelan[30]	USA	Estimate cost from insurance database for musculoskeletal injuries	Costs associated with chiropractic care were lower than medical care; both of these were lower than combined care
Legorreta[31]	USA	Retrospective comparison of expenditure of individuals with and without insurance cover for chiropractic care	Members with chiropractic insurance cover had lower total healthcare expenditure (US$1463 vs US$1671 per member per year)
Korthals-de Bos[32]	Netherlands	Evaluation of cost-effectiveness of three approaches to neck pain care	Spinal manipulation is more cost-effective than physiotherapy or care by general practitioners
Stano[33]	USA	Compare 1 year costs for back pain treated either medically or by chiropractors	Average costs of chiropractic were higher than for medical care (US$214 vs US$123)

uniform overall picture as to the question, does CAM save money or cause extra expenditure?

Systematic reviews

Systematic reviews could in principle overcome this confusion. Several such projects have recently become available (Table 5.6.4).[34–38] Canter indicates that CAM in the UK, when subjected to proper cost-effectiveness analysis, does represent an additional healthcare cost.[38] For acupuncture[28] and spinal manipulation[27,29] the cost per Quality of Life Adjusted Years (QALY) relative to usual care is between £6000 and £10 000 depending on the exact assumptions made. Policy makers must judge whether the typically small increases in quality of life achieved are worth the extra expenditure. Even though cost per QALY may compare favourably with other more expensive treatments, such as surgery, there is a ceiling to the incremental quality of life which can be achieved with any modality. It should also be noted that cost effectiveness studies are typically less rigorous than RCTs and do not use blinding and placebo controls. The effectiveness side of the equation may therefore include a hefty slice of non-specific effect.

Collectively, these reviews fail to bring sufficient clarity. They do, however, emphasise two important points: we need better quality data and we must focus our research questions.

Comment

The rigorous cost-evaluation of CAM has only just begun. The complexity of the subject and the heterogeneity as well as the paucity of reliable studies currently prevents any firm conclusions. It is likely that this area of research will have a profound impact on the future of CAM.

Table 5.6.4 **Systematic reviews of cost evaluations**

First author	n	Type of studies included	Conclusion	Comment
White[34]	34	Any type of cost evaluation, including retrospective studies	Retrospective studies suggested savings, prospective studies suggested extra cost	Need for more rigorous studies was identified
Kernick[35]	5	Controlled trials of manipulation for back pain with basic economic evaluation	No clear indication that manipulation associated with less cost than other treatments	Not strictly speaking a systematic review
Hulme[36]	19	Any form of cost evaluation	No conclusion regarding cost. A CAM sensitive approach is required	Aim was to see whether existing methodologies are adequate for CAM
Thompson-Coon[37]	28	Any type of prospective economic analysis	No firm conclusions are possible	Data-set included 27 cost-effectiveness analyses
Canter[38]	4	UK cost-effectiveness studies	CAM in the UK probably represents an additional cost	Very limited data restricted to acupuncture and spinal manipulation only

n – number of studies included

REFERENCES

1　Ernst E, White A R. The BBC survey of complementary medicine use in the UK. Complement Ther Med 2000;8:32–36

2　Thomas K S, Nicholl J P, Coleman P. Use and expenditure on complementary medicine in England – a population based survey. Complement Ther Med 2001;9:2–11

3　Harris P, Finlay I G, Cook A, Thomas K J, Hood K. Complementary and alternative medicine use by patients with cancer in Wales: a cross sectional survey. Complement Ther Med 2003;11:249–253

4　Ramsey S D, Spencer A C, Topolski T D, Belza B, Patrick D L. Use of alternative therapies by older adults with osteoarthritis. Arthritis Rheum. 2001;45:222–227

5　Patterson R E, Neuhouser M L, Hedderson M M, Schwartz S M, Standish L J, Bowen D J, Marshall L M. Types of alternative medicine use by patients with breast, colon, or prostate cancer: predictors, motives, and costs. J Altern Complement Med 2002;8:477–485

6　Wasner M, Klier H, Borasio G D. The use of alternative medicine by patients with amyotrophic lateral sclerosis. J Neurol Sci 2001;191:151–154

7　Marstedt G, Moebus S. Inanspruchnahme alternativer Methoden in der Medizin. In:

Gesundheitsberichterstattung des Bundes Heft 9. Berlin: Verlag Robert Koch-Institut; 2002:1–32

8　Schäfer T, Riehle A, Wichmann H E, Ring J. Alternative medicine in allergies – prevalence, patterns of use, and costs. Allergy 2002;57:694–700

9　McKenzie J, Keller H H. Vitamin-mineral supplementation and use of herbal preparations among community living older adults. Can J Pub Health 2001;92:286–290

10　Shenfield G, Allen H. Survey of the use of complementary medicines and therapies in children with asthma. J Paediatr Child Health 2002;38:252–257

11　Yamashita H, Tsukayama H, Sugishita C. Popularity of complementary and alternative medicine in Japan: a telephone survey. Complement Ther Med 2002;10:84–93

12　Chrystal K, Allan S, Forgeson G, Isaacs R. The use of complementary/alternative medicine by cancer patients in a New Zealand regional cancer treatment centre. New Zealand Med J 2003;116:1–8

13　Nielsen J, Hansen M S, Fink P. Use of complementary therapy among internal medical inpatients. Prevalence, costs and association with mental disorders and physical diseases. J Psychosomatic Res 2003;55:547–552

14 Pucci E, Cartechini E, Taus C, Giuliani G. Why physicians need to look more closely at the use of complementary and alternative medicine by multiple sclerosis patients. Eur J Neurol 2004;11:263–267

15 Lafferty W E, Bellas A, Baden A C, Tyree P T, Standish L J, Patterson R. The use of complementary and alternative medical providers by insured cancer patients in Washington State. Cancer 2004;100:1522–1530

16 Murray J, Shepherd S. Alternative or additional medicine? An exploratory study in general practice. Soc Sci Med 1993;37:983–988

17 Fautrel B, Adam V, St-Pierre Y, Joseph L, Clarke A E, Penrod J R. Use of complementary and alternative therapies by patients self-reporting arthritis or rheumatism: results from a nationwide Canadian survey. J Rheumatol 2002;29:2435–2441

18 Ni H, Simile C, Hardy A M. Utilization of complementary and alternative medicine by United States adults. Med Care 2002;40:353–358

19 Al-Windi A. Determinants of complementary alternative medicine (CAM) use. Complement Ther Med 2004;12:99–111

20 Wolsko P M, Eisenberg D M, Davis R B, Ettner S L, Phillips R S. Insurance coverage, medical conditions, and visits to alternative medicine providers. Arch Intern Med 2002;162:281–287

21 Sharples F M C, van Haselen R, Fisher P. NHS patients' perspective on complementary medicine: a survey. Complement Ther Med 2003;11: 243–248

22 Metz R D, Nelson C F, LaBrot T, Pelletier K R. Chiropractic care: is it substitution care or add-on care in corporate medical plans? J Occup Environ Med 2004;46:847–855

23 Slade K, Chohan B P S, Barker P J. Evaluation of a GP practice based homeopathy service. Homeopathy 2004;93:67–70

24 Resch K L, Hill S, Ernst E. Use of complementary therapies by individuals with 'Arthritis'. Clin Rheumatol 1997;16:391–395

25 Eisenberg D M, Davis R B, Ettner S L, Appel S, Wilkey S, Van Rompay M, Kessler R C. Trends in alternative medicine use in the United States, 1990–1997: results of a follow-up national survey. JAMA 1998;280:1569–1575

26 Kominski G F, Heslin K C, Morgenstern H, Hurwitz E L, Harber P I. Economic evaluation of four treatments for low-back pain. Results from a randomized controlled trial. Med Care 2005;43:428–435

27 UK BEAM Trial Team. United Kingdom back pain exercise and manipulation (UK BEAM) randomised trial: cost effectiveness of physical treatments for back pain in primary care. BMJ 2004;329:1381

28 Wonderling D, Vickers A J, Grieve R, McCarney R. Cost effectiveness analysis of a randomised trial of acupuncture for chronic headache in primary care. BMJ 2004;328:747

29 Williams N H, Edwards R T, Linck P, Muntz R, Hibbs R, Wilkinson C, Russell I, Russell D, Hounsome B. Cost-utility analysis of osteopathy in primary care: results from a pragmatic randomized controlled trial. Fam Pract 2004;21:643–650

30 Phelan S P, Armstrong R C, Knox D G, Hubka M J, Ainbinder D A. An evaluation of medical and chiropractic provider utilization and costs: treating injured workers in North Carolina. J Manipulative Physiol Ther 2004;27:442–448

31 Legorreta A P, Metz D, Nelson C F, Ray S, Chernicoff H O, DiNubile N A. Comparative analysis of individuals with and without chiropractic coverage. Arch Intern Med 2004;164:1985–1992

32 Korthals-de Bos I B C, Hoving J L, van Tulder M W, Rutten-van Mölken P M H, Adèr H J, de Vet, H C W, Koes B W, Vondeling H, Bouter L M. Cost effectiveness of physiotherapy, manual therapy, and general practitioner care for neck pain: economic evaluation alongside a randomised controlled trial. BMJ 2003;326:911

33 Stano M, Haas M, Goldberg B, Traub P M, Nyiendo J. Chiropractic and medical care costs of low back care: results from a practice-based observational study. Am J Manag Care 2002;8:802–809

34 White A R, Ernst E. Economic analysis of complementary medicine: a systematic review. Complement Ther Med 2000;8:111–118

35 Kernick D, White A. Applying economic evaluation to complementary and alternative medicine. In: Getting health economics in practice. In Kernick De, ed. Oxford; Radcliffe Medical Press, 2002:173–180

36 Hulme C, Long A F. Square pegs and round holes? A review of economic evaluation in complementary and alternative medicine. J Altern Complement Ther Med 2005;11:179–188

37 Thompson-Coon J, Ernst E. Economic evaluation of complementary and alternative medicine –a systematic review. Perfusion 2005;18:202–214

38 Canter P H, Thompson-Coon J, Ernst E. Cost effectiveness of complementary medicine in the UK – a systematic review. BMJ 2005;331: 880–881

Postscript to the 1st edition

Our main aim has been to provide state-of-the-art information and evidence on CAM as a practical reference resource, in a way that is accessible to busy physicians and other healthcare professionals. Despite persistent suggestions that the RCT is not an appropriate or feasible method for testing CAM, we have found large numbers of RCTs that cover almost every form of therapy, demonstrating that CAM can be tested in a rigorous manner. As in all branches of medicine, inevitably some evidence is negative but the overriding conclusions are that some forms of CAM are frequently supported by evidence and therefore do have a role in modern healthcare.

The writing of this book has been a major, fascinating and novel task for us as authors and contributors. We have ourselves learnt a great deal from the experience. We intend to continue the project, to update and expand the evidence base. We recognise that there will inevitably be errors and omissions and that not all readers will agree with every recommendation we make. We invite your constructive criticism and feedback with a view to improving future editions of this book.

GENERAL TOPICS

Postscript to the 2nd edition: another epitaph

We have started this book with an epitaph and we end it with one – this time we say farewell to the lack of progress in CAM. We believe that CAM is not much different from other fields of medicine in that progress depends on meaningful research. For years, it seemed as though CAM was in hibernation. Research into CAM was slow, not meaningful for efficacy/safety questions, and often of dubious methodological quality. A vicious circle seemed to prevent CAM research from thriving: no research funds → no preliminary data → no 'acceptable' hypothesis → no research funds. The field was thus starved of highly qualified scientists who were willing to dedicate their career to CAM. Consequently huge gaps in our knowledge continued to exist. These gaps are now being filled at an unprecedented rate.

When we took on the task of updating this book we knew that it would be substantial. But we were surprised just how much the evidence-base of CAM had solidified in merely five years. Even though it was our policy to only cite the most essential studies, we had to add hundreds of new references to this text.

For both editions we evaluated what we call 'the weight of evidence' (see p 5), and this provides us with an easy measure to tell in which areas the evidence-base has become stronger (independent of the 'direction of the evidence', see p 5). In our first edition, we attributed maximum weight only to 29 interventions (Box 5.7.1).

Box 5.7.1
Interventions with maximum weight of evidence in the 1st edition of this book

Acupoint stimulation for nausea of pregnancy
Acupoint stimulation for postoperative nausea
Acupuncture for smoking cessation
Acupuncture for stroke
Biofeedback for constipation
Biofeedback for headache
Echinacea for upper respiratory tract infection
Evening primrose oil for atopic eczema
Exercise for depression
Fish oil for rheumatoid arthritis
Garlic for hypercholesterolaemia
Ginkgo for Alzheimer's disease
Ginkgo for intermittent claudication
Guar gum for hypercholesterolaemia
Guar gum for overweight

GENERAL TOPICS

Hawthorn for congestive heart failure
Horse chestnut for chronic venous insufficiency
Kava for anxiety
Oat fiber for hypercholesterolaemia
Peppermint for irritable bowel syndrome
Phytodolor for rheumatoid arthritis
Psyllium for hypercholesterolaemia
Relaxation for anxiety
Saw palmetto for benign prostatic hyperplasia
St John's wort for depression
Stress management for AIDS/HIV
Vitamin C for upper respiratory tract infection
Yohimbine for erectile dysfunction
Zinc for upper respiratory tract infection

In the new edition, the treatments which are judged to be associated with maximum 'weight' include, of course, the ones mentioned above plus the following 87 listed in Box 5.7.2.

Box 5.7.2
Interventions with maximum weight of evidence in the 2nd edition of this book

Acupuncture for asthma
Acupuncture for back pain
Acupuncture for cocaine/opiate dependence
Acupuncture for hay fever
Acupuncture for insomnia
Acupuncture for migraine
Acupuncture for nausea after chemotherapy
Acupuncture for neck pain
Acupuncture for osteoarthritis
Acupuncture for overweight
African plum for benign prostate hyperplasia
Allium vegetables for cancer prevention
Antioxidants for cancer prevention
Antioxidants for hepatitis
Aromatherapy for cancer palliation
Asian mixture for cancer palliation
Asian mixtures for cancer treatment
Ayurveda for diabetes
Ayurveda for rheumatoid arthritis
Biofeedback for hypertension
Biofeedback for insomnia
Biofeedback for migraine
Black cohosh for menopause
Butcher's broom for chronic venous insufficiency
Cannabinoids for cancer palliation
Chelation therapy for peripheral arterial occlusive disease

box continues

Chinese herbals for diabetes
Chitosan for overweight
Chondroitin for osteoarthritis
Chromium for diabetes
Chromium for overweight
Co-enzyme Q10 for hypertension
Devil's claw for back pain
Diet for rheumatoid arthritis
Enzymes for cancer palliation
Ephedra sinica for overweight
Exercise for AIDS/HIV
Exercise for back pain
Exercise for cancer palliation
Exercise for cancer prevention
Exercise for chronic fatigue syndrome
Fibre for constipation
Fibre for irritable bowel syndrome
Fish oil for diabetes
Fish oil for hypertension
Fish oil for ulcerative colitis
Garlic for hypertension
Glucosamine for osteoarthritis
Green tea for cancer prevention
Group behaviour therapy for smoking cessation
Guar gum for diabetes
Guided imagery for anxiety
Hypnotherapy for irritable bowel syndrome
Hypnotherapy for labour
Hypnotherapy for overweight
Iberogast for irritable bowel syndrome
Massage for anxiety
Meditation for anxiety
Melatonin for insomnia
Mistletoe for cancer treatment
Music therapy for anxiety
Oat for hypercholesterolaemia
Padma 28 for peripheral arterial occlusive disease
Peppermint/caraway for non-ulcer dyspepsia
Phyllanthus for hepatitis
Phytodolor for osteoarthritis
Psyllium for constipation
Psyllium for diabetes
Red clover for menopause
Relaxation for hypertension
Relaxation for insomnia
Relaxation for nausea after chemotherapy
SAMe for osteoarthritis
Sophora flavescens for hepatitis

Soy for hypercholesterolaemia
Soy for menopause
Spinal manipulation for neck pain
Tomato for cancer prevention
Valerian for insomnia
Vitamin E for congestive heart failure
Vitamin E for stroke
Water immersion for labour
Zinc for acne

But the term 'strong' tells us nothing about the question whether the evidence is 'positive' (indicating a treatment is effective) or 'negative' (suggesting a therapy does not work). In fact, for a number of the above treatments, the evidence was far from 'positive'. The therapies for which new data changed the overall direction of evidence in a 'positive' sense include those in Box 5.7.3. The therapies for which the new data changed the overall direction of evidence in a 'negative' sense include those in Box 5.7.4.

Box 5.7.3
Interventions for which new data changed the overall direction of evidence in a 'positive' sense

Acupoint stimulation for nausea of pregnancy
Acupuncture for alcohol dependence
Acupuncture for asthma
Acupuncture for constipation
Acupuncture for herpes zoster
Acupuncture for neck pain
Acupuncture for osteoarthritis
Acupuncture for tinnitus
African plum for benign prostatic hyperplasia
Autogenic training for depression
Biofeedback for alcohol dependence
Biofeedback for anxiety
Biofeedback for erectile dysfunction
Biofeedback for insomnia
Biofeedback for irritable bowel syndrome
Borage for atopic eczema
Buteyko for asthma
Cannabis for multiple sclerosis
Chaste tree for premenstrual syndrome
Chitosan for hypercholesterolaemia
Diet for atopic eczema
Exercise for fibromyalgia
Exercise for smoking cessation

box continues

Ginger for osteoarthritis
Green tea for cancer prevention
Homeopathy for anxiety
Homeopathy for chronic fatigue syndrome
Massage for anxiety
Massage for low back pain
Melatonin for insomnia
Music therapy for anxiety
NADH for chronic fatigue syndrome
Nettle for benign prostatic hyperplasia
Phyllantus for hepatitis
Psyllium for constipation
Red clover for menopause
Relaxation for migraine
Relaxation for nausea/vomiting after chemotherapy
Selenium for atopic eczema
Spinal manipulation for migraine
Thymus extract for hepatitis
Zinc for atopic eczema

Box 5.7.4
Interventions for
which new data
changed the overall
direction of evidence
in a 'negative' sense

Acupoint stimulation for nausea after chemotherapy
Acupoint stimulation for postoperative nausea
Acupuncture for cancer palliation
Acupuncture for cocaine/opiate dependence
Acupuncture for insomnia
Acupuncture for irritable bowel syndrome
Acupuncture for menopause
Acupuncture for stroke
Avocado-soybean unsaponifiables
Biofeedback for constipation
Black cohosh for menopause
Capsaicin for herpes zoster
Co-enzyme Q10 for hypercholesterolaemia
Devil's claw for osteoarthritis
Echinacea for prevention of upper respiratory tract infections
Echinacea for treatment of upper respiratory tract infections
Electrostimulation for drug/alcohol dependence
Evening primrose oil for atopic eczema
Fish oil for rheumatoid arthritis
Garlic for hypercholesterolaemia
Garlic for peripheral arterial occlusive disease
Ginger for postoperative nausea
Ginkgo for tinnitus

Homeopathy for anxiety
Homeopathy for asthma
Homeopathy for rheumatoid arthritis
Hypnotherapy for insomnia
Hypnotherapy for irritable bowel syndrome
Hypnotherapy for postoperative nausea
Liquorice for hepatitis
Massage for AIDS
Meditation for anxiety
Red vine leaf for chronic venous insufficiency
Red yeast rice for hypercholesterolaemia
Relaxation for rheumatoid arthritis
Selenium for hepatitis
Selenium for rheumatoid arthritis
Soy for menopause
Spinal manipulation for headache
Spinal manipulation for neck pain
Support group therapy for cancer treatment
Vitamin E for Alzheimer's
Yoga for depression

These lists show how important it is to not just consider the intervention but also the indication. For acupuncture or spinal manipulation, for instance, the evidence has become more 'positive' for some conditions and more 'negative' for others.

The book includes eight new indications. These are usually conditions for which we had previously felt that not enough evidence was available to merit an entry. Many condition chapters which had already been included in the first edition had to be extended considerably and much of the new evidence is 'positive' (Table 5.7.1).

Table 5.7.1 **Examples of conditions chapters that extended markedly**

Condition	Number of treatments in 1st edition	Number of treatments in 2nd edition
AIDS/HIV	13	21
Anxiety	14	22
Asthma	14	30
Cancer palliation	6	25
Hay fever	6	12
Hepatitis	13	26
Herpes simplex	3	11
Osteoarthritis	10	29
Overweight	5	17

We believe there is a good reason for putting the terms 'negative' and 'positive' in inverted commas. From the patients' point of view (a perspective we try to identify with), there is no such thing as a 'negative' or a 'positive' result. Even if the data clearly demonstrated lack of effectiveness for a specific intervention, this result would be positive – patients could then avoid this intervention and choose one that is backed by evidence! Patient choice is a good thing but it must be supported by evidence, if not choice degenerates to arbitrariness.

Progress in CAM is encouraging but there is, of course, still much room for improvement. Even in the USA (a country which many CAM researchers watch with envy for its relative affluence of CAM research funds) the money dedicated into this sector is minute in percentage terms: in 2004, the NHS spent US $117 million on CAM research which amounts to 0.42% of the institution's total research budget, a figure which is conspicuously similar to those from the UK.[1]

Improvement would also be desirable, we believe, in terms of research priorities. Complementary medicine is in danger of drowning in surveys, interview studies and similar projects. The authors typically state that their results will inform policy, alas we have hardly ever seen this happening (in many cases, this would also be undesirable as the methodological quality is often such that it might misinform policy). What policy makers foremost need and want is evidence on safety and efficacy.[2] Whatever CAM is, it is medicine which must be informed by medical research and not by sociological audit. Redirecting CAM research accordingly would, in our view, be an important service to our field.

We believe that, despite these limitations, this book is hugely encouraging. It demonstrates that progress is firmly on its way. Progress means more and better research. And good CAM research will always be aimed at improving the medical care of tomorrow's patients. We hope that our epitaph is not premature and that CAM research will soon impact on better care for patients.

REFERENCES

1 Ernst E. Why looking at complementary medicine receives so little funding. Pharm J 2005;274:557

2 van Haselen R, Fisher P. Evidence influencing British Health Authorities' decisions in purchasing complementary medicine. JAMA 1998;280:1564

Index

Notes Page numbers in **bold** denote main discussions (where necessary).
Page numbers in *italics* refer to tables